AF674770

Coronary Angioplasty

Evolved to Perfection

Coronary Angioplasty
Evolved to Perfection

Editor

Jagdish S Hiremath
DM DNB (Cardiology) FACC
Director, Cath Lab
Ruby Hall Clinic
Pune, India

Foreword

Emmanuel Manolas

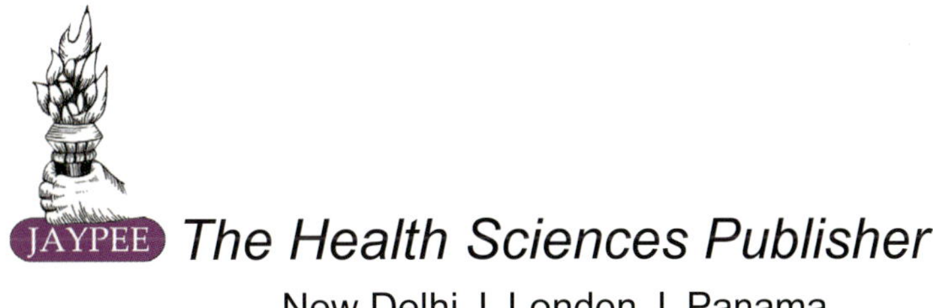

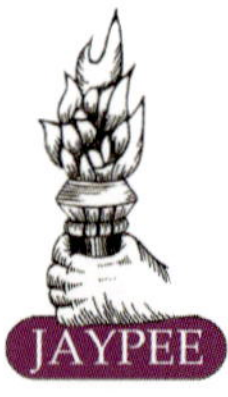

Jaypee Brothers Medical Publishers (P) Ltd.

Headquarters
Jaypee Brothers Medical Publishers (P) Ltd.
4838/24, Ansari Road, Daryaganj
New Delhi 110 002, India
Phone: +91-11-43574357
Fax: +91-11-43574314
E-mail: jaypee@jaypeebrothers.com

Overseas Offices
J.P. Medical Ltd.
83, Victoria Street, London
SW1H 0HW (UK)
Phone: +44-20 3170 8910
Fax: +44(0) 20 3008 6180
E-mail: info@jpmedpub.com

Jaypee-Highlights Medical Publishers Inc.
City of Knowledge, Bld. 235, 2nd Floor, Clayton
Panama City, Panama
Phone: +1 507-301-0496
Fax: +1 507-301-0499
E-mail: cservice@jphmedical.com

Jaypee Brothers Medical Publishers (P) Ltd.
17/1-B, Babar Road, Block-B, Shaymali
Mohammadpur, Dhaka-1207
Bangladesh
Mobile: +08801912003485
E-mail: jaypeedhaka@gmail.com

Jaypee Brothers Medical Publishers (P) Ltd.
Bhotahity, Kathmandu, Nepal
Phone: +977-9741283608
E-mail: kathmandu@jaypeebrothers.com

Website: www.jaypeebrothers.com
Website: www.jaypeedigital.com

Inquiries for bulk sales may be solicited at: jaypee@jaypeebrothers.com

Coronary Angioplasty: Evolved to Perfection

First Edition: **2017**

ISBN: 978-93-86261-96-0

Printed at Replika Press Pvt. Ltd.

Contributors

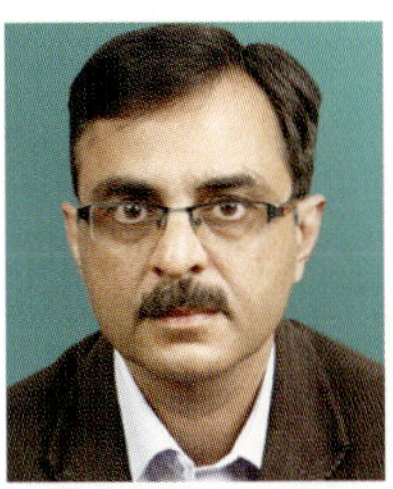

Aditya Kapoor
Professor
Department of Cardiology
Sanjay Gandhi Postgraduate Institute of Medical Sciences
Lucknow, Uttar Pradesh, India

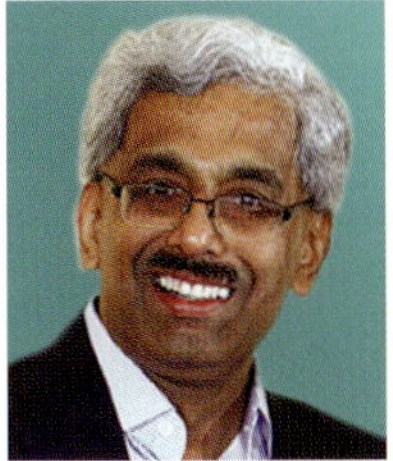

Ajit S Mullasari
Director and Head
Department of Cardiology
Institute of Cardiovascular Diseases
Madras Medical Mission
Chennai, Tamil Nadu, India

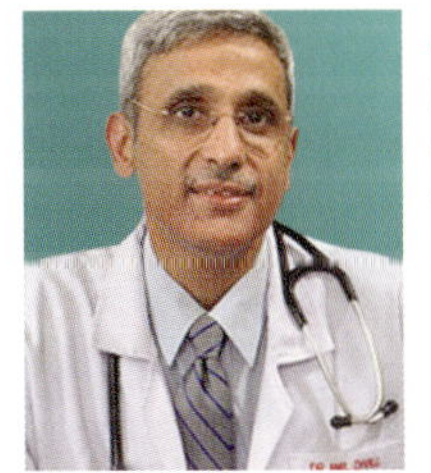

Anil Dhall
Director
Cardiovascular Sciences
Venkateshwar Hospital
New Delhi, India

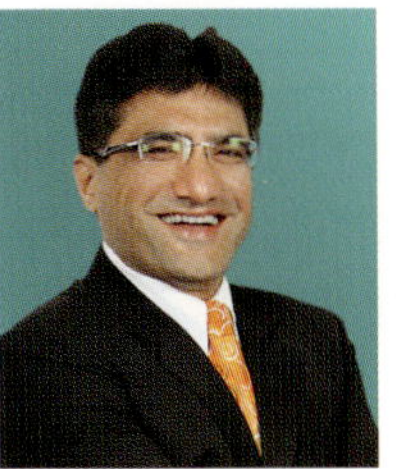

Anish Chandarana
Interventional Cardiologist
Care Institute of Medical Sciences (CIMS) Hospital
Ahmedabad, Gujarat, India

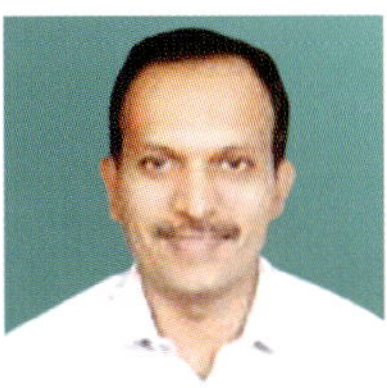

Chandrashekhar V Patil
Consultant Invasive and Noninvasive Cardiologist
Director, Cath Lab
Shri Sai Cardiac Center
Kolhapur, Maharashtra, India

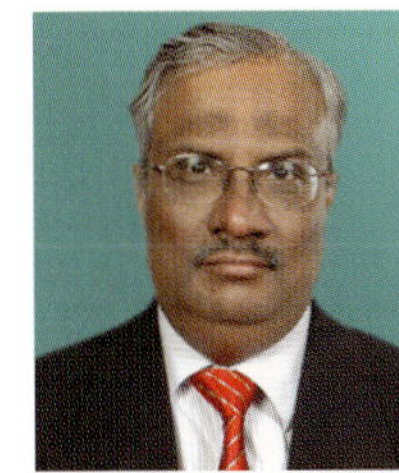

Chandrashekhar Makhale
Professor of Cardiology
Ruby Hall Clinic
Pune, Maharashtra, India

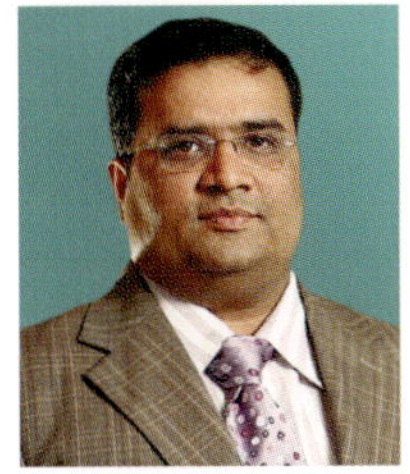

Cherukupalli Raghu
Director–Cardiologist
Aster Prime Hospitals
Hyderabad, Telangana, India

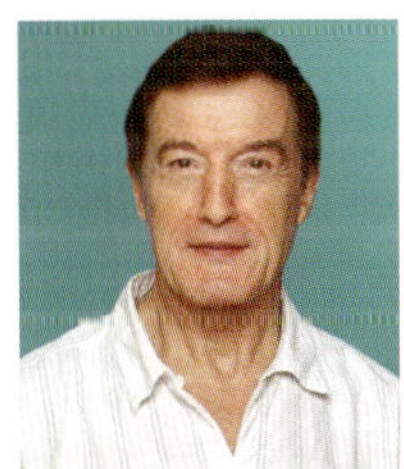

David Cumberland
Consultant Interventional Cardiologist
Prince Court Medical Center
Kuala Lumpur, Malaysia

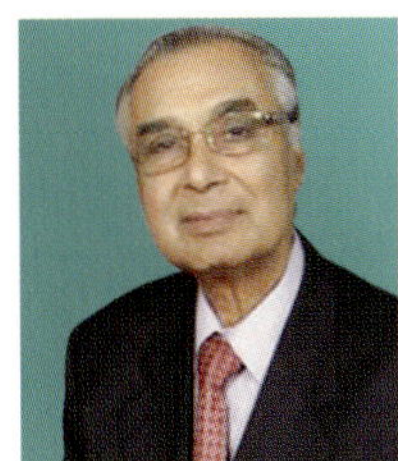

Dev Pahlajani
Head
Department of Cardiology and Interventional Cardiology
Breach Candy Hospital
Mumbai, Maharashtra, India

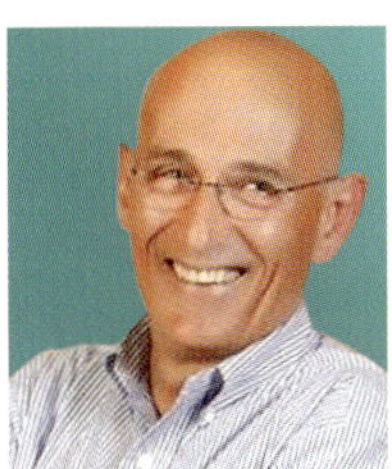

Imad Sheiban
Director
Cath Lab
Interventional Cardiologist
Pederzoli Hospital
Verona, Italy

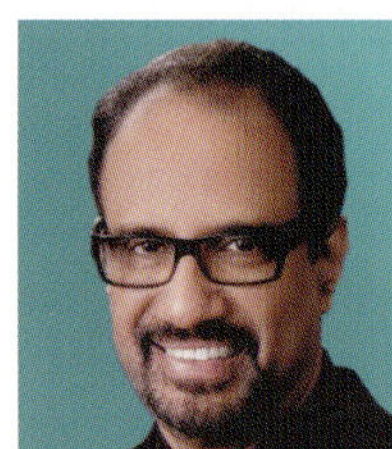

Jagdish S Hiremath
Director, Cath Lab
Ruby Hall Clinic
Pune, India

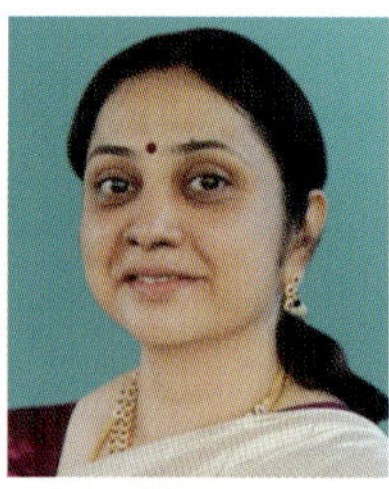

Lalita Nemani
Interventional Cardiologist
Prime Hospital
Hyderabad, Telangana, India

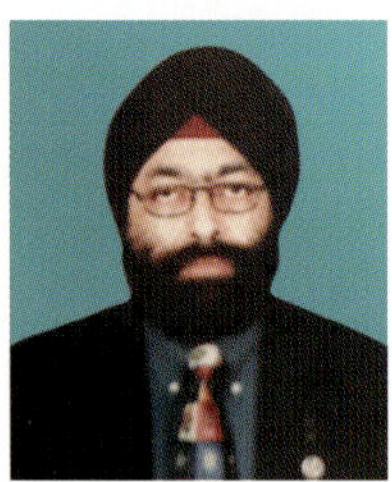

Jaskaran Singh Dugal
Head
Department of Cardiology
Jehangir Hospital
Pune, Maharashtra, India

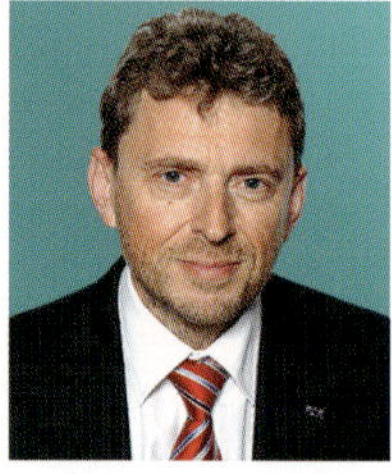

Maciej Lesiak
Director
Catheterization Laboratory
Karol Marcinkowski University of Medical Sciences
Poznań, Poland

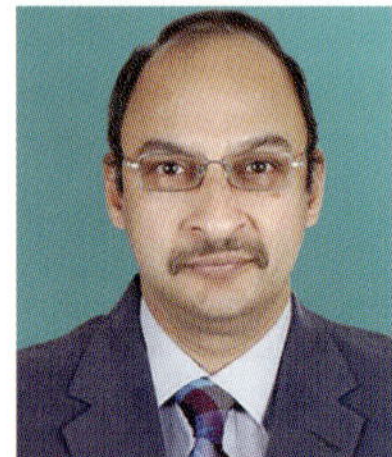

Kaushal Pandey
Consultant Cardiovascular Surgeon
Hinduja and Lilavati Hospital
Mumbai, Maharashtra, India

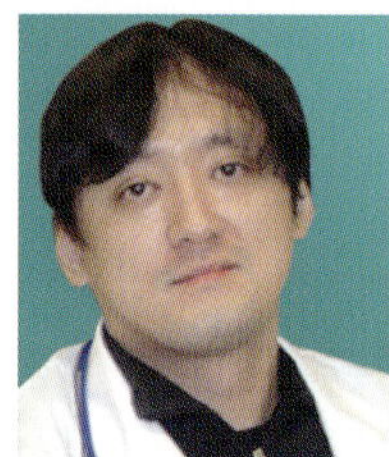

Masaki Tanabe
Head
Cardiovascular Department
Daini Okamoto General Hospital
Japan

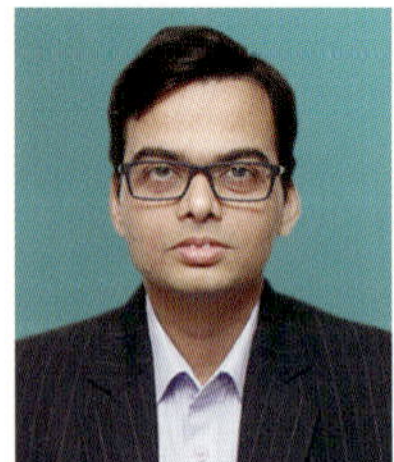

Kaushik Sheth
Interventional Cardiologist
Ruby Hall Clinic
Pune, Maharashtra, India

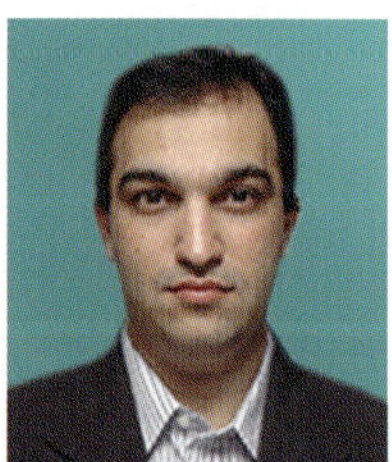

Piroze M Davierwala
Senior Consultant
Department of Cardiac Surgery
Heart Center
Leipzig, Germany

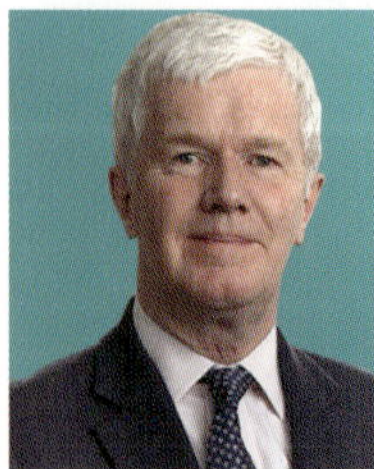

Keith D Dawkins
Global Chief Medical Officer and
Executive Vice President
Boston Scientific Corporation
Massachusetts, US

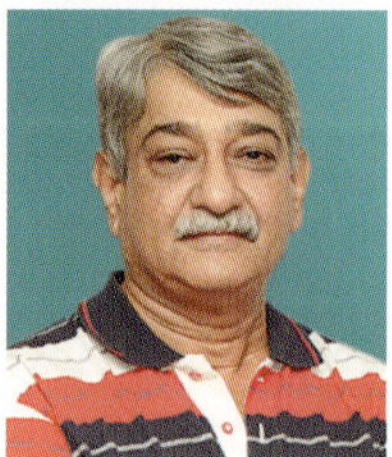

Rajendra G Bahaley
Surgeon and Consultant
Sports Medicine
Consultant
Cardiac Rehabilitation
Ruby Hall Clinic
Pune, Maharashtra, India

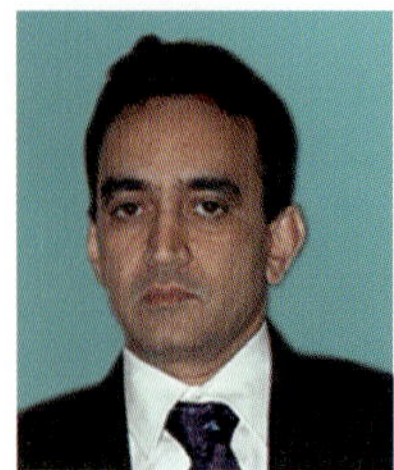

K Sarat Chandra
Consultant Cardiologist
Indo-US Superspeciality Hospital
Hyderabad, Telangana, India

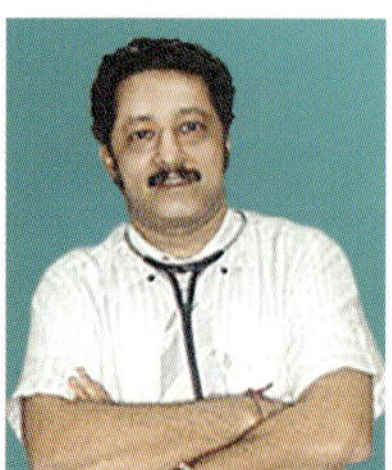

Rajiv G Bhagwat
Consultant Cardiologist
Dr Balabhai Nanavati Hospital
Shushruta Hospital
Mumbai, Maharashtra, India

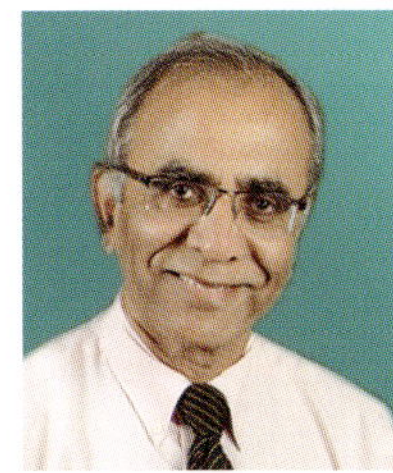

Shekhar Shriram Ambardekar
Honorary Cardiologist
Asian Heart Institute
SL Raheja Hospital
All India Institute of Diabetes
Mumbai, Maharashtra, India

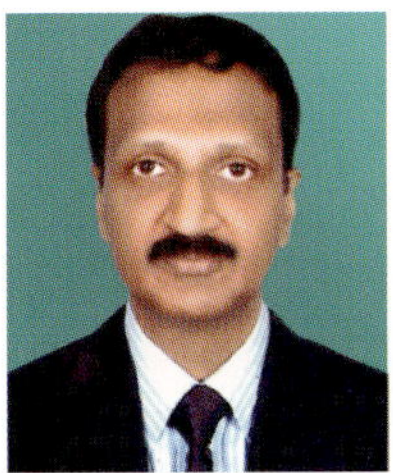

Tiny Nair
Head
Department of Cardiology
PRS Hospital
Thiruvananthapuram, Kerala, India

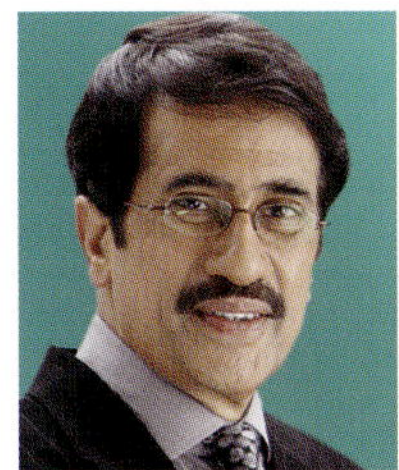

Shirish (MS) Hiremath
Director
Cardiac Cath Lab
Ruby Hall Clinic
Pune, Maharashtra, India

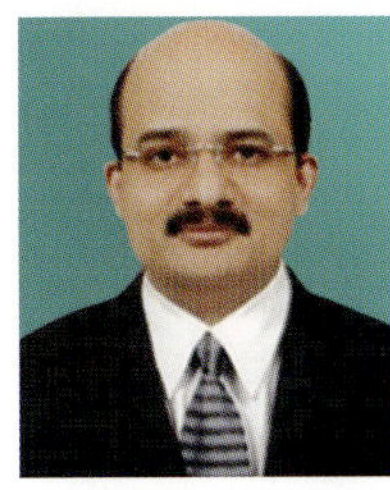

Vilas P Magarkar
Senior Consultant and Interventional Cardiologist
Seth Nandlal Dhoot Hospital
Aurangabad, Maharashtra, India

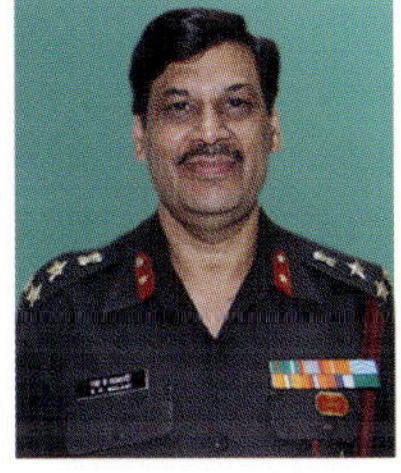

Susheel K Malani
Consultant
Department of Medicine and Cardiology)
Professor and Head
Department of Cardiology
Armed Forces Medical College
Military Hospital (Cardiothoracic Center)
Pune, Maharashtra, India

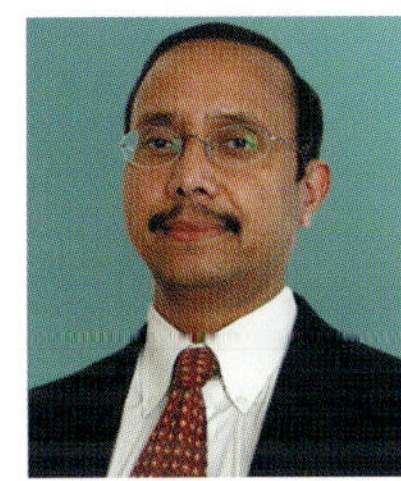

Y Chandrashekhar
Professor
Department of Medicine
University of Minnesota
Minnesota, USA

Co-Authors

Ajay Joshi

Ajit Mehta

Akshay K Mehta

Aleksander Araszkiewicz

Amit V Sharma

Anup Banerji

DS Chadha

Filippo Figini

Jaideep Rajebahadur

K Krishnakumar

Omkar Thopte

Omür Akhavuz

Paul F Chouinard

Pritika Gaur

Raveen Kandan

Ronak V Ruparelia

Salil Garg

S Nagendra Boopathy

Todd Drexel

Varun Nivargi

Foreword

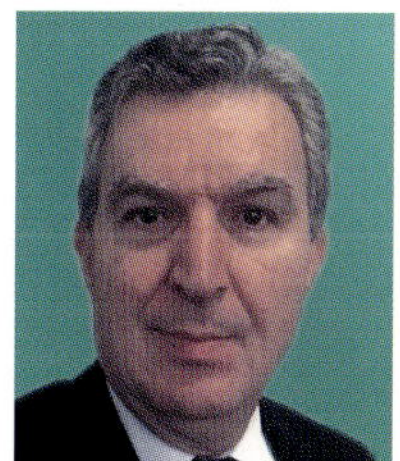

The year 2017 marks 40 years since Andreas Gruentzig performed the first percutaneous transluminal coronary angioplasty (PTCA), dilating a proximal left anterior descending (LAD) stenosis using an early bulky rather crude and nonsteerable balloon catheter.

Advances in technology and pharmacotherapy, a better understanding of the pathophysiology of the atherosclerotic plaque and improved imaging intravascular ultrasound (IVUS), and optical coherence tomography (OCT), have enabled an exponential increase in numbers and an expansion in indications for percutaneous coronary interventions. Percutaneous coronary intervention (PCI) has overtaken coronary artery bypass grafting (CABG) in most categories of coronary artery disease (CAD) requiring revascularization.

Many books have been published addressing various aspects of interventional cardiology, from how-to-do manuals to reviews of the most recent trials of interventions and pharmacotherapy.

In an ever-changing field, books are often quickly obsolete. *Coronary Angioplasty: Evolved to Perfection* focuses on percutaneous coronary intervention. The chapters, very useful to the 'beginners', are balanced with pathophysiology, and intervention in specific conditions, e.g. left main or during acute myocardial infarction (AMI).

Evolving and controversial areas of PCI are explored, from chronic total occlusions to left main and triple-vessel PCI. There are chapters devoted to fractional flow reserve (FFR) and its place in decision for PCI, imaging with IVUS and OCT, and to contrast nephropathy. Indications for PCI and potential complications are not forgotten. Bioresorbable stents are introduced and there is a look into future directions.

Structural, valvular heart disease, and electrophysiology, etc. are not covered, as these areas are well represented in a variety of the current texts.

Dr Jagdish S Hiremath should be congratulated for bringing together a group of authors with special interests in different areas of PCI, to create a meritable text.

Dr Jagdish S Hiremath has been part of the evolution of PTCA/PCI, from his time as cardiology fellow at Epworth Hospital, Melbourne, Australia, in 1987–88, when PTCA was in its infancy. It has been the most exciting era to be a cardiologist and those of us on this journey certainly feel privileged.

We have come a long way, where most coronary lesions can now be corrected percutaneously. It is now even more so, as now no longer a question of 'can this be done' but 'should it be done'. Gruentzig insisted on objective evidence of ischemia. Intervention must be evidence based. Are we improving prognosis? And, we must not lose sight of why a disease occurs rather than just correcting its effect.

This book will have wide appeal, good for beginners and also a useful text for experienced interventionalists, general cardiologists and physicians.

Emmanuel Manolas
Director
Victorian Cardiovascular Services
Epworth Hospital
Melbourne, Australia

Preface

On my own journey with coronary angioplasty, this book comes as a major milestone. Of course, I do hope to have miles and miles to go on this path, before I rest my gloves.

From the early fumbling steps in 1988 with balloon angioplasty in Epworth Hospital, Melbourne, Australia, under the guidance of Dr Emmanuel Manolas, to the present era of left main angioplasties, this has been a highly satisfying and evolving journey in various ways; as an interventionalist, as a human being, as a socialistic thinker and as a teacher. Coronary angioplasty, in itself, has almost reached its summit of excellence, hence the title *Coronary Angioplasty: Evolved to Perfection*.

The book shall unfold this evolution, shall present the present-day nitty-gritty and shall dare to have a peep into the future.

I must thank all the contributors, both from India and abroad, who responded promptly to my personal request, not just to help a colleague, a friend, a student, a brother but, more importantly, to help the primary purpose of dissemination of scientific knowledge about this revolutionary treatment. I appreciate their generous gift of effort and time and selfless sharing of their knowledge and expertise and I shall always remain indebted to them.

I also appreciate M/s Jaypee Brothers Medical Publishers (P) Ltd, New Delhi, India, for understanding the demands of time on a practicing interventional cardiologist. Their professional well-oiled machineries and the expert team, made it easy for me to focus mainly on the area of content, while they took care of the rest.

I would be failing in my duty if I do not thank my personal "JSH" (I am known as JSH in cardiology circles) team (Aruna Murali in particular) for bearing and grinning my onslaughts!

It is my immense pleasure and pride to present this monograph on coronary angioplasty. It is slated to be a reference book for all cardiologists and hopefully a Bible for younger cardiologists. I am optimistic to the point of being overconfident!

I hope, you will be as happy reading it as I am, making it!

Jagdish S Hiremath

Contents

CHAPTER

1

Evolution of Coronary Angioplasty

David Cumberland, Raveen Kandan

HISTORY

It could be said that the specialty of inter-ventional cardiology was born in 1966, when Rashkind produced an atrial septal defect with a balloon catheter in an infant with transposition of the great arteries.[1] On the other hand this chapter is going to confine itself to coronary intervention, whose prehistory straddles this period but which really started a little later.

Selective coronary angiography occurred unintentionally for the first time in 1958, when Mason Sones saw an aortogram catheter slip into the right coronary artery during contrast injection (Fig. 1.1);[2,3] much to everyone's surprise the patient survived. Sones favored the brachial cutdown, an approach which survived well into the 80s and early 90s, but has since been largely replaced by percutaneous entry.

Melvin Judkins (1967) used the percutaneous femoral route pioneered by Seldinger and designed the well-known and still oft-used Judkins catheters for selective angiography.[4,5] It was also 1967 when Favaloro, who had worked with Sones at the Cleveland Clinic, performed the first saphenous vein coronary bypass graft.[6] Coronary angiography then became essential as a prerequisite for surgery.

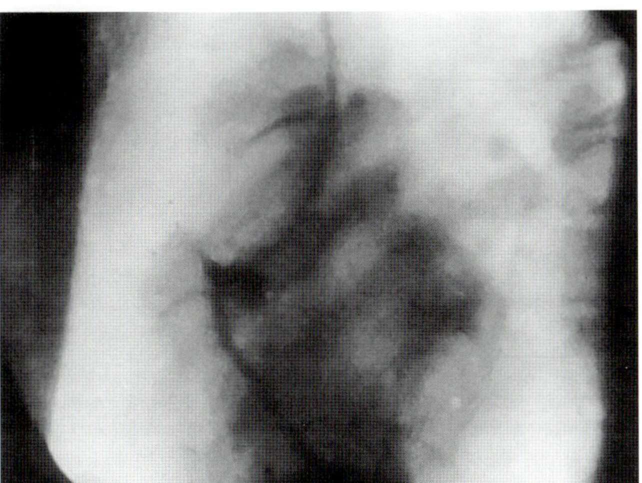

Fig. 1.1 The first selective coronary angiogram, by Mason Sones in 1958

Source: Ryan TJ. The coronary angiogram and its seminal contributions to cardiovascular medicine over five decades. Trans Am Clin Climatol Assoc. 2002;113:261-71

It was around that time that peripheral angioplasty was taking its first stuttering steps. In 1964, Charles Dotter in Portland, Oregon pushed a catheter through a femoral artery stenosis and restored blood flow[7]—his surgical colleague was not so impressed, indeed in future requests for femoral arteriography came the instruction "visualize but do not try to fix". This was called the "Dotter" technique; it was taken up in isolated centers in Europe, and the pushing of a catheter through a narrow conduit became verbalized as "dottering". The problem of course was that to make a 3 mm hole required a 9 French catheter. Despite this, even in 1964, Dotter predicted that his technique would eventually be applied to the coronary arteries.

The breakthrough came when Andreas Grüntzig in Zurich developed a catheter with a home-made cylindrical polyvinyl chloride (PVC) balloon. He tried this in peripheral arteries (Figs 1.2A to C)[8,9] (a testbed then, and for decades since, for eventual coronary application), in the coronary artery of dogs (1976),[10] intraoperatively in San Francisco with Richard Myler and colleagues (May 1977),[11] and then, the first successful percutaneous transluminal coronary angioplasty—and the true birth of percutaneous transluminal coronary angioplasty (PTCA), in a proximal left anterior descending (LAD) stenosis in September 1977 (Figs 1.3A to C).[12] Grüntzig demonstrated his first four patients at the AHA in November 1977. It is interesting that the fourth patient had an unprotected left main stem stenosis.[13] This patient died a few weeks later, so Grüntzig realized the importance of very careful patient selection to guide the early development of his method.

Richard Myler in San Francisco performed the first PTCA in the United States in early 1978—he was a pivotal figure worldwide in the development of PTCA, in training and in new developments, for many years thereafter. He was also a

Figs 1.2A to C Andreas Grüntzig's first peripheral angioplasty with his new balloon catheter in 1974: (A) pre; (B) post; (C) Maintained patency after 2 years

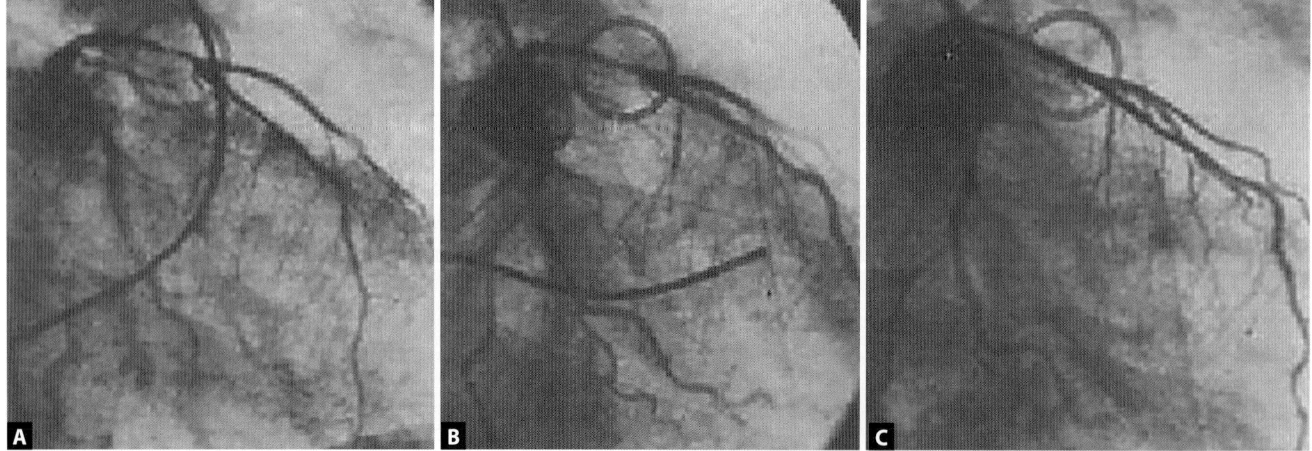

Figs 1.3A to C Angiogram of the first successful percutaneous transluminal coronary angiography (PTCA) by Grüntzig in September 1977, with follow-up at 1 month
Source: EAPCI textbook

really good man, and will be missed by many interventionists who have benefited from his guidance and friendship (Fig. 1.4).

In the early days the indications were a single isolated lesion in a patient with good left ventricular function and who was suitable for coronary bypass surgery. Dedicated surgical standby was needed then because the incidence of emergency bypass was not inconsiderable.[14] Some surgeons quipped that PTCA stood for "Procedure Terminating in Cardiac Arrest".

In clinical practice in the early 80s a local isolated lesion was relatively rarely seen; indeed in the UK to get one or two suitable cases per week was regarded as impressive. The equipment was crude and angiography not yet digitally enhanced; the guide catheter was 9 or 10 F and the first coronary balloon catheters had a short fixed wire at the tip (Fig. 1.5). They were available from Schneider Medintag in Zurich—you could buy them only after attending one of Grüntzig's courses. This was another pioneering aspect of his development of the method: live demonstrations of a new

Fig. 1.4 In the early days, and on a sunny day in Zurich: Andreas Grüntzig atop his scooter, with Richard Myler at the front and Simon Stertzer behind

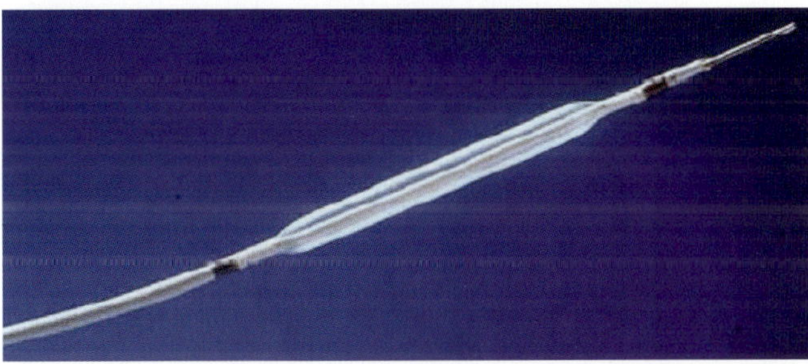

Fig. 1.5 The first coronary angioplasty catheters, with a 20 mm long balloon and a short fixed wire at the tip—Schneider Medintag offered them with a straight wire or J shaped tip versions
Source: EAPCI textbook

technique from the catheter lab to a lecture theater. Such live demonstrations took place in many parts of the world in the early years of percutaneous coronary intervention (PCI) to help people start up, e.g. in Pune from 1987. Such demonstrations remain a tradition to this day.

The 1980 course was the last in Zurich before Grüntzig moved to Atlanta; it was also noteworthy because the pioneers of interventional cardiology were there: Sones, Judkins, Dotter and Grüntzig (Fig. 1.6). Also present were Richard Myler, Kurt Amplatz and others. At that time everyone's experience was summarized on a blackboard, and the numbers were small.

In the UK, by 1981/82 a few centers had started. The British Coronary Angioplasty Group (BCAG) was formed so that we could all learn from each other; the first meetings consisted of a small group of colleagues huddled around a cine viewer in a Sheffield hotel. Angio-based sharing of experience, good and bad, continues to provide invaluable training for all. The BCAG grew rapidly, and in 1987 became formalized into the British Cardiovascular Intervention Society (BCIS) associated with the British Cardiac Society; it thrives to this day as the premier force for training, data collection and research in UK interventional cardiology.

In 1982, John Simpson introduced the removable intracoronary guidewire, over which balloon catheters could be separately passed.[15] This improved safety because the lesion and anatomy could be better visualized, and re-crossing the lesion after dilatation, known from the start to be dangerous, proved a lot safer. The wires were difficult to see, but advances in wire technology were swift.

An over-the-wire balloon catheter needed (at that time) a long enough guidewire for exchange whilst maintaining its position in the distal vessel. Extension attachments were devised, with varying success. For a time the so-called Kaltenbach technique was favored by some; a 300 cm long wire was used at the start without a bulky balloon catheter preloaded in the guide catheter.[16] Angiographic visualization of progress was good, though as can be imagined handling was a bit cumbersome. On the other hand multiple balloon catheter exchanges were possible.

Then the system which is in universal use today was conceived, simple in retrospect as with many good ideas. Tassilo Bonzel in Germany and Paul Yock in the US separately realized that if the guidewire lumen exited the shaft of the balloon catheter near enough to the distal end to allow its removal and exchange over a standard length wire, this would facilitate the use of multiple catheters, whilst allowing initial "bare wiring" of the lesion.[17] Also PTCA could now be done with a single operator; hitherto there had been a division of labor between the guide catheter handler/balloon catheter pusher, and the "wirer". This change meant that unless trainees in interventional cardiology were allowed to be at the "top end" they would only become adept at making encouraging noises and using the inflation device. Uptake of Bonzel's "monorail" or Yock's "rapid exchange" system was rapid in Europe, but was delayed in the US, at least partly for patent reasons. The system has of course allowed for easy exchange of not only balloon catheters but also the various other adjunctive devices—to which we now turn.

In the mid-80s, coronary intervention was developing apace but there were still very significant limitations: complications, including emergency CABG, had been going down with experience and better gear but acute closure of the vessel was still a problem. Restenosis was common, especially if one was adventurous and strayed into diffuse disease or total occlusions—technical capability in terms of achieving success in adverse lesions was not matched by usefulness in

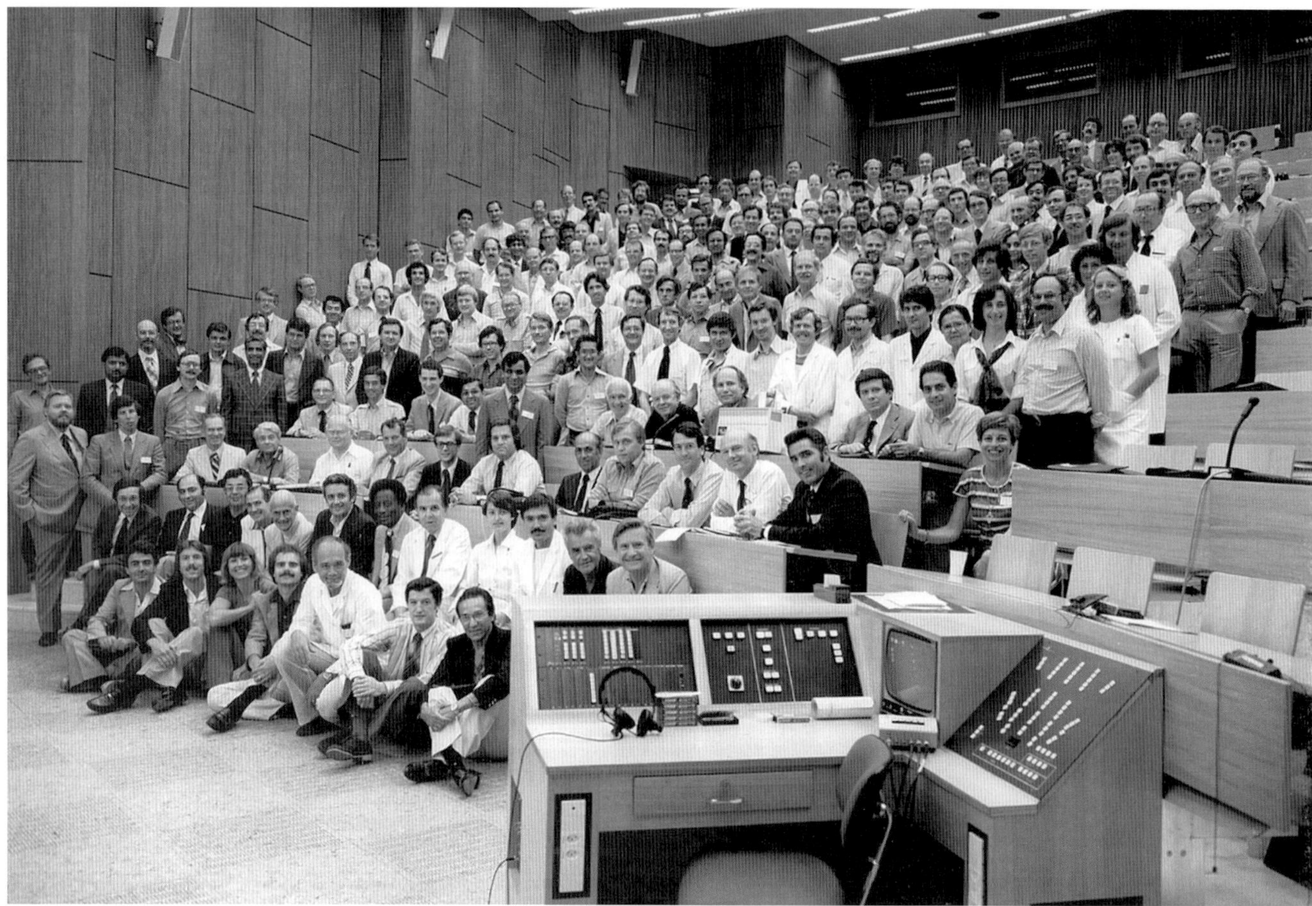

Fig. 1.6 "Class" photograph of the 1980 PTCA course; this course was notable because it was the last before Grüntzig moved to Atlanta, and because the pioneers of cardiovascular intervention were there:
Grüntzig himself, third from right on second row from the front
Charles Dotter, eighth from right, second row
Melvin Judkins, ninth from right, third row
Mason Sones, fourth from right, fourth row
Richard Myler, seventh from right, second row
And others—one of the authors (DCC) is seated on the floor, second from right, first row

terms of maintained patency. Chronic occlusions were being recanalized, and a few stiffer tip wires were being developed, but success was achieved in less than half of attempts.

And so we entered the new device era. It was hoped that modification and/or debulking of the plaque before balloon dilatation by an energetic device might reduce restenosis (Figs 1.7A to D).[18] The main candidates were as follows:

- Directional coronary atherectomy, comprising a housing within which lay a cutter to excise plaque through an eccentric aperture, was tried. In the event several randomized trials, even after technical and procedural improvements, showed no real benefit in restenosis or acute closure. It probably did help in very eccentric lesions in big arteries, which were notoriously difficult to dilate to good effect.
- The Rotablator, not without its technical challenges and complications, also failed to live up to its hope in reducing restenosis in diffuse disease. Of course it is still useful, and has had something of a renaissance, in resistant, calcified and/or diffuse disease, particularly as nowadays this is more readily tackled.
- Lasers seemed exciting and futuristic—the stuff of Star Wars—but they also failed to affect restenosis. Indeed lasers associated with thermal effect tended to increase the risk of acute closure. There is still the occasional protagonist for the use of excimer lasers in resistant lesions or perhaps crossing total occlusions, but most laser machines are gathering dust.
- Energy of some sort was thought as the possible answer to boring our way through chronic total occlusions. The

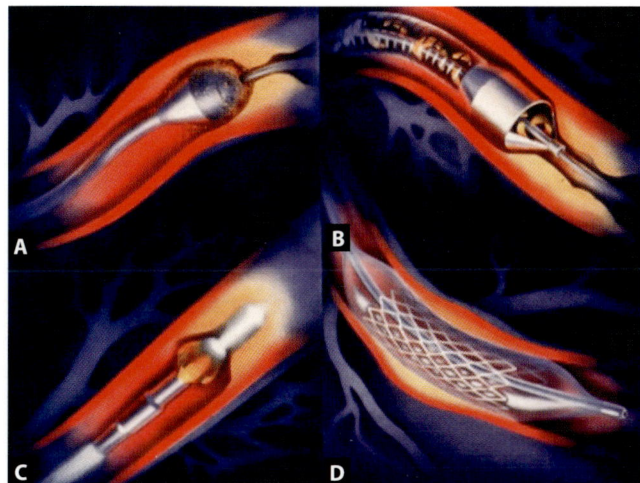

Figs 1.7A to D Some of the "new devices" being tried from the mid-80s: (A) Rotational atherectomy; (B) Directional atherectomy; (C) Laser tipped probe; (D) The stent

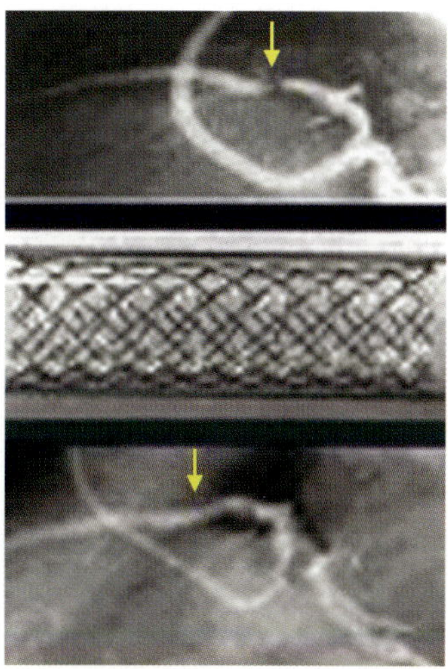

Fig. 1.8 The first human coronary stent implantation, by Jacques Puel using the self-expanding wallstent
Source: EAPCI textbook

Rotacs catheter had a slowly rotating olive shaped tip; it succeeded in a few cases but not consistently so, as did probes powered by lasers or therapeutic ultrasound.

The device which of course triumphs over all is the stent. Development started in the mid-80s and in 1986 Jacques Puel implanted the first coronary stent, in this case the stainless steel self-expanding Wallstent (Fig. 1.8).[19] Soon afterwards the Palmaz balloon expandable slotted tube gained clinical exposure. It was very stiff, so much so that it was only available in 7 mm length. Schatz, working with Palmaz, was responsible for the single short straight connector between two Palmaz components; thus the famous 15 mm Palmaz Schatz stent was born (Fig. 1.9).

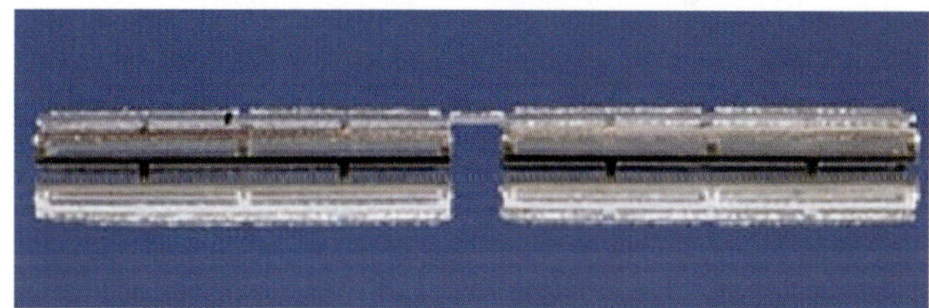

Fig. 1.9 The Palmaz Schatz stent, comprising two separate modules with a short connector between, the whole being 15 mm long
Source: EAPCI textbook

Gary Roubin, working with a particularly inventive radiologist, Cesar Gianturco, developed a premounted stent comprising an interdigitating coil, the Gianturco Roubin stent. In the early 90s both stents were clearly able to treat acute closure and to scaffold the vessel if a threatening looking dissection occurred—the incidence of emergency bypass surgery and periprocedural myocardial infarction (MI) plummeted (Fig. 1.10).[20,21] The Gianturco Roubin was flexible and easy to use, especially in a hurry, but it turned out to be not as good as the Palmaz Schatz in terms of restenosis. It was a very useful stent in its day though, because the alternative was the radially strong but relatively stiff Palmaz Schatz.

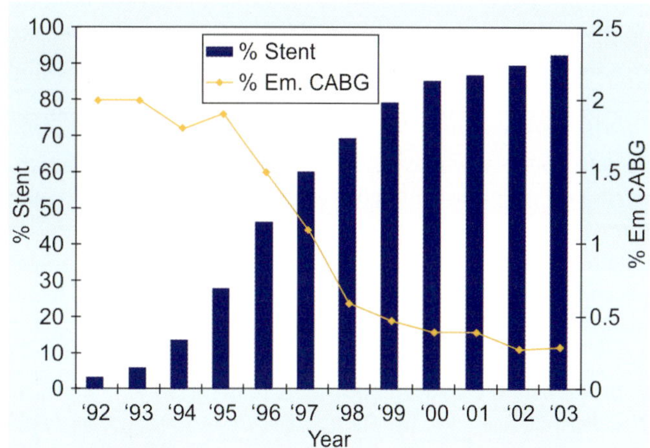

Fig. 1.10 Data from the audit returns of the British Cardiovascular Intervention Society up to 2003, showing declining need for emergency coronary artery bypass grafting (Em-CABG) after PTCA in-line with the increasing practice of stent implantation.
Source: Dr Peter Ludman and BCIS

The gap between these two extremes was progressively filled by developments from enthusiastic interventionists and by Industry. Notably in Rotterdam, dedicated stent meetings comprised a "stent line-up" at which protagonists of new designs could describe their putative advantages. At one of these, Guagliumi showed marvelous angioscopic videos of several implanted stent types with a rousing background of classical music; this was memorable. Also memorable was the spoof presentation by Kiemeneij (later better known as the pioneer of the radial approach to PCI) on his "BIC" stent, which was actually the spring from a ballpoint pen.

Some stents came premounted but many had to be manually crimped onto a chosen balloon by the operator (one trick was to cut a Palmaz Schatz in half if a very short stent was wanted). The variability in crimping success and the sometimes aggressive maneuvers needed to get a stent to the right place resulted in it occasionally parting company with the balloon, and in some cases the stent was lost somewhere in the patient, never to be found. Luckily it seemed an innocuous, though probably underreported event; the main thing was to try maintaining the dislodged stent on the angioplasty equipment until it could be withdrawn distal to the great vessels.

At last, in 1994 restenosis, the Achilles heel of angioplasty, was shown to be significantly modulated by stent implantation—as shown in the Benestent and Stress trials.[22,23] This was at the price of significant bleeding complications associated with the anticoagulation regimes used, but nevertheless it was a major step forward. It was realized that acute recoil and/ or negative remodeling, major components of restenosis, could be abolished by a metallic scaffold; the other major component, neo-intimal hyperplasia, still occurred, indeed was sometimes encouraged by the stent.

Remarkable advances in the technology of stent design and delivery systems, including more recently the use of alloys such as cobalt chromium, have allowed stenting to be the default strategy in most vessels, even in adverse anatomy. Backup from guide catheters is still needed, but buddy wires, extra support wires, etc are much less so nowadays; the years learning the skills of guide catheter manipulation and optimal guide catheter shapes when using comparatively crude equipment can still occasionally bear fruit in challenging cases.

The problem of stent thrombosis is, gratifyingly mainly in retrospect nowadays, interesting. The risk was known, as it was seen in clinical practice and reported; at the time the obvious way to minimize this risk appeared to be aggressive anticoagulation consisting of the use of almost every anticoagulant known to man. This turned out to be mistaken, being only partially effective at best and causing many bleeding complications. It turned out that the best approach, as is now well known, is dual antiplatelet therapy. The French Registry discovered this first, using aspirin and ticlopidine, reporting its 30-day results in 1996.[24] Antonio Colombo in Milan also made a major contribution, teaching us to implant stents properly and showing that without high-pressure postdilatation underdeployment on ultrasound was common. This probably particularly applied to the stent he used, the Palmaz Schatz, because its expansion characteristics were unruly, but the advice to ensure thorough implantation holds good today—in fact this is being advised with renewed emphasis with the advent of resorbable scaffolds.

The superiority of dual platelet therapy over anticoagulation was established by several randomized controlled trials,[25,26] and ticlopidine was replaced by clopidogrel, a more pleasant drug (and of course since by prasugrel and ticagrelor). This was a great relief after the harrowing days of aggressive anticoagulation. The topic of dual antiplatelet therapy, far from becoming simpler, has become more complex with better agents and better stents changing the balance of risk and benefit. Stent thrombosis (thrombus horribilis) was to rear its ugly head again during the next big phase in intervention—drug-eluting stents (DES), as discussed later.

So stents remarkably reduced the problem of acute or threatened closure and the need for emergency bypass surgery. As experience grew it was clear that restenosis in many lesion types was significantly reduced—but by no means abolished, and sometimes diffuse**,** aggressive and/or refractory instent restenosis was seen. Intracoronary brachytherapy came on to the scene to abolish the proliferative vascular reaction to our efforts, and for a time we welcomed radiation physicists and their equipment into our catheterization labs. Local radiation could be effective, especially in repeatedly recurrent or diffuse restenosis, but its usefulness was compromised by a tendency to late catch-up recurrence, thrombosis and difficulties with dose distribution.

Neointimal hyperplasia, the substance of restenosis, was studied extensively by the vascular biologists and those amongst us with such expertise, both by *in vitro* experiments and in animal models.[27-29] A wide array of likely drug candidates were put forward; some appeared successful in animal models when given systemically but only in clinically unrealistic doses, and systemic drug therapy was uniformly unsuccessful in clinical trials as far as restenosis was concerned. During the 90s the notion of achieving high local doses of an agent with little or no systemic effect by local drug delivery seemed appealing, and there was an array of ingenious drug delivery devices, such as porous balloons and needles. Though it could be shown in animal models that agents could be transferred into the vessel wall, convincing evidence of an effect was elusive, even though many biologically plausible agents were tried. So something else had to be done. Polymer coatings on stents emerged as the most promising way for local sustained elution and delivery, and polymer chemists worked with vascular biologists to produce biocompatible coatings tailored for elution of specific agents, including sophisticated ones such as antisense oligonucleotides to growth factors, all designed to quench the vascular response to injury.[30]

The day was won, first by sirolimus, the (predominantly) immunosuppressive agent, first isolated on Easter Island,

and temporally a close second, the antimitotic drug paclitaxel derived from the Pacific Yew. The Ravel trial, a multicenter double-blinded randomized clinical trial, revealed remarkable results[31,32]: at six months there was no instance of restenosis in the sirolimus eluting BX Velocity stent (to become known as the Cypher) compared with 26% with the bare metal stent, and at that time there was no adverse safety signal. Perhaps no one would have believed these amazing results if it had been a single center study, but this was a well performed multicenter trial in association with the renowned clinical research organization, Cardialysis, so its scientific credentials were faultless. Indeed Patrick Serruys and his group in Rotterdam and Cardialysis have over the years added remarkably to the body of knowledge in coronary intervention by the collection and thorough analysis of data.

So another new era had begun. Dr Renu Virmani, a cardiovascular pathologist, warned us of unbridled enthusiasm because healing of the vessel wall was clearly delayed by these drugs, and she had seen pathological evidence of this. She was proven right when in 2007, the SCAAR Scandinavian Registry study scared us all by showing a relatively high incidence of late (after 30 days) and very late (after one year) thrombosis in DES, seldom seen with bare metal stents.[33] This considerably dampened enthusiasm, so yet again, as in the history of many new drugs and new methods in medicine, enthusiasm turned into scepticism and reflection. The problem was blamed on delayed healing, partly due to the drug and partly to the persistent presence of polymer irritating the vessel wall. Again researchers—polymer chemists, vascular biologists and clinicians, have worked with industry to mitigate this problem by develop developing better polymers (including biodegradable ones), better drug elution profiles and stents with thinner struts, combined with prolongation of dual antiplatelet therapy. Current data show a very low incidence of stent thrombosis with DES, especially with sirolimus and its analogs—at least as safe as bare metal stents, even in complex patient and lesion subsets.

For many years the notion of completely resorbable stents has been mooted, because of the appeal of not having a permanent implant interfering with normal vasomotion and potentially encouraging neoatherosclerosis. Also the possibility of not interfering with future coronary bypass graft implantation sites is appealing. Completely resorbable polymer scaffolds incorporating drug (sirolimus or an analog) are now in clinical use. Two are on the European and other world markets, and have been shown to be statistically noninferior to modern DES—though there does appear to be a tendency to somewhat higher thrombosis rates with the bioresorbable scaffold. Modern drug eluting stents have been very forgiving, but resorbable scaffolds in their current form, with relatively thick struts and different expansion characteristics, demand meticulous implantation. Attention to this, and to advances in the devices themselves, may well prove that they are as safe as DES, and it is hoped they live up to their promise.

Local drug delivery has taken an interesting turn in the form of the drug-eluting balloon (DEB). Though this is currently limited to paclitaxel because of its lipophilicity and thus residence time in the tissues, the DEB does reduce recurrent in-stent stenosis and appears to have a role in small vessels. Some protagonists recommend its use in many other situations, such as side branches of bifurcations, in diffuse disease, even in vessels traditionally amenable to stent implantation. Clinical experience and the results of trials will be very interesting in this field.

What of imaging? The radiographic equipment has transformed, and nowadays so much can be done with just angiographic guidance. Intravascular ultrasound imaging has taught us much about the amount and type of disease we are dealing with (sometimes frighteningly so), and has revealed a lot about the vascular response to our maneuvers. It is rather expensive for everyone to use routinely, but is a fine tool in selected cases, such as borderline stenosis of the left main stem, or for assessing calcification and for determining the thoroughness of stent deployment if there is doubt. Optical coherence tomography has come on the scene to give even finer detail, for example about strut apposition, healing and strut coverage, and is following IVUS in becoming not just a research tool but probably being actually useful in selected cases. Fiberoptic angioscopy had its day as was mentioned earlier intriguing pictures of the vessels' interior could be seen, but it was technically challenging to obtain a clear fiel, and its subjectivity rather inhibited its usefulness as a research tool.

In the early days measurement of the distal coronary pressure was attempted via the balloon catheter lumen to assess the angioplasty result, partly because angiographic assessment was so murky until the balloon catheter had been removed, but it was not very reliable. The assessment of intracoronary hemodynamics changed with the excellent work on fractional flow reserve by de Bruyne and Pijls; available since the mid-90s its usefulness is now cemented by (a) clinical data from thorough clinical trials[33,34] and (b) marked improvement in the handling and reliability of the guidewire (a challenge in the early days). The concept of instantaneous flow reserve, without the need for inducing hyperemia, is intriguing and data from comparative clinical trials are awaited.

Certain patient and lesion subsets deserve individual attention, as they have evolved tremendously.

ACUTE CORONARY SYNDROME

Elective angiography and PCI took a dive with the publication of the Courage trial in 2007, because it indicated that overall there is no benefit of intervention over optimal medical therapy in stable coronary artery disease.[35] It was at about this time that the spectre of stent thrombosis with drug eluting stents arose, so cardiac surgeons became inclined to view interventional cardiologists with renewed suspicion. Of course optimal medical therapy can be difficult to achieve in routine practice, and patients with limiting angina do benefit from PCI, but it is clear that the main, and thoroughly established, role of PCI is in acute coronary syndromes. In many countries the logistic challenges of providing a 24-hour primary PCI service have been commendably overcome, transforming the management and outcomes of ST elevation myocardial infarction (STEMI). Early intervention in Non-STEMI, especially in patients with highrisk features, is well characterized. There was a period when GPIIb/IIIa platelet receptor inhibitors were regarded as de rigueur in this context, but selective use is now the norm.

INTRACORONARY THROMBUS

Following on from ACS, extensive intracoronary thrombus remains a challenge. Thrombolytics can work but of course increase bleeding, and intracoronary thrombectomy catheters have limited success in the presence of much clot; they too have had their prime time after earlier trials suggested they should be routinely used in AMI, subsequent ones indicating that selective application is the best approach.[36] Self expanding stents probably have some role here, but there is still much work to be done, perhaps in the local application of energy to enhance or to provide thrombolysis. For example, locally delivered therapeutic ultrasound deserves further investigation as a potentially useful player in this field.[37]

CHRONIC TOTAL OCCLUSIONS

Chronic total occlusions (CTO) have been attempted since the beginnings of coronary angioplasty, but success rates have rocketed with ingenious techniques, and a remarkable (and somewhat confusing) range of guidewires and accessories to aid the process. Our Japanese colleagues have contributed, and continue to contribute, immensely to this field. Just achieving primary success is no longer merely a temporary triump, now that DES provide good sustained patency. There is a lot to be said for a dedicated CTO operator or two in every center, as happens in some places.

MULTIVESSEL AND LEFT MAIN DISEASE

Unprotected left main stenosis, even though as discussed earlier was treated by balloon angioplasty in the very early days was a no-go area for many years, but the Syntax trial and subsequent studies have shown that PCI can be safe and effective in this condition[38,39] The Syntax trial, reporting in 2009, compared the paclitaxel eluting Taxus stent to coronary bypass surgery in left main and/or multi-vessel disease. As usual, the need for repeat revascularization was higher after PCI then CABG, but the gap was narrower than in previous stent versus surgery trials, and subgroup analysis has shown that patients with relatively localized, and yet true multivessel disease, can be well managed by PCI. Also from this study, the Syntax score, a brave and somewhat useful attempt to quantify the extent and adversarial characteristics of the disease, further enhanced by the inclusion of clinical characteristics, has emerged.[40] Studies using the score continue, and the results with later generation DES are very likely to be better than with the Taxus stent. The interface between PCI and CABG continues to evolve, and the evidence base generally swings ever more in favor of PCI-fuelled also by patient preference. Our cardiac surgical colleagues have been invaluable supporters, especially in the relatively dark days of not infrequent complications, and remain so in their collaboration to provide the optimum care to patients in their lifetime of coronary disease.

BIFURCATIONS

In the early days true bifurcation lesions were attacked with two separate guide catheters armed with separate wires and balloon catheters, which was quite a performance. Ingenious variations on the double stenting theme are in use, and depend on the vascular anatomy and operator skills/preferences, but interestingly the best approach in many applications is still to "keep it simple", with stenting of the side branch only if deemed necessary.

CONCLUSION

Inevitably some events, devices and important people have been missed out, but we hope this gives a balanced overview of major developments in coronary intervention, and how we have got where we are today. Many lessons have been learned, not just in the technical and clinical development of PCI, but also how to develop new techniques and how to teach them. The remarkable status of current coronary intervention, and the benefits it provides to patient care, are testament to the efforts of clinicians, industry, engineers, vascular biologists and, last but most important of all, patients. Without their trust and participation in clinical trials the massive and evolving evidence base we enjoy today would not have been possible.

REFERENCES

1. Rashkind WJ, Miller WW. Creation of an atrial septal defect without thoracotomy. A Palliative Approach to Complete Transposition of the Great Arteries. JAM. 1966;196:991-2.
2. Sones FM, Shirey EK, Proudfit WL, Westcott RN. Cine-coronary arteriography. Circulation. 1959;20:773-4.
3. Ryan TJ. The coronary angiogram and its seminal contributions to cardiovascular medicine over five decades. Trans Am Clin Climatol Assoc. 2002; 113:261-71.
4. Seldinger SI. Catheter replacement of the needle in percutaneous arteriography; a new technique. Acta Radiol. 1953;39(5):368-7.
5. Judkins MP. Selective coronary arteriography. Radiology. 1967;89:815-24.
6. Favaloro RG. Saphenous vein autograft replacement of severe segmental coronary artery occlusion: operative technique. Ann Thorac Surg. 1968;5:334-9.
7. Dotter CT, Judkins MP. Transluminal treatment of arteriosclerotic obstruction. Description of a new technique and a preliminary report of its application. Circulation. 1964;30:654-7.
8. Grüntzig A, Hopff H. Perkutane Rekanalisation chronischer arterieller mit einem neuen Dilatationskatheter. Dtsch Med Wochenschr. 1974;99(49):2502-1.
9. Cumberland DC. Percutaneous transluminal angioplasty: a review. Clin Radiol. 1983;34(1):25-3.
10. Grüntzig A, Riedhammer HH, Turina M, Rutishauser W. Eine neue Methode zur perkutanen Dilatation von Koronarstenosen—tierexperimentelle Prüfung. Verh Dtsch Ges Kreislaufforsch. 1976;42:282.
11. Grüntzig J. Der Pionier der kardialen Ballondilatation: Andreas Grüntzig, mein Bruder. Kardiologieforum. 2008;2:54-63.
12. Grüntzig AR, Senning Å, Siegenthaler WE. Nonoperative dilatation of coronary-artery stenosis: percutaneous transluminal coronary angioplasty. N Engl J Med. 1979;301(2):61.
13. Grüntzig A, Turina M, Schneider J. Transluminal dilatation of coronary-artery stenosis. Lancet. 1978;1:263.
14. Turina M, Grüntzig A, Krayenbühl C, Senning A. The role of the surgeon in percutaneous transluminal dilatation of coronary stenosis. Ann Thorac Surg. 1979;28(2):103-12.
15. Simpson JB, Baim DS, Robert EW, Harrison DC. A new catheter system for coronary angioplasty. Am J Cardiol. 1982;49:1216-22.
16. Kaltenbach M. The long wire technique—a new technique for steerable balloon catheter dilatation of coronary artery stenoses. Eur Heart J. 1984;5:1004-9.
17. Bonzel T, Wollschläger H, Just H. A new catheter system for the mechanical dilatation of coronary stenoses with exchangeable intracoronary catheters, fast flow of the contrast agent and improved control. Biomed Tech (Berl). 1986;31:195-200.
18. Waller BF. "Crackers, breakers, stretchers, drillers, scrapers, shavers, burners, welders and melters"—the future treatment of atherosclerotic coronary disease? A clinical-morphologic assessment. J Am Coll Cardiol. 1989;13(5):969-98.
19. Puel J, Joffre F, Rousseau H. Endoprothèses coronaires dans la prévention de la restenose post dilatation. Resultats préliminaires. Arch Mal coeu. 1987;80:1311-2.
20. Serruys PW, Strauss BH, Beatt KJ, Bertrand ME, Puel J, Rickards AF, Meier B, Goy J, Vogt P, Kappenberger L, Sigwart l. Angiographic follow-up after placement of a self-expanding coronary-artery stent. N Engl J Med. 1991;324:13-7.
21. Roubin GS, Cannon AD, Agrawal SK, Macander PJ, Dean LS, Baxley WA, Breland J. Intracoronary stenting for acute and threatened closure complicating percutaneous transluminal coronary angioplasty. Circulation. 1992;85:916-27.
22. Serruys PW, de Jaegere P, Kiemeneij F, Macaya C, Rutsch W, Heyndrickx G, Emanuelsson H, Marco J, Legrand V, Materne P, Belardi J, Sigwart U, Colombo A, Goy JJ, van den Heuvel P, Delcan J, Morel MA. A comparison of balloon-expandable-stent implantation with balloon angioplasty in patients with coronary artery disease. Benestent Study Group. N Engl J Me. 1994;331:489-95.
23. Fishman D, Leon M, Baim D. A randomized comparison of coronary-stent placement and balloon angioplasty in the treatment of coronary artery disease. The STRESS trial. N Engl J Me. 1994;331:496-501.
24. Karrillon GJ, Morice MC, Benveniste E, Bunouf P, Aubry P, Cattan S, Chevalier B, Commeau P, Cribier A, Eiferman C, Grollier G, Guerin Y, Henry M, Lefevre T, Livarek B, Louvard Y, Marco J, Makowski S, Monassier JP, Pernes JM, Rioux P, Spaulding C, Zemour G. Intracoronary stent implantation without ultrasound guidance and with replacement of conventional anticoagulation by antiplatelet therapy. 30-day clinical outcome of the French multicenter registry. Circulatio. 1996;94:1519-27.
25. Schömig A, Neuman F, Kastrati A. A randomized comparison of antiplatelet and anticoagulant therapy after the placement of coronary stents. N Engl J Me. 1996;334:1084-9.
26. Bertrand ME, Legrand V, Boland JP. Randomized multicenter comparison of conventional anticoagulation vs. antiplatelet therapy in unplanned and elective coronary stenting. The FANTASTIC study. Circulation. 1998;98:1597-603.
27. Herrman JP, Hermans WR, Vos J, Serruys PW. Pharmacological approaches to the prevention of restenosis following angioplasty. The search for the Holy Grail? (Part I). Drugs. 1993;46(1):18-52.
28. Herrman JP, Hermans WR, Vos J, Serruys PW. Pharmacological approaches to the prevention of restenosis following angioplasty. The search for the Holy Grail? (Part II). Drugs. 1993;46(2):249-62.
29. Feldman LJ, Riessen R, Steg PG. Prevention of restenosis after coronary angioplasty: towards a molecular approach? Fundam Clin Pharmacol. 1995;9(1):8-16.
30. Gunn J, Cumberland DC. Stent coatings and local drug delivery: state of the art. Eur Heart J. 1999;20:1693-700.
31. Morice MC, Serruys PW, Sousa JE, Fajadet J, Ban Hayashi E, Perin M, Colombo A, Schuler G, Barragan P, Guagliumi G, Molnàr F, Falotico R; RAVEL Study Group. Randomized Study with the Sirolimus-Coated Bx Velocity Balloon-Expandable Stent in the Treatment of Patients with de Novo Native Coronary Artery Lesions. A randomized comparison of a sirolimus-eluting stent with a standard stent for coronary revascularization. N Eng J Me. 2002;346:1773-80.
32. Lagerqvist B, James SK, Stenestrand U, Lindback J, Nilsson T, Wallentin L. Long-term outcomes with drug-eluting stents versus

bare-metal stents in Sweden. N Eng J Med. 2007;356(10):1009-19.
33. Tonino PAL, De Bruyne B, Pijls NHJ, et al. Fractional flow reserve versus angiography for guiding percutaneous coronary intervention. N Engl J Med. 2009;360:213-24.
34. De Bruyne B, Pijls NHJ, Kalesan B, et al. Fractional flow reserve-guided PCI versus medical therapy in stable coronary disease. N Engl J Med. 2012;367:991-1001.
35. Boden WE, O'Rourke RA, Teo KK, Hartigan PM, Maron TJ, Kostuk WJ, Knudtson M, Dada M, Casperson P, Harris CL, Chaitman BR, Shaw L, Gosselin G, Nawaz S, Title LM, Gau G, Blaustein AS, Booth DC, Bates ER, Spertus JA, Berman DS, Mancini GB, Weintraub WS; COURAGE Trial Research Groul. Optimal medical therapy with or without PCI for stable coronary disease. N Engl J Med. 2007;356:1503-16.
36. Jolly SS, Cairns JA, Yusuf S, Meeks B, Pogue J, Rokoss MJ, Kedev S, Thabane L, Stankovic G, Moreno R, Gershlick A, Chowdhary S, Lavi S, Niemelä K, Steg PG, Bernat I, Xu Y, Cantor WJ, Overgaard CB, Naber CK, Cheema AN, Welsh RC, Bertrand OF, Avezum A, Bhindi R, Pancholy S, Rao SV, Natarajan MK, ten Berg JM, Shestakovska O, Gao P, Widimsky P, Džavík V; TOTAL Investigators. Randomized trial of primary PCI with or without routine manual thrombectomy. N Engl J Me. 2015;372(15):1389-9.
37. Hamm CW, Steffan W, Terres W, de Scheerder I, Reimers J, Cumberland DC, Siegel RJ, Meinertz T. Intravascular Therapeutic Ultrasound Thrombolysis in Acute Myocardial Infarction. The American Journal of Cardiology. 1997;80:200-4.
38. Serruys P, Morice M, Kappetein A, Colombo A, Holmes D, Mack M, Ståhle E, Feldman T, van den Brand M, Bass E, Van Dyck N, Leadley K, Dawkins K, Mohr F; SYNTAX Investigators. Percutaneous coronary intervention versus coronary artery bypass grafting for severe coronary artery disease. N Eng J Med. 2009;360:961-72.
39. Morice MC, Serruys PW, Kappetein AP, Feldman TE, Stahle E, Colombo A, Mack MJ, Holmes DR, Torracca L, van Es GA, Leadley K, Dawkins KD, Mohr F. Outcomes in patients with de novo left main disease treated with either percutaneous coronary intervention using paclitaxel-eluting stents or coronary artery bypass graft treatment in the Synergy Between Percutaneous Coronary Intervention with TAXUS and Cardiac Surgery (SYNTAX) trial. Circulatio. 2010;121:2645-53.
40. Dawkins KD, Morel MA, Serruys PW. Counting the score: the SYNTAX Score and coronary risk. EuroInterventio. 2009;5:33-5.

CHAPTER

2

An Overview of the History and Fundamentals of Coronary Stent Design

Keith D Dawkins, Paul F Chouinard

TIMELINE OVERVIEW

Originally demonstrated in 1986 in a series of 19 patients for the treatment of restenosis, abrupt vessel closure and deterioration of coronary artery bypass grafts,[1] the use of coronary stents is now common place in percutaneous coronary angioplasty. Since the placement of the first expandable stents in human coronary arteries, the field of coronary stenting has been continuously evolving. Advances in technique and technology, and refinement of design have led to multiple ground breaking advances in the field through clinical research. Among the most notable early developments included the following:

1986: Placement of first self-expanding stent in human coronary artery.[2]

1987: Placement of first balloon-expanding stent (Palmaz-Schatz) in human coronary artery.[3]

1994: Publication of the BENESTENT[4] and STRESS[5] studies, demonstrating a reduction in restenosis rate with Palmaz-Schatz stent placement in comparison to balloon angioplasty alone.

2002–2003: Publication of RAVEL[6] and SIRIUS[7] trials demonstrating a reduction in restenosis and revascularization with sirolimus-eluting stents in comparison to bare metal stents.

2003–2004: Publication of TAXUS I and TAXUS IV trials demonstrating a reduction in restenosis and revascularization with paclitaxel-eluting stents in comparison to bare metal stents.

After the introduction of the first balloon-expandable stents in coronary use in the mid-1980s, and more significantly, after the findings of BENESTENT and STRESS demonstrated improved outcomes over simple balloon angioplasty alone, there was a proliferation in the number of available bare metal stents introduced on the market. This boom in balloon-expandable stent design resulted in many products that would prove to be short-lived, but it also gave rise to the coronary stent businesses of the three predominant players in today's US market, namely Guidant (the vascular interventions business of which was acquired by Abbott Laboratories), AVE (which was acquired by Medtronic), and Boston Scientific.

STENT TECHNOLOGIES

Deployment Mechanisms

As early as 1964, Dotter described the concept of a Silastic endovascular splint to maintain the diameter of an expanded vessel.[8] As the first metallic stents emerged in the mid-1980s they fell within two operating mechanisms, self-expanding and balloon expandable. Self-expanding stents are set to an expanded diameter and then compressed within a catheter for delivery to the vessel. The stent is released from the catheter, allowing the stent's elastic restoring force to cause the stent to expand within the vessel, and exert outward force from within the vessel. In contrast, balloon expandable stents rely upon plastic deformation of the stent structure for their expansion within the vessel. Balloon expandable stents are placed over a balloon and typically affixed onto the balloon by crimping or some other mechanical means. Upon delivery to the target location, the expansion of the balloon causes plastic deformation within the stent structure so as to establish an expanded stent diameter and create a scaffold by which to hold the vessel in an opened state (Figs 2.1A and B).

Self-Expanding

The first stent to be placed within a human coronary artery was made of braided tubular mesh of elastic wire,[2] whereby the diameter of the stent is defined in an expanded state, and then compressed to a smaller diameter and constrained

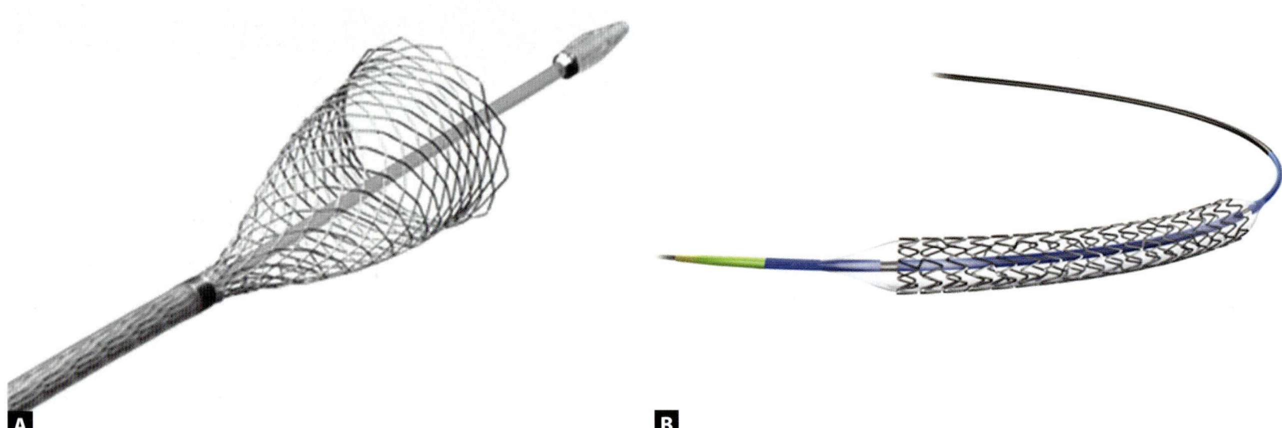

Figs 2.1A and B Examples of the self-expanding and balloon expandable stent deployment mechanisms. (A) Wallstent; (B) Element

within a sheath. The stent is then either advanced from the sheath, or the sheath withdrawn over the surface of the stent, so as to allow the stent to expand by its own elastic properties to appose the vessel. Such a mechanical construct is the basis of the Wallstent, which although no longer in use for coronary stenting, remains in widespread use for other stenting applications to this day. A second coronary stent to be designed using a self-expanding deployment mechanism was the radius stent.[9] The Radius stent employed Nitinol, an alloy of nickel and titanium which has a high degree of recoverable strain.[10] Cut from a tube of Nitinol and shaped to a pre-set expanded diameter, the radius stent was compressed within a delivery catheter which was used to deliver the stent to the target location where it would be allowed to expand within the vessel. Similar to the Wallstent, self-expanding Nitinol stents are no longer in common use for coronary stenting applications. However, Nitinol stent technology forms the basis of most self-expanding stents in current clinical use for peripheral stenting applications.

In coronary use, self-expanding stents failed to gain traction in comparison to their balloon expandable counterparts for several reasons. Self-expanding stents require a constraining member (tube, catheter, sheath, membrane, etc.) on the outside of the stent to hold it in the collapsed condition for delivery. This added component on the outside of the stent increases catheter profile and impacts catheter flexibility in comparison to balloon-expandable stents which typically require no exterior covering. Braided stents such as the Wallstent are subject to substantial length changes upon deployment, in comparison to most balloon expandable stents, presenting a challenge in correctly sizing the stent for the intended length. Also, early self-expanding Nitinol stents such as Radius exhibited a tendency to "jump" from the catheter upon deployment, posing a challenge for deployment accuracy. These challenges have been effectively addressed in peripheral stenting applications, but self-expanding stents have yet to gain a significant foothold in coronary use.

Balloon Expandable

In current interventional cardiology practice, virtually all stents available are balloon expandable. Stents are shaped, formed or machined into tubular lattice structures that can be affixed to a balloon, and subsequently expanded by application of outward force from the balloon. In contrast to self-expanding stents, in which materials and designs are selected to allow a large amount of recoverable strain by elastic deformation, balloon expandable stents utilize designs and materials which achieve plastic (permanent) deformation at low strains.[11] As such, a balloon expandable stent can be crimped onto a balloon without significant elastic recoil, which is necessary to achieve securement of the crimped stent to the balloon. Similarly, once expanded by the balloon within the vessel, the stent maintains its expanded diameter without excessive deployed recoil, and thus sufficiently maintains its expanded diameter. Once deployed, the stent resists inward forces from the stented vessel, so as to maintain a patent lumen.

Fabrication Methods

Multiple fabrication methods have been employed in the manufacture of stents.[12,13] For the purposes of categorization, most stents are manufactured by employing one or more of the following methods.

Braided Wire

Braided wire stents such as the Wallstent are created by an interwoven lattice of helical springs. For example, a braided stent might be made up of approximately 20 wires evenly spaced around the perimeter of the stent, half of which traverse the stent in a right-handed helix, and half of which traverse the stent in a left-handed helix. At the points where the wires coincide, one wire crosses to the outside of the stent lumen, and the other crosses to the inside of the stent lumen. A pattern of over and under crossing points produces an interwoven tube in which each helical element is held in place by other wires. The wires are typically made from a spring alloy which allows the tubular structure to be elongated in length with a corresponding reduction in diameter, placed within a delivery catheter and subsequently deployed from the catheter into a vessel (Fig. 2.2).

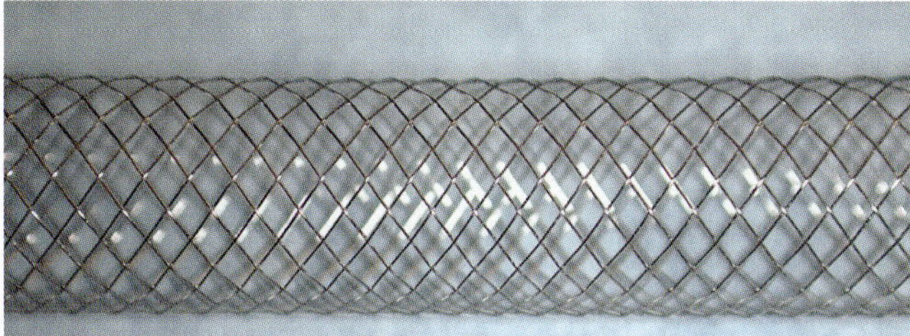

Fig. 2.2 Braided wire stent in the deployed (expanded) state

Knitted Wire

While the Wallstent is made from a woven construct (a braid), the Strecker stent was formed using a knitted configuration, with interlaced loops of tantalum wire making up a cylindrical tube (Fig. 2.3).

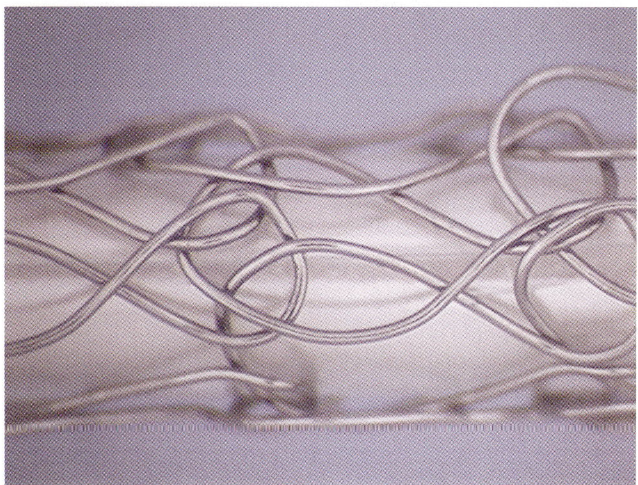

Fig. 2.3 Balloon expandable knitted wire stent. Strecker stent shown in the crimped state

Formed Wire

Multiple stent constructs have been made from formed wire. The first coronary stent to be approved for use in the United States, the GR Flex stent, was made using a single stainless steel wire formed into a series of reversing undulations around the stent circumference.[14] The resulting structure was a "clamshell"-like structure, which was wrapped around a balloon catheter and opened by balloon dilation. Multiple other formed wire stents have been evaluated over the years, but one noteworthy wire stent in current use is the integrity stent.[15] The integrity stent is made from a wire that is formed into a sinusoidal pattern. The formed wire is then wrapped in a helical configuration to form a cylinder, and adjacent apices of the formed wire are welded together in particular locations to create the stent (Fig. 2.4).

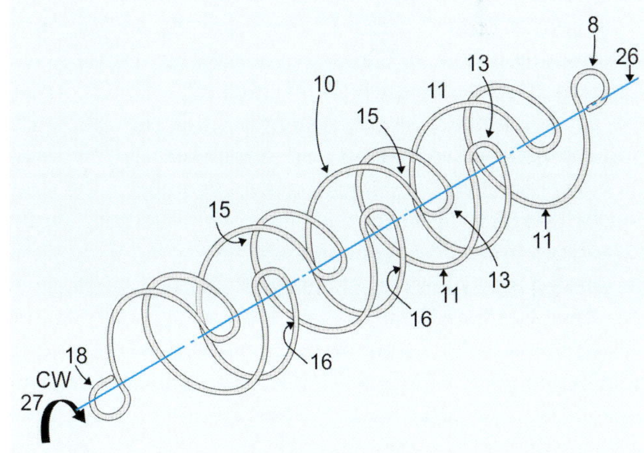

Fig. 2.4 Patent drawing of Gianturco-Rubin (GR) Flex stent

Soldered or Welded Sheet, Hoops, Wire, etc.

A number of stents have been designed using soldering or welding to create attachments within the stent pattern. The original stent designed by Palmaz utilized solder to adjoin wire.[3,16] The NIR stent utilized welding to adjoin opposite edges of a sheet together in order to form a tube.[16] Also, the AVE—Medtronic coronary stents (e.g. GFX, S540, S670, driver, integrity) have utilized welding to attach adjacent peaks of wire to create the desired structure. With the exception of the integrity stent which is formed from a sinusoidal wire, the other mentioned Medtronic stents are formed from wire rings or hoops.[15] The hoops are formed into an undulating circular sinusoid, and the formed hoop segments are placed in series and welded together in locations so as to create a cylindrical stent (Figs 2.5A and B).

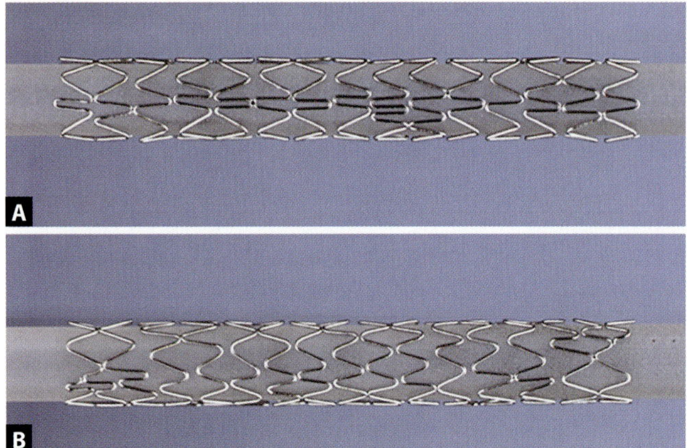

Figs 2.5A and B Examples of welded wire hoop (A) and sinusoidal wire (B) stents in the expanded state

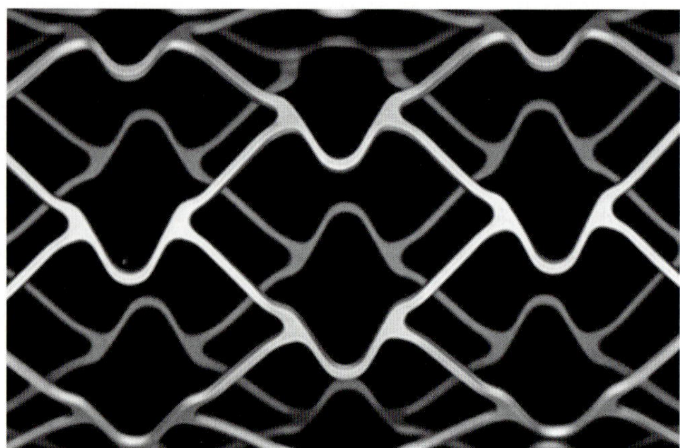

Fig. 2.6 Example of stent fabricated from a sheet prior to being formed into a cylindrical shape and welded

Machined from Sheet

Although stents are typically fabricated into a tubular shape for delivery within the vessel, some stents may be manufactured from a flat sheet and subsequently rolled into a tubular form. Flat sheet can be machined by electrical discharge manufacturing (EDM), water jet cutting, laser cutting or etching, so as to create the stent pattern in a flat form. The flat pattern is then rolled to form a cylinder and welded at its edges to form a tubular structure (Fig. 2.6).

Machined from Tube

The predominant method of fabricating coronary stents is machining the stents from a tube. Typically, laser-cutting equipment is used to cut the stent pattern from a metal tube, although other techniques (EDM, etching, water jet) may also be used. Once the stent is cut from a tube, the stents are typically polished to remove any nonuniformities or heat-affected regions from the laser, to create a smooth, uniformly polished surface. Cutting the stent from a tube confers certain advantages in the design and manufacture of the stent. First, the use of a tube allows for "seamless" construction, in which the tube is fabricated from drawing a hollow cylindrical metal bar machined from a solid bar, to progressively smaller and smaller diameters.[11] The result is a metal tube with consistent material characteristics throughout its cross-section, without regions affected by high-temperature processes such as welding. By machining the stent pattern from a tube rather than forming from a wire, the designer is free to vary the shape or width of any feature within the stent, rather than being constrained by working with features of constant width, as is typically the case with wire. Of the many of laser-cut coronary stents in use today, examples include the Boston Scientific Promus PREMIER and SYNERGY stents and Abbott Vascular Xience and Multi-Link stents (Figs 2.7A and B).

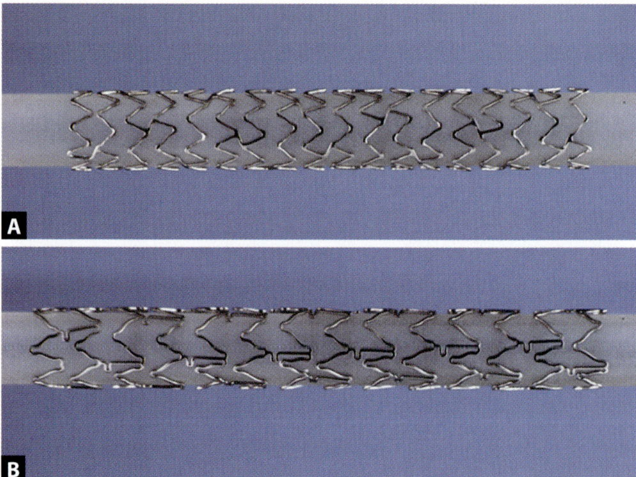

Figs 2.7A and B Examples of stents fabricated from tube, shown in the expanded state. (A) Promus Element stent and (B) Xience V stent

Balloon Expandable Stent Materials

One of the most fundamental decisions to be made in mechanical design is the selection of appropriate materials. In the design of a balloon expandable coronary stent, a number of important factors need to be considered, including the followings:

Biocompatibility

The implant must be accepted by the surrounding tissues in the implanted environment.

Corrosion Resistance

The material must be capable of withstanding the implant environment and maintain its stability over time. Conversely, for a resorbable stent, the material must allow for a controlled resorption by the body.

Strength

The materials selected must allow for the design of an implant with small dimensions but sufficient strength to hold the vessel open.

Stiffness

An ideal material will have very little strain (deformation) for a given amount of stress (force applied). In this way, a stent can be designed with minimal elastic recoil after expansion.

Ductility

In order to maximize the diameter to which the implant can be expanded, the material must be sufficiently ductile. That is, the material should withstand a large amount of deformation or strain before eventual fracture.

X-ray Attenuation

In order to be visible under fluoroscopy, typically referred to as radiopaque, the material selected must sufficiently attenuate the passage of X-rays through the implant.

Permanent Metals

From the first described use of the Palmaz experimental expandable stent in 1985 until the early 2000s, most balloon expandable stents were made from stainless steel. Some notable exceptions include the use of platinum-iridium alloy and the use of tantalum wire several early stents, but most first-generation balloon expandable stents which gained widespread commercial acceptance were made from 316L stainless steel. This alloy found favor as a biomaterial for stent design due to its combination of corrosion resistance, biocompatibility, ductility and strength.[17] However, the continuous drive to improve the performance of stents drove an effort to determine a more idealized material for the construction of stents. Such a material would allow for the construction of thinner, lower profile stents while maintaining strength and radiopacity. In order to achieve these seemingly contradictory goals, new materials needed to be designed and/or selected.[17]

Improved alloys for stent design required increased yield strength so as to provide adequate strength with smaller struts, and also increased density so as to provide adequate radiopacity with smaller struts. Two commercially-available alloys, commonly referred to as L605 and MP-35N were selected by several stent manufacturers to achieve these objectives. These cobalt-based alloys were used previously in other biomedical applications, but were later adopted for stent design due to their density and mechanical characteristics. MP-35N is the material used in present-day Medtronic coronary stents such as Driver and Integrity. L605 is the material used in present-day Abbott Vascular stents such as Xience.

Most conventional engineering alloys, including 316L, MP35N and L605 were originally designed to meet mechanical and environmental requirements, and not necessarily all requirements for the design of a stent, such as radiopacity. Accordingly, such conventional alloys are not necessarily optimized for stent design purposes. Another approach to selecting a material to enable thinner-strut stents was to design a specialty stainless steel alloy which provides for both increased strength and radiopacity. In one such design effort, a platinum enriched stainless steel was developed. In the alloy described by O'Brien et al.[17] a specialty alloy later branded by Boston Scientific as Platinum-Chromium or PtCr was created by substituting platinum for a significant amount of the nickel and iron which is present in 316L stainless steel. The resulting alloy has increased yield strength and ultimate tensile strength compared to 316L and higher density and lower nickel content than 316L, MP-35N and L605.[17] Platinum-Chromium alloy is the material used in present-day Boston Scientific stents such as Promus PREMIER and Synergy (Table 2.1 and Fig. 2.8).

Bioabsorbable Materials

The use of biostable (permanently implanted) metallic stents revolutionized the practice of interventional cardiology, and the continuous refinement of stent technology in the 30 years since its first use has dramatically improved patient outcomes. However, from the early days of coronary stenting, the question has been raised whether stents should be a permanent implant, or whether a more ideal solution would be a temporary scaffold to support the vessel, followed by resorption of the scaffold structure by the body.[18] The notion of a resorbable scaffold is based on the premise that mechanical scaffolding is no longer needed after approximately six months, once the neointimal response is complete and the vessel has healed following the procedure.[19]

Unlike the permanent metals which have been selected due to their mechanical properties and biostability, materials suitable for bioresorbable scaffold design must be at once biocompatible, sufficiently strong and deformable, and also absorbable by the body. Furthermore, the degradation byproducts of the stent must themselves be biocompatible within the window of local tissue concentrations, and capable of being safely metabolized and/or eliminated by the body. This design requirement significantly constrains the list of

Table 2.1 Typical compositions of alloys used in designs of balloon-expandable coronary stents

Element	*316L*	*PtCr*	*L605*	*MP35N*
Chromium	18	18	20.00	20.00
Nickel	14	9	10.00	35.00
Molybdenum	2.25–3.0	2.43–2.83	—	9.0–10.5
Tungsten	—	—	15.00	—
Platinum	—	33	—	—
Titanium	—	—	—	1.0 max
Manganese	2.0 max	0.05 max	1.5±.05	0.15 max
Iron	Bal	Bal	3.00 max	1.0 max
Cobalt	—	—	Bal	Bal
Boron	—	—	—	0.015 max
Carbon	0.030 max	0.003—0.023	0.10±.05	0.025 max
Oxygen	—	—	—	—
Nitrogen	0.10 max	0.010 max	—	—
Phosphorus	0.025 max	0.010 max	0.040 max	0.015 max
Sulfur	0.010 max	0.0007 max	0.030 max	0.010 max
Silicon	0.75 max	0.10 max	0.40 max	0.15 max
Copper	0.50 max	0.02 max	—	—

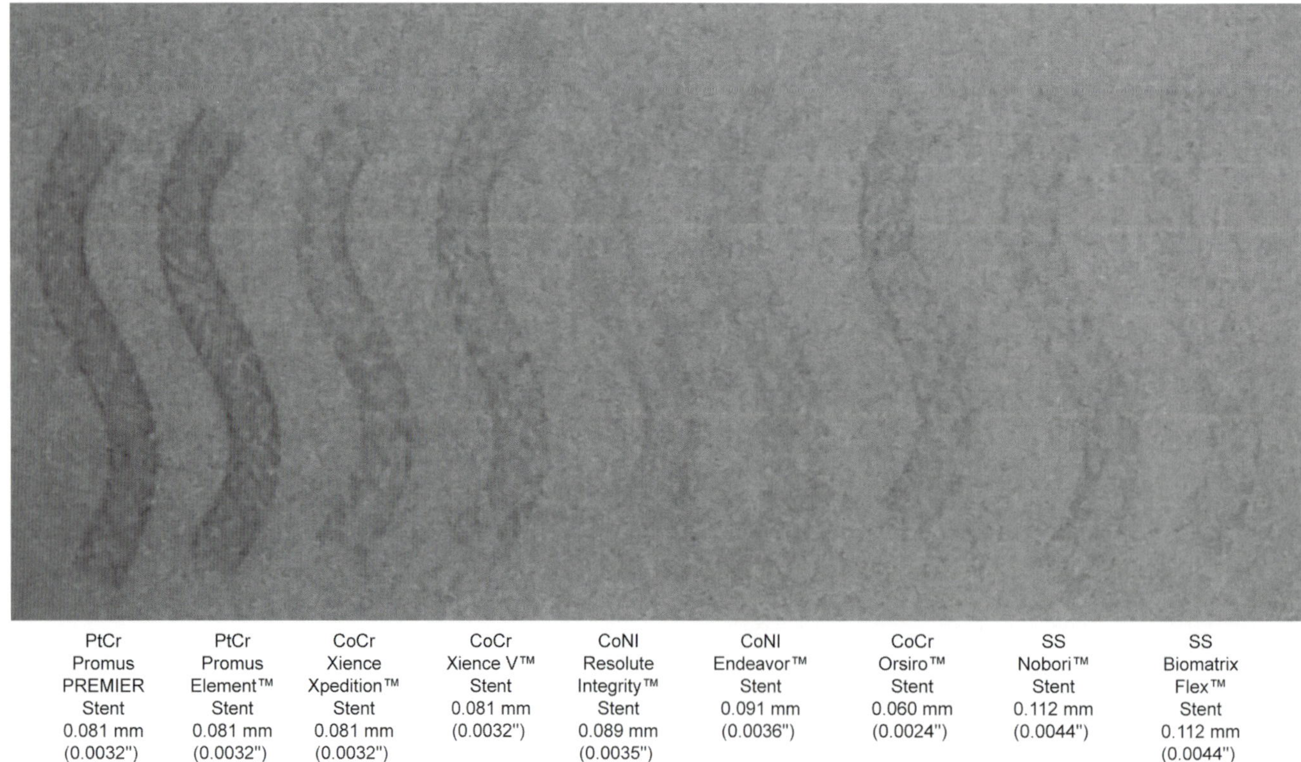

Fig. 2.8 Radiopacity images of stents of varying composition and thickness, imaged through a thickness of copper to simulate body mass

candidate materials. The available materials with which to design a resorbable scaffold have significantly lesser strength and radiopacity than the permanent metals in use today, and accordingly first-generation resorbable scaffolds are significantly more bulky and/or less strong than present-day permanent metallic stents. Because of these limitations, the development of an optimized bioabsorbable material and scaffold design remains an active area of development today (Fig. 2.9).

Two basic classes of materials have been developed for use as a resorbable stent material—bioabsorbable metals and bioabsorbable polymers. Among the metallic materials considered for resorbable stent design are magnesium alloys and pure iron.[10] Polymer materials utilized or considered for resorbable stent design include polymers and copolymers of lactic acid, glycolic acid and caprolactone.[10] Perhaps most notably, Poly (L-lactide) (PLLA) is the material used in the design of the Abbott Vascular Absorb bioresorbable vascular scaffold (BVS).[20] The Absorb stent is commercially available in European markets, and is currently under review for pre-market approval by the US FDA. In its pivotal trial for US approval, the Absorb stent met its noninferiority endpoint at one year, however, the acute performance and adverse outcomes were numerically worse than the permanent-metallic control device. The readiness for this and other first-generation resorbable scaffolds to replace the highly-refined permanent metallic stents of today is a topic of debate.[21]

The concept of a resorbable stent has inherent appeal for several reasons, including the potential restoration of vasomotor tone, positive arterial remodeling, the preservation of surgical options for potential future CABG, and the absence of a foreign body long-term. Balanced against these potential benefits are the limitations that result from designing a stent from the lesser-strength bioabsorbable materials currently available. The promise of this emerging technology has yet to be fully realized, and only time will tell whether fully resorbable scaffolds evolve to a point where they can replace permanent metallic stent usage as a workhorse product.

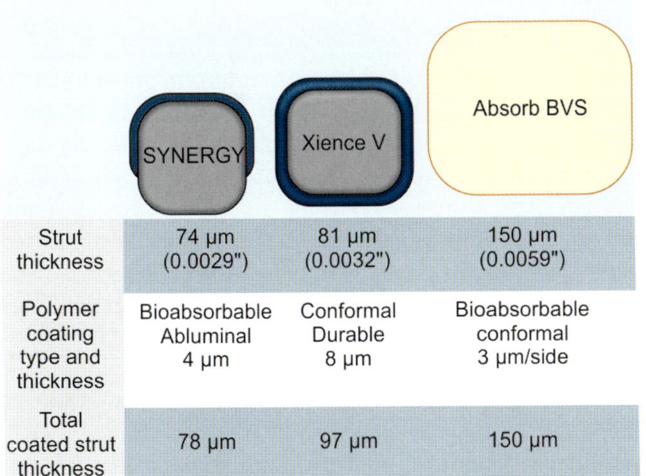

Fig. 2.9 Illustration of the relative strut thicknesses of present-day metallic stents (SYNERGY and Xience stents) and of the Absorb BVS resorbable polymer stent

PERFORMANCE REQUIREMENTS

Engineering and design require the pragmatic consideration of multiple sometimes contradictory performance requirements so as to arrive at a solution which strikes a favorable balance. In the design of coronary stents, the following basic performance requirements must be considered.

Deliverability to the Target Location

High among the list of requirements for a stent system is its ability to be routed safely to the intended treatment location. Some of the key components of deliverability are the following:

Flexibility

The ability of the crimped stent and distal end of the catheter to flex around a curve is needed in order to traverse tortuous anatomy. Multiple test methods have been developed to characterize the flexibility of a catheter. These include pure bend stiffness tests, distal tip flexibility tests, and tracking tests to directly measure the force required to traverse a catheter around a tortuous path.

Pushability

Pushability refers to the efficiency with which a push force applied at the proximal end of the catheter is transmitted to the distal end of the catheter. Stent delivery catheters are typically an assembly of multiple components in series, each of which is designed and selected to transmit the applied force at the catheter shaft outside the body through the shaft in the aorta, around the aortic arch, through the coronary anatomy to the tip of the device. An ideal catheter provides high flexibility in the intracoronary portions, and also high pushability so as to transmit the force to the tip.

Profile

The profile of the stent system refers to the diameter of the catheter at locations critical for its ability to cross a lesion. The most frequently-used measure of catheter profile is the crossing profile, which is the largest diameter between the catheter distal tip and the proximal end of the crimped stent.

Expandability at Target Location

Once placed at the target location, which can be confirmed by fluoroscopic visualization of either the stent, or the radiopaque markers on the catheter which flank the stent, the catheter and stent must be capable of expanding the stent to its targeted location within the vessel.

Deployment Pressure

The catheter is designed to achieve its labeled nominal diameter at a pre-specified pressure. This requires the careful design of the balloon diameter and compliance, and evaluation in combination with the stent to confirm correct sizing.

Compliance

The compliance of the balloon refers to the change in balloon diameter over a range of pressure. The radial stiffness of the balloon is tailored so as to achieve the desired degree of diameter growth within a specified pressure range.

Foreshortening

More correctly described as deployed length change, foreshortening refers to the change in stent length that may occur from the crimped state to the expanded state, expressed as a percentage of the crimped length. Some stents, particularly braided stents, are predisposed to shorten upon deployment,[22] and foreshortening is a term commonly used to describe this length change. Most contemporary balloon-expandable coronary stents undergo relatively little length change in comparison to braided stents.

Recoil

When the stent is opened with the balloon, the stent undergoes a brief elastic deformation before being plastically deformed to the larger diameter. Likewise, when the balloon is deflated, the stent undergoes elastic recoil before it reaches equilibrium at its new diameter. The difference in the stent diameter while pressurized by the balloon, and the stent diameter in the relaxed deployed state, expressed as a percentage of the pressurized diameter, is the deployed stent recoil. In stent design, an objective is to minimize the recoil of the stent, so as to maximize the preserved diameter resulting from expansion, and to avoid the need for unnecessary over-dilation to achieve the desired result.

Postdilatation Diameter

Balloon expandable stents are typically designed to accommodate a range of deployed diameters, so that complete apposition of the stent to the vessel wall can be achieved by postdilatation if it is not achieved with the initial stent deployment. In order to allow some flexibility in sizing the stent to the target vessel, some degree of over-sizing is incorporated within the stent design. This allows the operator to adjust the diameter of the stent with post-dilatation balloons within specified limits in the event of vessel taper or mis-sizing the selected stent, for example.

Scaffolding of the Vessel

Once deployed within the vessel, the primary mechanical role of the stent is to provide mechanical support or scaffolding to the vessel. The stent must exhibit sufficient strength so as to resist vessel recoil, and sufficient surface coverage so as to prevent plaque ingress into the stented lumen (Figs 2.10A and G).

Conformability

Conformability typically refers to the ability of the stent to adapt or conform to the native curvature of the vessel in which it is placed. Ideally, a stent will not force a curved vessel to straighten, but rather the stent will conform to the curvature of the vessel. This minimizes the stress that the stent places on the vessel, and minimizes potential flow disruptions that may occur particularly at the ends of a curved stented vessel segment.[23] One typical measure of conformability is the bending stiffness of the expanded stent, or the bending torque required to achieve a given stent curvature. A stent with high conformability will exhibit a low bending stiffness.

Minimize Vessel Injury

The process of mechanically dilating a stenotic vessel by balloon angioplasty is frequently injurious to the vessel. Part of the rationale for placing a stent is to address the acute injury that is caused by the angioplasty procedure. As such, the balloon and stent should be designed so as to minimize the degree of injury caused by the procedure. One important design consideration by which vessel injury can be minimized is by controlling the degree to which the balloon body (the cylindrical portion of the balloon) extends beyond the edges of the stent. It is important that the balloon be precisely sized to the stent. The balloon body must extend to both ends of the stent, so as to achieve complete stent expansion. However, the length of the balloon extending beyond the stent ends should be minimized, and the compliance of the balloon carefully designed so as to limit any injury that may result from the unconstrained balloon outside the stent. Another means by which a stent minimizes vessel injury is to retain its mechanical structure for the duration of its implant life; the

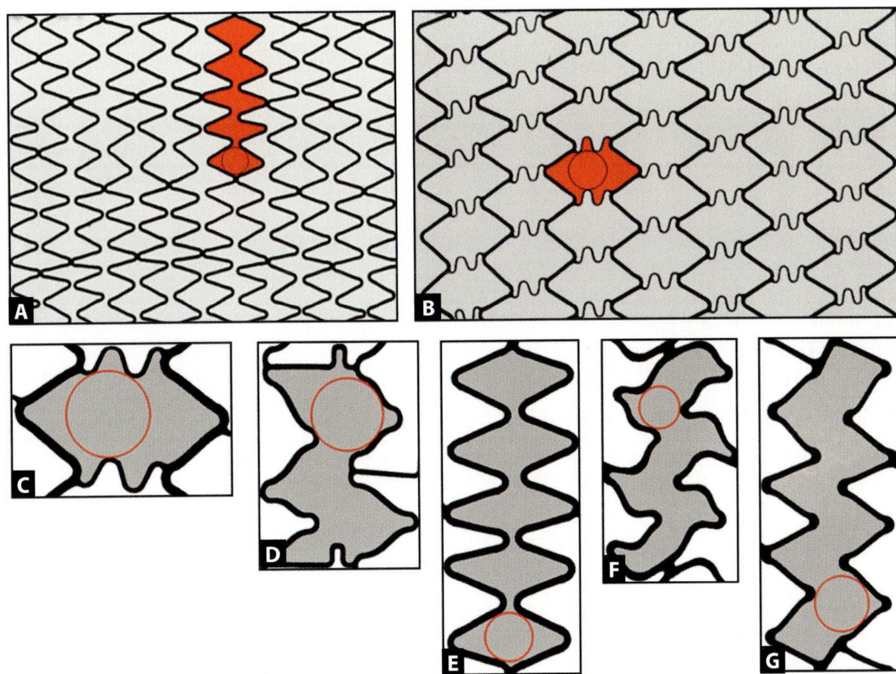

Figs 2.10A to G Scaffolding images of various balloon expandable coronary stents. Images (A) and (B) depict open-cell and closed-cell geometry, respectively, in which closed cell designs have connections between each peak and a peak of an adjacent segment. Cell areas are shaded in red, and the largest circle which can be inscribed within the cell is also shown. The inscribed circle diameter is one measure of scaffolding. Images C-G depict the representative scaffolding of the Cypher (C), Xience V (D), Endeavor (E), TAXUS Liberté (F) and TAXUS Element (G) 3.0 mm stents

stent design should minimize the risk of fatigue fracture when exposed to physiologic distensions.

Minimize Disruption of Flow

The purpose of angioplasty is to restore flow to the coronary vascular bed by dilating narrowed vessels. The placement of a stent serves the purposes of holding up flow-limiting dissections and preventing flow-limiting recoil. However, the struts of the stent themselves are a potential impediment to blood flow,[24] and minimizing the flow disturbances caused by the stent is a design goal. Additionally, the change in vessel curvature that can result from the increased bending stiffness of a stent can result in modified flow shear stress in proximity to the ends of the stent.[23] In order to minimize both of these potential stent-related flow disruptions, stents are designed with an objective to minimize stent wall thickness and minimize bending stiffness, so as to minimize any stent-related disruption of flow. Stents should be appropriately deployed so as to prevent any unnecessary flow disruption from mal-apposed struts (Fig. 2.11).[24]

Combat Restenosis

The introduction of coronary balloon angioplasty in 1977 and the introduction of coronary stents in 1986 have been described as two revolutions in interventional cardiology.[25] With the introduction of drug eluting stents in 1999 came the third revolution in interventional cardiology, and the promise of significantly curtailing the restenosis response which had limited the success of bare metal stents. Prior to the introduction of bare metal stents, plain balloon angioplasty had a restenosis rate of about 30–40%, and with the advent of bare metal stents, the rate was reduced significantly to about 20–30%.[4,5] However, the success of stenting procedures was still significantly limited by the threat of restenosis. Two clinical trials evaluating restenosis rate in thin-walled bare metal stents in comparison to thicker-walled stents found a significantly reduced rate of restenosis in the thin-walled cohort,[35,36] adding further reason to pursue thin-walled stents as a design goal. However, even with the reduced rate of restenosis found with the remarkably thin 50 micron stent group, the restenosis rate was still in the 15–20% range.[35,36] The introduction of antiproliferative drug coatings on the stent has significantly curtailed the rates of restenosis to <10%.[7,26] Drug eluting stents (DES) were immediately adopted for the vast majority of stenting procedures upon their introduction to the market. In addition to the restenosis-limiting benefit of drug coatings, reduced stent thickness is still pursued as a means to limit restenosis and to speed healing.[37,38]

With the advent of drug-eluting stents, the optimization of the stent as a drug-delivery vehicle became a focus of research

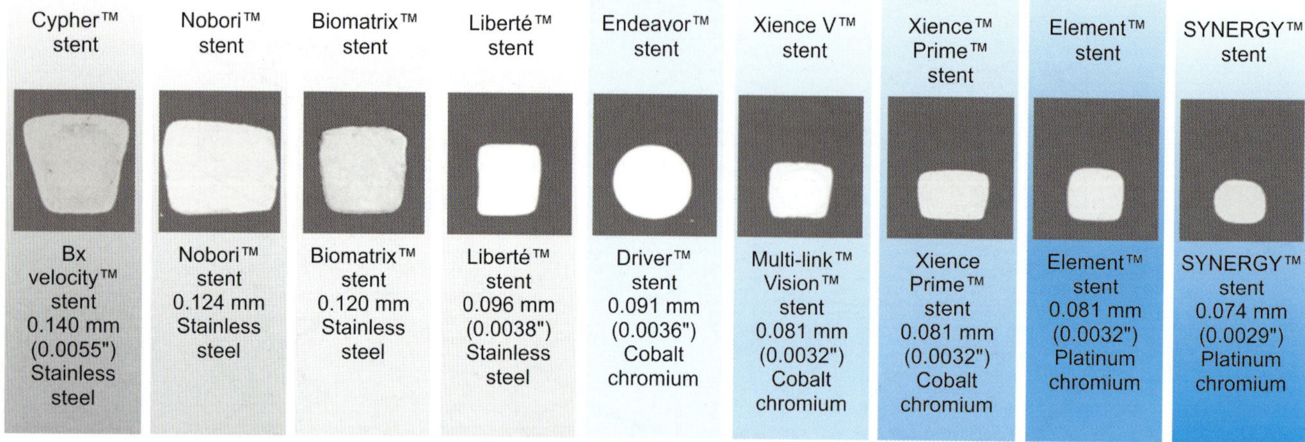

Fig. 2.11 Representative cross-sections of stent struts, illustrating the difference in strut dimensions from earlier thicker strut designs (Cypher, Express) to more recent thin strut designs (Xience, Element, Synergy)

and development efforts. Most DES utilize a polymer/drug mixture as the stent coating, in which the polymer provides a stable matrix for the drug and modulates the release of the drug over a period of time. In most cases, the polymer in the coating is a permanent polymer, which remains present on the surface of the stent after drug release is complete. Typically, these coatings are conformally applied to the stent, with each stent strut enveloped by the coating. Examples of DES utilizing a conformal coating with a permanent polymer include Cypher, TAXUS, Endeavor, Resolute, XIENCE and Promus. Over the years since the introduction of Cypher, a number of different drug delivery formulations and methods have been explored, including bioabsorbable polymer coatings, polymer-free coatings, struts with reservoirs for drug delivery, and abluminal coatings.[33] As an example of a stent which incorporates some of these new technologies, the Synergy DES utilizes an ultrathin abluminal coating designed to deliver the drug everolimus to the vessel tissue with an absorbable polymer/drug matrix.

The design of pharmaceuticals and coatings formulations and processes are the subject of extensive research and development,[27,28] and are not discussed in detail here. However, with respect to the requirement of the stent to allow for the reduction of restenosis, one requirement of the stent is that it must be a suitable substrate for the application of drug coatings. The specific requirements which define the stent's suitability for coating depend on the coating formulation and method of coating application. Some design elements which may be important for the application and adherence of a coating include stent surface energy, stent edge radius, and stent feature radii. Another design aspect regarding the use of the stent as a drug delivery vehicle is the uniformity with which the stent applies the drug coating against the surface of the vessel.[29,30] The development of stents with a more uniform

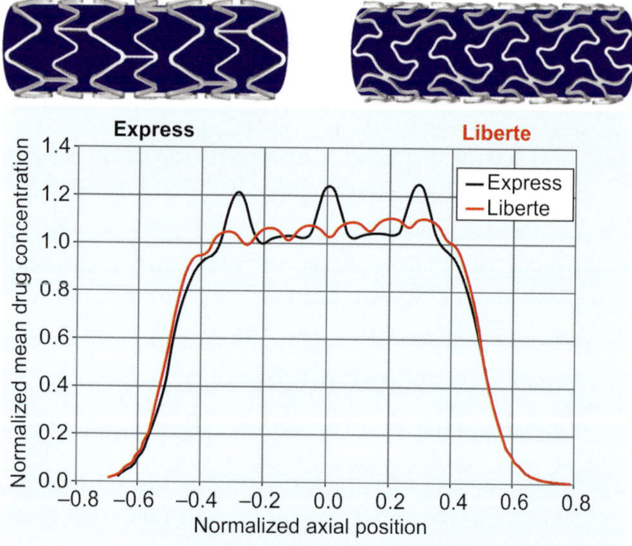

Fig. 2.12 Computer modeling of drug distribution within vessel as a function of vessel axial position for two different stent designs. The Express stent modeling predicts greater fluctuation in drug concentration whereas the Liberté stent modeling predicts a more uniform distribution of drug throughout the length of the stented vessel

distribution of struts to support the vessel lumen may also result in a more uniform application of the drug-eluting surface to the vessel wall (Figs 2.12 and 2.13).

Promote Healing

Ultimately, the performance goal of a stent is to restore flow to the stented vessel and to preserve that restored flow indefinitely. The advent of drug-eluting stents brought about a dramatic reduction in stent restenosis, thereby preserving

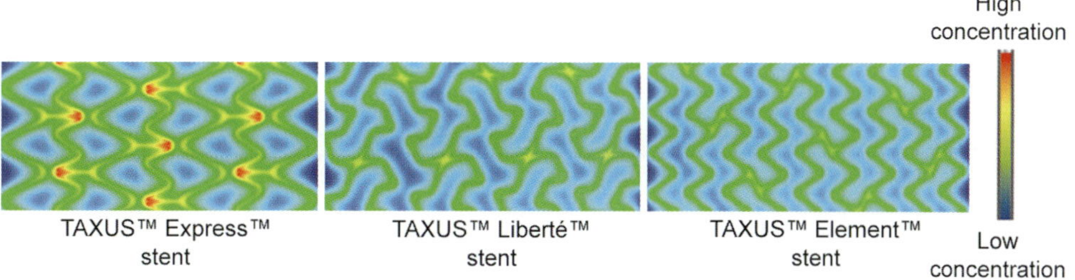

Fig. 2.13 Computer modeling of drug distribution as a function of axial and circumferential position relative to the stent pattern of three different stent designs. Note the more uniform distribution of drug for the more contemporary Element stent design as compared to that of the first generation Express drug-eluting stent

vessel cross-sectional area for flow by significantly reducing the degree of intimal hyperplasia. However, the presence of the drug coating was also found to bring about a delay in the healing response, with a greater likelihood of incomplete strut endothelialization in DES as compared to BMS, which may result in an increase in late stent thrombotic events.[30,31] This led to new guidelines for extended duration of dual antiplatelet therapy (DAPT), so as to reduce the likelihood of this newly increased late-term risk.[32] The recognition of the increased late stent thrombosis risk spurred a number of experimental approaches to improve the healing characteristics of the stent, with varied results. Numerous surface treatments, pro-healing surfaces, polymer-free drug delivery, bioresorbable polymer drug delivery, and other approaches have been investigated as means to provide an improved healing outcome and lessen the need for long-term DAPT therapy.[33]

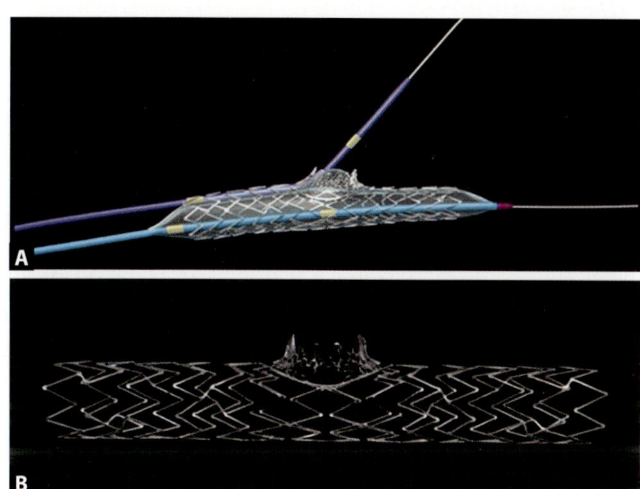

Figs 2.14A and B TAXUS Petal stent system in the deployed state on the delivery catheter (A) and after removal of the delivery catheter (B)

Special Purpose Requirements

In addition to the above requirements which apply to all coronary stents, a number of specialty-purpose stents have been designed to be especially suited for particular situations, such as bifurcation stenting or coronary ostium stenting. One example of a specialty bifurcation stent is the Petal stent (investigated as TAXUS Petal), which incorporated a specially-designed side feature which provides scaffolding to the sidebranch ostium and allow for sidebranch stenting if necessary. The Petal stent was designed for a particular clinical application, but several technical and practical challenges, in combination with the refinement of bifurcation clinical technique, have forestalled the commercialization of this technology. For one, the alignment of the Petal side feature with the bifurcation incorporated the use of a secondary guidewire to align the stent axially and rotationally with the sidebranch. This second wire creates the potential for wire entanglement with the delivery catheter. Although this is a potential difficulty with any two-wire procedure, the requirement to align the stent with the bifurcation may increase the potential for this difficulty with a rotation-specific stent. The development of a bifurcation-specific stent with a sidebranch feature requires specialized balloons, specialized catheters and stent design, with significant investment to develop each of these technologies. Meanwhile, bifurcation stenting technique with conventional stents has become more refined and simplified, raising the question of whether the development of specialty stents is indeed worthwhile.[34] The bifurcation stent serves as an example of the factors which must be considered in determining whether to invest the significant resources required to bring a product to market. Technical challenges, time to market and opportunity cost, competing technologies, and the potential for evolving technique or an emerging disruptive technology must be included in the calculus of whether to develop a product (Figs 2.14A and B).

DESIGN OPTIMIZATION

The progression of available materials and stent design over time has resulted in significant refinement of stents over the years since the introduction of the Palmaz-Schatz stent. Over time, stents have become thinner, more visible, and much more conformable and deliverable than their predecessors. In combination with the groundbreaking advance that drug eluting stent coatings represent, the current state of the art in coronary stents allows for the treatment of more challenging cases with better outcomes than ever before.

As a case example of the design of a coronary stent, the following is a description of some of the fundamentals employed in the design of the Promus PREMIER and SYNERGY stent systems.

Product Matrix

The development of a stent product line should start with an understanding of the user's needs and requirements of the product. One important aspect of this starting point is an understanding of the range of vessels sizes intended to be addressed by the product. For example, the intended use range of a coronary stent might call for stent diameters from 2.25–4.00 mm, and lengths from 8 mm to 38 mm or more. Furthermore, the increments in diameter and length can be determined, so as to provide physicians with the ability to treat all vessels within the range of diameters and lengths.

Stent Models

Once the range of diameters and lengths has been determined and the product requirements defined, one of the next important aspects of stent design is to determine whether the performance requirements of the product are the same for all sizes, or if there are unique requirements for smaller/larger or shorter/longer stents. Most stent product lines use two or more unique stent designs (stent models) to cover the range of diameters within the product matrix. For example, the express stent product line utilized two stent models to cover the range of diameters (Workhorse and Large Vessel), the Liberté stent product line consisted of three models (Small Vessel, Workhorse and Large Vessel), and the Element and Premier product lines consist of four models (Small Vessel, Small Workhorse, Workhorse and Large Vessel). Each stent model is optimized for the range of diameters for which it is designed. For a given stent design, certain performance characteristics are optimized at the minimum use diameter, while others are optimized at the maximum use diameter, and so determining the number of stent models requires determining the desired performance parameters and confirming that those requirements are met across the range of use diameters indicated for the product (Fig. 2.15).

Designing for Expansion

Fundamentally, each stent is designed for two use states—the crimped state on the catheter, and the deployed state in the vessel. In the crimped state, the objective is to minimize crimped stent profile and maximize flexibility. In the expanded state, the objective is to optimize the other performance parameters that are required for the device as implanted. Furthermore, the design goal to maximize postdilatation diameter plays a role in the early stages of stent design. In order to achieve a given postdilated diameter, the structural elements of the stent must be capable of being deformed to achieve that diameter. One means of designing for this maximum diameter is by calculating the total undulation length required of the stent. Total undulation length refers to the distance that is traversed through the stent pattern in one full circumference. In order to achieve a given diameter of expansion without elongating the structural elements

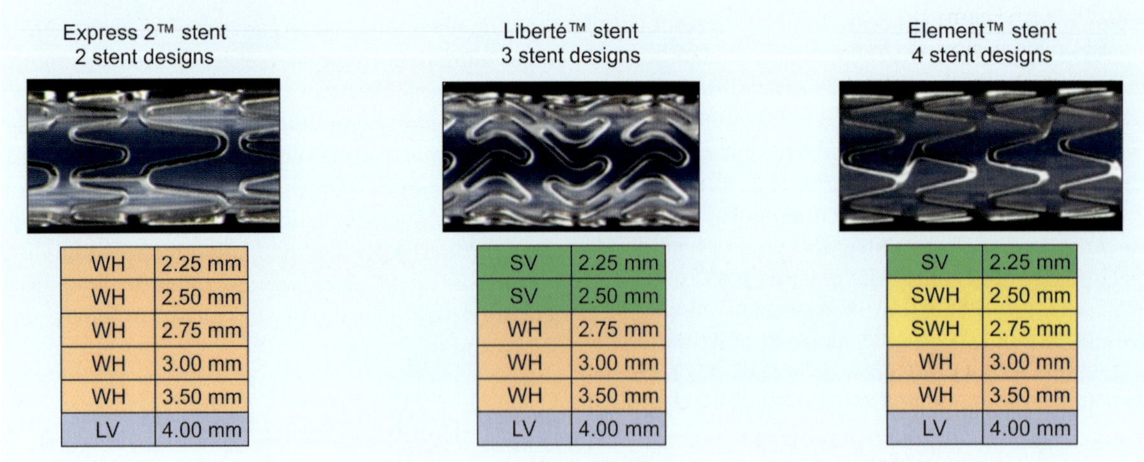

Fig. 2.15 Examples of stent design model matrix for three different product lines, to provide stents designed for specific diameter ranges

themselves, the total undulation length must meet or exceed the circumference of the maximum intended diameter.

Most balloon expandable stents can be generalized as having struts, peaks and connectors or junctions. Struts are the generally linear or curvilinear beams which at their ends are joined with another beam with a different trajectory. The stent features at which the struts are connected are referred to by some as crowns, but for the purposes of this publication will be referred to as peaks. Often times, the peaks are arc-shaped, but may be other shapes as well. The combined length of the struts and the peaks which encircle one full circumference of the stent is the total undulation length.

Designing for Radial Strength

One of the most important performance characteristics of a stent is its ability to resist vascular recoil forces and the intrusion of plaque. Along these lines, stents are designed so as to provide the maximum degree of strength—or resistance to compression—that can be achieved within the other performance targets and limitations. One way that this is achieved is by selecting materials which have high inherent strength. Beyond material selection, stent strength is determined by finer points of stent geometry and design.

One key early decision in designing a stent is to determine how many struts and peaks should make up one circumference. Logically, for a stent with a given undulation length, a stent with fewer struts in one circumference will have correspondingly longer struts than another stent with more struts in one circumference. So, the designer must decide whether having a smaller number of longer struts or a larger number of shorter struts is in the best interest of meeting the design objectives. For example, in the Element and Premier product lines, the Small Vessel, Small Workhorse and Workhorse stent models utilize 16 struts (8 strut pairs) in each segment, whereas the Large Vessel stent model utilizes 10 strut pairs in each segment.

A second key decision in the design of a stent is the number of circumferential repeats in a given length of stent. Most stents are either made up of a number of "segments" or "rings" or of a number of helical windings. If the struts and peaks which encircle the circumference join at the ends to make an enclosed structure, then the stent is made up of segments. The Premier and Synergy stents are made up of segments. The number of segments which make up a given length of stent contributes to the radial strength of the stent. Given that each segment resists radial compression, the number of segments of a given design per unit length should be maximized in order to maximize the radial strength of the stent.

In addition to the number of segments, the radial strength of a stent is determined by several key factors. Among the most significant factors contributing factors to radial strength are strut length, width and thickness, peak width, strut distension and material mechanical strength. Strut distension is a function of the total undulation length, the number of struts in a circumference and the diameter change from the expanded state to a compressed state. Similarly, strut length is generally a function of undulation length and the number of struts in the stent circumference. The other factors of peak width, strut width and strut thickness can be modified by changes in dimension. Strut width and strut thickness are both important contributors to stent radial strength, strut width being the more impactful of the two. However, strut width can only be increased to a point—beyond which point a strut that is significantly wider than it is thick may not deform in the desired manner when the stent is deployed (Fig. 2.16).

For reasons discussed earlier, thinner struts are preferred for optimizing healing and blood flow. And the introduction of radiopaque materials allows for the use of thinner materials while maintaining visibility. As a result, it is generally desirable to minimize the thickness of the struts. However, given that both strut width and thickness contribute to stent radial strength, making the stent thicker is in the interest of radial strength. This is at odds with other design goals and is reconciled by having more struts of smaller dimensions, rather than fewer struts of larger dimensions.

As a result of these various considerations, a balance is generally found wherein strut widths and thickness are approximately equal, the number of struts in the circumference is maximized, and the number of segments per unit length is maximized to produce a stent which has maximum radial strength and minimum wall thickness.

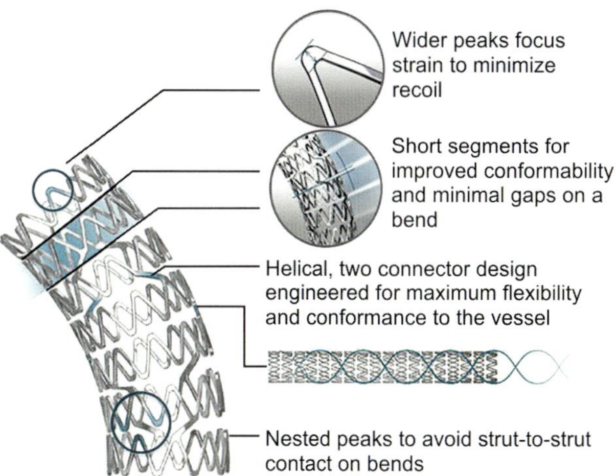

Fig. 2.16 An illustration of several of the key considerations in the design of the Element and Promus PREMIER product lines

Designing for Deliverability

A great many design fundamentals are considered when designing a delivery catheter for a stent system. These design aspects are not within the scope of this chapter. However, the stent itself also contributes to the deliverability of the stent delivery system, and so deliverability is of interest as an important aspect of stent design. Likely the most important consideration for stent design with respect to deliverability is its ability to be crimped to a small outer diameter or profile. The crimped profile of a stent is a function of the stent thickness, and of the combined circumferential dimensions of the struts and peaks when reduced to the diameter of the unexpanded balloon. This in turn is a function of the dimension and number of struts and peaks in one circumference, and of the degree to which these features are aligned in the crimped state. Another important stent contribution to deliverability is the bending stiffness of the stent in the crimped condition. The factors which are important for this vary by the specific design in question, but may include wall thickness, segment length, and connector count and configuration.

Designing for Scaffolding

One of the fundamental requirements of a stent is to provide adequate scaffold, or support to the vessel or lesion which is expanded. Radial strength accounts for one important aspect of scaffolding. Another important consideration is the uniformity of the supporting structure across the inner surface of the vessel. Sometimes simply referred to as "scaffolding", a stent should provide uniformly distributed support to the stented vessel, so that there are no large areas which are left unsupported. Unlike the early Palmaz-type stents which had large diamond-shaped openings between struts, and therefore relatively large spaces of unsupported vessel, most current stents have a staggered strut configuration or generally parallel "in-phase" sinusoidal structures intended to confer more uniform scaffolding to the vessel.

Designing for Conformability

It is desirable to minimize the degree to which a stent causes a curved vessel to straighten. As such, the bending stiffness of the stent should be minimized. Early stent designs such as the Palmaz-Schatz and Cypher were exceedingly stiff by today's standards. These early stents employed a "closed cell" configuration, in which each peak of each segment was attached to or continuous with another peak of an adjacent segment. Given that every peak was connected throughout the stent structure, the bending strain was accommodated almost entirely by the connectors between segments. In the case of the Palmaz-Schatz stent, there was a link bridging an otherwise rigid structure, so that the stent could accommodate some degree of curvature by bending like a hinge about the link. In the case of the Cypher stent, the connectors themselves were capable of some degree of flexion, but the stent overall still had a high degree of stiffness. Contemporary stents, such as the Multi-Link, Driver, Integrity, Premier and Synergy, utilize an "open cell" configuration, generally with 1–3 junctions between segments, and accordingly offer a

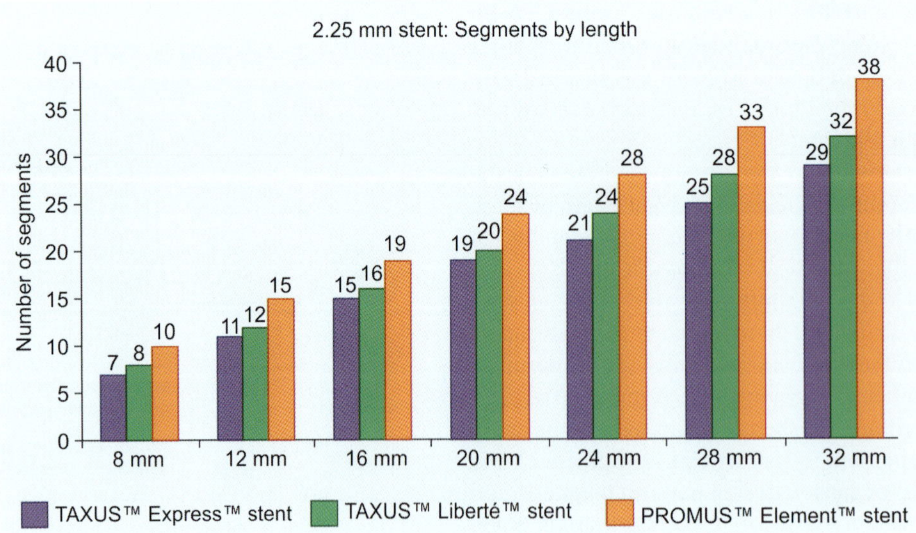

Fig. 2.17 The number of segments as a function of stent length for the Express, Liberté and Element stent product lines. Note the increase in the number of segments, which in combination with low bending stiffness generally correlates with the ability of the stent to smoothly conform to curved vessels

much lower bending stiffness than earlier stent designs. Generally, bending stiffness decreases dramatically with a reduced number of connectors, and so two connector stent designs typically have much lower bending stiffness than even a 3 connector stent design. One additional factor in designing a stent for conformability is the number of segments per unit length. In general, the greater the number of segments, the more uniformly the stent can conform to the curvature of the vessel (Fig. 2.17).

Developing an Optimized Stent

The process of designing a stent product line requires determining the optimized performance of multiple performance parameters. As a practical matter, optimization requires determining the relative importance of various performance parameters (outputs), understanding the contribution of design factors (inputs) to these performance parameters, and seeking to determine the combination of design inputs that maximizes the outputs in total. Due to the complex interactions between the multiple design inputs, multiple design solutions can be determined to satisfy the design requirements. Furthermore, product design and refinement is an ongoing process, with new technologies and evolving clinical practice continuously influencing the array of potential optimized design solutions. Consequently, a stent that may have been considered optimized ten years ago is not considered adequate by today's standards and the development of the optimized stent is an ongoing pursuit.

CONCLUSION

The development of the coronary stent has been one of the most important advances in the history of interventional cardiology. Globally, more than 6 million stents are implanted annually (2015), of which more than 5 million are drug-eluting stents. Through the vision of early pioneers and the diligence of many clinicians, designers and engineers over years of optimization, today's coronary stents deliver excellent outcomes. The history of stent design, like the history of interventional cardiology in general, has been marked with significant advances resulting in the highly-refined products of today.

REFERENCES

1. Sigward U, Puel J, Mirkovitch V, Joffre F, Kappenberger L. Intravascular stents to prevent occlusion and restenosis after transluminal angioplasty. N Engl J Med. 1987;316:701-6.
2. Puel J, Joffre F, Rousseau H, Guermonprez B, Lancelin B, Morice MC. Self-expanding coronary endoprosthesis in the prevention of restenosis following transluminal angioplasty. Preliminary clinical study. Arch Mal Coeur. 1987;8:1311-2.
3. An Expert Interview with Dr Julio Palmaz: Part I—Serendipity and the Stent. *http://www.medscape.com/viewarticle/474644*
4. Serruys PW, de Jaegre P, Kiemeneij F, et al., for the Benestent Study Group. A comparison of balloon-expandable-stent implantation with balloon angioplasty in patients with coronary artery disease. N Engl J Med. 1994;331:489-95.
5. Fischman DL, Leon MB, Baim DS, et al., for the Stent Restenosis Study Investigators. A randomized comparison of coronary-stent placement and balloon angioplasty in the treatment of coronary artery disease. N Engl J Med. 1994;331: 496-501.
6. Morice MC, Serruys PW, Sousa JE, et al. A randomized comparison of a sirolimus-eluting stent with a standard stent for coronary revascularization. N Engl J Med. 2002:346:1773-80.
7. Moses JW, Leon MB, Popma JJ, et al. Sirolimus-eluting stents versus standard stents in patients with stenosis in a native coronary artery. N Engl J Med. 2003:349:1315-23.
8. Dotter CT, Judkins MP. Transluminal treatment of arteriosclerotic obstruction. Description of a new technic and a preliminary report of its application. Circulation. 1964;30:654-70.
9. Hirayama A, Kodama K, Adachi T, Nanto S, Ohara T, Tamai H, et al. Angiographic and clinical outcome of a new self-expanding intracoronary stent (RADIUS):results from multicenter experience in Japan. Catheter Cardiovasc Interv. 2000;49(4):401-7.
10. Mani G, Feldman MD, Patel D, Agrawal CM. Coronary stents: a materials perspective. Biomaterials. 2007;28:1689-710.
11. Poncin P, Proft J. Stent tubing; understanding the desired attributes. Proceedings of the Materials & Processes for Medical Devices Conference. Sanjay Shrivastava, editor, pp. 253-9.
12. Sangiogi G, Melzi G, Agostoni P, Cola C, Clementi F, et al. Engineering aspects of stents design and their translation into clinical practice. Ann Ist Super Sanita. 2007;43(1):89-100.
13. Stoeckel D, Bonsignore C, Duda S. A survey of stent designs. Min Invas Ther & Allied Technol. 2002;11(4);137-47.
14. Current State of Coronary Stenting. Kutryk MJB, Serruys PW (Eds). Fourth Thoraxcenter Course on Coronary Stenting (Barjesteh van Waalwijk van Doorn & Co's, 1997).
15. Lee SWL, Chan MPH, Chan KKW. Acute and 16-month outcomes of a new stent; the first-in-man evaluation of the Medtronic S9 (Integrity) stent. Catheterization and Cardiovascular Interventions. 2011;78:898-908.
16. Bonsignore C in SMST-2003: Proceedings of the International Conference on Shape Memory and Superelastic Technologies. AR Pelton, T Duerig (Eds) (Pacific Grove, Calif); 2003. pp. 519-28.
17. O'Brien BJ, Stinson JS, Larsen SR, Eppihimer MJ, Carroll WM. A platinum-chromium steel for cardiovascular stents. Biomaterials. 2010;31:3755-61.
18. Agrawal CM, Haas KF, Leopold DA, Clark HG. Evaluation of poly(L-lactic acid) as a material for intravascular polymeric stents. Biomaterials. 1992;13(3):176-82.
19. Colombo A, Karvouni E. Biodegradable stents "fulfilling the mission and stepping away". Circulation. 2000;102:371-3.
20. Ellis SG, Kereiakes DJ, Metzger DC, Caputo RP, Rizik DG, Teirstein PS, et al., for the ABSORB III Investigators. Everolimus-eluting bioresorbable scaffolds for coronary artery disease. N Engl J Med. 2015;373(20):1905-15.

21. Byrne RA. Bioresorbable vascular scaffolds—will promise become reality?. N Engl J Med 2015;373(20):1969-71.
22. Jedwab MR, Clerc CO. A study of the geometrical and mechanical properties of a self-expanding metallic stent—theory and experiment. Journal of Applied Biomaterials. 1993;1:77-85.
23. Wentzel JJ, Whelan DM, van der Giessen WJ, et al. Coronary stent implantation changes 3D vessel geometry and 3D shear stress distribution. J Biomech. 2000;33:1287-95.
24. Kolandaivelu K, Swaminathan R, Gibson WJ, Kolachalama VB, et al. Stent thrombogenecity early in high-risk interventional settings is driven by stent design and deployment and protected by polymer-drug coatings. Circulation. 2011;123:1400-9.
25. Iqbal J, Gunn J, Serruys PW. Coronary stents: historical development, current status and future directions. British Medical Bulletin. 2013;106:193-211.
26. Stone GW, Ellis SG, Cox DA, Hermiller J, O'Shaughnessy C, Mann JT, et al. A polymer-based, paclitaxel-eluting stent in patients with coronary artery disease. N Engl J Med. 2004;350: 221-30.
27. Daemen J, Serruys PW. Drug-eluting stent update 2007 Part I: A survey of current and future generation drug-eluting stents: Meaningful advances or more of the same?. Circulation. 2007;116:316-28.
28. Chen Y, Robertson K. PROMUS Element Plus®: A drug-eluting stent. In: S. Lyu & R. Siegal (Eds.), Drug-device combinations for chronic diseases. Hoboken, NJ: John Wiley & Sons, Inc. 2015. pp. 214-40.
29. Hwang CW, Wu D, Edelman ER. Physiological transport forces govern drug distribution for stent-based delivery. Circulation. 2001;104:600-5.
30. Garg S, Serruys PW, Coronary stents current status. J Am Coll Cardiol. 2010;56:S1-42.
31. Joner M, Finn AV, Farb A, Mont EK, Kolodgie FD, Ladich E, et al. Pathology of drug-eluting stents in humans. J Am Coll Cardiol. 2006;48:193-202.
32. Smith SC, Feldman TE, Hirshfeld JW, Jacobs AK, Kern MJ, King SB, et al. A report of the American College of Cardiology/ American Heart Association task force on practice guidelines. J Am Coll Cardiol. 2006;47:e1-121.
33. Garg S, Serruys PW, Coronary stents looking forward. J Am Coll Cardiol. 20a10;56:S43-78.
34. Rizik DG, Klasses KJ, Hermiller JB. Bifurcation coronary artery disease: current techniques and future directions (Part 2). J Invasive Cardiol. 2008;20(3):135-41.
35. Kastrati A, Mehilli J, Dirschinger J, Dotzer F, et al. Intracoronary stenting and angiographic results Strut thickness effect on restenosis outcome (ISAR-STEREO) trial. Circulation. 2001;103:2816-21.
36. Pache J, Kastrati A, Mehilli J, et al. Intracoronary stenting and angiographic results: Strut thickness effect on restenosis outcome (ISAR-STEREO-2) trial. J Am Coll Cardiol. 2003;41:1283-8.
37. Turco MA, Ormiston JA, Popma JJ, et al. Reduced risk of restenosis in small vessels and reduced risk of myocardial infarction in long lesions with the new thin-strut TAXUS Liberte stent. J Am Coll Cardiol Intv. 2008;1:699-709.
38. Kereiakes DJ, Cannon LA, Ormiston JA, et al. Propensity-matched patient-level comparison of the TAXUS Liberte and TAXUS Element (ION) paclitaxel-eluting stents. Am J Cardiol. 2011;108:828-37.

CHAPTER

3

Percutaneous Coronary Intervention

Dev Pahlajani, Akshay K Mehta

INTRODUCTION

Before scheduling a patient for percutaneous coronary intervention (PCI) an interventional cardiologist must use his knowledge and clinical wisdom to decide whether: a patient needs PCI that will improve his/her clinical outcome such as death, myocardial infarction (MI), stroke and weigh it against the risk of the procedure. Of particular concern is the risk of bleeding, stroke MI and need for emergency coronary artery bypass surgery.

INDICATIONS

PCI is indicated for patients with:

Stable angina with: (1) Refractory to optimum medical treatment with definite evidence of inducible myocardial ischemia on stress test or myocardial perfusion scan; (2) Significant lesion (>70%) or fractional flow reserve of > 0.8 in an artery supplying a large area of myocardium.

Unstable angina particularly patients with intermediate or high Thrombolysis in Myocardial Infarction (TIMI) risk score of 3 or more.

Primary PCI in acute MI is the most important and rewarding indication. It should be performed within 6 hours after chest pain with door to balloon time of less than 90 minutes.

Post-coronary Artery Bypass Grafting Recurrence of Angina

Unexplained arrhythmia or cardiac failure to rule out coronary artery disease.

Symptoms or signs of restenosis following PCI:

- Patients need revascularization but having high European System for Cardiac Operative Risk Evaluation (EuroSCORE) for CABG
- Unsuitable anatomy for CABG or diffuse disease where PCI of 1 or 2 vessels would offer symptomatic relief to the patient
- High-risk coronary anatomy

CONTRAINDICATIONS

- Absence of symptomatic or objective evidence of myocardial ischemia
- Bleeding diathesis and bleeding disorder.
- Active bleeding from any organ
- Advanced liver disease deranging the coagulation profile
- High international normalized ratio (INR) of more than 2, low platelet count of less than 75000-80000
- *Evidence of infection*: High fever > 99°F or WBC count > 10,000 with raised polymorphs
- Noncompliant patient due mental disorder like dementia or severe musculoskeletal deformities
- Unable to take dual antiplatelet therapy due to gastrointestinal bleeding
- Multiple restenosis patients are better treated with CABG
- Renal dysfunction though not absolute contraindication needs careful monitoring of creatinine and proper preparation of the patient with hydration therapy and nephrologist consult should a need for dialysis arise following PCI.
- While these are general indications and contraindications an interventional cardiologist must be familiar with the guidelines and recommendations to select the appropriate therapy.

GUIDELINES

Guidelines for the Performance of Percutaneous Transluminal Coronary Angioplasty were first published in 1982 in Circulation.[1] The first ACC/AHA Task Force report on guidelines for coronary balloon angioplasty was published in 1988.[2]

The current guidelines from the European Society of Cardiology (2014) and the ACCF/AHA/SCAI Practice Guidelines (2011) are in consensus. In addition, Appropriate Use Criteria for Coronary Revascularization were published in 2009 and updated in 2012.[3,4]

The Chapter discusses the latest recommendations on Indications for performance of PCI and when it needs to be avoided.[5,6]

The objective of revascularization in patients with coronary artery disease (CAD) is to:

- Improve survival and/or
- Relieve symptoms.

PCI BASED ON ANATOMIC LESION

In patients with stable ischemic heart disease (SIHD), "significant" stenosis defined as ≥70% diameter narrowing (≥50% for left main CAD).

Contemperorary practice also relies on physiological assessment by measuring fractional flow reserve (FFR), to decide whether revascularization is indicated. Coronary stenoses with FFR ≤0.80 is considered to be "significant."[7,8]

Syngery between PCI with TAXus and Cardia Surgery (SYNTAX) scores are used as surrogate for estimating the extent and complexity of CAD and are particularly employed for SIHD patients with unprotected left main and complex CAD. The preferred way is the heart team approach wherein the interventional cardiologist and cardiac surgeon get the opportunity to discuss revascularization options with the patient. Calculation of Society of Thoracic Surgeons (STS) score and the SYNTAX score have been shown to predict adverse outcomes in patients undergoing coronary artery bypass graft (CABG) and PCI, respectively, calculation of these scores is employed to assist the revascularization decisions.

SYNTAX score is based on the location, severity, and extent of coronary stenoses, with a low score indicating less complicated anatomic CAD.

- Low score is defined as ≤22
- Intermediate 23 to 32
- High ≥33.

Significance of Syntax Score

At 12-month follow-up, the primary endpoint was similar for CABG and DES in those with a low SYNTAX score. However, major adverse cardiac events (MACE) occurred more often after PCI than after CABG in those with an intermediate or high SYNTAX score. On 3 years of follow-up, deaths were more frequent in the 3-vessel CAD treated with PCI than in those treated with CABG (6.2% versus 2.9%). The differences in MACE between those treated with PCI or CABG increased with an increasing SYNTAX score.[6,9]

The SYNTAX II score, which is a combination of anatomical and clinical factors [age, creatinine clearance, left ventricular (LV) function, gender, chronic obstructive pulmonary disease, and peripheral vascular disease] is a better predictor of long-term mortality in patients with complex three-vessel or left main (LM) coronary artery disease (CAD).[10]

In addition to the above, appropriateness of revascularization in stable CAD depends on:

- Severity of angina (asymptomatic, Canadian Cardiovascular Society [CCS] Class I, II, III, or IV)
- Extent of ischemia on noninvasive testing and the presence or absence of other prognostic factors, such as congestive heart failure, depressed left ventricular function, or diabetes
- Extent of medical therapy.[3,4]

Consider the following for PCI, in patients with left main CAD:

- PCI may considered over CABG in patients with significant stenosis (≥50% diameter stenosis) when
- Anatomic conditions associated with a low risk of PCI procedural complications and a high likelihood of good long-term outcome (e.g. a low SYNTAX score [≤22], ostial or trunk left main CAD); or those with low-intermediate SYNTAX score of <33, bifurcation left main CAD)
- Clinical characteristics that predict a significantly increased risk of adverse surgical outcomes (e.g. moderate-severe chronic obstructive pulmonary disease, disability from previous stroke, or previous cardiac surgery; STS-predicted risk of operative mortality ≥5%, or even if > 2% and not amenable to CABG).[9,11]
- When survival can be improved in patients with UA/NSTEMI when the patient is not a candidate for CABG.[12]
- For better survival outcomes in patients with acute STEMI when distal coronary flow is less than TIMI (Thrombolysis in Myocardial Infarction) grade 3, and PCI can be performed more rapidly and safely than CABG.[13]

PCI should not be attempted in patients with Left main CAD[14]:

In stable patients with significant (≥50% diameter stenosis) unprotected left main CAD who have unfavorable anatomy for PCI and who are good candidates for CABG.

However, data from several recent trials indicates that left main ostial or shaft disease could be tackled by PCI with comparable results versus CABG. Inpatients with left main bifurcation and high EURO or STS score that would indicate high risk of CABG, PCI could be fair alternate form of revascularization.

Consider the following for PCI, in patients with non-left main CAD:

In survivors of SCD, who would benefit from PCI and are not candidates for CABG.

In those with multivessel lesions or lesion in proximal CAD, the usefulness may vary. However, such patients who have unacceptable angina despite *guideline-directed medical therapy* (GDMT) with stenosed vessel amenable to PCI; It may be performed to improve symptoms.

Also for patients with previous CABG and extensive anterior wall ischemia the benefits of PCI are not known. However, if in the patients with previous CABG, if unacceptable angina despite *guideline-directed medical therapy* (GDMT). PCI may be performed to improve symptoms.

Factors that favor PCI over CABG include limited areas of ischemia causing symptoms, suitable PCI targets, and a patent graft to the LAD artery, poor CABG targets, and co-morbid conditions.

PCI should not be attempted in patients with non-left main CAD:

If patient does not have significant stenoses, that <70% diameter of non-left main coronary artery is stenosed, Or FFR is >0.80, no or only mild ischemia on noninvasive testing or when it involves only the left circumflex or right coronary artery, or subtends only to a small area of viable myocardium.[15,16]

PCI for symptom improvement must not be performed in patients who do not meet the anatomical (≥50% diameter left main or ≥70% non-left main stenosis diameter) or physiological (e.g. abnormal FFR) criteria.

Chronic Total Occlusions

PCI of a chronic total occlusion (CTO) should be attempted only by expert operators when appropriate clinical indications exist with favorable anatomy.[17]

Saphenous Vein Graft

PCI is not recommended for chronic saphenous vein graft (SVG) occlusions.[18]

SPECIAL PATIENT CLASSES

Elderly

PCI has been found to be equally beneficial in elderly as in younger populations. In fact with higher absolute benefit, however, they carry higher risk of adverse outcomes such as major bleeding and stroke and thus need careful consideration of the benefits and risks.[19]

Diabetes

For patients with diabetes, those who need revascularization of multivessel CAD or have complex and extensive CAD, PCI may be considered carefully and may be restricted for patients who are not candidates for CABG.[20] Diabetes is also an important risk factor for the development of contrast-induced AKI.

Women

They tend to have more risk factors (including hypertension, advanced age, elevated cholesterol, and more significant and diffuse CAD) compared with men, hence need careful risk benefit analysis.[21]

Severe Renal Dysfunction

Even for patients with severe renal dysfunction CABG may have better survival outcomes than PCI.[22] If PCI is performed the GFR must be estimated and dosages of renally cleared medications should be adjusted.

Dual Antiplatelet Therapy (DAPT) for Non-compliant Patients

PCI with coronary stenting (BMS or DES) is avoided in patients who would be unable to tolerate/comply with DAPT for the appropriate duration of treatment based on the type of stent implanted.[23]

Absence of On-site Cardiac Surgery Capabilities

PCI may be performed, if adequate planning has been done and rigorous clinical and angiographic criteria are used for proper patient selection.

It should be avoided, if proven plan for rapid transport to a cardiac surgery operating room in a nearby hospital or when appropriate hemodynamic support capability for transfer is not available.

PCI IN SPECIFIC CLINICAL SITUATIONS

UA/NSTEMI

For patients with refractory angina/electrical and hemodynamic instability early PCI may be considered.

However, in patients with extensive comorbidities (e.g. liver or pulmonary failure, cancer), medical therapy may be opted over invasive strategy.

ST-elevation Myocardial Infarction

PCI may be considered for following cases with STEMI:

- All patients of STEMI who are candidates for primary PCI
- Those with severe heart failure or cardiogenic shock who are suitable candidates for revascularization.[24]
- Those with moderate to large area of myocardium at risk or those with evidence of failed fibrinolysis
- Within 3–24 hours of initiating fibrinolytic therapy in a hemodynamically stable patient.

Primary PCI of the infarct artery should preferably be performed:

- Within 12 hours of onset of STEMI.
- Within 90 minutes of first medical contact as a system's goal. Within 120 minutes of first medical contact as a system's goal.
- In patients with STEMI who develop severe heart failure or cardiogenic shock and are suitable candidates for revascularization as soon as possible, irrespective of time delay.[21]
- In patients with STEMI having contraindications to fibrinolytic therapy with ischemic symptoms for less than 12 hours.[6,24,25]
- In patients with STEMI, within 12–24 hrs after symptom onset, if there is clinical and/or electrocardiographic evidence of ongoing.[6]

PCI should not be performed:

- If risks of primary PCI outweigh the benefits
- If the patient refuses invasive care[6]
- In a non-infarct artery at the time of primary PCI in patients with STEMI without hemodynamic compromise.[26]
- In a totally occluded infarct artery of greater than 24 hours after STEMI in an asymptomatic patients with 1- or 2-vessel disease, if the patients is hemodynamically and electrically stable and does not have evidence of severe ischemia.

REFERENCES

1. Williams DO, Gruntzig A, Kent KM, et al. Guidelines for the performance of percutaneous transluminal coronary angioplasty. Circulation. 1982;66:693-4.
2. Guidelines for percutaneous transluminal coronary angioplasty. A report of the American College of Cardiology/American Heart Association Task Force on Assessment of Diagnostic and Therapeutic Cardiovascular Procedures (Subcommittee on Percutaneous Transluminal Coronary Angioplasty). Circulation. 1988;78:486-502
3. Patel MR, Dehmer GJ, Hirschfield JW, et al. ACCF/SCAI/STS/ AATS/AHA/ASNC 2009 Appropriateness Criteria for Coronary Revascularization: A Report of the American College of Cardiology Foundation Appropriateness Criteria Task Force, Society for Cardiovascular Angiography and Interventions, Society of Thoracic Surgeons, American Association for Thoracic Surgery, American Heart Association, and the American Society of Nuclear Cardiology. Circulation. 2009;119:1330-52
4. Patel MR, Dehmer GJ, Hirschfield JW, et al. ACCF/ SCAI/ STS/ AATS/ AHA/ ASNC/ HFSA/ SCCT 2012. Appropriate Use Criteria for Coronary Revascularization Focused Update. A Report of the American College of Cardiology Foundation Appropriate Use Criteria Task Force, Society for Cardiovascular Angiography and Interventions, Society of Thoracic Surgeons, American Association for Thoracic Surgery, American Heart Association, American Society of Nuclear Cardiology, and the Society of Cardiovascular Computed Tomography. J Am Coll Cardiol. 2012;59(9):857-81
5. Windecker S, Kolh P, Alfonso F, et al., 2014 ESC/EACTS Guidelines on myocardial revascularization: web addenda The Task Force on Myocardial Revascularization of the European Society of Cardiology (ESC) and the European Association for Cardio-Thoracic Surgery (EACTS) Developed with the special contribution of the European Association of Percutaneous Cardiovascular Interventions (EAPCI). European Heart Journal *doi:10.1093/eurheartj/ehu278b.https://www.escardio.org/static_file/Escardio/Guidelines/publications/PCIMR-Web%20addenda.pdf*
6. Levine GN, Bates ER, Blankenship JC, et al. ACCF/AHA/SCAI Practice Guideline 2011 ACCF/AHA/SCAI Guideline for Percutaneous Coronary Intervention. Circulation. 2011;124: e574-e651. *http://circ.ahajournals.org/content/124/ -23/e574.full.*
7. Beller GA, Ragosta M. Decision making in multivessel coronary disease: the need for physiological lesion assessment. J Am Coll Cardiol Intv. 2010;3:315-7.
8. Tonino PA, Fearon WF, De Bruyne B, et al. Angiographic versus functional severity of coronary artery stenoses in the FAME study fractional flow reserve versus angiography in multivessel evaluation. J Am Coll Cardiol. 2010;55:2816.
9. Morice MC, Serruys PW, Kappetein AP, et al. Outcomes in patients with de novo left main disease treated with either percutaneous coronary intervention using paclitaxel-eluting stents or coronary artery bypass graft treatment in the Synergy between Percutaneous Coronary Intervention with TAXUS and Cardiac Surgery (SYNTAX) trial. Circulation. 2010;121:2645-53.
10. Farooq V, van Klaveren D, Serruys PW, et al. Anatomical and clinical characteristics to guide decision making between coronary artery bypass surgery and percutaneous coronary intervention for individual patients: development and validation of SYNTAX score II. Lancet. 2013;381(9867):639-50.
11. Kim YH, Park DW, Kim WJ, et al. Validation of SYNTAX (Synergy between PCI with TAXUS and Cardiac Surgery) score for prediction of outcomes after unprotected left main coronary revascularization. J Am Coll Cardiol Intv. 2010;3:612-23.
12. Shahian DM, O'Brien SM, Filardo G, et al. The Society of Thoracic Surgeons 2008 cardiac surgery risk models: part 1—coronary artery bypass grafting surgery. Ann Thorac Surg. 2009;88 (1 Suppl):S2-22.
13. Lee MS, Bokhoor P, Park SJ, et al. Unprotected left main coronary disease and ST-segment elevation myocardial infarction: a contemporary review and argument for percutaneous coronary intervention. J Am Coll Cardiol Intv. 2010;3:791-5.
14. Park SJ, Kim YH, Park DW, et al. Randomized Trial of Stents versus Bypass Surgery for Left Main Coronary Artery Disease. N Engl J Med. 2011;364:1718-27.
15. Davies RF, Goldberg AD, Forman S, et al. Asymptomatic Cardiac Ischemia Pilot (ACIP) study two-year follow-up: outcomes of patients randomized to initial strategies of medical therapy versus revascularization. Circulation. 1997;95:2037-43.
16. Tonino PA, De Bruyne B, Pijls NH, et al. Fractional flow reserve versus angiography for guiding percutaneous coronary intervention. N Engl J Med. 2009;360:213-24.
17. de Labriolle A, Bonello L, Roy P, et al. Comparison of safety, efficacy, and outcome of successful versus unsuccessful percutaneous coronary intervention in "true" chronic total occlusions. Am J Cardiol. 2008;102:1175-81.

18. Al-Lamee R, Ielasi A, Latib A, et al. Clinical and angiographic outcomes after percutaneous recanalization of chronic total saphenous vein graft occlusion using modern techniques. Am J Cardiol. 2010;106:1721-7.
19. de Boer SP, Westerhout CM, Simes RJ, et al. Mortality and morbidity reduction by primary percutaneous coronary intervention is independent of the patient's age. J Am Coll Cardiol Intv. 2010;3:324-31.
20. Magnuson EA, Farkouh ME, Fuster V, et al. Cost-effectiveness of percutaneous coronary intervention with drug eluting stents versus bypass surgery for patients with diabetes mellitus and multivessel coronary artery disease Results From the FREEDOM Trial. Circulation.2013;127:820-31
21. Singh M, Rihal CS, Gersh BJ, et al. Mortality differences between men and women after percutaneous coronary interventions. A 25-year, single-center experience. J Am Coll Cardiol. 2008;51:2313-20.
22. Ix JH, Mercado N, Shlipak MG, et al. Association of chronic kidney disease with clinical outcomes after coronary revascularization: the Arterial Revascularization Therapies Study (ARTS). Am Heart J. 2005;149:512-9.
23. McFadden EP, Stabile E, Regar E, et al. Late thrombosis in drug-eluting coronary stents after discontinuation of antiplatelet therapy. Lancet. 2004;364:1519-21
24. Hochman JS, Sleeper LA, Webb JG, et al. Early revascularization in acute myocardial infarction complicated by cardiogenic shock. SHOCK Investigators. Should We Emergently Revascularize Occluded Coronaries for Cardiogenic Shock. N Engl J Med. 1999;341:625-34.
25. Borgia F, Goodman SG, Halvorsen S, et al. Early routine percutaneous coronary intervention after fibrinolysis versus standard therapy in ST-segment elevation myocardial infarction: a meta-analysis. Eur Heart J. 2010;31:2156-69.
26. Toma M, Buller CE, Westerhout CM, et al. Non-culprit coronary artery percutaneous coronary intervention during acute ST-segment elevation myocardial infarction: insights from the APEX-AMI trial. Eur Heart J. 2010;31: 1701-7.

CHAPTER

4

Coronary Angioplasty for the Beginners

Jagdish Hiremath

INITIAL MUSINGS

Writing this chapter for beginners gives me immense pleasure because to follow the journey of a beginner to competency, is a joy of sorts. Like parents, teachers need to be alert and noninterfering; passing on the doctrine without curbing instincts and new ideas. A few pleasant parental guiding tips are all that are needed for a toddler to become a sprinter one day. The hand skills of angioplasty can be learnt and developed but the mindset of a coronary interventionist needs "special nurturing". It is the mindset that loses/wins many games for the him/her.

If you are reading this chapter, it is given that you are already on the path of the fascinating journey of coronary angioplasty. You either have recently qualified as a coronary interventionist or will do so in a few years. Let your enthusiasm, passion, hunger for knowledge and keenness to do a good job, remain unabated—even after many decades. The world's best operators do have the maturity of experience but what separates them from the rest is the "beginner" in them who is still alive within, even at the twilight of their careers.

When you begin your stint in the Cath lab as a student or as a young interventionist, think whether you would be able to do each and every job in the Cath lab, be it shifting an obese patient on and out of the table, calming an anxious patient, or doing a cardioversion. Reflect upon whether you can be a good second in command? Can you do the nurse's job of preparing hardware and setting the trolley or handle the console and do the technician's job?

SETTING THE TONE

It begins by doing simple things meticulously and flawlessly like arterial punctures, sheath removals, bedside echocardiograms and periprocedural pharmacological management. A few visits to the patient with the rehabilitation expert also help in expanding your horizon and making you into a complete coronary interventionist.

When observing a senior, junior or the world's best interventionist, observe everything, right from how prepercutaneous coronary intervention (pre-PCI) angiograms are studied, interaction with patients and relatives, hand scrub procedure, respect for radiation protection of patient and performers, economization of contrast and radiation. Observe how they treat each and every person in the Cath lab and how they use the changing room.

Be aware of how tempers get lost, how fear is hidden, how behaviors differ in simple and complex cases, how rules get trampled, how success gets celebrated and failure gets underplayed. Watch documentation and periprocedural management. It is also important to see how he looks after his own cardiac health and other personal aspects.

When you observe closely, each person can teach you something about coronary angioplasty, good or bad.

TAKE BACK AND APPLY

There is ample opportunity these days to observe live cases or recorded inbox video and visit higher centers as observer. It is very easy to get fascinated by the leading operators. On the way back from many conferences one returns dejected and disheartened seeing the enormous gap between what you see happening in the world and your own work. It is the same feeling when you see very expensive branded items in the world's best shops. But remember, world leaders have toiled hard to reach these heights. Instead of just getting plainly fascinated or dejected, jot down take home messages or points, that you can apply in your day to day practice. Finally everything matters in giving good results, including the work atmosphere and culture, finances and legal weather.

Categorize your observations into those that are relevant immediately and start using them. Retain the others which you think are important but you cannot apply today and set them aside for another day.

DECISIONS GALORE

Every angiography needs to be viewed from various angles. The syntax score, calcium, tortuosities, ectasia, aneurysm, collaterals, area supplied by the concerned artery, viability of the myocardium, length of the lesion. These types of observations are all often discussed. These points are scientific; they are indispensable and should be on top of the discussion. But also of importance is to visualize the artery/lesion/coronary circulation before percutaneous transluminal coronary angioplasty (PTCA) is performed. Visualize/imagine your best result and your worst result (inadequate expansion/loss of side branches, failure to recross in bifurcation) for that particular anatomy.

Only if the possibility of a good result is significantly higher than failure, go ahead with angioplasty. In doing so think of the stents used, costs involved, ability to continue DAPT. Finally think of how the best acute result would look at the end of 6 months. If you are convinced in your mind that all the "negativities" are in single digit (less than 10%) your case to perform angioplasty is made. Think of the difference made to the patient by putting 6 stents with metal jacket/two stents for criticality/surgery before taking the call. Debate this in your mind and discuss with seniors. Such observations will also differentiate between the decision to do a simplistic inferior job or a complex complete job. Numbers, finances, individual pride and ego have no role to play in this decision making process. All should aim at a perfect result but sometimes attempting an anatomically perfect result can spoil your painting [Excessive post dilatation leading to rupture).

In short, visualize the coronary angiography anatomically, clinically with risk benefit ratio, cost effectiveness and then come to a conclusion and decision. Remember we are not mere cosmetic plumbers. The procedure is performed (or not performed) to give decent acute and long-term "clinical" result. If a young interventionist is not confident of performing a distal left main bifurcation with low syntax score, involving a competent senior should be preferred over surgery.

BEYOND HAND SKILLS

Coronary angioplasty, unlike many other medical procedures is performed in the brain as the "what to do" is dominates over the "how to do" in coronary angioplasty.

A person with even average hand skills complimented by a sound thinking mind is better than a person with a superb hand but an average brain. If your decision to perform PTCA is sound, your homework adequate, your hardware selection perfect, most intervention would be successful with average hand skills. A scientifically resilient thought process (of plan B and C) will win you some more games. Of course, if these are coupled with exceptional hand skills, you become a world leader.

Observing lives cases with a panel of experts gives the opportunity to know different thought processes. All the thoughts are based on science and their variation explains one the vagaries of PTCA. Many times panelists give better suggestions than what the main operator has thought of, because performer is engrossed in performing. This highlights why it is mandatory to go into a case with full mind preparations and covering all your tracks.

A beginner may be short of experience but need not be short in theory. Case by case reading or reading for a proposed case will be of immense help. One becomes a practical genius only after going through the beginning stages as a theoretical idiot. Many good operators are not good in theory but that does not mean you can be successful without studying hard. Whatever knowledge you get by reading is your weapon in every case. Knowing in depth about hardware, nuances of every aspect, makes you a better performer. Knowledge about medicolegal aspects also is available at touch of a button. The younger tech-savvy generation should be very quick with statistics, guidelines, recent updates because unlike in the earlier days, these need not be known by heart or remembered.

Coronary angioplasty is a field which tests the operators' mettle in many ways. It is not enough to be a nonemotional smoothly operating professional who goes about his job like a mathematical task. One has to be a sensitive human who will be aware of the pain, cold or the full bladder that an awake patient feels. Utmost respect to tissues must be nurtured to prevent preventable complications. Growth of the interventionist as a human being (physical, mental, social, spiritual and financial growth) helps him becoming complete.

Apparently highly technical decisions can get influenced by the "background music" (background of the person) in the mind of the operator. A little above average intelligence, good hand skills, clear eyes, empathy in heart makes a world leader in this field, not just a technocraft.

WELCOME TO A FASCINATING WORLD

Welcome to this fascinating world of coronary angioplasty. Pursue your journey with the innocence of a child and let the child remain intact always. Follow science for correctness and learn from personalities about successful incorrectness. Coronary angioplasty is a supreme field of the science and art of medicine and often is ridiculed as the commerce of medicine.

Your efforts and toil of many years long training has earned you this privilege of being a interventional cardiologist. Approach this task with utter sincerity, humility backed by a solid scientific mind and one day you will be scaling new heights!

REFERENCE

The book of experience!

CHAPTER

5

Periprocedural Use of Drugs for Routine Percutaneous Coronary Intervention

Shekhar Shriram Ambardekar, Amit V Sharma

ARMAMENTARIUM FOR THE INTERVENTIONIST: ARE WE BATTLE SAVVY ENOUGH?

Percutaneous coronary intervention (PCI) usually with stenting, has become the standard treatment for acute coronary syndromes (ACS). Besides optimal stenting technique, antiplatelet therapy with antithrombotics is necessary to avoid catastrophic stent thrombosis and to ensure a successful long-term result after PCI. Both antiplatelets and antithrombotics are evolving fields and numerous questions remain regarding which agents in which combinations will best achieve the goal of a successful PCI.

Drug therapy in the cath lab, can be largely divided into the following:

- Antiplatelets
- Antithrombotics
- Adjuvant therapy.

ANTIPLATELETS

Aspirin

Irreversible cyclo-oxygenase inhibitor that blocks platelet synthesis of thromboxane A2 therapy reducing platelet aggregation.

Aspirin administered at the time of PCI, was associated with an extraordinary 75% reduction in the relative risk of acute thrombotic events compared with placebo. Aspirin treated patients experienced a remarkably large (>80%) relative reduction in myocardial infarction (MI) in the following 6 months (compared with placebo).[1]

The American College of Cardiology Foundation (ACCF), the American Heart Association (AHA) and the European Society of Cardiology ST-elevation myocardial infarction (ESC STEMI) guidelines recommend aspirin 162–325 mg to be given before primary PCI and continued indefinitely thereafter. If ticagrelor is used as the second antiplatelet agent, the dosage of aspirin for maintenance therapy should be 81 mg daily.[2,3]

Clopidogrel

The P2Y12 receptor inhibitor therapy is an important component of antiplatelet therapy in patients undergoing PCI. It is basically a pro-drug that takes up to 6 hours to have maximal effect after the loading dose.

While the PCI cure trial[4] showed that pretreatment with 300 mg, loading dose of clopidogrel before PCI reduced cardiovascular death MI by 30% after 1 month as compared to aspirin alone, the ARMYDA-2 trial demonstrated more rapid onset of action and more potent inhibitory effect with a loading dose of 600 mg clopidogrel.[5]

The ACCF/AHA and ESC STEMI guidelines recommend clopidogrel 600 mg loading dose as early as possible during primary PCI with 75 mg, maintenance dose for at least 1 year 300 mg loading dose should be given if no previous loading dose has been given and patient is to undergo PCI within 24 hours of fibrinolysis.

A 600 mg loading dose is to be given if the patient has not received a previous loading dose or if PCI is taking place after 24 hours of fibrinolysis.[6]

The use of higher maintenance dose (150 mg daily) has been proposed in patients with high thrombotic risk (e.g. in diabetic, recurrent MI, complex lesions, etc.). However, no studies have established short- or long-term benefit of 150 mg daily maintenance dose.

Cilostazol

Phosphodiesterase inhibitor, approved by Food and Drug Administration (FDA) for treatment of intermittent claudication. It reportedly has a synergistic action with clopidogrel to inhibit platelet aggregation by increasing platelet cyclic adenosine monophosphate (AMP). In the

OPTIMUS-2 study, cilostazol augmented platelet inhibition when added to dual antiplatelet therapy (DAPT) after PCI.[7] However, neither the ACCF/AHA nor the ESC guidelines have any recommendations for triple antiplatelet therapy.

Prasugrel

Thienopyridine that inhibits ADP-induced platelet aggregation more rapidly (onset of action <1 hour).

In the TRITON TIMI 38 trial, patients who underwent PCI had a significant 19% risk reduction in cardiovascular death, nonfatal MI or nonfatal stroke when treated with prasugrel as compared with clopidogrel. The benefit is somewhat negated, however by 39% increased risk of major bleeding with prasugrel compared to clopidogrel.[8]

A periprocedural loading dose of 60 mg and a post-PCI daily maintenance dose of 10 mg, is advocated. Both ACCF/AHA and ESC guidelines have class I recommendations for prasugrel use doing PCI with doses as mentioned above.

Ticagrelor

Ticagrelor is a novel, reversible ADP receptor inhibitor that has a more rapid onset and more pronounced platelet inhibition than clopidogrel. In patients with ACS undergoing PCI ticagrelor (180 mg loading, 90 mg twice daily maintenance dose) compared to clopidogrel (300–600 mg loading, 75 mg daily), significantly reduced cardiovascular events without increasing the overall risk of major bleeding.[9]

In the PLATO trial at 1 year, cardiovascular death, MI or stroke had occurred in 9.8% of patients receiving ticagrelor as compared with 11.7% of those receiving clopidogrel (a significant 16% relative risk reduction, $p < 0.001$). Lower rates of stent thrombosis were observed with ticagrelor. Although, there was no significant difference in the overall rate of major bleeding in this study, ticagrelor was associated with significantly higher rates of fatal intracranial hemorrhage.[10]

The ACCF/AHA and ESC STEMI guidelines recommend ticagrelor use doing PCI as a class I indication with a loading dose of 180 mg followed by maintenance dose of 90 mg twice daily for at least 1 year with drug-eluting stent (DES) and bare-metal stent (BMS) and beyond one year (Class II b recommendation).

Cangrelor

Most recent addition to the antiplatelet armamentarium. It is a fast acting, potent intravenous P2Y12 inhibitor having rapid onset and offset of antiplatelet activity.

In the Champion Phoenix study, cangrelor, in conjuction with bivalirudin when compared to clopidogrel, significantly reduced ischemic events at 48 hours including stent thrombosis, without increasing major bleeding.[11]

Glycoprotein IIb/IIIa Inhibitors

Platelet aggregation requires the activation of GpIIb/IIIa receptor on platelet suface. Blocking the GPIIb/IIIa receptor inhibits platelet aggregation and reduces thrombus formation.

Abciximab

The EPIC and EPILOG trial established the benefit of using abciximab in high-risk patients with unstable angina, demonstrating lower ischemic event rates and mortality at 30 days, abciximab has been studied in three class of patients.

1. *Low-risk stable patients:* The ISAR-REACT study enrolled low risk stable patients and detected no benefit of Gp IIb/IIIa blockade. Subsequently, the same drug regimen was tested in stable diabetic patients in the ISAR-SWEET study, which showed no benefit from abciximab.
2. *High-risk ACS (non-STEMI):* The ISAR-REACT-2 study[12] randomized 2022 high risk patients with ACS undergoing PCI to receive abciximab or placebo in addition to aspirin and clopidogrel 600 mg loading dose. The incidence of the primary end point (death/MI/urgent TVR) at 30 days was significantly reduced by 25% in the abciximab group. The CAPTURE study required abciximab to be given 18–24 hours before PCI and it showed decrease rate of death, MI and urgent intervention.[13]
3. *STEMI:* CADILLAC was the largest trial, which did not show a benefit of abciximab over placebo in patients undergoing PCI. The study had the limitation that half of the patients did not receive a stent and more importantly randomization occurred following coronary angiography. This resulted in the enrolment of a low-risk population.

   The BRAVE-3 trial showed that abciximab did not help in reducing the infarct size in patients with acute STEMI undergoing primary PCI after pretreatment with 600 mg clopidogrel at 1 year after stenting.[14]

Eptifibatide

It has been evaluated in patients with unstable angina/NSTEMI with a decreased rate of death/nonfatal MI at 30 days compared with placebo, although with an increased risk of bleeding (PURSUIT trial).[15]

Tirofiban

The RESTORE trial was studied in patients with ACS undergoing PCI treated with heparin with addition of tirofiban or placebo. Treatment with tirofiban resulted in reduction of mortality and MI.[16]

In the PRISM-PLUS trial tirofiban in addition to heparin (in ACS patients) was associated with a decreased mortality,

MI or refractory ischemia when compared to heparin alone at 7 days, 30 days up to 6 months.[17]

Present Recommendations for Gp IIb/IIIa Inhibition

The use of this drug class is now showing steady decline with the advent of newer anti-thrombotic and antiplatelets (bivalirudin, prasugrel and ticagrelor). According to the 2013 ACCF/AHA STEMI guidelines Gp IIb/IIIa inhibitors such as abciximab, high bolus tirofiban or double bolus eptifibatide have a class II a recommendation for use at the time of primary PCI in patients with STEMI who are receiving unfractionated heparin (UFH).

The precatheterization use of Gp IIb/IIIa inhibitors (in ambulance/ED) to patients with STEMI for whom primary PCI is intended is a class IIB recommendation. The intra-coronary use of abciximab doing PCI is a class IIb recommendation. For unstable angina/NSTEMI patients, the GP IIb/IIIa inhibitors have got a class II a recommendation for use in both pre-PCI and during PCI (ACCF/AHA 2012 guidelines). Thus the benefit of Gp IIb/III a inhibitors is predominantly in patients undergoing PCI especially high-risk troponin positive, diabetic patients.

Postprocedure Antiplatelet Therapy

Percutaneous coronary interventions (PCI), whether with balloon angioplasty alone (POBA) or with stent make the patient susceptible to thrombosis at the site of endothelial injury. Most of these patients could present with ST elevation MI with high mortality rates. The period of the risk of thrombosis gradually decreases as the stent is fully endothelialized.[18] Hence, stent thrombosis frequently presents as 'acute' and 'subacute, thrombosis. However at times, 'late' and 'very late' thrombosis are witnessed. This risk of thrombosis can be drastically reduced by using dual antiplatelet therapy (DAPT). DAPT generally consists of combination of *aspirin* and a P2Y12 receptor blocker. Duration of DAPT generally is designed to eliminate the risk of thrombosis totally. However, it is not advised to prescribe DAPT indefinitely since that would increase the risk of hemorrhage.

Chances of thrombosis are higher with drug eluting stents (DES) than with bare metal stents (BMS). Second generation stents (everolimus and zotarolimus-eluting stents) promote endothelial healing earlier than with older generation (paclitaxel and sirolimus-eluting) stents.

However, the decision regarding the duration of DAPT is also dictated by certain patient factors. Prolonged DAPT must be avoided in patients with relatively high bleeding risk. These factors include: history of cerebrovascular transient ischemic attack or stroke, age ≥ 75 years, propensity to bleed (recent or recurrent gastrointestinal bleeding, active peptic ulcer disease, severe hepatic impairment), body weight <60 kg, or concomitant use of medications that increase risk (oral anticoagulants or nonsteroidal anti-inflammatory drugs [NSAIDs]).[19]

Considering the above, the duration of DAPT must be individualized, taking into account the benefits (prevention of ischemic events) and risks (bleeding).

It is generally advisable to continue DAPT for a period of 12 months after PCI. It is reasonable to continue DAPT for additional 18 months in patients with lower risk of bleeding and higher chances of thrombosis (older generation stents, complex procedures, multiple stents, previous history of stent thrombosis) with the newer stents now having bioabsorbable polymers that get fully absorbed after 3 months (evolve II data), the risk of polymer-induced inflammation is negated, promoting speedier healing, thereby which the duration of DAPT has been tested for 3 months post-PCI.

In patients with higher risk of bleeding, DAPT should be given at least for one month when BMS is used. With newer generation drug-eluting stents DAPT duration should at least be three months preferably six months.

For guiding duration of DAPT, recently the investigators of the DAPT trial proposed a decision tool to identify which patients would likely benefit from continuing dual antiplatelet therapy beyond one year. The DAPT score predicts the combined ischemic and bleeding risks taking into consideration some patient factors (age, history of smoking within the last two years, prior MI or PCI, history of heart failure or left ventricular ejection fraction <30%, MI at presentation, stenting of a vein graft, or stent diameter <3 mm). With a lower DAPT score, there is a greater increase in bleeding and smaller reduction in ischemia. At a higher score, there is a greater reduction in ischemia and small increase in bleeding. The DAPT investigators concluded that patients with a score <2 have greater harm than good from continued therapy beyond 12 months, while those with a score of 2 or more derive benefit from treatment for an additional 18 months.[20]

After the period of DAPT is over, single antiplatelet drug (generally aspirin) is continued lifelong. Patients who are intolerant to aspirin can be given a P2Y12 receptor blocker (generally clopidogrel).

Noncardiac surgery after recent coronary stent placement is associated with increased risk of adverse cardiac events. The proinflammatory and prothrombotic conditions during surgery may increase the baseline risk of stent thrombosis even in the presence of DAPT if a significant percent of struts are not endothelialized. Consequently, it is desirable to delay elective surgery as long as possible after coronary stent placement. For patients with DES undergoing noncardiac surgery, current guidelines recommend the following:

(1) elective surgery after DES implantation should be delayed until completion of 1 year of DAPT. In presence of newer generation DSE one antiplatelet can be temporarily withheld for surgery after 3–6 months of the PCI procedure, in these patients, a platelet P2Y12 receptor blocker should be discontinued for as brief a period as possible continuing aspirin or (2) if the surgery is urgent, the surgery should be performed without cessation of APT. In presence of BMS, a delay in surgery and temporary cessation of APT after 4–6 weeks from stent placement can be permissible.[21]

During the course of DAPT, there may be occasions when one needs to change over from one platelet P2Y12 receptor blocker to another. In patients who are already on clopidogrel, one may consider switching over to prasugrel or ticagrelor if the patient develops thrombosis or if the patient shows allergic manifestations with clopidogrel. When the switch over is due to higher risk of thrombosis, loading dose of prasugrel or ticagrelor should be given followed by the maintenance dose. If the changeover is not due to thrombosis risk but for intolerance, no loading is required. Maintenance dose can be directly started.

At times one may have to switch over from prasugrel or ticagrelor to clopidogrel. Such situation may arise either due to increased bleeding risk or due to cost constraints. While stopping prasugrel and starting clopidogrel, no loading dose is required. Whereas while changing over from ticagrelor to clopidogrel, loading dose of clopidogrel is required as antiplatelet effect of ticagrelor is reversible and is of short duration.

ANTITHROMBOTICS

Unfractionated Heparin

Time tested therapy for pre-PCI use in patients with ACS on the cath table.

This has been the antithrombin agent of choice during PCI, one of the main advantages being the ability to monitor the anticoagulant effect peri- and postprocedure.

Low Molecular Weight Heparin (LMWH)

Clinical studies published over the years have consistently shown that PCI can be safely performed in patients who are receiving standard doses of enoxaparin. In the SYNERGY trial, in patients assigned to enoxaparin and undergoing PCI within 8 hours of the last subcutaneous injection, no additional anticoagulation (neither enoxaparin nor UFH) was to be given. For those who received the last enoxaparin dose 8 or more hours before the PCI an additional intravenous bolus of 0.3 mg/kg of enoxaparin was to be given before the procedure. The trial found no difference in ischemic complications during PCI between patients treated with enoxaparin and those treated with UFH—including abrupt closures and no difference in 30 day mortality or MI.[22]

The safely and efficacy of enoxaparin in percutaneous coronary intervention patients (STEEPLE) trial, revealed that patients in the enoxaparin group had a significant reduction in the rate of non-CABG related bleeding compared with UFH[23] Overall Enoxaparin has the following advantages over UFH.

- Predictable pharmacological activity.
- Lack of need for monitoring anti-coagulation.

Fondaparinux Sodium

Fondaparinux is a synthetic selective factor X A inhibitor, unlike both UFH and LMWH, fondaparinux does not interact with other plama proteins (including factor IIa) thus resulting in a more predictable pharmacological profile.

The fifth Organization to Assess Strategies for Ischemic Syndromes (OASIS-5) compared low dose FONDAPARINUX (2.5 mg once daily, subcutaneous route) with enoxaparin in patients with unstable angina/NSTEMI of the 6238 patients who underwent PCI (PCI cohort) from this group, the ischemic events (death/MI/stroke) had a similar incidence in both groups (at 9 days/30 days/6 months) and there was a significant reduction incidence of major bleeding in the fondaparinux group. This trial clearly demonstrated the net clinical benefit of fondaparinux in the PCI cohort

However, it did raise a caution with patients (receiving fondaparinux) showing increased incidence of guide catheter thrombosis.[24]

In the OASIS-6 trial, in patients with STEMI not undergoing primary PCI fondaparinux significantly reduced mortality and re-infarction, without increasing the bleeding complications. In the subgroup that underwent primary PCI, guiding catheter thrombosis occurred more often with fondaparinux than control with no significant difference in bleeding at 9 days.[25]

Bivalirudin

Acute coronary syndromes result from platelet activation and initiation of the coagulation cascade, most often following plaque rupture. Due to the central role of thrombin in clot formation, direct thrombin inhibitors were developed to block the prothrombotic effects of thrombin without an increase in hemorrhagic events. The advantages of bivalirudin include direct inhibition of thrombin (without co factor), has no circulating inhibitors and no threat of heparin-induced thrombocytopenia.

The Randomized Evaluation in PCI Linking Angiomax to Reduced Clinical Events (REPLACE-2) trial demonstrated bivalirudin to be noninferior to heparin plus Gp IIb/IIIa

Table 5.1 2014 European Society of Cardiology and European Association of Cardiothoracic Surgery guidelines on myocardial revascularization

Recommendations for PCI class	*Class*	*Level*
Treatment with 600 mg clopidogrel is recommended in elective PCI patients once anatomy is known and decision to proceed with PCI preferably 2 hours or more before the procedure	I	A
Pretreatment with clopidogrel may be considered in patients with high probability for significant CAD	IIb	C
In patients on a maintenance dose of 75 mg clopidogrel, a new loading dose of 600 mg or more may be considered once the indication for PCI is confirmed	IIb	C
Antiplatelet therapy during PCI		
ASA is indicated before elective stenting	I	B
ASA oral loading dose of 150–300 mg (or 80–150 mg IV) is recommended if not pre-treated.	I	C
Clopidogrel (600 mg loading dose or more, 75 mg daily maintenance dose) is recommended for elective stenting.	I	A
GP IIb/IIIa antagonists should be considered only for bail-out.	IIa	C
Antiplatelet therapy after stenting		
DAPT is indicated for at least 1 month after BMS implantation	I	A
DAPT is indicated for 6 months after DES implantation	I	B
Shorter DAPT duration (<6 months) may be consider after DES implantation in patient with high bleeding risk	II b	A
Life-long single antiplatelet therapy, usually ASA, is recommended	I	A
Instruction of patients about the importance of complying with antiplatelet therapy is recommended.	I	C
DAPT may be used for more than 6 months in patients at high ischemic risk and low bleeding risk	IIb	C
Anticoagulant therapy		
Unfractionated heparin 70–100 U/kg	I	B
Bivalirudin (0.75 mg/kg bolus, followed by 1.75 mg/kg/hour for up to 4 hours after the procedure) in case of heparin-induced thrombocytopenia	I	C
Bivalirudin (0.75 mg/kg bolus, followed by 1.75 mg/kg/hour during the procedure) in patients at high bleeding risk	II a	A
Enoxaparin IV 0.5 mg/kg	IIa	B

blockade in reducing ischemic complications associated with PCI while significantly reducing the role of major in-hospital bleeding.[26]

The ACUITY study revealed that bivalirudin alone and with GP IIb/III a inhibition, compared to heparin plus a Gp IIb/IIIa inhibitor were associated with noninferior 30 days rates of the primary endpoint of death and myocardial infaction with a significant low bleeding in bivalirudin alone group.

Thus, the results from ACUITY support the use of bivalirudin when compared to treatment with heparin and Gp IIb/III a inhibitor with similar incidence of ischemic events yet significantly less major bleeding complications.[27]

However, the HEAT-PPCI investigators revealed a lower rate of MACE in heparin treated group, with an increased MACE (re infarction/TLR) in bivalirudin treated group.[28]

The MATRIX trial in ACS patients undergoing invasive management showed that bivalirudin was not superior to UFH on MACE end-points but did exhibit a significant reduction in risk of cardiovascular death and with a significant reduction in nonaccess site bleeding.[29]

Summarizing the 2013 ACCP/AHA recommendations for management of STEMI.

Bivalirudin 0.75 mg/kg IV bolus, then 1.75 mg/kg/hr infusion (with or without pretreatment with UFH) is preferred over UFH + Gp IIb/III a receptor antagonist in patients at high risk of bleeding.

Table 5.1 Summarizes these recommendations.

ADJUVANT TREATMENT IN THE LABORATORY

Basically comprises pharmacologic adjuncts in treatment of no reflow phenomenon ('the Achilles heel' in primary angioplasty !)

The no-reflow phenomenon following PCI is associated with significant cardiac consequences due to myocardial ischemia caused by inadequate distal microvascular flow and poor myocardial perfusion.[31]

No-reflow predicts a poor functional recovery and impaired ventricular remodeling, and its persistence—

Table 5.2 Pharmacologic adjuncts to limit no-reflow

Category/drug	*Mechanism of action*	*Advantages/disadvantages*
Adenosine	Activation of mitochondrial K ATP channel in myocardium	Requires rapid, multiple bolus administration Depresses SA and AV nodal conduction First, second or third degree AV block sinus bradycardia possible
Diltiazem	Slow L- type CCB	IC diltiazem can cause type I second degree AV block occasionally
Nicardipine	Slow, L-type CCB	Stronger vasodilating effect. Greater coronary blood flow velocity than diltiazem or verapamil. Longer duration of action. Minimal negative chronotropic and dromotropic effects
Verapamil	Slow, L-type CCB	Prolongs AV nodal effective refractory period, bradyarrhythmias when used IC
Nicorandil—Potassium channel agent and nitric oxide donor	Acts on ATP sensitive K^+ channels	May be effective via intravenous route in addition to IC, augmented effect of adenosine in small studies
Simvastatin (HMG-Co A reductase inhibitors)	Activation of mitochondrial K-ATP channel in myocardium, upregulation of nitric oxide	Tachycardia, hypertension, myocardial ischemia, palpitations, flushing
Epinephrine (alpha and beta adrenoreceptor agonist)	Activates adenyl cyclase	
Abciximab/Tirofiban (glycoprotein IIb/III a receptor inhibitor)	Block platelet aggregation	Reduce platelet plugging during reperfusion
Nitroprusside—Nitric oxide donor	Activation of guanylyl cyclase by free radical nitric oxide	Very rapid onset; IC administration appears safe. Cyanide toxicity possible

despite attempted treatment—is associated with a high incidence of ongoing or recurrent acute coronary syndrome (ACS) as well as increased short-term mortality.[32]

A range of pharmacologic adjuncts have been evaluated to limit no-reflow, including adenosine, diltiazem, nicardipine, verapamil, nitroprusside, glycoprotein antiplatelet medications, soluble factor antagonists, anti-endothelins and others. Most await large-scale, randomized, controlled trials to confirm their roles and define optimal regimens (Table 5.2).[33]

Other Adjuvant Drugs

Beta Blockers

Some nonrandomized studies showed lower rates of CK MB rise in patients on beta blockers going for PCI than those not on beta blockers. Thirty day and one year mortality rates after the procedure also favored use of pre-PCI use of beta blockers.[34,35] Some studies suggested that rates of coronary stenosis after PCI could be brought down by using intracoronary beta blockers during the procedure.[36] One year outcomes after PCI were shown to be significantly better in patients given inracoronary propranolol during procedure compared to placebo in a study.[37]

Many patients undergoing PCI for stable CAD are generally on beta blockers as part of their medical treatment. Those who are not, are the patients who for some reason cannot tolerate them.

Calcium Channel Blockers

This group of drugs has been found to be useful in "no reflow" situation after successful stenting of the epicardial vessel. This is considered to be due to extensive thromboembolism of 'small vasculature'. Calcium channel blockers are potent vasodilators and therefore help restoring high grade TIMI flow.[38]

These drugs were also shown to reduce rates of restenosis.[39,40] However, after the entry of drug eluting stents CCBs are no longer considered for this purpose.

Angiotensin Converting Enzyme Inhibitors

Apart from their beneficial effects on ventricular remodeling and myocardial function, these drugs have been shown to reduce restenosis of the stented vessels by some studies.[41,42] However, these findings were not confirmed by a large randomized trial.[43] With drug-eluting stents which have been proved to be extremely useful for this purpose, ACE inhibitors are no more considered for their effect on coronary vascular reactivity.

Statins

Statins have been proved to be of great benefit in management of the entire spectrum of coronary disease. All patient undergoing PCI should be given high doses of statin. This was aptly shown by a large meta analysis.[44] Authors of this study concluded that high-dose statin pretreatment leads to a significant reduction in periprocedural myocardial infarction and 30-day adverse events in patients undergoing percutaneous coronary intervention. This strategy should be considered in all patients with planned percutaneous coronary intervention.

Local Anesthetic

Coronary interventions are generally done under local anesthesia. 10–20 mL of 2% xylocaine is used for femoral route while 1–2 mL of the anesthetic is sufficient for radial access.

Cocktail for Radial Procedures

Combination of 100 μg of nitroglycerin and 1.25–2.5 mg of verapamil prevents radial artery spasm. This increases the comfort level for the patient as well as the operator for smoother procedure.

Apart from these drugs the other drugs which can have significant impact on hemodynamics must be had handy during every PCI procedure. Vagolytics such as atropine, inotropes such as dobutamine and dopamine, vasopressors such as noradrenaline, diuretics, etc should be available during the cath lab procedures to promptly correct hemodynamic abnormalities which may sometimes be witnessed during complex PCI procedures. Nitroglycerin, nicorandil can be required to treat coronary spasm and angina. Analgesics and midsedatives may be required by some apprehensive patients especially for procedures taking long time.

Thus, apart from the hardware that is used for coronary interventions, use of certain drugs is essential part of these procedures. Basic knowledge of these drugs helps in obtaining optimal result from the interventions.

REFERENCES

1. Schwartz L, Bourassa MG, Lesperance J, Aldridge HE, Kazim F, Salvaton VA, Henderson M, Bonan R, David PR. Aspirin and dipyridamole in the prevention of restenosis after percutaneous luminal coronary angioplasty. N Engl J med. 1988;318:1714-9.
2. Patrick T O'Gara, Frederick G Kushner, Deborah D Ascheim, Donald E Casey 2013. ACCF/ AHA guideline for the management of STEMI Executive summary= A report of the ACCFF/AHA Task Force on Practice Guidelines. J Am Coll Cardiol. 2013;61(4): 485-510.
3. Steg PG, James SK, Atar D, Badano LP, Lundquist CB, Borger MA. ESC guidelines for the management of acute myocardial infarction in patients presenting with STMI; Eur Heart J. 2012;33:25, 69-619.
4. Mehta SR, Yusuf S, Peters RJG, et al. Effects of pretreatment with clopidogrel and aspirin followed by long term therapy in patients undergoing PCI. (the PCI-CURE study) Lancet. 2001;358: 527-33.
5. Patti G, Lolonna G, Pasceri V, Pepe LL, Montinaro A, Disciascio G, Randomised trial of high loading dose of clopidogrel for reduction of periprocedural MI in patients undergoing coronary intervention results from the ARMYDA- 2 study. Circulation. 2005;111:2099-106.
6. Patrick T, O'Gara, Frederick E Kushner, Deborah D, Ascheim, Donald E, Cosey. 2013. ACCFF/AHA guideline for the management of STEMI Executive Summary. Circulation. 2013;127:529-55.
7. Angiolillo DJ, Capranzano P, Goto S, Aslam M, Desai B, Charlton RK, Suzuki Y, Box LC, Shoemaker SB, Zenni MM. A randomised study assessing the impact of cilostazol on platelet function profiles in patients with DM and CAD on dual antiplatelet therapy: results of the OPTIMUS-2 study. Eur Heart J. 2008 Sep;29(18):2202-11.
8. Wiviott SD, Braunwald E, Mc Cabe CH, Montalescot G, Ruzyllo W, Gottheb S, Neumann FJ, Ardissino D, De servi S, Morphy SA, Antman EM. Prasugrel versus clopidogrel in patients with ACS. N Engl J Med. 2007;357:2001-15.
9. Wallentin L, Becher RC, Budaj A, Cannon CP, Emanuelsson H, Held C, Horrow J, Husted S for the PLATO investigators, Ticagrelor versus clopidogrel in patients with ACS. N Engl J Med. 2009;361:1045-57.
10. Cannon C, Hamngton R, James S, Ardissino D, Becher R, Emanvelsson H, Husted S. The Platelet inhibition and patient outcomes (PLATO) investigators. Ticagrelor compared with clopidogrel in acute coronary syndromes. Patients with a planned invasive strategy (PLATO), A randomised double blind study. Lancet. 2010;375:283-93.
11. White H, Bhatt DL, Gibson M, Hamm CW, Stone GW. Outcomes with Cangrelor versus clopidogrel on a background of Bivalirudin: Insights from the CHAMPION PHOENIX study: J AM Coll Cardwl Intv. 2015;8(3):424-33.
12. Kastrati A, Mehilli J, Neumann FJ, Dotzer F, TenBerg J, et al. Abciximab in patients with ACS undergoing PCI after Clopidogrel pretreatment: the ISAR-REACT 2 randomised trial. JAMA. 2006;295:1531-8.

13. Randomised placebo controlled trial of abciximab before and during coronary intervention in refractory unstable angina. The CAPRURE study Lancet. 1997;349:1429-35.
14. Schulz S, et al. One year clinical outcomes with abciximab in acute myocardial infarction results of the BRAVE-3 randomised trial. Clin Res Cardiol. 2010;99(12):795-802.
15. PURSUIT Trial Investigators. Inhibition of platelet Gp II b/III a with eptifibatide in patients with ACS. N Eng J Med. 1998;339: 436-43.
16. The RESTORE Investigators. Effects of platelet Gp IIb/IIIa blockade with Tirofiban on adverse cardiac events in patients with unstable angina or acute MI undergoing coronary angioplasty. Circulation. 1997;96:1445-53.
17. Inhibition of the platelet glycoprotein IIb/III a with tirofiban in unstable angina and non q wave myocardial infarction. PRISM-PLUS study investigators. N Engl J Med. 998;338:1488-97.
18. Airoldi F, Colombo A, Morici N, et al. Incidence and predictors of DES thrombosis during and after discontinuation of Thienopyridine treatment. Circulation. 2004;116:745.
19. Ducrocq G, Amarenco P, Labreuche J, et al. A history of stroke. TIA indicates high risks of cardiovascular event and hemorrhagic stroke in patients with CAD. Circulation. 2013:127:730.
20. Mauri L, Kereiakes DJ, et al. DAPT Study Investigators: 12 or 30 months of dual antiplatelet therapy after drug-eluting stents. N Engl J Med. 2014;371(23):2155.
21. Hawn MT, Graham LA, et al. Risk of major adverse cardiac events following non-cardiac surgery in patients with coronary stents. JAMA. 2013;310(14):1462-72.
22. White HD, Kleiman NS, Mahaffey KW, et al. Efficacy and safety of Enoxaparin compared with UFH in high risk patients with non-ST segment elevation, acute coronary syndrome undergoing PCI in the SYNERGY trial. Am Heart J. 2006;152(6): 1042-50.
23. Montalescot G, White HD, Gallo R, et al. Enoxaparin versus unfractioned heparin in elective PCI. N Eng J Med. 2006;355(10): 1006-17.
24. Yusuf S, Mehta SR, Chrolavidus S, et al. Comparison of Fondaparinux and Enoxaparin in acute coronary Syndromes. N Eng J Med. 2006; 354(14):1464-76.
25. Yusuf S, Mehta SR, Chrolavidus S, et al. Effects of Fondaparinux on mortality and re-infarction in patients with acute ST segment elevation MI. The OASIS-6 randomized trial. JAMA. 2006;295(13): 1519-30.
26. Lincoff AM, Bittl JA, et al. Bivalirudin and provisional glycoprotein IIb/IIIa blockade compared with heparin and planned Gp IIb/IIIa blockade during PCI: REPLACE-2 randomised trial JAMA. 2003;289(7):853-63.
27. Stone GW, McLaurin B, Cox D, et al. Bivalirudin for patients with Acute Coronary Syndromes (For the ACUITY Investigators) N Eng J Med. 2006;355:2203-16.
28. Shahzad A, Kemp J, Mars C, Wilson K, Koom C, Cooper R. HEAT-PPCI: An open label, single centre, randomised controlled trial. The LANCET. 2014;384(9957):1849-58.
29. Valgimigli M, Frigoli E, Leonardi S. Bivalirudin or unfractionated heparin—in acute coronary syndromes: N Eng J Med. 2015;373:997-1009.
30. O'Gara PT, Kushner F, Ascheim DD. ACCF/AHA guideline for the management of STEMI. Circulation. 2013;127.
31. Piana RN, Paik GY, Moscucci M, et al. Incidence and treatment of "no-reflow" after percutaneous coronary intervention. Circulation. 1994;89:2514-8.
32. Eeckhout E, Kern MJ. The coronary no-reflow phenomenon: A review of mechanisms and therapies. Eur Heart J. 2001;22: 729-39.
33. Pharmacological adjuncts evaluated for prevention or reversal of no reflow phenomenon in the setting of PCI Jl. Invasive Cardiol. 2008.
34. Sharma SK, Kini A, Marmur JD, et al. Cardio protective effect of beta blocker therapy in reducing creatinine kinase MB elevation after coronary intervention: Benefit is extended to improvement in intermediate term survival. Circulation. 2000;102:166-72.
35. Chan AW, Quinn MJ, Bhatt DL, et al. Mortality benefit of beta blockade after successful elective percutaneous coronary intervention. J Am Coll Cardiol. 2002;40:669-75.
36. Jackson JD, Muhlestein JB, Bunch TJ, et al. Beta blockers reduce the incidence of clinical restenosis; Prospective study of 4840 patients undergoing percutaneous coronary revascularisation. Am Heart J. 2003;145:87-881.
37. Uretsky BF, Birnbaum Y, Osman A, et al. Dista myocardial protection with intra coronary beta blocker when added to a GpIIb/IIIa latelet receptor blocker during percutaneous coronary intervention improves clinical outcome. Catheter Cardiovasc Interv. 2008;72:488-97.
38. Umemura S, Nakamura S, Sugiura T, et al. The effect of Verapamil on restoration of myocardial perfusion and functional recovery in patients with angiographic no reflow after primary percutaneous coronary intervention. Nucl Med Commun. 2006;27:247-54.
39. Yamazaki T, Taniguchi I, Kurusi T, et al. Effect of Amlodipine on vascular responses after coronary stenting compared with an angiotensin converting enzyme inhibitor. Circ J. 2004;68: 328-33.
40. Bestehorn HP, Neumann FJ, Buttener HJ, et al. Evaluation of the effect of oral verapamil on clinical outcome and angiographic restenosis after percutaneous coronary intervention. The randomised, double blind, placebo controlled, multicenter Verapamil Slow Release for Prevention of Cardiovascular Events After Angioplasty (VESPA) trial. J Am Coll Cardiol. 2004;43: 2160-5.
41. Okimoto T, Imazu M, Hayashi T, et al. Quinapril with high affinity to tissue angiotensin converting enzyme reduces restenosis after percutaneous transcatheter coronary intervention. Cardiovasc Drugs Ther. 2001;15:323-9.
42. Deftereos S, Giannopoulos G, Kossyvakis C, et al. Effect of Quinapril on in stent restenosis and relation to plasma apoptosis signalling molecules. Am J Cardiol. 2010;105:54-8.
43. Does the new angiotensin converting enzyme inhibitor Cilazapril prevent restenosis after percutaneous transluminal coronary angioplasty? Results of the MERCATOR study. A multicenter, European Research Trial with Cilazapril after angioplasty to Prevent Transluminal Coronary Obstruction and Restenosis (MERCATOR) study group. Circulation.1992;86: 325-7.
44. Patti G, Cannon CP, Murphy SA, et al. Clinical benefit of statin pretreatment in patients undergoing percutaneous coronary intervention. A collaborative patient-level meta-analysis of 13 randomized studies. Circulation. 2011;123:1622-32.

CHAPTER

6

Hardware for Coronary Angioplasty

Susheel K Malani, DS Chadha

INTRODUCTION

The first coronary balloon angioplasty was done by Andreas Gruntzing way back in 1977. Since then the field of percutaneous coronary intervention (PCI) has witnessed a sea change in development of better hardware and techniques to ensure enhanced safety and efficacy. The purpose of this chapter is to review the available hardware for PCI except chronic total occlusion which is dealt separately.

GUIDE CATHETERS

An ideal guide catheter serves as a conduit for contrast media delivery and pressure measurement apart from providing coaxial alignment and support for device passage to the target site.[1,2] Guide catheters have a stiffer shaft, larger luminal diameter, and a shorter, nontapered and less angulated tip compared to diagnostic catheters. They are available in a variety of shapes and sizes. For proper guide catheter selection one has to take into consideration access site (transfemoral/transradial), the size and configuration of the aortic root and arch, the coronary artery side (right vs. left), lesion location (ostium/distal), lesion morphology (discrete, diffuse or chronic total occlusion) graft vessel affected, and the need for catheter support.[1,2]

Guide Catheter: Basic Structure

Guiding catheters are generally composed of 3 layers.[1,2] The outer layer consists of either polyurethane or polyethylene for overall stiffness. The middle layer is composed of a wire matrix for torque generation. The inner coating is of Teflon for smooth passage of balloon catheters and stents. There are 3 basic components of a guide catheter, a hub for connection, a shaft of variable size, length and stiffness, and a tip with an end-hole (Fig. 6.1).

The standard length of a percutaneous coronary intervention guide catheter is 100 cm (centimeter) while shorter (80–90 cm) catheters are useful for PCI of chronic total occlusion (CTO). Length of the guide catheter can be shortened by removing a segment of the proximal shaft, and by capping with a flared, short one size smaller sheath.

The size of the guide catheter is defined by the outer diameter measurement, and is commonly expressed in French size.[1,2] Catheter size is determined by the outer diameter measurement, whereas sheath size is determined by the inner diameter measurement (Fig. 6.2). The most commonly used size is 6F. Smaller sized guides are used for the radial intervention while larger-sized catheters which provide better support with improved visibility are used for CTO and bifurcation angioplasties. Larger guide catheters in addition facilitate the delivery of bulkier devices, and imaging catheters while performing complex angioplasties.[3,4] However larger guiding catheters are associated with higher rates of vascular complication and often compromise antegrade perfusion (which manifests as pressure damping when engaging the coronary ostium). Table 6.1 summarizes the accommodating

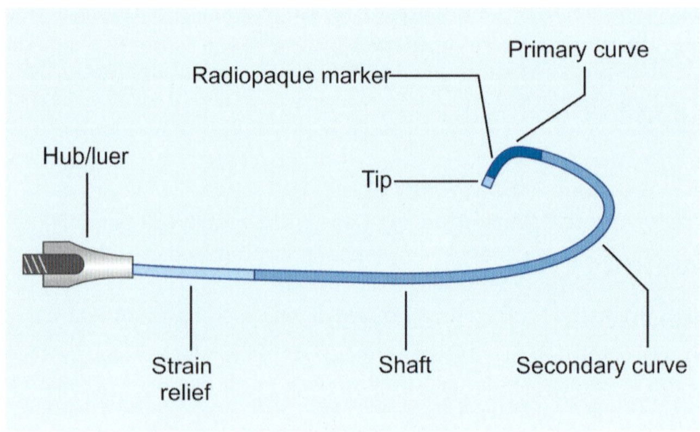

Fig. 6.1 Components of a guide catheter

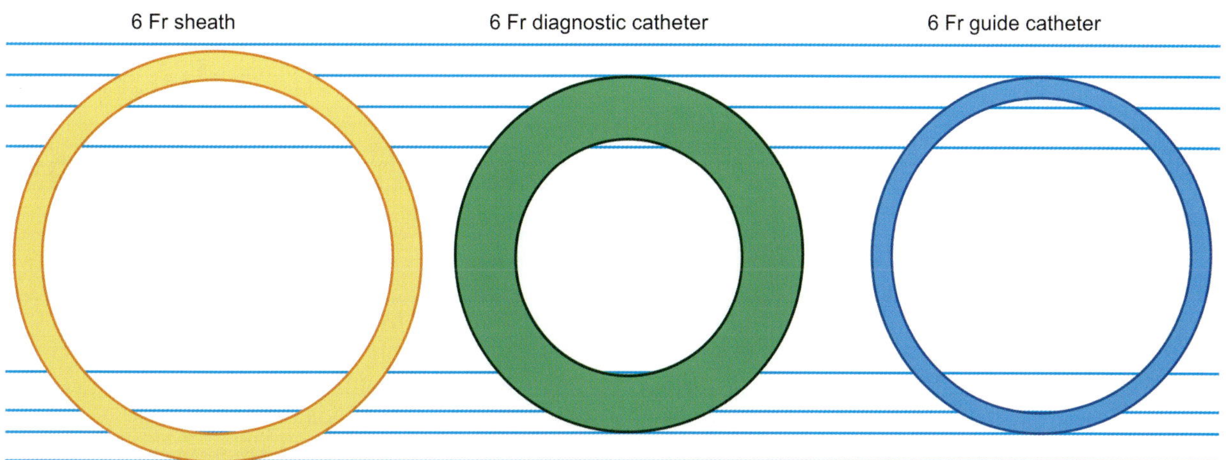

Fig. 6.2 Difference in the inner and outer diameter of 6 French sheath, diagnostic catheter and guide catheter size is determined by the outer diameter while the sheath size is determined by the inner diameter

Table 6.1 Guide catheter and their accommodating capacity for various devices used for percutaneous coronary interventions

	Inner lumen size	*Accommodating capacity for the PCI device*
1	5 Fr (1.42–1.50 mm)	All coronary balloons, most coronary stents (BVS up to 3 mm), rotablator burr 1.25 mm, microcatheters, IVUS catheter.
2	6 Fr (1.73 1.83 mm)	Two rapid exchange balloons for kissing balloon angioplasty, thrombus aspiration catheter 6 Fr, BVS above 3 mm, OCT catheter, covered stents above 4 mm, Rotablator burr 1.5 mm, cutting balloon, 6 Fr guideliner.
3	7 Fr (1.98–2. 08 mm)	Rotablator burr 1.75 mm, simultaneous 2 stent deployment, thrombus aspiration catheter 7 Fr, crusade twin pass catheter along with rapid exchange balloon catheter for balloon trapping technique.
4	8 Fr (2.24–2.30 mm)	Rotablator burr 1.75 mm, Corsair microcatheter + IVUS catheter, 02 over the wire balloon catheters

Abbreviations: PCI, percutaneous coronary interventions; Fr, French; BVS, bioabsorbable vascular scaffold; IVUS, intravascular ultrasound; OCT, optical coherence tomography

capacity of different size of guiding catheters. Catheters with side holes are helpful while doing cases with ostial stenosis as antegrade perfusion is maintained. Catheters with side holes require higher dose of contrast and contrast escaping through the side holes may result in suboptimal opacification of the artery.[1,2] Side hole guiding catheters are generally not recommended while performing fractional flow reserve (FFR) measurement. Tables 6.2 and 6.3 describes the properties of commonly used guiding catheters.

COMMONLY USED GUIDING CATHETERS

Judkins Catheters

Judkins catheters were among the earliest catheters developed for coronary angiography.[5] The Judkins left (JL) curve catheter is designed with its curves fitting the aortic root and allowing it to engage the LMCA ostium. The length (ranging from 3.5 to 6 cm) of the segment between the primary and secondary curves determines the curve size of a Judkins catheter. In the majority of patients with normal body habitus and normal size of aortic root, Judkins left and right 4 cm curves will provide good coronary engagement. For coronary cannulation from the left radial/brachial artery approach, a Judkins left catheter with a secondary curve 0.5 mm (millimeter) smaller than required for femoral approach is generally better suited. The Judkins right catheter is shaped to enter into the right coronary artery with a small amount of clockwise rotation from both femoral and radial approaches. A Judkins catheter can be carefully manipulated to "deep seat" into the vessel to provide "active support". The Judkins catheter is suitable for noncomplex lesions or left main stenosis when good catheter support is not critical.[1,2,5]

Amplatz Catheters

Amplatz catheters by resting against the back wall and aortic cusp provide strong "passive support" for the angioplasty.[6] The Amplatz left catheter is useful for 'down going' left circumflex and for right coronary artery (RCA) with

Table 6.2 Properties of guiding catheters used for the native right and left coronary artery intervention

Catheter description	*Sizes*	*Remarks/Applications*
Left coronary		
Judkins left (JL)	3.0, 3.5, 4.0, 4.5, 5.0, 6.0	Standard left coronary artery (LCA) intervention, shorter curve for left anterior descending (LAD), larger for left circumflex (LCX). Useful in left main and ostial LAD intervention
Back up catheters (Voda (VL), EBU, XB	3.0, 3.5, 3.75, 4.0, 4.5, 5.0	Excellent backup support from contralateral aortic wall. Useful for tortuous and angulated vessels and calcific or total occlusions.
Right coronary		
Judkins right (JR)	3.0, 3.5, 4.0, 4.5, 5.0, 6.0	Standard right coronary artery (RCA) intervention, bypass graft
Back up catheters [VR (Voda Right), ECR]	3.0, 3.5, 3.75, 4.0, 4.5, 5.0	Excellent backup support from contralateral aortic wall. Useful for tortuous and angulated vessels and calcific or total occlusions, Shepherd's Crook RCA
Double Loop Aran75 (DA75), Double Loop Arani 90 (DA90)		Excellent backup support from contralateral aortic wall, useful for tortuous and angulated vessels and calcific or total occlusions, Shepherd's Crook RCA
Amplatz left	1.0, 1.5, 2.0, 2.5, 3.0, 4.0	Shepherd's Crook RCA, high anterior RCA, all saphenous venous grafts, excellent backup support
Amplatz right	1,2,3	RCA and right saphenous venous graft with inferior origin
Three dimensional Right catheter (3DRC)		Used mainly to cannulate RCA with posterior or superior take-off

Table 6.3 Properties of miscellaneous and radial guiding catheters

Catheter description	*Sizes*	*Remarks/Applications*
Miscellaneous guides		
Multipurpose	MPA1- MPA2 with 45-60° primary curve; MPB1 - MPB2 with 80° primary curve	Useful for downward pointing bypass graft to RCA or inferior pointing native RCA.
Hockey stick (HS)		RCA with inferior takeoff, right SVG with inferior takeoff
Internal mammary artery (IMA) catheter		Catheter is rotated anticlockwise to engage left internal mammary artery (IMA), and clockwise for right IMA also useful for upward-pointing RCA
Bypass grafts guides (LCB or RCB)		Left sided or right sided saphenous vein graft (SVG) with horizontal or slightly superior takeoff
ElGamal (ELG)	0.75, 1.0, 2.0	Horizontal or slightly superior RCA takeoff, left SVGs
Radial		
Barbeau, Kimney, Fadajet, Ikari, MAC, SherpaNX, Sheathless Guides		Standard femoral guides can also be used.

anterior origin in the right coronary cusp. It is also useful for engaging a horizontal or superior take-off saphenous vein graft (SVG) or RCA. These catheters are best avoided in patients with ostial lesions as they tend to engage deeply the coronary ostia. Extra caution is needed when disengaging an Amplatz catheter from the coronary ostia as they tend to dissect the ostia if not disengaged properly. To disengage, the catheter is advanced downward gently to prolapse the tip out of the ostium, before being rotated to remove the tip completely. A word of caution: unlike the Judkins catheter, pull back of this catheter may cause it to dive deeper into the vessel.[1,2,6]

Extra Back-up Catheters

These catheters are more commonly used for left coronary artery (LCA) intervention, the variable anatomy (origin and orientation) of RCA makes their coxial alignment less predictable.[1,2,7] These catheters with their long tip from a fairly straight line with the left main coronary artery (LMCA) axis or the proximal part of the RCA and provide a hybrid of "active" and "passive" supports. The long secondary curve provides a large area of contact between the catheter and the aortic wall and increases the resistance to displacement further stabilizing the catheter. The Voda catheter (Boston Scientific was the first extra back-up curve catheter marketed in the early 1990s.[8] The other extra back-up catheters include the EBU (Medtronic), XB (Cordis), Q-Curve and CLS® Curve (Boston Scientific).[1,2] In normal-sized aortic root, the LMCA can usually be cannulated using XB 3.5 or EBU 3.5–3.75.

Other Special Catheters

The multipurpose guide catheter has a slight bend (MPA1 and MPA2 with 45–60° primary curve; MPB1 and MPB2 have 80° primary curve) some distance from the tip. It is most useful for the downward-pointing bypass graft to the RCA.[1,2,9] Occasionally, it is also used to cannulate the high LMCA take-off or inferior-pointing native RCA. The internal mammary artery (IMA) catheter has a more angulated (80° primary curve) tip, which facilitates the engagement of the IMA with an anticlockwise rotation from femoral approach.[1,2,9] This catheter is also useful for upward-pointing RCA. The left coronary bypass (LCB) catheter has the reach needed for cannulating left-sided grafts which are usually superior and to the left of the native LCA ostium. The three dimensional right catheter (3DRC) is used mainly to cannulate a RCA with posterior or superior take-off.[10] It has multiple curves leading to a three-dimensional configuration, and consequently does not require much manipulation to cannulate the right coronary artery as is normally done with the JR catheter. Arani catheter; the double angle 90° curve sits on ascending aorta in S configuration and is therefore useful for RCA with horizontal take-off.[11] The primary and secondary curve provides two contact points on the opposite side of aorta thus providing tremendous back-up support. XBR and XBRCA catheters have been developed specifically for the inferior and superior take off of RCA respectively.[1,2,12]

GUIDE CATHETER SELECTION FOR RADIAL INTERVENTION

The angle of radial approach to coronary/bypass graft ostia is different from the femoral approach hence many catheters for transfemoral intervention (TFI) do not provide optimal coaxial engagement while performing transradial intervention (TRI), especially when using the right radial approach.[9,13,14] The radial artery has a tendency for spasm which further limits the catheter size available for TRI. Left TRI can be performed using standard guide catheters developed for TFI.[13-15] While using the right radial artery, most of the TFI catheters can also be used but the catheter support is generally less. In order to provide better back up support using the contralateral aortic wall a number of modified long-tip catheters (Ikari, Kimny, Power Backup, Fajadet, etc.) have been developed for right TRI.[13-15] However for proper catheter selection additional anatomical factors to be taken into consideration include the position of origin of the brachiocephalic trunk from the aortic arch, and subclavian-brachiocephalic tortuosity.[13-15,18]

For the left coronary artery while using a Judkins catheter via right RA, it is recommended either to downsize by 0.5 cm from what is used for femoral approach. Back up support available for Judkins while using radial approach is much lesser than that available while using femoral approach.[9,13-15] While using extra back up catheters from the right radial approach one needs to push these catheters towards the left coronary sinus over a 0.035" guidewire making a large J-shaped loop in the sinus of Valsalva for engaging the left coronary ostia.

For the right coronary artery the Judkins right catheter in sizes similar to TFI is the catheter of first choice for noncomplex or ostial RCA lesions.[9] If extra back up is required, long tipped catheters can be used taking care not to dissect the coronary ostium. Internal mammary artery TRI is usually performed using an IMA or JR catheter via ipsilateral radial access while SVG TRI is performed from the left radial approach using standard catheters such as JR, LCB, AL, or multipurpose. From the right radial approach, Judkins right and Amplatz right catheters can be used to engage SVG to left coronary arteries.[1,2] Cannulation of inferior-pointing SVG to the right coronary artery can be performed using a multipurpose catheter.[9,10]

Radial artery diameter and its tendency to spasm is the major limitation of TRI. Spasm of radial artery may lead to its occlusion. A major predictor of occlusion is a larger ratio of sheath diameter to radial artery diameter. Though the use of a smaller (e.g., 5 Fr) sheath or catheter is associated with lower radial occlusion or stenosis rate but these guides provide reduced catheter support with poor angiographic visualization and restricts use of adjunctive devices. Sheath less guide catheters (Eaucath sheathless guide, Asahi Intec, Japan) are now available which do not require an introducer sheath.[16] This reduces the equipment size within the radial lumen by ~2 Fr. While using this system a 7.5 Fr guide has internal diameter similar to a conventional 7 Fr guide catheter but an outer diameter smaller than a 6 Fr sheath. These catheters have hydrophilic surface coating to facilitate catheter movement in the radial artery, aiming to reduce patient discomfort and arterial spasm.

GUIDE CATHETER FOR SAPHENOUS VEIN GRAFTS AND LEFT INTERNAL MAMMARY ARTERY INTERVENTIONS

For saphenous vein graft (SVG) interventions, JR guiding catheter is usually chosen. However, for abnormal take-offs or abnormal positions of graft, AL1 or MP guiding catheter may be more appropriate. Left or right coronary bypass (LCB/RCB) catheters have also been found to be useful for SVG cannulation. LCB catheter is designed for left coronary venous bypass grafts.[1,2,17] Its tip has 90° primary and 70° secondary bend. It is shaped much like a cobra catheter. RCB catheter is designed for right coronary venous bypass grafts, its tip and secondary bends approximate 120°. It is shaped much like a JR catheter with a shallower tip bend. Multipurpose A-1 may also be useful in this situation since it has a straight tip which often falls into right coronary bypass grafts easily.

CORONARY GUIDEWIRE

Coronary guidewires are fundamental to any coronary intervention. The wide selection of available guidewires can on most of the occasions be confusing and often leads to random selection. In the current chapter we will provide an overview for guidewire selection.

Basic Performance Requirements

As with the guide catheter the proper selection of guidewire is critical to the success of the interventional procedure.[19-21] Guidewire serves as a rail over which balloon catheters, stents, and other devices are threaded. The choice of the wire is often dictated by the clinical circumstances wherein one selects a wire with specific features to solve patient-specific problems. Success of the angioplasty depends on the ability of the guidewire to be maneuvered through the coronary anatomy (steerability), around curves (trackability), and with favorable control of the guidewire tip by rotation of the opposite end of the guidewire (torquability).[19,20] Guidewires must not only be visible throughout their length but they also should have lubricity as they interact directly with the vessel wall. Most operators select "workhorse" guidewires (softer tips and medium support) for a majority of cases. It is important for the operator to keep in mind that selection of any guidewire other than a workhorse type is usually a compromise and is fraught with complications. Every departure from the safe workhorse type guidewire should be made keeping in mind the coronary anatomy and thorough knowledge of the characteristics of the wire.[1-4,19,20]

Basic Guidewire Structure

The principle components of a coronary guidewire include: (1) the central core, (2) the more flexible guidewire tip, and (3) a coating. Central core is the longest portion of the guidewire forming its backbone extending from the proximal to the distal part where it begins to taper.[19,20] The central core material is usually made of stainless steel (supportive with good torque control), nitinol (excellent flexibility) or high tensile stainless steel. The core diameter is usually from 0.010" to 0.18" with 0.014" being the most common size. Larger diameters provide better support for the devices. Tip at the distal end of the wire may be tapered or non-tapered and has a diameter of 0.008" to 0.014". Distal tip style could be either core to tip style (the core wire extends from the proximal end of the wire to its tip) or shaping ribbon style (the core wire stops short of the tip making the tip more shapeable and flexible) (Figs 6.3A to D). In some of the Asahi wires a hybrid composite tip style has been introduced wherein the core to tip design is strengthened by the twist wire running parallel to core wire. The tip of the wire is covered by spring coil or polymer cover or micro cut nitinol sleeve. Polymer cover provides increased lubricity and trackability to the wire. The outer coating of the wire provides a smooth and non interactive surface to the wire. Proximal shaft of the wire is usually covered with PTFE or Teflon. The distal tip of the wire could have either a hydrophilic (slip coat or hydrocoat which makes the wire more slippery on contact with water thereby enhancing its lubricity and trackability) or a hydrophobic cover (silicon based coating which repels water and gives a good tactile feel of the lesion).[19,22] Hydrophilic wires are less thrombogenic and negotiate tortuous lesions well (Figs 6.4A to D).

CHARACTERISTICS AND CLASSIFICATION OF GUIDEWIRES

It is prudent to understand the design and composition of guidewire as this will assist in appropriate guidewire selection based on the morphology of the coronary lesion. No single guidewire has all desirable characteristics to be suitable for a given coronary lesion. Table 6.4 lists the properties of the most commonly used wires in the cath lab. Guidewires can be classified based on tip flexibility (floppy/soft, intermediate, stiff), tip coating (hydrophilic, hydrophobic, no coating), tip style (one-piece core-to-tip, two-piece core with shaping ribbon), tip tapering (tapered, untapered), core construction material (stainless steel, nitinol, high-tensile stainless steel), device support (light, moderate support, extra support), and

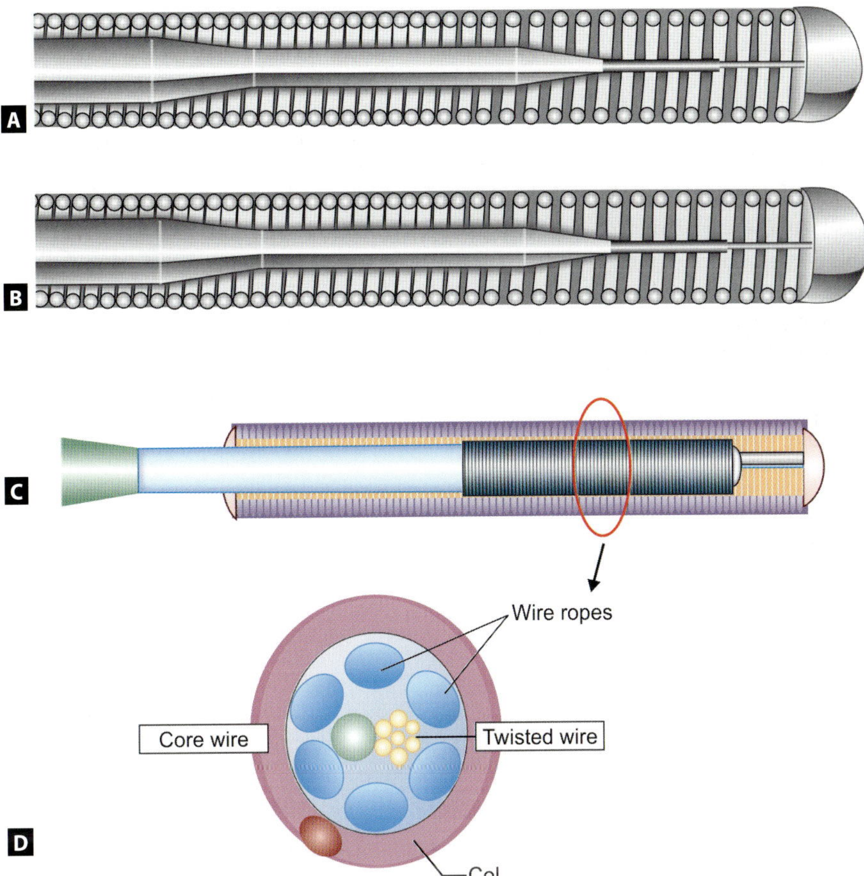

Figs 6.3A to D Distal tip design of the guidewire. Core to tip one piece design where the tapered core reached the distal end of the wire (A), shaping ribbon design the core stops just short of the distal tip (B), composite core is a hybrid design introduced by Asahi where the core wire is strengthened by the twist wire running in parallel (C), cross section of composite wire (D)

target lesion type (workhorse/frontline wires), CTO (chronic total occlusion) wires, wires for tortuous lesions, etc. There are other specific purpose guidewires, e.g. pressure wire, marker wire (with markers or length indicators), rotablator wire, wiggle wire, etc.[19,22]

Tip load of the guidewire tip determines its flexibility/stiffness and is usually measured and expressed as tip load. This is the force required for buckling or bending the wire tip. The "penetration force" of a wire depends on both the tip load and the cross-sectional area of the wire tip. Guidewires with greater tip load are stiffer and have greater penetration force and pushability. Tapered guidewires compared to untapered wire with similar tip load have greater penetration force.[23] Guidewire shaft support, a major factor involved in device delivery is determined by the properties of the core of the wire (diameter, construction material and pattern of core tapering of the wire). Shaft support is measured as the force required for bending the guidewire at different distances from the guidewire tip. The stiffer the shaft, the greater is the support provided for device passage through a tortuous and calcified lesion.[19,20]

Workhorse Guidewires

Workhorse guidewires form the bulk of guidewires used in any catheterization laboratory as they are suitable for the majority of lesions. A workhorse guidewire should possess a flexible tip that can be easily shaped and should be easily maneuverable into the desired position.[19,20,21] It should have lubricity and support is essential for the smooth passage of device. It should also have good torque transmission to the distal tip and should provide good tactile response. Needless to say that it should be able to track through a tortuous and angulated lesion without causing damage to the artery. The wire tip should retain the shape, or have the ability to be reshaped for multivessel/multilesion percutaneous coronary interventions (PCI). Workhorse guidewires generally have a tip load that ranges from 0.5–1.0 g, with a shaft providing light or moderate support.[19,20]

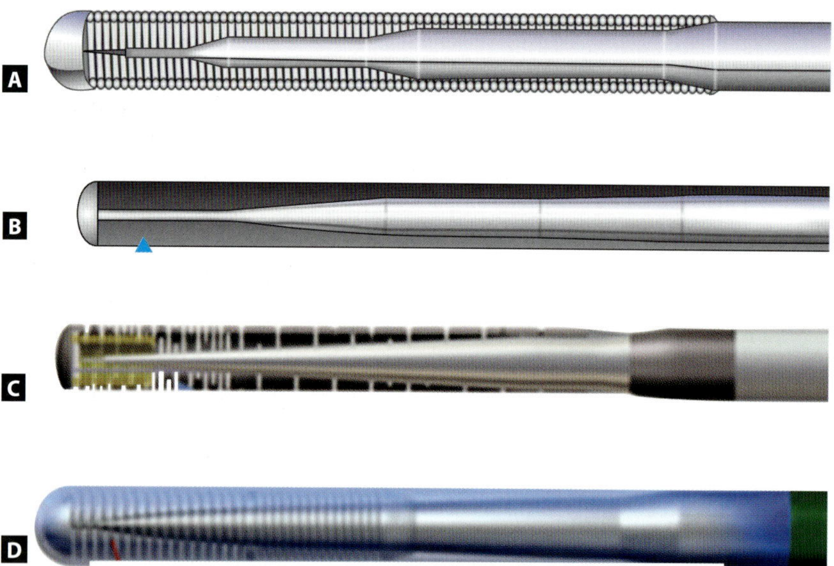

Figs 6.4A to D Distal tip covers of the guidewires. In spring coil design the distal end of the wire has a spring coil: (A) Polymer cover replaces the spring coil in other wires providing increased lubricity and trackability; (B) micro cut nitinol replaces the spring coil in some wires (C) While polymer cover is put over the spring coil in others (D)

Table 6.4 Composition and design of the various components of the guidewire

Nomenclature	*Manufacturer*	*Core material*	*Tip type*	*Tip radiopacity*	*Tip style*	*Tip coating type*
Balance middle weight	Abbott	Elastinite nitinol	Spring coil	3 cm	Shaping ribbon	Hydrophilic
Whisper	Abbott	Tru Torque Steel	Polymer over coil	3 cm	Core to tip	Hydrophilic
Cougar-XT	Medtronic	Nitinol	Spring coil	3 cm	Shaping ribbon	Hydrophilic
Fielder	Asahi Intec	Tru Torque Steel	Polymer over coil	3 cm	Core to tip	Hydrophilic
Fielder XT series	Asahi Intec	Tru Torque Steel	Polymer over coil	16 cm	Composite core	Hydrophilic
Gaia	Asahi Intec	Tru Torque Steel	Spring coil	3 cm	Composite core	Hydrophilic
Sion Blue	Asahi Intec	Tru Torque Steel	Spring coil	3 cm	Composite core	Hydrophobic
Sion Black	Asahi Intec	Tru Torque Steel	Polymer over coil	3 cm	Composite core	Hydrophilic
Runthrough NT	Terumo	Proximal, stainless steel; Distal, Nitinol	Stainless steel coils	3 cm	Shaping ribbon	Hydrophilic
Cross IT	Abbott	Durasteel	Spring coil	3 cm	Core to tip	Hydrophilic
Progress	Abbott	Durasteel	Polymer/spring coil	3 cm	Core to tip	Hydrophilic except distal tip
Pilot	Abbott	Durasteel	Polymer over coil	3 cm	Core to tip	Hydrophilic
Conquest	Asahi Intec	Tru Torque Steel	Spring coil	3 cm	Core to tip	Hydrophilic
Miracle	Asahi Intec	Tru Torque Steel	Spring coil	3 cm	Core to tip	Hydrophobic
Provia	Medtronic	Stainless steel	Spring coil	3 cm	Core to tip	Hydrophilic

Extra Support Guidewire

Extra support guidewires provide additional rail support for device delivery in tortuous and calcified vessels. These guidewires generally have soft tips, stiffer shaft and a shorter core tapering properties which make them less steerable. Some disadvantages of these guidewires include causing "pseudostenoses" and guidewire bias in a tortuous vessel. At an acute bend, the stiff wire shaft can cause "cheese-cutter" effect by burying into intima/plaque.

Guidewires for Totally Occluded Lesions

There has been considerable technological advancement in chronic total occlusion (CTO) guidewires. Additional properties are required for CTO guidewires to traverse the microchannel, or to penetrate the hard fibrous cap and plaque.[22-24] To achieve these goals, most of the CTO guidewires have the following design features:

- A joint less core which is usually made of stainless steel, with larger core diameter and shorter tapering for increased support and torque transmission
- Tip style is that of the one-piece core-to-tip design for better torque transmission
- Presence of polymer cover in some to enhance lubricity

Understanding the design and properties of the chosen CTO wire is of the utmost importance for procedural success. choice of the wire is determined not only by the lesion characteristics but also by the technique to be used for wiring ("controlled drilling" vs. "penetration" vs. "sliding") as different CTO wires have different strengths and weaknesses. Needless to say that in CTO PCI, more than one wire or one wiring technique is usually employed.[22-24]

Controlled Drilling Strategy

This technique involves controlled rotational tip motion with gentle forward probing. Operators using this technique usually start with a guidewire with moderate tip stiffness (e.g., Asahi Miracle series, Medtronic Persuader 3 and 6, Abbott Hi-Torque Progress 40, 80 and 120). These guidewires have either hydrophilic or hydrophobic coating providing good tactile feedback. Progressively stiffer wires may be used if greater penetration force is required. Long CTO with tortuosity is best approached using the drilling or sliding technique.[24]

Penetration Strategy

Heavily calcified CTO entry cap or obstructive material may require the use of a very stiff guidewire with a tapered end (e.g, Asahi Conquest Pro 8-20, Medtronic Persuader 9, Medtronic ProVia 15, Abbott Progress 140T and 200T) to achieve passage. In such cases penetration technique is used with stiffer guidewires compared to drilling technique. In this technique aggressively directed forward probing motion with minimal rotation of tip achieves the desired result. The wire tip movement has to be more precise. This technique is most suitable for shorter straight CTO with an identified near target. Stiffer wires have reduced tactile response and a higher risk of perforation or subintimal entry.[24]

Sliding Strategy

In this strategy hydrophilic guidewires with polymer cover (e.g., Asahi Fielder series, Abbott Pilot series, Abbott Whisper series) are used in softer, less calcified CTOs encountered in crossing subtotal occlusion or intrastent total occlusion. Most of these lesions have intraluminal microchannels, varying in size from 100–500 µm, which often run within and parallel to the thrombosed parent vessel. These micro channels provide a potential passage for the guidewire to "slide through" the CTO. Lubricious wires (hydrophilic coating, polymer cover) with a tapered tip (e.g., Asahi Fielder XT) are best suited for this purpose. The wire typically advances with minimal resistance and tactile feedback, however carries a high risk of subintimal entry.[23-25]

Shaping the Wire Tip

A bend at the guidewire tip makes its manipulation easier in the coronary tree. The wire tip can be shaped using a guidewire introducer or a needle, or by manipulating it gently between the thumb and the index finger.[19,20] Excessive force should not be applied during this as it can damage the structure and integrity of the wire in addition a large bend increases the risk of wire prolapse. For the majority of non-CTO lesions, a simple J-curve with a gentle distal bend is usually sufficient. A double-bend configuration is useful for steering into steeply angled vessels.[19,20] For hydrophilic wire it is recommended to wet the wire to activate the hydrophilic coating before shaping. Proper shaping of the wire in CTO lesions will prevent entering the subintimal space. A small tip curvature is usually sufficient while using the sliding technique. For "drilling" and "penetrating" strategies, a commonly applied shape consists of a short tip curve at a distance of 0.5–2 mm from tip along with a secondary proximal curve sited 3–5 mm from the tip. However the distal wire tip is dictated essentially by the morphology of the lesion and the anatomy of the coronary artery with lesion. Use of a microcatheter may allow an adaptable change to the secondary curvature of the CTO guidewire.

BALLOON ANGIOPLASTY CATHETER PLATFORMS AND BALLOON ANGIOPLASTY PROCEDURE

Balloon catheters are an integral part of coronary interventions.[26] Table 6.5 summarizes the commonly used terms for balloon angioplasty. Broadly speaking there are three platforms of balloon angioplasty (BA) catheters:

Table 6.5 Commonly use terms for balloon angioplasty

S No	*Term*	*Definition*
1.	Balloon diameter	Nominal inflated balloon diameter measured at a specified pressure
2.	Balloon length	Typically refers to the working length or the length of the straight body section
3.	Nominal pressure	Refers to the pressure at which when balloon is inflated it achieves the listed balloon diameter. It is usually 6–12 atm
4.	Mean burst pressure	It is the average pressure where 50% of balloons will burst (usually measured at body temperature)
5.	Rated burst pressure	The pressure below which 99.9% of the balloons will not burst upon single inflation
6.	Balloon profile	It is the maximum diameter of the balloon when mounted on a catheter in its deflated and wrapped condition or the smallest hole through which the deflated wrapped balloon can pass
7.	Balloon compliance	It is an index of stretchability and is defined as the change in balloon diameter per atmosphere of inflation pressure
8.	Trackability	Refers to the ease of tracking a balloon over the guidewire up to the target lesion
9.	Creep	Refers to tendency of a balloon to enlarge after serial inflations at the same pressure. More compliant balloons are generally associated with more creep
10.	Pushability	Refers to the ability to advance the balloon across the lesion

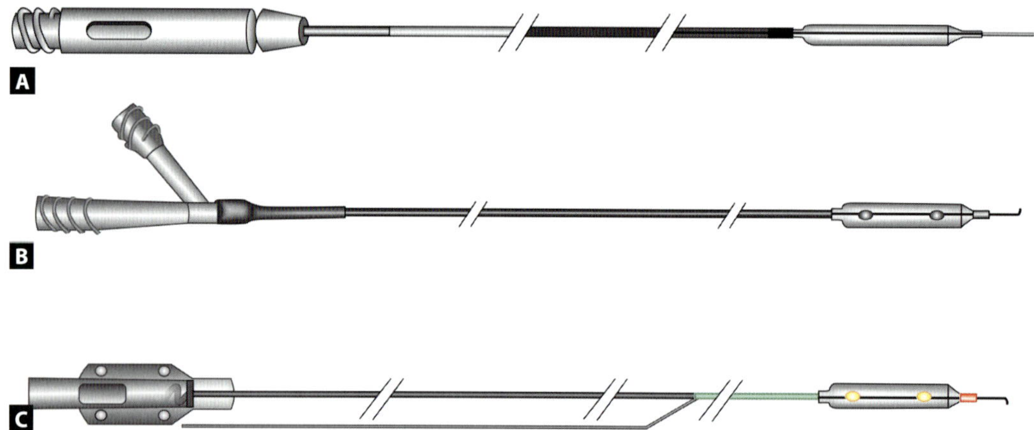

Figs 6.5A to C The construction characteristics of balloon catheter systems (A) Fixed wire platform with single inflation lumen with a spring tip wire affixed to the distal end of the balloon. (B) Over-the-wire (OTW) platform with dual lumens (guidewire and inflation) throughout entire length of catheter. (C) Rapid exchange (RX) platform with single inflation lumen throughout length of catheter with short wire lumen at distal end of the catheter

- Fixed wire
- Over-the-wire (OTW)
- Rapid exchange (RX) (Figs 6.5A to C).

Fixed Wire BA Catheters

The fixed-wire design of balloon catheter was the first platform used for BA. It consists of a balloon catheter with a short segment of coronary guidewire at the distal end of the balloon. These platforms are no longer in production.

Over-the-wire Balloon Catheter

The over-the-wire (OTW) platform consists of a dual-lumen catheter with the balloon at the distal end and a "Y" hub proximally.[27] The vertical limb of the Y hub is the central lumen of the catheter for the coronary guidewire. The angled limb of the Y hub is the balloon lumen for connection to the inflation device. The balloon catheter is advanced with the coronary guidewire loaded in the central lumen into the guiding catheter. The guidewire is then advanced into the coronary artery, and the balloon catheter is advanced along the wire to provide support for the wire as it is advanced through tortuous segments.

The OTW platforms have the advantage of allowing exchange of the coronary guidewire once the balloon catheter is in the artery. Additionally, the central lumen can be used for intracoronary drug delivery or contrast injection to ensure intraluminal position of the balloon. The major disadvantage of the OTW is that it requires two operators for delivery and exchange of the balloon. This platform also requires the use of a 300 cm guidewire.

With OTW systems the guidewire can be lengthened with an extension wire connected firmly to the proximal end of the normal guidewire (known as a docking extension). Instead of docking extension many operators use an indeflator and "saline flush method" to "blow out" the OTW balloon system. Balloon is withdrawn until its proximal hub is at the limit of the guidewire; an indeflator is then attached to the proximal end of balloon catheter and inflated to 20 atm (atmosphere) with touhy kept open. This action propels the balloon system backwards and out of the O-ring without disturbing the position of the intracoronary guidewire. Another option for OTW balloon exchange is the trapping balloon technique. In this the balloon is pulled back into the guiding catheter within the ascending aorta, then a standard rapid exchange balloon is passed into the guiding catheter and placed more distal to OTW balloon and inflated to trap the guidewire against the inner wall of the guiding catheter. Thereafter the OTW balloon is safely withdrawn.[27,28]

Rapid Exchange (RX) Balloon Catheter

The RX platform has a single balloon lumen hub proximally, and dual lumens distally, with one for the balloon and the other a separate short-wire lumen. With RX platforms, the coronary guidewire is first advanced across the lesion. Once in place, the balloon catheter is then advanced to the desired location.[27,28] Unlike the OTW platform, the RX platform can be performed with a single operator. As a result, the RX platform is the most popular platform for coronary balloons.

Another advantage of RX platforms is that they are generally lower profile, and in many cases, two RX balloons (for kissing inflations) can be advanced through a 6F guiding catheter. The disadvantage of the RX platform is that it does not allow for wire exchanges and delivery of intracoronary medications via the balloon catheter.

Preparation of Balloon Catheter

Preparation of balloon involves removing the residual air in the balloon and replacing it with a mixture of diluted contrast for fluoroscopic visualization during balloon inflation. A 20 cc syringe partially filled with diluted contrast is used for this purpose. A negative pressure created by the syringe upon attaching it to the balloon withdraws the air in the balloon catheter. The balloon can be visualized under fluoroscopy by the radi-opaque markers at the ends of the balloon. Once appropriate position is confirmed with contrast injection, a balloon inflation device filled with diluted contrast is connected to the balloon lumen at the hub of the balloon catheter and the balloon is inflated and deflated under fluoroscopy.[26]

Balloon Catheter Inflation Kinetics

Coronary balloons are available in multiple diameters (1.2–5.5 mm, occasionally in quarter sizes) and lengths (6–30 mm) so that an appropriate-sized balloon can be selected to match the length and diameter of the lesion. For standalone BA using standard balloons, the final balloon chosen generally has a diameter-to-artery ratio of 1.0:1–1.2:1. Ratios <1.0:1 may result in a greater degree of restenosis, whereas ratios >1.2:1 may result in acute complications.[26-28] Balloons have characteristic inflation parameters labeled on a prepackaged inflation chart with the balloon. Definition of the important terms used in the balloon angioplasty describing various kinetics of balloon are given in Table 6.5.

In general, balloons are inflated to the nominal pressure, although the operator may choose to inflate to a lower pressure if the balloon is oversized or a higher pressure if the lesion is resistant to balloon inflation. The time that the balloon is inflated is also variable. For standalone balloon angioplasty inflation times are generally long (~1 minute) depending on patient's tolerance of ischemia. BA for treatment of coronary perforation or dissection may also require longer inflation times (up to 10 minutes with perfusion balloons). In the modern era, however, predilation BA is usually performed with shorter inflation times (10 15 seconds) since elastic recoil and dissection are usually addressed by coronary stent placement.

SPECIFIC BALLOON ANGIOPLASTY DEVICES

Compliant Versus Noncompliant Balloons

Standard coronary balloons are manufactured from polyethylene, polyethylene terephthalate, or nylon, with a balloon wall thickness of <0.005 inches. They are coated with a friction resistance coating (usually silicone) for increased ease of delivery across severely narrowed lesions. Standard coronary balloons are labeled compliant or noncompliant, based on their inflation profile.[26]

The compliance of a balloon refers to the change in balloon diameter with inflation pressure. Compliant balloons expand to larger diameters as inflation pressures are increased beyond the nominal pressure. Compliant balloons have the advantage of being more flexible and deliverable. Compliant balloons are generally used for predilation of lesions prior to delivery of other devices (i.e. stents).

Noncompliant balloons have the advantage of being able to be inflated to high pressures while maintaining relatively constant diameter. These balloons are stiffer than compliant balloons and hence less deliverable. Because of their ability to achieve high pressures with consistent balloon diameter, noncompliant balloons are ideal for resistant lesions and post-dilation of stents for maximum expansion and apposition.[26]

Perfusion Balloons

The perfusion balloon has side holes that allow blood to enter the catheter lumen proximal to the balloon and exit via side holes distal to the balloon when the balloon is fully inflated, allowing antegrade flow to the distal vessel and thereby minimizing ischemia. Most perfusion balloons can provide 40–60 cc/min of blood flow to the coronary vessel distal to the balloon. These balloons are no longer being produced.

Plaque-incising Balloons

Plaque-incising balloons are coronary balloon catheters that have the ability to cut into coronary plaque using either blades mounted on the balloon itself or fine wires attached to the balloon that score the plaque as the balloon is inflated. These devices requiring lower inflation pressure allow predictable cutting of the coronary plaque and resulting in controlled dissections. In general, the cutting element makes these devices stiffer and more difficult to deliver compared to standard compliant balloons.[29]

An advantage of plaque-incising balloons is that they prevent balloon slippage (watermelon seeding) in very tight lesions or in lesions with slippery surfaces such as in-stent restenosis (ISR). The presence of the cutting element anchors the balloon at the site of the lesion, minimizing damage to otherwise nondiseased coronary segments. The presence of the cutting element makes careful balloon sizing a must, as over sizing may lead to coronary perforation.[29]

The first plaque-incising balloon developed was the cutting balloon (Boston Scientific Corporation, Natick, MA) (Figs 6.6A and B). These balloons play an important role in the ostial lesions and patients with instent restenosis. Despite theoretical advantages of the plaque-incising balloon concept, a large randomized clinical trial comparing cutting balloon angioplasty (CBA) with standard BA failed to show a clear, long-term benefit of CBA.

Drug-eluting Balloons

Drug eluting balloons (DEB) could offer a viable alternative to drug eluting stents (DES) in the treatment of coronary artery disease. The concept behind the technology of DEB is based on rapid delivery of drug into the arterial tissue.[30] These balloons may also offer a valuable new option to treat patients in whom stent implantation is not desirable—including small vessels, in-stent restenosis, bifurcation side-branch, and possibly acute ST-elevation MI. Currently 4 DEBs are available: (B Braun's SeQuent™ Please, Medrad Interventional's Cotavance™ with Paccocath technology, Eurocor's DIOR™ paclitaxel-coated and Invatec's IN.PACT™ Amphirion paclitaxel-eluting balloon). The "SeQuent™ Please" drug eluting balloon delivers drugs directly to the lesion during angioplasty.

CORONARY STENTS

Historical Perspective

In 1986, the first coronary WallstentTM implantation ushered in a new era in interventional cardiology with the purpose of circumventing the 2 major limitations of balloon coronary angioplasty viz early acute occlusion and late restenosis.[31]

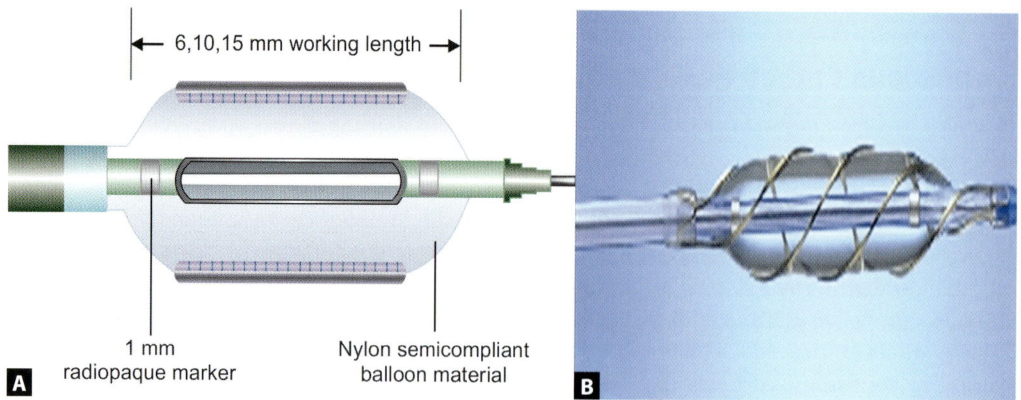

Figs 6.6A and B Plaque incising balloons (A) standard semicompliant cutting balloon with linear atherotomes mounted on it, (B) scoring semicompliant balloon within a helical nitinol cutting element

Improvements in stent technology have contributed to the widespread adoption of percutaneous coronary intervention (PCI) for the treatment of an ever-expanding variety of CAD scenarios. Ulrich Sigwart has been credited with the concept and realization of endoluminal stenting, a procedure that has revolutionized coronary and peripheral arterial revascularization. Julio Palmaz, an interventional vascular radiologist, is known for inventing the balloon-expandable stent, for which he received a patent filed in 1985. This patent has been included on the list of the 10 most important inventions of all times. The Palmaz-Schatz stent got approved in 1994, within 4 years of Food and Drug Administration approval, the balloon expandable stent was used in 80% of PCI. Since inception, stent design has undergone constant refinement, including the development of drug-eluting stents (DESs) and bioabsorbable vascular scaffold (BVS).

Bare-metal stents were the first devices used for coronary stenting. Interestingly, although these devices reduced rates of restenosis compared with balloon angioplasty, in-stent restenosis (ISR) continued to develop in 20–30% of lesions. DESs are composed of a metallic stent, a polymer-based drug delivery platform, and a pharmacologic agent (typically an immunosuppressant and/or antiproliferative compound). The goal of DES technology is to minimize PCI-related vascular inflammation and cellular proliferation thus reducing ISR.[32,33] Indeed, early trials of the first generation DES (sirolimus eluting stents [SES] and paclitaxel-eluting [PES]) demonstrated markedly reduced rates of ISR (5%–10%), heralding the DES revolution that followed. Although these stents have advanced our treatment of obstructive coronary disease, ISR and stent thrombosis (ST) presented important limitations. PES and SES have been complimented with development of everolimus eluting stents (EES) and zotarolimus eluting stents (ZES). Improvement of the stent design, strut thickness and replacement of steel with cobalt chromium and platinum chromium as stent platform along with biodegradable polymer has led to further reduction of restenosis rates. The advent of DESs has undoubtedly improved outcomes in patients undergoing PCI.[32,33]

Bioresorbable materials are also being used to construct the actual stents, with the intent of providing mechanical support initially when elastic recoil and constrictive remodeling are of concern but then getting absorbed and disappearing thereafter.[34] Hence, they offer the theoretical advantage of reducing long-term risks associated with existing metallic struts including stent fracture, impaired vessel homeostasis, and neoatherosclerosis, while allowing for computed tomography evaluation of stented coronaries and providing graft targets for surgical revascularization if needed. Overall, although the theoretical gains of bioresorbable stents are certainly enticing, we await the results of ongoing randomized trials to better characterize any potential advantages over existing stenting systems and ensure equivalent safety profiles.[34]

A detailed discussion on the stents can be found in some other section of this book.

ANCILLARY HARDWARE

Coronary angioplasty in addition to the above mentioned hard ware does require the assistance of miscellaneous hardware like imaging catheters (optical coherence tomography, intravascular ultrasound), intra- aortic balloon pump, thrombus aspiration catheter (used for aspiration of thrombus in patients with thrombus laden coronary arteries) and atherectomy devices (rotablator and tornus device). These devices have been discussed in detail in some other section of this textbook.

REFERENCES

1. Meier B. The guiding catheter: the most underrated asset to coronary angioplasty. J Invasive Cardiol. 2005;17:642-3.
2. Mishra S, Bahl VK. The choice of guiding catheter. Indian Heart Journal. 2009;61:80-8.
3. Levine GN, Bates ER, Blankenship JC, et al. 2015 ACC/AHA/SCAI Focused update on primary percutaneous coronary intervention for patients with ST-elevation myocardial infarction: an update of the 2011 ACCF/AHA/SCAI guideline for percutaneous coronary intervention and the 2013 ACCF/AHA guideline for the management of ST-elevation myocardial infarction: a report of the American College of Cardiology/American Heart Association Task Force on clinical practice guidelines and the Society for Cardiovascular Angiography and Interventions. Circulation. 2016;133(11):1135-47.
4. Dehmer GJ, Blankenship JC, Cilingiroglu M, et al. SCAI/ACC/AHA Expert consensus document: 2014 update on percutaneous coronary intervention without on-site surgical backup. Catheter Cardiovasc Interv. 2014;84(2):169-87.
5. Judkins M, Judkins E. Coronary arteriography and left ventriculography: Judkins technique. In: King SI, Douglas JJ (Eds). Coronary Arteriography and Angioplasty. New York: McGraw-Hill. 1985. pp. 182-217.
6. Amplatz K, Formanek G, Stanger P, et al. Mechanics of selective coronary artery catheterization via femoral approach. Radiology. 1967;39:1040-7.
7. Takahashi S, Saito S, Tanaka S, et al. New method to increase a backup support of a 6 French guiding coronary catheter. Catheter Cardiovasc Interv. 2004;63:452-6.
8. Mehta S, Margolis JR, Traktman M, et al. Voda guiding catheter is superior to Amplatz guiding catheter for performing left circumflex PTCA. J Invasive Cardiol. 1994;6(7):229-33.
9. Ikari Y, Nagaoka M, Kim JY, et al. The physics of guiding catheters for the left coronary artery in transfemoral and transradial interventions. Journal Invasive Cardiol. 2005;17:636-41.
10. Nader RJ. Clinical Review of the Cordis 6F 3DRC VISTA BRITE TIP® Guiding Catheter. Clinical Update 2003;2E: 800-1148-51.

11. Clark DA. Risks and benefits of the Arani curve guiding catheter for stenting of the right coronary artery: the value of experience. Cath Cardiovasc. Interven. 1998;39(1):96.
12. Myler RK, Boucher RA, Cumberland DC, et al. Guiding catheter selection for right coronary artery angioplasty. Cath Cardiovasc Diag. 1990; 19(1): 58-67.
13. Sahu U. Selection of hardware and cath lab preparation for transradial approach. Indian Heart J. 2010;62(4):267-72.
14. Benamer H. Transradial approaches for coronary angiography and PTCA in obese patients. Indian Heart J. 2008;60:A 36-7.
15. Abhaichand RK. Choice of transradial catheters. Indian Heart J. 2008;60:A 18-21.
16. D'Souza MS, Hendryc, et al. Use of the sheathless guide catheter during routine transradial percutaneous coronary intervention: a feasibility study. Cather Cardiovasc Interv. 2010;75:596-602.
17. Douglas JS. Percutaneous interventions in patients with prior coronary bypass surgery. In: Topol EJ (Eds). Textbook of Interventional Cardiology. pp. 317-44.
18. Ochiai M, Ikari Y, Yamaguchi T, et al. New long-tip guide catheters designed for right transradial coronary intervention. Catheter Cardiovasc Interv. 2000;49:218-24.
19. Mishra S, Bahl VK. Curriculum in cath lab: coronary hardware-part II guidewire selection for coronary angioplasty. Indian Heart J. 2009;61: 178-85.
20. Erglis A. Tools and techniques: coronary guidewires. Euro Intervention. 2010;6:168-9.
21. Bonzel T. The monorail technique. In: Bertrand ME, (Ed). The Evolution of Cardiac Catheterization and Interventional Cardiology. ESC/Iatric Press; 2006. pp.97-104.
22. Karatasakis A, Tarar MN, Karmpaliotis D, et al. Guidewire and microcatheter utilization patterns during antegrade wire escalation in chronic total occlusion percutaneous coronary intervention: Insights from a contemporary multicenter registry. Cath Cardiovasc Interv. 2016 May 17. doi: 10.1002/ccd.26568. [Epub ahead of print].
23. Green P, Monga S, Ramcharitar S, et al. Tools and techniques - clinical. Update on coronary guidewires 2016: chronic total occlusions. EuroIntervention. 2016;11(9):1077-9. doi: 10.4244/EIJV11I9A216.
24. Maeremans J, Knaapen P, Stuijfzand WJ, et al. Antegrade wire escalation for chronic total occlusions in coronary arteries: simple algorithms as a key to success.J Cardiovasc Med (Hagerstown). 2015 Nov 21. [Epub ahead of print].
25. Sianos G, Werner GS, Galassi AR, et al. Recanalisation of chronic total coronary occlusions: 2012 consensus document from the Euro CTO club. EuroIntervention. 2012;8:139-14
26. Mishra S, Bahl VK. Curriculum in cath lab: coronary hardware-part III balloon angioplasty catheters. Indian Heart J. 2009;61:335-41.
27. Jahnke T, Schafer JP, Bolte H, et al. Retrospective study of rapid-exchange monorail versus over-the-wire technique for femoropopliteal angioplasty. Cardiovasc Intervent Radiol. 2008;31(5):854-9
28. Amighi J, Sabeti S, Dick P, et al. Impact of the rapid-exchange versus over-the-wire technique on procedural complications of renal artery angioplasty. J Endovasc Ther. 2005;12(2): 233-9.
29. Ajani AE, Kim HS, Castagna M, et al. Clinical utility of the cutting balloon. J Invas Cardiol. 2001;13:554-7.
30. Unverdorben M, Vallbracht C, Cremers B, et al. Paclitaxel-coated balloon catheter versus paclitaxel-coated stent for the treatment of in-stent restenosis" (PEPCAD II-ISR) study. Circulation. 2009;119:2986-94.
31. Muller DWM. Coated stents and local drug delivery for the prevention of restenosis. In: Topol's Textbook for Interventional Cardiology. 4th. edn, Published by Saunders. 2003. pp. 649-73.
32. Claessen BE, Henriques JP, Dangas GD. Clinical studies with sirolimus, zotarolimus, everolimus, and biolimus A9 drug-eluting stent systems Curr Pharm Des. 2010;16(36): 4012-24.
33. Bangalore S, Toklu B, Amoroso, et al. Bare metal stents, durable polymer drug eluting stents, and biodegradable polymer drug eluting stents for coronary artery disease: mixed treatment comparison meta-analysis. BMJ. 2013;8:347.
34. Brie D, Penson P, Serban MC, et al. Bioresorbable scaffold—a magic bullet for the treatment of coronary artery disease? Int J Cardiol. 2016;215:47-59. Epub 2016 Apr 12.

CHAPTER

7

Fractional Flow Reserve

Y Chandrashekhar, Todd Drexel

INTRODUCTION

Traditionally, presence of ischemia on a noninvasive test or angiographic stenosis of >70% for nonleft main coronary artery (non-LMCA) and 50% or more for LMCA lesions, have been used to guide coronary revascularization. However, noninvasive testing for ischemia has limitations (including modest specificity and positive predictive values) that limit its precision;[1] while commonly accepted and a major reason for intervention, evidence for a well proven strong benefit after treating small to moderate ischemia is lacking.[2] Similarly, angiography has long been recognized as imprecise and prone to wide interobserver variability.[3] Finally, there is little outcome data after intervening for ischemia deduced with traditional strategies like angiography.

Ischemia ultimately is a reduced tissue level perfusion but methods to measure blood flow at tissue level are difficult in clinical practice. Fractional flow reserve (FFR) is a measurement that can bridge this gap between deducing ischemia (reduced blood flow) from anatomy and need for intervention. It measures the pressure drop across a lesion during maximal vasodilatation (when pressure becomes proportional to flow) to approximate the degree of reduced flow as a consequence of a given lesion, thus more precisely assessing the physiological significance of the lesion.[4] Lesions with uncertain hemodynamic significance, stenoses in the 40–80% range, can be better defined with the use of FFR and FFR based intervention has been repeatedly shown to improve prognosis.[5-8] It is especially useful in evaluating lesions in patients coming to the catheterization lab without noninvasive testing for ischemia or for lesions that do not show ischemia-territory concordance, or when there is concern for a false negative test. Not surprisingly, FFR is currently the most objective invasive measurement predicting the potential benefits of revascularizing lesions or leaving them alone. Both the American College of Cardiology/American Heart Association (ACC/AHA) and the European Society of Cardiology (ESC) endorse its use for evaluating of stable ischemic heart disease.[9,10] and many have argued that FFR should be the standard gatekeeper for intervention in stable ischemic heart disease—functional percutaneous coronary intervention (PCI).[11] We provide a brief overview of FFR and the data to support its use in guiding coronary revascularization.

BASIC CORONARY PHYSIOLOGY AND INTRAVASCULAR MEASUREMENTS

Coronary arteries have three main regions of structural resistance and flow. The large epicardial conduit arteries (>0.5 mm) are conduit vessels that have little resistance to flow (<10% of overall resistance) and no significant drop in pressure along these segments. These arteries supply the pre-arterioles (0.1–0.5 mm in diameter) that are located just proximal to the myocardium. The prearterioles provide flow to the arterioles and then capillary arteries (<0.1 mm). The prearterioles, arterioles and capillary arteries are referred to as the microcirculation. The microcirculation in normal arteries accounts for 90% or more of the coronary resistance. One fascinating facet of the coronary microcirculation is its ability to maintain flow in presence of a range of perfusion pressures—called autoregulation. Animal studies have long shown that regional myocardial function is still preserved during severe coronary hypotension provided coronary blood flow is maintained.[12] Autoregulation is accomplished by sensing flow, shear and metabolic signals like adenosine during ischemia. Autoregulation reduces vascular resistance distal to the site of flow reduction (or pressure drop) and allows for increased flow, thus protecting against ischemia. There is however a limit to this and as stenoses progress, the microcirculation eventually becomes maximally dilated and this dilatory reserve is exhausted. This partly explains why hemodynamically significant stenosis, may not be detectable via rest indices of flow and only becomes apparent under hyperemia. Ischemia (reduced flow) thus needs to then be defined taking into account the autoregulation.

Two important concepts (Fig. 7.1) help understanding our diagnostic strategies in CAD. Gould et al. showed that rest myocardial blood flow remains normal till the epicardial stenosis is over 85% but falls at >50% epicardial stenosis under hyperemia.[13] Classically, reduced coronary flow at peak hyperemia is thus considered the *sine qua non* of ischemia. Others postulated that the ratio of flow in the stenotic vessel to flow if there were no stenosis[14] would quantify the severity of an anatomic stenosis and possibly relief after revascularization. This did not gain acceptance in day-to-day practice as it is difficult to measure flow. While easier methods to indirectly estimate ratio of rest to hyperemic flows were developed, most of these used surrogates (like Doppler velocities) for flow. Since pressure is reasonably proportional to flow during maximal vasodilation (abolishing autoregulation), pressure ratio between the coronary pressure distal to a stenosis and aortic pressure (a surrogate of proximal pressure) during maximal coronary vasodilation was introduced as a viable surrogate of the ratio of rest to hyperemic flow, thus ushering in the FFR era.[4] In the usual conditions when it does not violate several physiological assumptions (microvascular resistance is constant and that we achieve maximal steady state vasodilation at the time of measurement), this measure—FFR has been shown to reliably predict stenotic lesions that are ischemic and benefit from treatment.

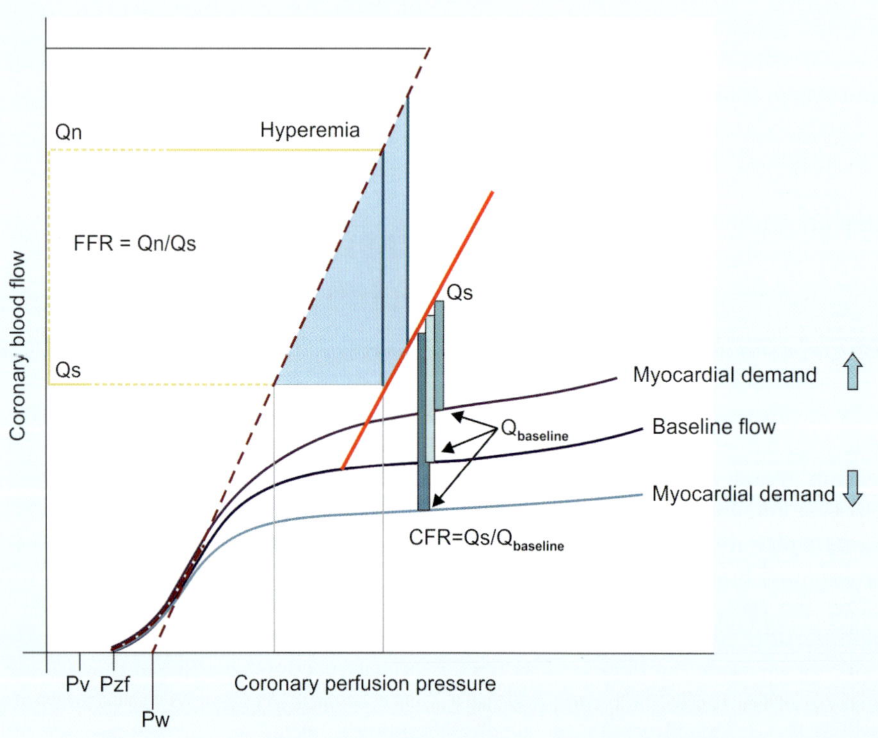

Fig. 7.1 Simplified cartoon about coronary physiology for understanding FFR. Normally, coronary flow is maintained at a rather constant level over a wide range of perfusion pressures (baseline flow curve) – called autoregulation. Increased myocardial demand (e.g. tachycardia or increased inotropy) shift this curve upwards (purple curve) while reduced myocardial demand or intrinsic microcirculation disease shifts it down (blue curve). Since CFR is the ratio of hyperemic flow (with or without stenosis – Qs or Qn) to resting flow (Qbaseline, bars with various shades of blue), it is affected by both reduced vasodilatation due to microvascular pathology as well as change in resting blood flow due to tachycardia, increased contractility or hypertension. FFR on the other hand not affected by basal flow; since it is a ratio of Qs/Qn and is expressed as a ratio of pressures proximal and distal to the lesion, change in perfusion pressures (solid vertical blue lines) does not affect Qs/Qn to a large extent. It is obvious that maximal vasodilatation is needed for accurate FFR

Abbreviations: Pv, venous pressure; Pw, wedge pressure; Pzf, zero flow intercept; Qn, peak hyperemic flow in normal vessels; Qs, peak hyperemic flow in stenotic vessels; dotted red line, pressure vs. flow relation during hyperemia in normal vessels; solid red line, pressure vs. flow relation during hyperemia in stenotic vessels.

Source: van de Hoef TP, et al. Fractional flow reserve as a surrogate for inducible myocardial ischaemia. Nature Rev Cardiol. 2013;10:439-52 and Bishop AH, Samady H. Fractional flow reserve: critical review of an important physiologic adjunct to angiography. Am Heart J. 2004;147:792-802 and Ref #4.

The standard equation for FFR across the myocardial bed is

$$Qs/Qn = \frac{[(P_{distal}-P_{venous})/R]}{[(P_{aorta}-P_{venous})/R]}$$

Where Qs and Qn are flows with and without stenosis; R is resistance; P_{distal} and P_{aorta} are pressures after and before the stenosis and P_{venous} is the pressure in the receiving end—usually the RA pressure but can be wedge pressure too if known and especially if particularly high—using pulmonary artery wedge pressure instead of RA pressure for P_{venous} gives FFR (across the coronary bed) instead of FFR (across the myocardial bed). Since resistance is thought to be constant and venous pressure is thought to be minimally influencing the ratio (even in most degrees of RA pressure seen clinically), both are disregarded and the formula is simplified to

$$Qs/Qn = \frac{[P_{distal}]}{[P_{aorta}]}$$

Of course, collateral flow is assumed to be negligible in most clinical situations but FFR contribution from the collateral flow can be derived by subtracting FFR (across the coronary bed) from FFR (across the myocardial bed).

Fraction flow reserve (FFR) has some inherent advantages. It is 1.0 in a normal vessel irrespective of heart rate, hemodynamics or contractility since it is not dependent on the level of basal or hyperemic blood flow, unlike the CFR. In addition, FFR is a specific for the site of the epicardial stenosis, unlike noninvasive imaging which provides territorial information. FFR decreases in proportion to severity of stenosis and has been validated against noninvasively determined ischemia in single vessel disease. Values <0.75 (suggesting that the lesion has reduced flow to 75% of the normal nonstenotic artery) had sensitivity (identification of reversible ischemia) and negative predictive value of 88%, the specificity and positive predictive value of 100%, and accuracy of 93%. Moving FFR cut off value to <0.80 increase sensitivity without significant degradation of specificity and has a 95% negative predictive accuracy.[15]

LIMITATIONS OF ANGIOGRAPHY AS THE GATEKEEPER FOR INTERVENTIONS

Assessing the functional significance of intermediate coronary lesions is difficult and visual angiographic inspection is still the main pathway to PCI but has been shown to be inaccurate even when there is ischemia with noninvasive imaging (Figs 7.2A and B) and does not correlate with the reactive hyperemic response.[16] Various methods have been used to improve its performance in assessing the hemodynamic significance of coronary lesions including quantitative coronary angiography (QCA). Quantitative coronary angiography analyses of lesion severity by either percent area stenosis or percent diameter stenosis but it too was found to be inaccurate in identifying the hemodynamic significance of coronary lesions in the setting of multivessel or diffuse coronary artery disease.[17] Evaluation of discrete lesions with QCA did show a better correlation

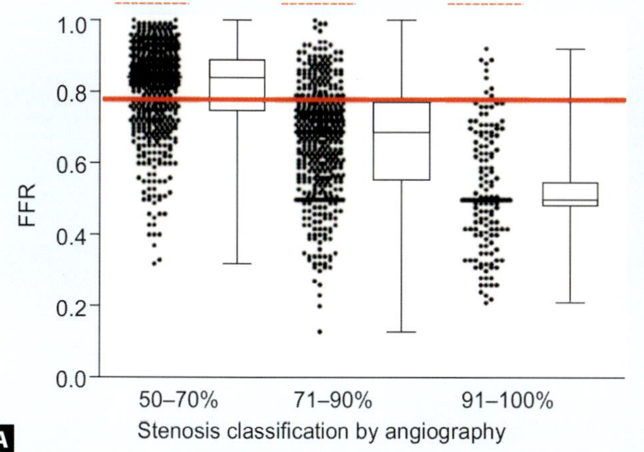

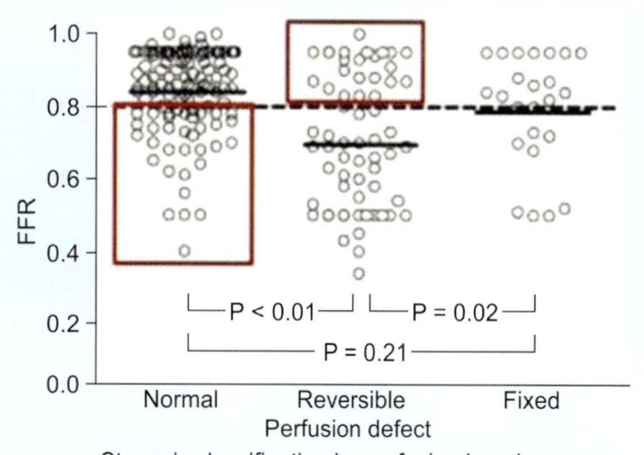

Figs 7.2A and B (A) Discordance between angiographic stenosis and FFR; (B) Myocardial perfusion imaging and FFR. There is significant error with both angiography and MPI in predicting flow limiting stenosis, especially in multivessel CAD. It is our belief that PCI in intermediate lesions should not be performed unless there is evidence for abnormal FFR. Documented > moderate ischemia might be enough to intervene without a FFR but widely believed and accepted, evidence for this is strategy is less than robust in absence of well controlled RCTs and will be clarified with on going studies.

Source: Pijls NH, Tanaka N, Fearon WF. Functional assessment of coronary stenoses: can we live without it? Eur Heart J. 2013;34:1335-44.

Source: Lotfi A, Jeremias A, Fearon WF, et al. Expert consensus statement on the use of fractional flow reserve, intravascular ultrasound, and optical coherence tomography. Cathet Cardiovasc Intervent. 2014;83:509-18.

with hemodynamic significance, but still only provides stenosis quantification of diameter and area.[18] In addition, QCA-determined diameter stenosis does not correlate well with exertional functional class.[19] Recent studies evaluating revascularization of stable ischemic heart disease, including COURAGE[20] and SYNTAX[21] among others have raised questions regarding better identification of lesions that will benefit from revascularization.

Fraction flow reserve has further shown the fallacy of angiography (Figs 7.2 and 7.3). Only 46% of the 1329 stenoses thought to be significant by angiography in the FAME study, were functionally significant after FFR. 2/3rd of the 50–70% stenosis and surprisingly, 20% of the even 71–90% (a group where cardiologists think they are very accurate for detecting significant stenosis) had FFR > 0.8 leading to calls for FFR even in lesions up to 90%.[22] Not surprisingly, FFR changes revascularization strategy decided initially on an angiogram alone in nearly half the cases without negatively affecting events in the deferred group.[23] Left main lesions are often underestimated while stenosis in the rest of the bed is often over estimated.[11] Unfortunately, FFR use is still miniscule; in a study of 61,874 patients with intermediate coronary stenosis, only 6.1% had FFR (largely limited to rather lower risk patients) compared to 20.3% for IVUS—nearly 3/4th had PCI with an angiography alone.[24] despite strong data for its routine use and a call for "functional angioplasty," using concordance between lesion and site of ischemia or proving need for revascularization with FFR seems appropriate.

Unlike with angiography, FFR has not been extensively compared with other anatomic imaging like IVUS and OCT. Most studies have tried to predict FFR based on anatomic imaging (IVUS and OCT) but the MLD or MLA correlation with FFR has been modest, especially in non- LMCA lesions. In addition, there are no data looking at revascularization guided by FFR vs anatomic or plaque imaging like IVUS or OCT although some are in the initial stages.[25]

CLINICAL METHODS TO STUDY CORONARY PHYSIOLOGY

Myocardial ischemia can also occur via pathology at any level in the coronary circulation, including at the microcirculation level; other comprehensive methods have been developed to isolate and localize pathologic segments within the coronary bed as etiology of ischemia. These can be divided as those based on flow and those based on pressure and there is a hot debate whether flow based indices triumph pressure based one in comprehensive evaluation of coronary circulation.[26] It might be that a combination of both might provide the best diagnostic and prognostic information in symptomatic CAD.[27]

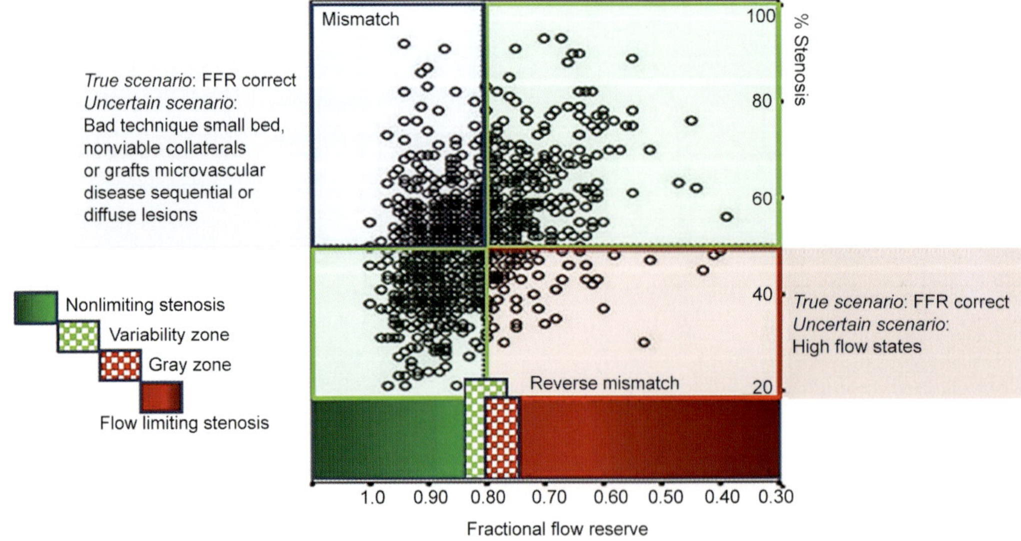

Fig. 7.3 FFR predicts a risk continuum and triages angiographic stenosis into prognostic subsets. However, before concluding FFR is correct and making major decisions on such a value it is absolutely necessary to make sure that the technique is proper and all physiologic variables are accounted for (blue and pick text boxes), In addition, there is a variability in FFR measurements around an FFR of 0.8 (green hatched box) and value between 0.75–0.80 are a technically gray zone (wider in LMCA lesions)

Source: Composite figure with background scattergram data from Johnson NP, et al. Circ Cardiovasc Imaging. 2013;6:817-32.

Flow Indices

Coronary flow reserve (CFR) was a precursor to FFR and evaluated the change in coronary flow distal to a diseased segment with induction of hyperemia. Coronary flow is measured with Doppler sensors or with thermodilution techniques. Accurate flow measurements require the Doppler sensor be positioned five to ten times the artery diameter distal to the lesion for a measurement within a laminar flow segment. Average flow velocities in the left coronary are approximately 30 cm/sec and are about 15–20% less in the right coronary artery.[28] CFR is a ratio of coronary flow in the coronary segment distal to the diseased segment during hyperemia to its resting flow. Coronary flow reserve values greater than 3.0 are considered in the normal range, values less than 2.0 is indicative of ischemia and values between 2.0 and 3.0 require additional evaluation or clinical correlation. The CFR values are highly position-dependent and poor signal may be seen in 15% of the studies. Tachycardia (increases basal flow and decreases CFR), hypertension (decreases maximal vasodilation and decreases CFR), aortic stenosis (decreases maximal vasodilation and decreases CFR) and diabetes (increases basal flow and decreases CFR) can confound measurements. CFR is often discordant with FFR since it assesses the entire bed (epicardial + microvascular bed) while FFR is a lesion specific measurement. CFR is thought to have significant advantage over FFR in predicting prognosis in some studies[29]—patients with normal FFR but abnormal CFR had higher event rates compared to normal FFR and CFR groups but those with abnormal FFR and normal CFR did not show such high risk. However, its superiority in planning interventions is not yet established in RCTs. It is thus not routinely used to assess functional significance.

Two indices of microvascular resistance are currently available—hyperemic microvascular resistance (HMR) which uses a Doppler flow velocity sensor and the index of microcirculatory resistance (IMR) using thermodilution. High resistance measured by either has been associated with worse prognosis in ACS and may add to the information obtained from FFR. These indices evaluate the coronary microvasculature to better characterize myocardial resistance.[30] and can be simplistically thought of as CFR—FFR and can be impaired independent of epicardial stenosis (FFR). IMR, the better known index, is the ratio of the mean distal coronary pressure to the coronary flow. Coronary flow is often estimated using the mean transit time based on thermodilution measurements.[31] The IMR assessment may help identify microvascular obstruction as the etiology of angina and diastolic dysfunction in patients without obstructive coronary artery disease. There is data that it helps triage FFR or CFR better and might identify high risk subsets in patients with FFR > 0.8, a group that traditionally is thought to have low risk.[32]

Pressure Indices

Fractional flow reserve is the ratio of the pressure in a coronary artery distal (Pd) to a diseased segment to the pressure in the aorta (Pa) and assumes a negligible venous pressure. Non-negligible venous pressures result in underestimation of the FFR value.[33] The FFR assessment is based on Poiseuille's law with the assumption that the flow, viscosity and radius do not change during rest and hyperemia, or maximal flow. Traditionally, accurate FFR measurements require induction of hyperemia which adds expense, complexity and variability of vasodilation. Hyperemia-independent methods of FFR evaluation based on resting indices like the instantaneous wave-free pressure ratio (iFR) while not as comprehensive as FFR, are useful in certain situations. The "wave-free" period of the diastolic phase in the cardiac cycle has the least amount of dynamic pressure change and resistance and can approximate FFR without needing hyperemia.[34] but the cut-off value of hemodynamic significance is slightly different between the two methods.[34,35] iFR has been proposed as a triage system for guiding the use of FFR.[36]

Technique of Fractional Flow Reserve

Fractional flow reserve requires direct pressure wire or NAVVUS catheter access to the segment of artery distal to the lesion, appropriate anticoagulation and hyperemia. Hyperemia can be induced by a variety of medications and routes of administration. Typically, adenosine is used as the pharmacologic agent for most studies and is administered either as a bolus intracoronary injection or as a continuous intravenous infusion. It acts via the A2 receptor on coronary endothelial and smooth muscle cells and reliably induces potent vasodilation and increases in coronary blood flow. Papaverine was one of the preferred medications used to induce hyperemia, especially in Europe, until a risk of torsade de pointes made it fall out of favor. Sodium nitroprusside and nitroglycerin can be used to induce hyperemia, but are used for slow flow or no reflow incidences in the setting of an acute myocardial infarction and are not typically used for measurement of FFR. Dipyridamole and dobutamine are other options to induce hyperemia, but are not routinely used for FFR measurement. Contrast also has an effect on coronary blood flow and in fact was one of the first agents used to study coronary physiology, can increase flow from 1.5 to 4.0 times greater than resting flow but is not used for FFR.

Adenosine is administered either systemically via intravenous route or intracoronary through the cardiac catheter. The dose of adenosine is directly correlated to coronary blood flow with larger doses causing increased flow and more prolonged hyperemia. Intravenous and intracoronary FFR measurements have excellent correlation and are reproducible regardless on the route of administration.

The intravenous adenosine dose is 140 µg/kg/min and is a continuous infusion throughout the FFR evaluation. The peak effect occurs around one minute and the duration of effect lasts for about 1 minute after discontinuation of the infusion. A decrease in blood pressure of approximately 10–20% and a corresponding increase in heart rate should be expected. Patients often develop an angina-like sensation in the chest and throat as well as dyspnea that is an effect of adenosine and is not associated with ischemia. The continuous infusion allows for ease in evaluating serial lesions with a pullback of the catheter and assessment of the change in FFR over the coronary length of interest. Conduction abnormalities are less common with systemic administration of adenosine, but caution should be taken in patients with bronchoconstrictive lung disease for concern of bronchospasm.

Intracoronary administration of adenosine is the alternative method for evaluating FFR with adenosine. The peak effect occurs within 10 seconds and the duration of action is typically less than 20 seconds. Adenosine is delivered as a bolus injection and the dose varies between the right and left coronary arteries. A dose of adenosine 40 µg given as a bolus is often used as the starting dose for the right coronary artery, and a dose of 60 µg bolus is used for the left coronary artery. The dose may then be titrated in 20–30 µg increments; some older protocols used a maximum dose of 150 µg or until conduction delays prohibit further titration. Conduction delays are more common with right coronary injections, but are transient and typically benign. While some advocate very high doses, it appears that 100 µg in the RCA and 200 µg in the LCA have the best maximum hyperemia to risk profile. Serial lesion evaluations require separate bolus injections as the duration of effect does not allow for pullback curve data collection. Even though IV and IC adenosine produce roughly equivalent hyperemia, some have recently questioned whether IV adenosine is a good method for FFR; investigators have noted difficult in consistently obtaining a stable Pd/Pa ratio, variability in pattern of pressure changes and timing of the measurement.[37,38] Lowest distal/aortic pressure ratio without wave artifacts seems to increase reproducibility. IC adenosine is making a comeback given less variability, rapid onset of maximal hyperemia, validated dosing for assured vasodilation; on the other hand, short duration of action with difficulty in obtaining pressure pullback curves for localization of stenotic sites in diffuse CAD and a higher chance of heart block are a disadvantage for IC adenosine.

Papaverine is an opium alkaloid vasodilator that acts on the phosphodiesterase inhibitor PDE10A receptor. Papaverine was administered as an intracoronary bolus with a right coronary dose of 10 mg and a left coronary dose of 15 mg. The peak effect occurred in 30–60 seconds and had a similar duration of 30–60 seconds. The prolonged effect allowed for a pullback evaluation of serial lesions with a single injection of papaverine. Unfortunately, papaverine resulted in a transient QT prolongation and, in a small percentage of patients, caused ventricular tachycardia and even torsade des pointes requiring electrical cardioversion. Thus, papaverine is no longer used for induction of hyperemia and FFR assessment.

CLINICAL SUPERIORITY OF FRACTIONAL FLOW RESERVE IN REVASCULARIZATION DECISIONS

The goal of an FFR evaluation is to better quantify the hemodynamic significance of a coronary artery lesion or segment of disease to help define the potential benefit of revascularization. Measuring pressure gradients across coronary artery lesions to assess stenosis severity is not a new concept. Andreas Gruentzig measured pressure gradients across lesions to guide effectiveness of balloon angioplasty treatments.[39] The three main studies that have established the current use of FFR are DEFER, FFR versus Angiography for Multivessel Evaluation (FAME) and FAME II. These studies showed that (1) the safety of foregoing revascularization in lesions that appeared angiographically significant, but had non-significant FFR measurements; (2) the benefit of using FFR rather than an angiographic-only assessment to guide revascularization; and (3) the benefit of revascularizing lesions that were significant by FFR in comparison to medical therapy alone. The general trend seems to be that benefit of PCI over medical therapy alone varies inversely with FFR value (Fig. 7.4).

One of the first questions studied was the safety of deferring PCI based on a FFR strategy in patients (n = 325) with moderate single vessel CAD and no inducible ischemia (negative or not done) who were scheduled for PCI–the DEFER trial.[5] Patients with FFR > 0.75 were randomly assigned to deferral (n = 91) or performance (n = 90) of PTCA. 144 with FFR < 0.75 acted as the PCI reference group. Event-free survival (all-cause mortality, myocardial infarction, CABG, coronary angioplasty and any procedure-related complication necessitating major intervention or prolonged hospital stay) was similar between both the FFR > 0.75 groups (92% vs 89% at 12 months and 89% vs 83% at 24 months) but was better than the reference group (80% at 12 months and 78% at 24 months), presumably because the latter had more disease. Angina relief was similar between the deferral and performance groups (49% vs 50% at 12 months and 70% vs 51% at 24 months) but was significantly higher in the reference group (67% at 12 and 80% at 24 months). This trial clearly identified a group of patients, thought to need PCI based on clinical and angiographic criteria, which could safely avoid PCI. Similar findings were noted at the 5 years[40] and now 15 years follow-up.[41] Death and MI were very low (<1% a year) and most events were revascularization.

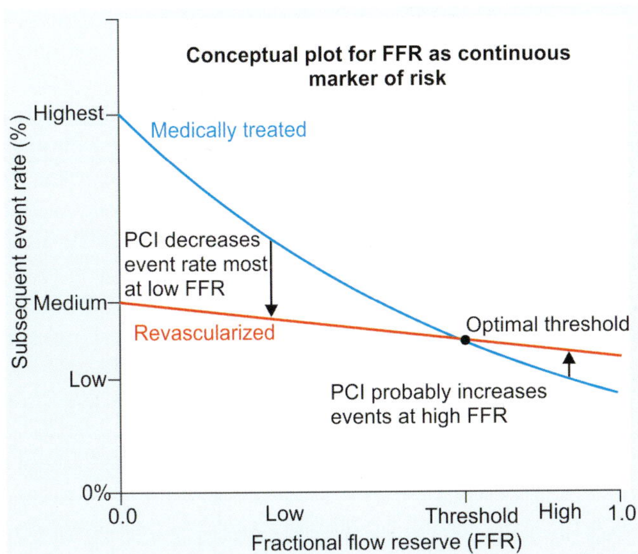

Fig. 7.4 FFR is often treated a 0.75 to 0.80 and is used as a "go-no go" decision maker. However, risk with a given FFR as well as benefit is a continuous curve with increasingly lower values correlating with higher benefit post revascularization. A lower value of FFR (in the range of 0.66) may be associated with the best benefit and those over 0.80 while thought to be low risk, do have events
Source: Ref. 66

There was a signal, albeit not reaching statistical significance, towards slight excess in death and MI if PCI was performed in the FFR > 0.75 group; interestingly at 15 years, MI rates were 14% in this group vs 2% in the deferred group with 70% of the events localized to the target vessel.[41] This study showed that a deferral strategy of revascularization for coronary lesions that did not have prior evidence of ischemia and did not have a significant FFR value was an acceptable alternative to revascularization.

The benefit of using FFR rather than an angiographic-only assessment to guide revascularization in multivessel disease, including both stable and unstable angina patients (n=1005 patients with >50% lesion in at least two major epicardial coronary arteries) and with the use of 1st generation drug coated stents was assessed in the initial FAME trial.[6] Patients with recent STEMI, large NSTEMI, cardiogenic shock, LMCA lesions, previous CAB, technically difficult coronary anatomy were excluded. Similar number of vessels were intervened in both groups (2.7 vs 2.8) but with less total stents/patient, less contrast use and an approximately $675 per patient cost savings with FFR. Both the primary end point (death, MI, and repeat revascularization at 1 year -13.2% vs 18.3%) and the secondary end point (death or MI at 1 year-7.3% vs 11.1%) were lower in the FFR-guided group but angina relief was not different (81% vs 78%). A 2-year follow-up data showed continued benefit in terms of death or MI but revascularization rate, MACE and angina relief were similar. Patients with FFR values greater than 0.8 that were deferred for revascularization had rates of myocardial infarction and revascularization of 0.2% and 3.2%, respectively, at two years. One important finding was that most MIs in the FFR guided group were not from deferred lesions once again proving that the strategy of leaving these alone is wise. A sub study looking at patients with ACS alone should results similar to the main trail, even though the overall event rates were higher in this group.[42] This trial demonstrated that FFR-guided revascularization in multivessel coronary artery disease decreased the composite of death, myocardial infarction and repeat revascularization.

Around this time, there was increasing evidence that PCI did not affect hard end points in patients with stable CAD, even if multivessel and having moderate ischemia[20] but that study did not use FFR to identify lesions needing therapy with certainty. The benefit of revascularizing lesions that were significant by FFR in comparison to medical therapy alone was evaluated in the FAME II trial.[7] This study randomized patients with stable coronary artery disease and hemodynamically significant lesions with FFR values of 0.80 or less to either both revascularization and optimal medical therapy or to optimal medical therapy alone. Recruitment was stopped early secondary to a large difference in the rate of primary end-point occurrence between groups. The primary end-point was a composite of death, myocardial infarction and urgent revascularization at one year and occurred in 4.3% of the revascularization group and 12.7% in the optimal medical therapy alone group ($p < 0.001$). The difference in the primary outcome was driven by urgent revascularization that occurred in 1.6% of the revascularization group and 11.1% of the optimal medical therapy alone group. The difference persisted at the two year follow up with the primary end-point occurring in 8.1% of the revascularization group and 19.5% of the optimal medical therapy alone group.[43] No significant difference in death or myocardial infarction between groups at one-year or two-year follow-up evaluations. A landmark analysis comparing the rate of death and myocardial infarction between eight days and two years showed a significantly decreased rate in the revascularization group (4.6%) compared to the medical therapy alone group (8.0%). This trial showed the benefit of revascularizing lesions with FFR values of 0.80 or less in comparison to optimal medical therapy alone. It also showed that leaving "angiographically significant" lesions alone if the FFR was >0.8 (nearly 25% of the screened population) was associated with a low event rate (3% in the registry arm). While this trial is very conclusive and shows that even hard points may be modified with an FFR guided strategy, there was a criticism about stopping the trial early which prevented clear data on hard end points, overestimation the benefit and the probity of emphasizing landmark analysis when the main intention to treat trial did not show a benefit. A recent meta-analysis[8] of 49, 517 patients (4 prospective and 3 retrospective studies) showed that FFR-guided PCI was associated with both lower MACE as well as MACCE; surprisingly, odds ratio for hard end points (OR: 1.71–2.05) was greater than for repeat revascularization (OR: 1.25, 95% CI 1.09–1.44). It is also important to note that most of the FFR < 0.8 patients treated medically did not have an event and about 10% of those in the > 0.8 group have MACE suggesting that while FFR is the best tool we have, it is far from perfect in predicting who will have an event. These studies, as a group, have established the role of FFR in clinical decision making and it is now believed that "physiologic stenting" is the way to go.

FFR IN SELECTED CLINICAL POPULATIONS

There are many other reported used of FFR that are promising but not yet tested in randomized trials.

Left main coronary lesions may be triaged with FFR. These are often difficult to assess based on angiographic appearance alone. Left main lesion angiographic-FFR mismatches were identified to occur with 35% of angiographic stenoses greater than 50% having FFR values greater than 0.80 and up to 40% of angiographic stenoses less than 50% having FFR values of 0.80 or less.[44] Fractional flow reserve was used to guide left main revascularization in a group with equivocal angiographic stenoses and the five-year survival rates were not statistically different between the deferred group (FFR greater than 0.80) and the group with hemodynamically significant lesions (FFR of 0.80 of less) who underwent surgical revascularization.[45] 5 of the 7 available studies have used a FFR cut off of < 0.75 while 2 used < 0.80 and nearly all have used IV adenosine. A meta-analysis of six different cohorts with left main stenoses and FFR-guided revascularization further supports the use of FFR to identify those lesions that will benefit from revascularization and those that can safely be deferred.[46] LMCA lesions are often associated with LAD-LCX bifurcation involvement and this might overestimate the FFR—a lower cutoff value (<0.75) is thus suggested and the wire is often placed in the nonstenosed vessel. FFR > 0.85 is thought to represent nonsignificant stenosis even in presence of complex lesions.[47]

Serial lesions along the same vessel can make individual lesion assessment difficult, but not impossible. An accurate assessment of lesion significance requires maximal flow across the lesion, which is inhibited by either proximal or distal stenoses that also limit flow. The summed contribution of all lesions can be characterized by the traditional FFR assessment calculated as the ratio of distal to aortic pressures. Experimental methods have been validated and include measuring the pressures between stenoses and the coronary occlusion wedge pressure in addition to the aortic and distal coronary pressures.[48] The need to obtain occlusion pressure limits it use but a strategy of dilating the stenosis with the largest pressure drop followed by re-evaluating has been found to be effective[49] and deferring PCI based on this strategy seemed safe.

Fractional flow reserve can be used to assess the effectiveness of percutaneous coronary interventions (Figs 7.5A and B).

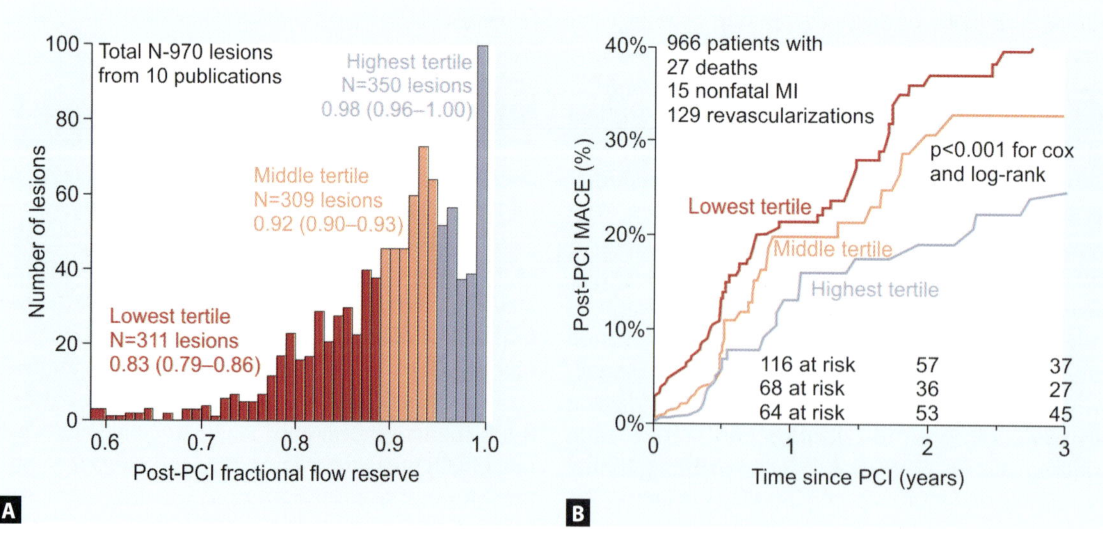

Figs 7.5A and B FFR predicts post-PCI outcomes. (A) Distribution of post–PCI FFR values (B) and survival. Low post-PCI value predicts higher clinical events on follow up.
Source: Ref. 66.

A registry evaluating 750 patients with FFR following angiographically successful bare metal stent revascularization showed that FFR predicts future adverse events.[50] The FFR value measured immediately following stent implantation was directly related to the risk of adverse events. Major adverse cardiovascular events (MACE) occurred in 4.9% of patients with an FFR greater than 0.95, but occurred in 29.5% of patients with an FFR less than 0.80. Similar findings were shown for FFR assessments following drug eluting stent implantation. A retrospective evaluation of 80 patients showed a one-year MACE rate of 12.5% in patients with an FFR less than 0.90 and only 2.5% in patients with an FFR greater than 0.90.[51]

In addition to evaluating the stented vessel immediately following revascularization, FFR has been used to assess side branches within a stented segment that have ostial lesions or lesions that developed from stenting the parent vessel. Side branch lesions within stented segments often appear to have a greater severity of stenosis than is actually present. An evaluation of side branch lesions within stented segments by FFR showed that only 27% of lesions with angiographic stenosis severity greater than 75% had FFR values less than 0.75.[52] The FFR measurement was successful in 97% of side branch lesions indicating that the FFR wire is nearly always capable of crossing the stent struts to access the side branch artery. While attractive and feasible, there is little convincing data either way. In one experience, FFR of jailed side branch did not affect cardiac event rates but reduced number of complex PCIs, a procedure that has poor results. Similarly, FFR post side branch PCI is not very predictive of good outcome at this time.[53,53a]

In-stent restenosis has also been evaluated for hemodynamic significance with FFR. Similar to native lesions, in-stent lesions have been shown to be poorly characterized by angiography alone.[54] Native and in-stent lesions with angiographically similar stenosis severities were compared with FFR using quantitative coronary angiography.[55] Although stenosis severity was similar between groups with a mean stenosis of approximately 52%, the measured FFR was significantly lower in the in-stent restenosis group. The FFR value was less than 0.75 in 48% of the in-stent restenosis lesion group compared to 26% of the native lesion group.

Fractional flow reserve has also shown to be useful in identifying arteries to target for surgical revascularization (Fig. 7.6). The use of FFR-guided coronary artery bypass graft revascularization has been shown to be associated with a fewer number of graft anastomoses and lower rate of on-pump operations in comparison to angiographic-only guided revascularization.[56] The FFR-guided group also had a significantly greater graft patency rate at three years. Another study assessed graft patency at one year in patients where the surgeon was blinded to FFR values and found occluded grafts in 8.9% of grafts bypassing functionally significant lesions and 21.4% of grafts bypassing nonsignificant lesions.[57] Finally, myocardial perfusion was evaluated by near infrared fluorescence complex angiography and perfusion analysis immediately follow surgical revascularization and found no change in perfusion following grafting in 24% of arterial and 22% of saphenous vein grafts indicating that the lesions were not hemodynamically significant.[58] These data support the use of FFR to help guide surgical revascularization as well as percutaneous revascularization.

Saphenous vein graft lesion significance can be complex, but many lesions can be characterized with FFR. Complexity arises with saphenous vein graft lesions as the vessel

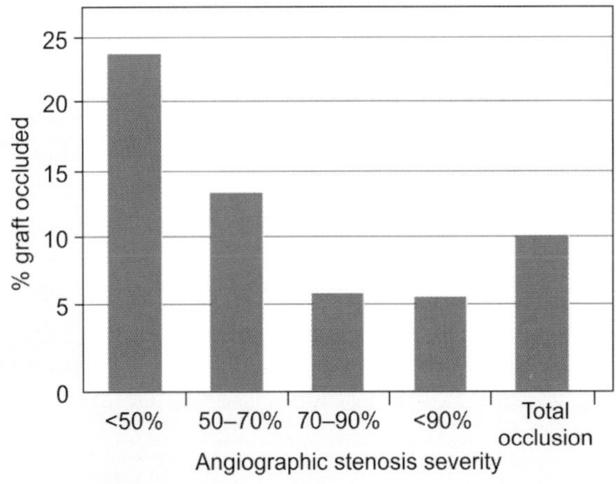

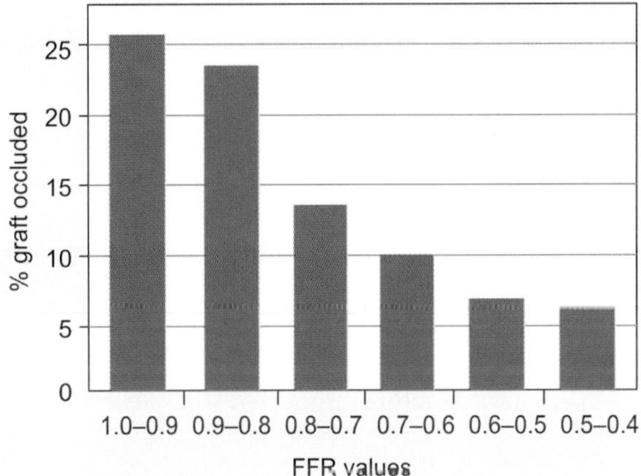

Fig. 7.6 FFR not only triages stenosis for optimum PCI outcomes but also better predicts outcomes after CAB. An FFR measured degree of stenosis predicts 1-year graft patency better than % diameter stenosis measurements. This may be because hemodynamically nonsignificant lesions have a higher incidence of graft closure when bypassed

Source: Kern MJ, Samady H. Current concepts of integrated coronary physiology in the catheterization laboratory. J Am Coll Cardiol. 2010;55:173-85.

segment distal to a graft lesion may have as many as three sources of blood supply. The distal graft receives blood from the graft itself and, in some cases, from the native artery, collateral arterial supply or both. Nonetheless, a small study evaluating vein graft lesion significance with FFR less than 0.75 in comparison to myocardial perfusion imaging found a sensitivity of 50%, specificity of 75%, positive predictive value of 33%, negative predictive value of 85% and accuracy of 70%.[59]

Microcirculatory dysfunction during a ST elevation myocardial infarction limits the utility of FFR in assessing coronary lesions but may have a role for lesions in nonculprit vessels. Wedge pressure can affect the results but there does not seem to be a major difference between immediate FFR values and those five weeks later in nonculprit vessels.[60] Less is known about FFR use in the setting of a non-ST segment elevation myocardial infarction (NSTEMI). The FAMOUS-NSTEMI trial evaluated NSTEMI patients and compared revascularization rates between angiographic-guided and FFR-guided randomized groups.[61] The angiographic-guided group had higher rates of initial revascularization (87%) and revascularization at one-year (87%) compared to the FFR-guided group with initial and one-year revascularization rates of 76% and 79%, respectively; health outcomes and quality of life were however not different at 1 year. Subgroup studies of the FAME trial also showed a similar benefit of FFR. Additional data evaluations from this study will help better characterize the utility of FFR in the setting of NSTEMI events.

LIMITATIONS OF FRACTIONAL FLOW RESERVE

Limitations of FFR are generally related to the tools used to obtain the data. Compared to standard coronary wires, pressure wires have been considered by many operators to provide poor support making maneuverability difficult. The pressure wires also tend to kink easier than typical coronary wires. Calibration of the pressure wire must be performed properly and maintenance of the calibration must be monitored as the wires have an inclination to undergo pressure signal drift. Guide catheter support must also be carefully monitored as guides can easily obstruct the coronary flow resulting in erroneous FFR values. Guide catheters with side holes should also be avoided. Care must be taken to avoid obstruction of coronary flow with the guide catheter, but still allow for adequate delivery of the hyperemic agent into the coronary artery (if given intracoronary) resulting in reduced hyperemia. While FFR has a continuous relation with ischemia, FFR 0.75–0.80 is a gray zone in terms of FFR stability and outcome, especially with values approaching 0.80.[62] Similarly, 0.75–0.85 is a grey zone for LMCA evaluation. Finally, FFR is not perfect and can even be false positive, especially in condition of high coronary flow. Normal CFR in this situation should lead one to suspect a nonsignificantly flow-limiting stenosis despite a low FFR and defer intervention.[63,64]

Conceptual issues remain with FFR even though that should not obscure its benefits and the need for widespread adoption. The debate whether CFR is better than FFR for predicting clinical outcomes especially if one withholds PCI is still unresolved. There is data that FFR > 0.8 group is not completely benign and that most patients with FFR < 0.8 do not have events. Interestingly, using CFR and IMR can further separate subsets with differing risk in this FFR > 0.8 population.[32] Plaque morphology is not accounted in FFR and intermediate lesions, thought to be at high risk for hard events like death and MI, may not be picked up by FFR alone[65]—this might be the reason why hard events are modified to a smaller extent with FFR guided PCI than soft events like future revascularization—newer modalities like OCT FFR/IVUS-FFR might help—this is being tested in trials like the FORZA study. Nevertheless, lesions with a necrotic core (an index of a high risk plaque) seem to have lower FFR than comparable lesions without a necrotic core[66] and future studies might fine tune our understanding about FFR and hard events. A lower level of 0.66 FFR cutoff value might better improve patient outcomes over optimal medical therapy.[67] A fact also noted in the FAME studies—future data might show that FFR might need a more nuanced approach than a simple *"go or no go"* strategy. This becomes even more relevant when considering that statins might improve FFR even without obvious change in angiographic lesion stenosis.[68]

CONCLUSION

There is excellent data that FFR is currently the best method to identify CAD that needs revascularization and helps optimize outcomes. In our opinion, nearly every intermediate lesion in patients with stable ischemic heart disease (IHD) coming for PCI (except for those with proven ischemia through other imaging) should demonstrate functional significance with FFR before being intervened upon. Despite clear advantages, FFR utilization is poor-over 50% of interventional cardiologists using FFR in less than 1/3 of their cases.[69] A study of 255 interventional cardiologists showed that 15% never used FFR, 55% used FFR in less than one-third of cases and only 10% used FFR in greater than two-thirds of their cases. A more recent survey shows a similar dismal picture.[24] Easier ways of obtaining FFR might help adoption but our first priority should be to encourage wider acceptance. Multiple studies are on the way, like the FAME 3 trial, comparing FFR-guided PCI with newer generation drug eluting stents with angiography guided CABG in patients with multivessel disease,[70] will provide more evidence for evidence based intervention and hopefully better outcomes.

REFERENCES

1. Patel MR, Peterson ED, Dai D, et al. Low diagnostic yield of elective coronary angiography. N Engl J Med. 2010;362:886-95.
2. Ischemia Trial. *https://www.ischemiatrial.org*
3. EJ Topol, SE Nissen. Our preoccupation with coronary luminology: The dissociation between clinical and angiographic findings in ischemic heart disease. Circulation. 1995;92:2333-42.
4. Pijls NH, van Son JA, Kirkeeide RL, De Bruyne B, Gould KL. Experimental basis of determining maximum coronary, myocardial, and collateral blood flow by pressure measurements for assessing functional stenosis severity before and after percutaneous transluminal coronary angioplasty. Circulation. 1993;87:1354-67.
5. Bech GJ, et al. Fractional flow reserve to determine the appropriateness of angioplasty in moderate coronary stenosis: a randomized trial. Circulation. 2001;103:2928-34.
6. Tonino PAL, et al. Fractional flow reserve versus angiography for guiding percutaneous coronary intervention. N Engl J Med. 2009;360:213-24.
7. De Bruyne, B. et al. Fractional flow reserve-guided PCI versus medical therapy in stable coronary disease. N Engl J Med. 2012;367:991-1001.
8. Zhang D, et al. Fractional flow reserve versus angiography for guiding percutaneous coronary intervention: a meta-analysis. Heart. 2015;101:455-62.
9. Fihn SD, et al. 2012 ACCF/AHA/ACP/AATS/PCNA/SCAI/STS guideline for the diagnosis and management of patients with stable ischemic heart disease: a report of the American College of Cardiology Foundation/American Heart Association task force on practice guidelines, and the American College of Physicians, American Association for Thoracic Surgery, Preventive Cardiovascular Nurses Association, Society for Cardiovascular Angiography and Interventions, and Society of Thoracic Surgeons. Circulation 2012;126:e354-471.
10. Windecker S. Cario Pulse: EuroPCR 2014: the 25th Official Congress of the European Association of Percutaneous Cardiovascular Interventions. Eur Heart J. 2014;35:2699.
11. Park SJ, Ahn JM, Kang SJ. Paradigm shift to functional angioplasty: new insights for fractional flow reserve- and intravascular ultrasound-guided percutaneous coronary intervention. Circulation. 2011;124:951-7.
12. Smalling RW, Kelley K, Kirkeeide RL, Fisher DJ. Regional myocardial function is not affected by severe coronary depressurization provided coronary blood flow is maintained. J Am Coll Cardiol. 1985;5:948-55.
13. Gould KL, Lipscomb K, Hamilton GW. Physiologic basis for assessing critical coronary stenosis: instantaneous flow response and regional distribution during coronary hyperemia as measures of coronary flow reserve. Am J Cardiol. 1974;33:87-94.
14. Young DF, Cholvin NR, Kirkeeide RL, Roth AC. Hemodynamics of arterial stenoses at elevated flow rates. Circ Res. 1977;41:99-107.
15. Pijls NH, De Bruyne B, Peels K, Van Der Voort PH, Bonnier HJ, Bartunek J, et al. Measurement of fractional flow reserve to assess the functional severity of coronary artery stenoses. N Engl J Med. 1996;334:1703-8.
16. White CW, et al. Does Visual interpretation of the coronary arteriogram predict the physiologic importance of a coronary stenosis? N Engl J Med. 1984;310:819-24.
17. Harrison DG, et al. The value of lesion cross-sectional area determined by quantitative coronary angiography in assessing the physiologic significance of proximal left anterior descending coronary arterial stenoses. Circulation. 1984;69:1111-9.
18. Wilson RF, Marcus ML, White CW. Prediction of the physiologic significance of coronary arterial lesions by quantitative lesion geometry in patients with limited coronary artery disease. Circulation. 1987;75:723-32.
19. Parisi AF, Folland ED, Hartigan P. A comparison of angioplasty with medical therapy in the treatment of single-vessel coronary artery disease. Veterans Affairs ACME Investigators. N Engl J Med. 1992;326:10-6.
20. Boden WE, et al. Optimal medical therapy with or without PCI for stable coronary disease. N Engl J Med. 2007;356:1503-16.
21. Serruys PW, et al. Percutaneous coronary intervention versus coronary-artery bypass grafting for severe coronary artery disease. N Engl J Med. 2009;360:961-72.
22. Lotfi A, Jeremias A, Fearon WF, et al. Expert consensus statement on the use of fractional flow reserve, intravascular ultrasound, and optical coherence tomography. Catheter Cardiovasc Interv. 2014;83:509-18.
23. Van Belle E, Rioufol G, Pouillot C, et al. Outcome impact of coronary revascularization strategy reclassification with fractional flow reserve at time of diagnostic angiography: insights from a large French multicenter fractional flow reserve registry. Circulation. 2014,129.173-85.
24. Dattilo PB, Prasad A, Honeycutt E, Wang TY, Messenger JC. Contemporary patterns of fractional flow reserve and intravascular ultrasound use among patients undergoing percutaneous coronary intervention in the United States: insights from the National Cardiovascular Data Registry. J Am Coll Cardiol. 2012;60:2337-9.
25. Burzotta F, Leone AM, De Maria GL, Niccoli G, Coluccia V, Pirozzolo G, et al. Fractional flow reserve or optical coherence tomography guidance to revascularize intermediate coronary stenosis using angioplasty (FORZA) trial: study protocol for a randomized controlled trial. Trials. 2014;15:140.
26. van de Hoef TP, Siebes M, Spaan JAE, Piek JJ. Fundamentals in clinical coronary physiology: why coronary flow is more important than coronary pressure. Eur Heart J. 2015;36:3312-9.
27. Escaned J, Echavarría-Pinto M. Moving beyond coronary stenosis: has the time arrived to address important physiological questions not answered by fractional flow reserve alone? Circ Cardiovasc Interv. 2014;7:282-4.
28. Kern MJ, et al. Fundamentals of translesional pressure-flow velocity measurements. Part II. Cathet Cardiovasc Diagn. 1994;31:137-43.
29. van de Hoef TP, van Lavieren MA, Damman P, et al. Physiological basis and long-term clinical outcome of discordance between fractional flow reserve and coronary flow velocity reserve in coronary stenoses of intermediate severity. Circ Cardiovasc Interv. 2014;7:301-11.

30. Fearon WF, et al. Novel index for invasively assessing the coronary microcirculation. Circulation. 2003;107:3129-32.
31. Martínez GJ, Yong ASC, Fearon WF, Ng MKC. The index of microcirculatory resistance in the physiologic assessment of the coronary microcirculation. Coron Artery Dis. 2015;26 (Suppl 1): e15-26.
32. Lee JM, Jung JH, Hwang D, et al. Coronary flow reserve and microcirculatory resistance in patients with intermediate coronary stenosis. J Am Coll Cardiol. 2016;67(10):1158-69.
33. Blows LJ, Redwood SR. The pressure wire in practice. Heart. 2007;93:419-22.
34. Sen S, et al. Development and validation of a new adenosine-independent index of stenosis severity from coronary wave-intensity analysis: results of the ADVISE (ADenosine Vasodilator Independent Stenosis Evaluation) study. J Am Coll Cardiol. 2012;59:1392-402.
35. Escaned J, et al. Prospective assessment of the diagnostic accuracy of instantaneous wave-free ratio to assess coronary stenosis relevance: results of ADVISE II international, multicenter study (ADenosine Vasodilator Independent Stenosis Evaluation II). JACC Cardiovasc Interv. 2015;8:824-33.
36. Samady H, Gogas BD. Does flow during rest and relaxation suffice? J Am Coll Cardiol. 2013;61:1436-9.
37. Johnson NP, Johnson DT, Kirkeeide RL, Berry C, DeBruyne B, Fearon WF, et al. Repeatability of fractional flow reserve (FFR) despite variations in systemic and coronary hemodynamics. J Am Coll Cardiol Intv. 2015;8(8): 1018-27.
38. Seto AH, Tehrani DM, Bharmal MI, Kern MJ. Variations of coronary hemodynamic responses to intravenous adenosine infusion: Implications for fractional flow reserve measurements. Catheter Cardiovasc Interv. 2014;84:416-25.
39. Aueron FM, Gruentzig AR. Percutaneous transluminal coronary angioplasty: indication and current status. Prim Cardiol. 1984;10:97-107.
40. Pijls NH, et al. Percutaneous coronary intervention of functionally nonsignificant stenosis: 5-year follow-up of the DEFER Study. J Am Coll Cardiol. 2007;49:2105-11.
41. Pijls NHJ. 15-year follow-up of the DEFER trial. Presented at: EuroPCR; May 19, 2015; Paris, France.
42. Sels JW, Tonino PA, Siebert U, et al. Fractional flow reserve in unstable angina and non-ST-segment elevation myocardial infarction experience from the FAME (Fractional flow reserve versus Angiography for Multivessel Evaluation) study. JACC Cardiovasc Interv. 2011;4:1183-9.
43. De Bruyne B, et al. Fractional flow reserve-guided PCI for stable coronary artery disease. N Engl J Med. 2014;371:1208-17.
44. Park SJ, et al. Visual-functional mismatch between coronary angiography and fractional flow reserve. JACC Cardiovasc Interv. 2012;5:1029-36.
45. Hamilos M, et al. Long-term clinical outcome after fractional flow reserve-guided treatment in patients with angiographically equivocal left main coronary artery stenosis. Circulation. 2009;120:1505-12.
46. Mallidi J, et al. Long-term outcomes following fractional flow reserve-guided treatment of angiographically ambiguous left main coronary artery disease: A meta-analysis of prospective cohort studies. Catheter Cardiovasc Interv. 2015;86:12-8.
47. Yong AS, Daniels D, De Bruyne B, et al. Fractional flow reserve assessment of left main stenosis in the presence of downstream coronary stenoses. Circ Cardiovasc Interv. 2013;6:161-5.
48. Pijls NH, De Bruyne B, Bech GJ. Coronary pressure measurement to assess the hemodynamic significance of serial stenoses within one coronary artery: validation in humans. Circulation. 2000;102:2371-7.
49. Kim HL, Koo BK, Nam CW, et al. Clinical and physiological outcomes of fractional flow reserve-guided percutaneous coronary intervention in patients with serial stenoses within one coronary artery. JACC Cardiovasc Interv. 2012;5:1013-8.
50. Pijls NH, Klauss V, Siebert U, et al. Coronary pressure measurement after stenting predicts adverse events at follow-up: a multicenter registry. Circulation. 2002;105:2950-4.
51. Nam CW, et al. Relation of fractional flow reserve after drug-eluting stent implantation to one-year outcomes. Am J Cardiol. 2011;107:1763-7.
52. Koo BK, et al. Physiologic assessment of jailed side branch lesions using fractional flow reserve. J Am Coll Cardiol. 2005;46:633-7.
53. Koo BK, Park KW, Kang HJ, et al. Physiological evaluation of the provisional side-branch intervention strategy for bifurcation lesions using fractional flow reserve. Eur Heart J. 2008;29:726-32.
53a. Lee BK, Choi HH, Hong KS, et al. Efficacy of fractional flow reserve measurements at side branch vessels treated with the crush stenting technique in true coronary bifurcation lesions. Clin Cardiol. 2010;33:490-4.
54. Lopez-Palop R, et al. Utility of the fractional flow reserve in the evaluation of angiographically moderate in-stent restenosis. Eur. Heart J. 2004;25:2040-7.
55. Krüger S, et al. Clinical significance of fractional flow reserve for evaluation of functional lesion severity in stent restenosis and native coronary arteries. Chest. 2005;128:1645-9.
56. Toth G, et al. Fractional flow reserve-guided versus angiography-guided coronary artery bypass graft surgery. Circulation. 2013;128:1405-11.
57. Botman CJ, et al. Does stenosis severity of native vessels influence bypass graft patency? A prospective fractional flow reserve-guided study. Ann Thorac Surg. 2007;83:2093-7.
58. Ferguson TB, et al. Fractional flow reserve-guided coronary artery bypass grafting: can intraoperative physiologic imaging guide decision making? J Thorac Cardiovasc Surg. 2013;146:824-35.e1.
59. Aqel R, Zoghbi GJ, Hage F, Dell'Italia L, Iskandrian, AE. Hemodynamic evaluation of coronary artery bypass graft lesions using fractional flow reserve. Catheter Cardiovasc Interv. 2008;72:479-85.
60. Ntalianis A, Sels JW, Davidavicius G, et al. Fractional flow reserve for the assessment of nonculprit coronary artery stenoses in patients with acute myocardial infarction. JACC Cardiovasc Interv. 2010;3:1274-81.
61. Layland J, et al. Fractional flow reserve vs. angiography in guiding management to optimize outcomes in non-ST-segment elevation myocardial infarction: the British Heart Foundation FAMOUS-NSTEMI randomized trial. Eur Heart J. 2015;36: 100-11.
62. Petraco R, Sen S, Nijjer S, et al. Fractional flow reserve-guided revascularization: practical implications of a diagnostic gray

zone and measurement variability on clinical decisions. JACC Cardiovasc Interv. 2013;6:222-5.
63. Johnson NP, Kirkeeide RL, Gould KL. Is discordance of coronary flow reserve and fractional flow reserve due to methodology or clinically relevant coronary pathophysiology? JACC Cardiovasc Imaging. 2012;5:193-202.
64. Echavarría-Pinto M, Escaned J, Macías E, et al. Disturbed coronary hemodynamics in vessels with intermediate stenoses evaluated with fractional flow reserve: a combined analysis of epicardial and microcirculatory involvement in ischemic heart disease. Circulation. 2013;128:2557-66.
65. Vorobiof G, Chandrashekhar Y, Narula J. Intermediate lesions: retrieving black from shades of gray. JACC Cardiovasc Interv. 2011;4:209-12.
66. Ahmadi A, Stone G, Leipsic J, Serruys P, et al. Association of coronary stenosis and plaque morphology with fractional flow reserve and outcomes. JAMA Cardiology. 2016;1(3):350-7.
67. Johnson NP, Tóth GG, Lai D, et al. Prognostic value of fractional flow reserve: linking physiologic severity to clinical outcomes. J Am Coll Cardiol. 2014;64:1641-54.
68. Kini AS, Baber U, Kovacic JC, et al. Changes in plaque lipid content after short-term intensive versus standard statin therapy: the YELLOW trial (reduction in yellow plaque by aggressive lipid-lowering therapy). J Am Coll Cardiol. 2013;62:21-9.
69. Hannawi B, Lam WW, Wang S, Younis GA. Current use of fractional flow reserve: a nationwide survey. Tex Heart Inst J. 2014;41:579-84.
70. Zimmermann FM, et al. Rationale and design of the fractional flow reserve versus angiography for multivessel evaluation (FAME) 3 trial: a comparison of fractional flow reserve-guided percutaneous coronary intervention and coronary artery bypass graft surgery in patients with multivessel coronary artery disease. Am Heart J. 2015;170:619-26.e2.

CHAPTER

8

Use of IVUS and OCT in Cath Lab

Imad Sheiban, Filippo Figini

BACKGROUND

Intravascular imaging modalities, mainly represented by Intravascular ultrasound (IVUS) and optical coherence tomography (OCT), are valuable tools that can overcome some of the limitations of simple contrast angiography (CA), such as:

- Poor reliability of visual estimation—but also of quantitative contrast angiography—in vessel sizing and assessment of lesion severity
- Possible underestimation of eccentric lesions
- Poor visualization due to superimposition of other vessels
- Foreshortening due to inadequate projections
- Impossibility to assess the vessel wall anatomy, apart for the presence of gross calcifications
- Inadequate visualization of stent struts
- Poor ability to distinguish some very different situations: e.g. thrombus, vessel wall calcification or dissection may all manifest with the same radiological sign of a "hazy lesion"

Accordingly, IVUS and OCT may have a distinct role in every part of diagnostic and interventional procedures:

- Before stent implantation, they can precisely assess reference vessel size, lesion severity ad characteristics
- They can assist in optimizing stent apposition and expansion
- They might disclose acute complications of percutaneous coronary intervention (PCI), such as edge dissections or intramural hematoma, which might go undetected based on simple angiography
- In case of stent failure (i.e. thrombosis or restenosis), they can disclose the causative mechanism (e.g. malapposition or struts fracture)

Indeed, several studies have demonstrated that IVUS- or OCT-guided PCIs are associated with better results compared to procedures performed with CA only.[1-9]

BASIC DIFFERENCES BETWEEN IVUS AND OCT

Both methods rely on backscattering of signal from the vessel wall, but they use different energies, i.e. ultrasounds and near-infrared light respectively. Despite providing a similar axial view of the vessel, they therefore have significant differences to keep in mind. First of all, OCT has a higher spatial resolution compared to IVUS (10–20 µm vs. 100–200 µm): hence, OCT is the method of choice to assess coverage of stent struts by endothelium, and can identify intimal ruptures more reliably compared to IVUS.[10] On the other hand, while OCT can visualize very clearly the endothelial boundary, it has a limited penetration power in the vessel wall (around 2 mm) compared to IVUS (4–8 mm). A partial exception to this rule is the presence of calcifications, that produce an acoustic shadowing with IVUS, but do not impair visualization of tissue behind the calcium by OCT.[11]

OCT requires contrast injection in order to clear the vessel lumen from blood, which can be a limitation in patients with renal impairment. Moreover, OCT is not ideal in evaluating the ostia of left main and right coronary artery, as adequate clearing of blood is difficult to obtain and because of the large diameter of these segments, often causing incomplete visualization of the vessel wall.

BASELINE VESSEL AND LESION EVALUATION

Basic Vessel Wall Anatomy

The normal vessel wall is composed by three layers: from the inside outwards, the tunica intima, the media and the adventitia, which are separated by the internal and external elastic laminae (Fig. 8.1). The media is a thin structure (generally around 200 μm) and tends to become thinner in presence of disease; the atherosclerotic plaque is instead comprised into the intima. The media is generally clearly evident at IVUS as a dark circle, and vessel diameter is measured up to its outer border (the external elastic membrane), while the lumen diameter and area are defined by the interface between blood (that produces a classical speckle image) and intima (Figs 8.2A and B). The difference between vessel area and lumen area represents the plaque area, which often is expressed as a percentage of vessel area (Fig. 8.3). When the vessel is diffusely diseased, some Authors recommend to choose stent size according to luminal diameter of the landing zone rather than to the actual vessel size derived from external elastic membrane (EEM) measure, in order to minimize the mismatch between the stented segment and the native vessel. Classically, an area with plaque burden <40% is chosen as an appropriate landing zone for stenting, as segments with greater amount of disease are more prone to thrombosis and restenosis.[12]

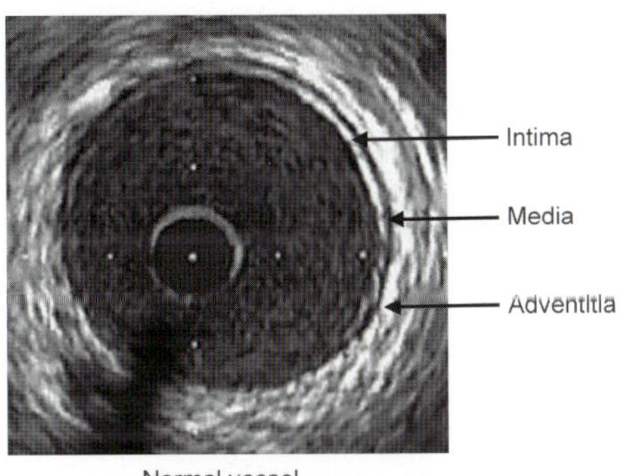

Fig. 8.1 Appearance of a normal vessel at IVUS. The three layers of the arterial wall appear well delineated

The same structures (Figs 8.4A and B) may be identified by OCT; however—due to its limited penetration power—OCT is often not able to visualize the media in presence of intimal plaques. Vessel size is usually determined based on the luminal diameter of a healthy segment close to the diseased segment (Fig. 8.5): therefore, OCT-derived vessel size could be in theory slightly underestimated compared to IVUS. On the other hand, good correlation between IVUS- and OCT-derived reference diameters—with no systematic error—has been shown in a clinical study.[13]

In order to get correct measurements, the IVUS or OCT probe has to be coaxial with the long axis of the vessels: indeed, in tortuous segments, vessel size can be overestimated by out-of-axis images.

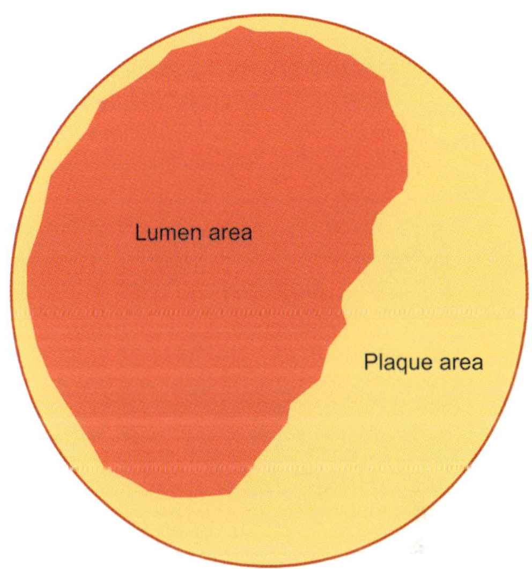

Fig. 8.3 Plaque area (in yellow) represents the difference between vessel area (defined by the external elastic lamina) and the lumen area (in red, defined by the interface between lumen and intima—see Fig. 8.2); it is often expressed as a percentage of vessel area

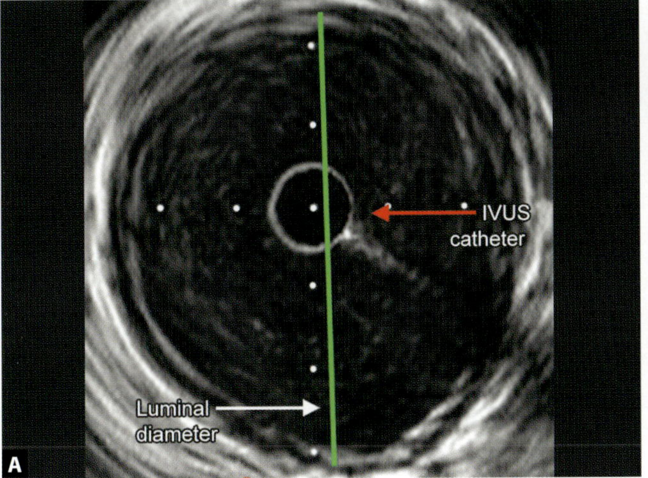

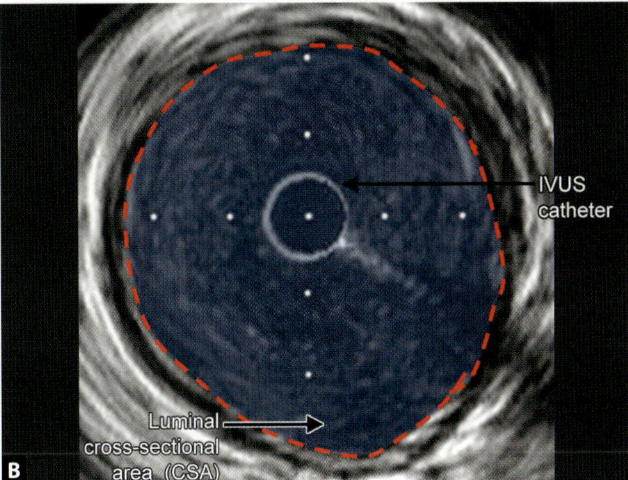

Figs 8.2A and B Luminal diameter and luminal cross-sectional area in a healthy vessel

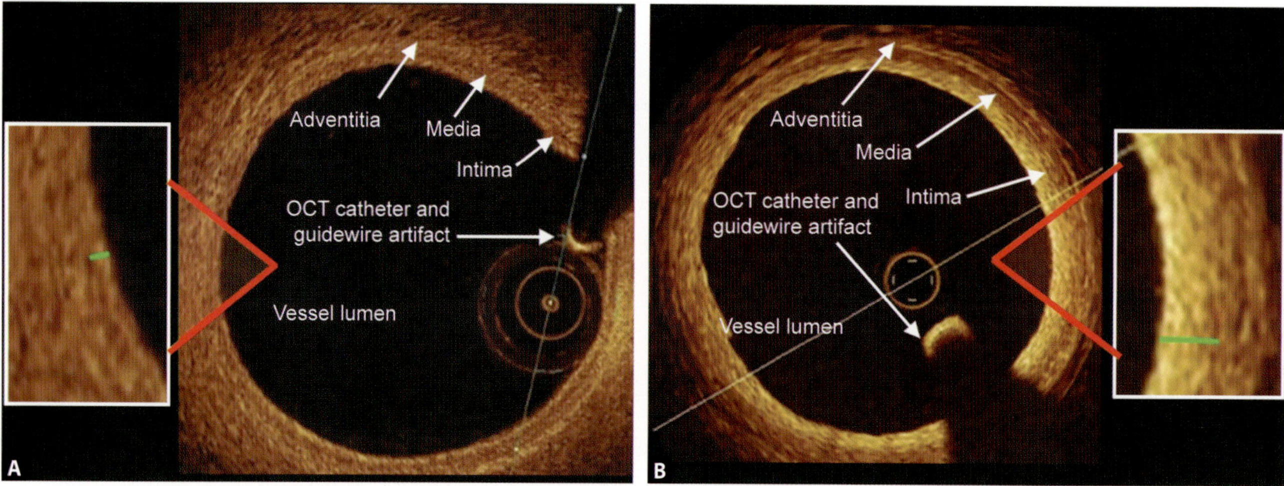

Figs 8.4A and B (A) Normal OCT findings: all three vessel wall layers are well defined. More detailed information and mesureaments can be performed and obtained by image magnification with high resolution images; (B) Moderate intimal hyperplesia can be easily observed (as compared to normal in A). Measurement of intimal thickness can be performed on the magnified segment. Compared to IVUS, OCT can provide more details due to high resolution images, but with reduced depth penetration.

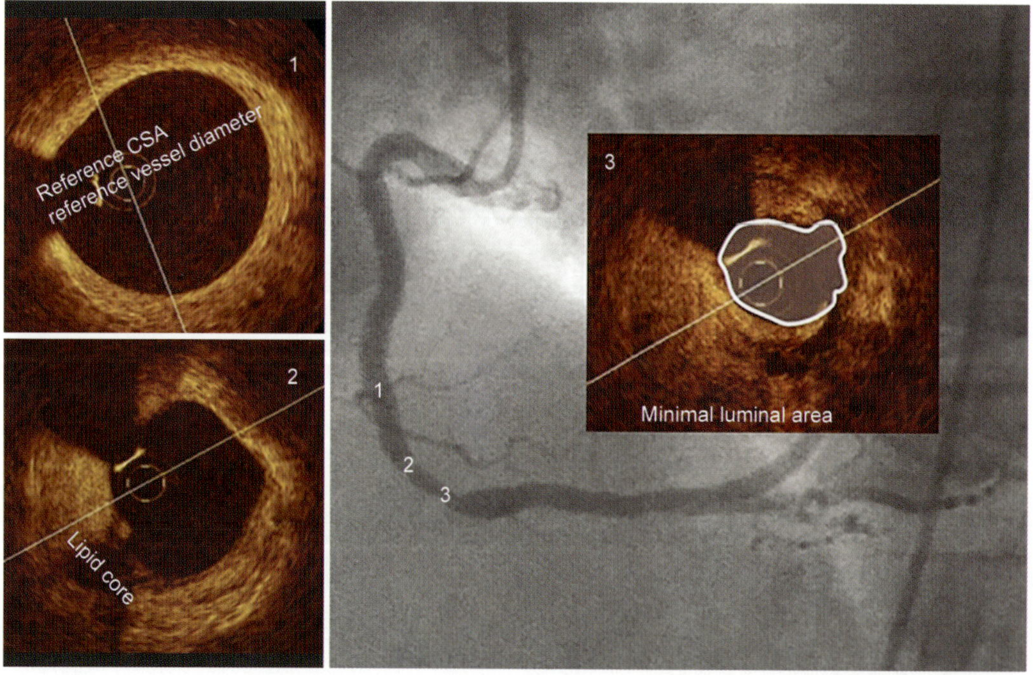

Fig. 8.5 Reference luminal area and vessel diameter, minimal luminal area and minimal vessel diameter can be obtained on OCT similarly to those obtained on IVUS. However, data on diagnostic performance of OCT in identifying significant stenosis on the basis of MLD are still to be defined

With both methods, correlation with angiographic images is paramount: in this respect, analysis of side branches is particularly useful. When left anterior descending artery (LAD) is imaged, the septal branches arise opposite to the pericardial film; diagonal vessels and left circumflex artery origin at 90° compared to septals. In the case of left circumflex (LCx) artery, major branches originate in only one direction; there is instead more variability in the orientation of vessels arising from right coronary artery (RCA).

Plaque Analysis

The majority of atherosclerotic plaques are composed mainly by fibrotic tissue, which has an IVUS appearance as bright as—or brighter—than the adventitia (Figs 8.6A to C). "Soft plaques" are instead darker than adventitia: their low echogenicity is due to the presence of a high lipid content (Figs 8.7A and B).

The assessment of calcifications is paramount in PCI planning; indeed, calcific plaques may require extensive lesion preparation (including rotational atherectomy), may preclude optimal stent deployment and predispose to worse acute and long-term outcomes.[14] Particularly important is the assessment of the radial extension of calcification: while focal spots can be easily displaced by balloons and stents, circumferential rings of calcium often preclude dilatation of the artery and may lead to stent underexpansion, increasing the risk of thrombosis and restenosis.[15]

At IVUS analysis, calcium is characterized by bright signal with acoustic shadowing (Figs 8.8 and 8.9). In contrast, at OCT calcific plaques appear as areas of low-intensity signal with sharp borders (Figs 8.10A to D); they should not be confused with lipid-rich necrotic core, which also is characterized by dark appearance at OCT, but compared to calcium is less well delineated, and is often covered by a bright fibrous cap. A fibrous cap <65 μm defines thin cap fibroatheroma (TCFA), which represents the anatomical feature of the vulnerable plaque.

IVUS is not able to characterize the thickness of the fibrous cap; the presence of echolucent material is considered indicative of lipid core (Figs 8.11A and B), but—compared to OCT—ultrasounds have a lower sensitivity in detecting

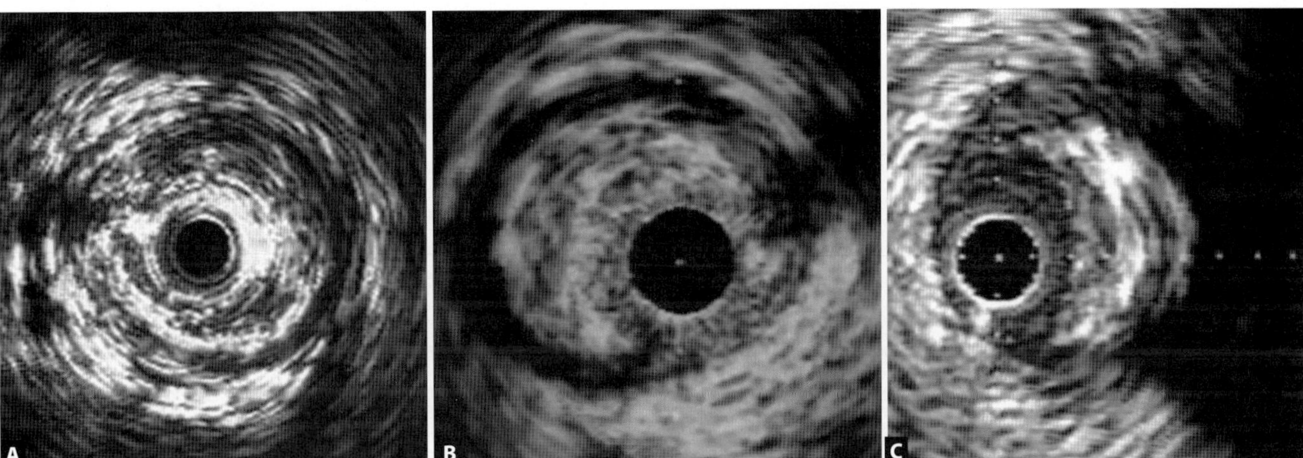

Figs 8.6A to C Fibrotic plaque—the majority of atherosclerotic plaques are fibrotic. Fibrotic plaque is as bright (A) or brighter (B) than the adventitia (hyperechogenicity is caused by fibrosis). Very fibrotic plaques may have a very high acoustic impedance, causing shadowing that could be misclassified as calcium (C)

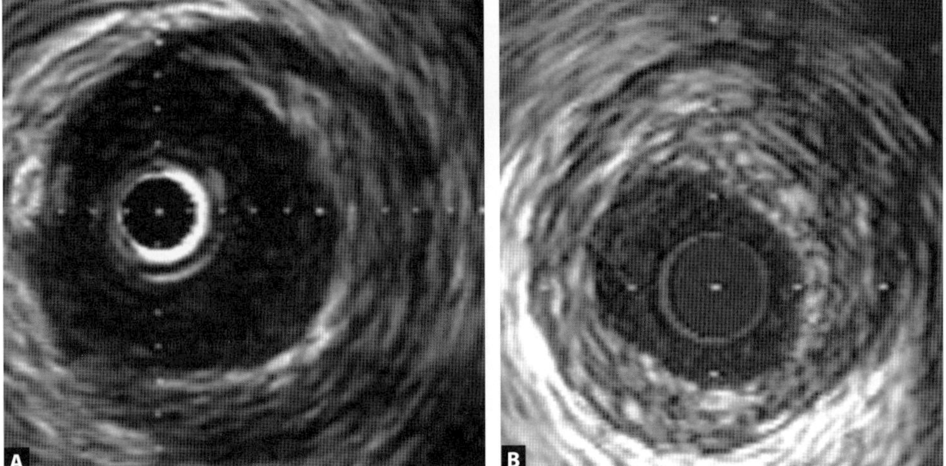

Figs 8.7A and B Soft plaque—"Soft" refers to the low echogenicity (less bright than adventitia), likely due to high lipid content in a mostly cellular plaque. Reduced echogenicity may be also due to intramural hematoma, thrombus and necrotic zone within the plaque

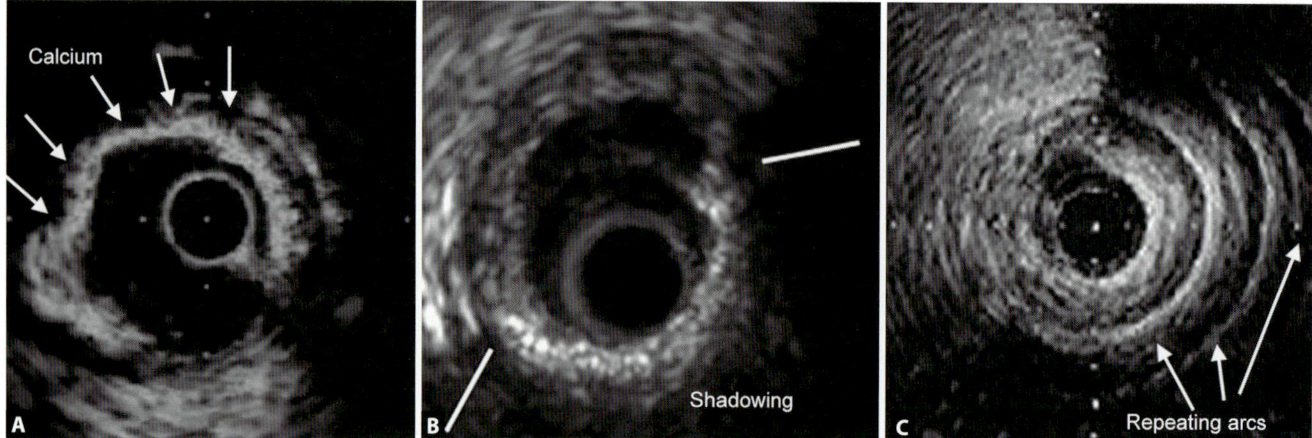

Figs 8.8A to C Calcified plaque—Calcium is detected as bright echoes (brighter than adventitia—A) and obstructs penetration of ultrasound waves (shadowing—B): only the luminal edge is detected. The oscillation of ultrasound waves between transducer and calcium (reverberation) can cause repeating arcs (C)

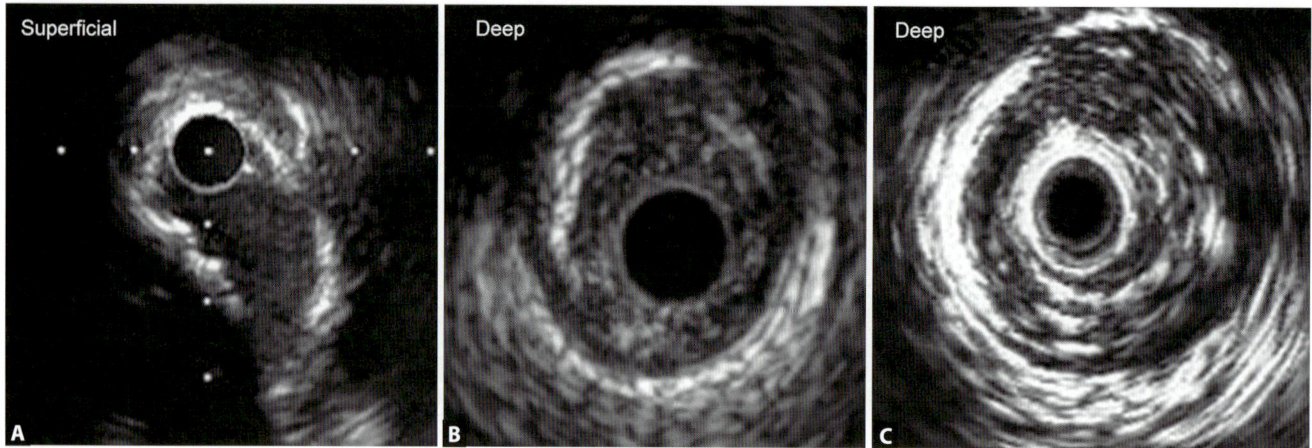

Figs 8.9A to C Location of calcium within the plaque is classified as superficial (when it is closer to the lumen than to the adventitia) and deep (when closer to the adventitia than to the lumen)

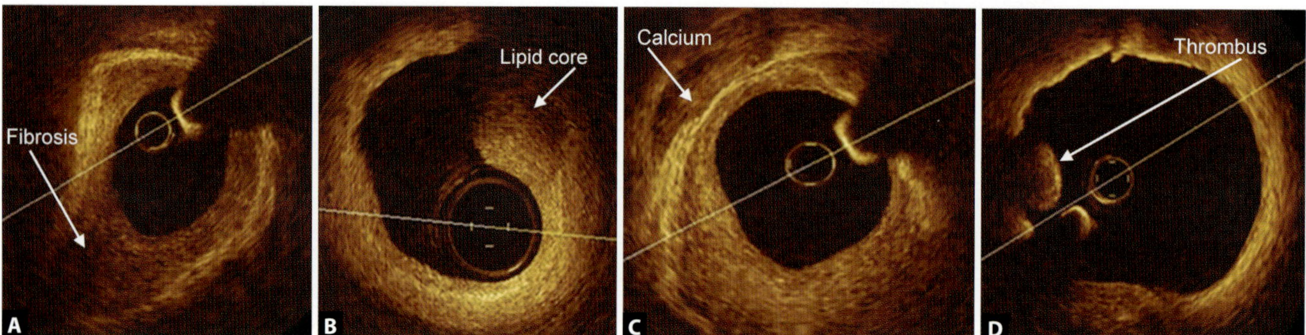

Figs 8.10A to D Plaque composition analysis by OCT: penetration of OCT is dependent on plaque composition

Figs 8.11A and B (A) Vulnerable plaque with a typical aspect of lipid core and fibrous cap; (B) IVUS finding in a vulnerable plaque, with reduced thickness and rupture of fibrous cap (arrow), often associated with ACS
Courtesy: Dr G Minz

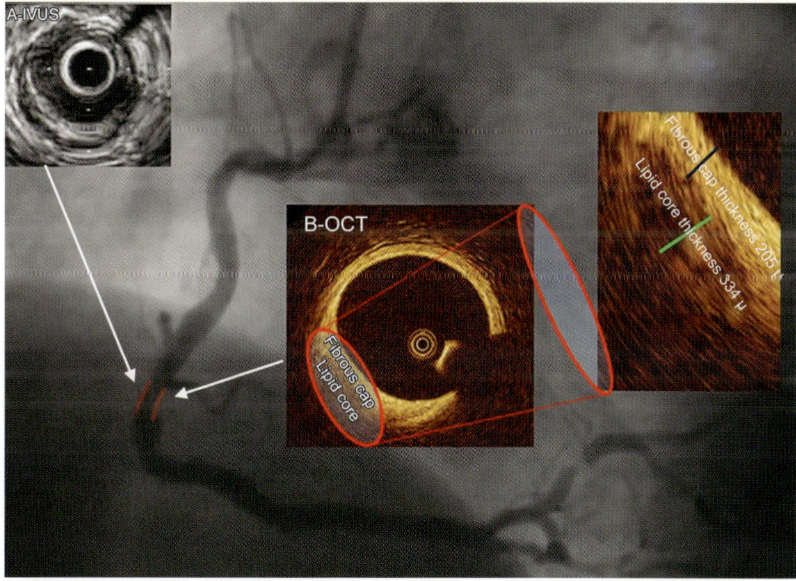

Fig. 8.12 Differences between IVUS and OCT in diagnostic capacities: same plaque on mid-RCA is examined by IVUS and OCT: (A) IVUS shows a small soft plaque, but no other details on plaque composition; (B) OCT shows a thick lipid core and a thick fibrous CAP. Both lipid core and fibrous cap can be precisely measured on OCT

lipid-rich plaques (Fig. 8.12).[16] In addition, OCT can show the presence of macrophages as highly reflective dots, often situated beneath the fibrous cap in vulnerable atheromas.[17,18]

Thrombus is detected as intraluminal mass, which is echolucent at ultrasounds; its signal is brighter for fresh thombi and tends to become darker for older and more organized material (Figs 8.13A to D). With OCT, red thrombi are visualized as high backscattering lesions with shadowing (which may mask the underlying plaque—Figure 8.10), while white thrombi have a low backscatter and a dense signal: however, generally red and white thrombi are mixed in the same lesion.[19]

The presence of TCFA, high necrotic core burden, plaque rupture or thrombus (Figs 8.14A and B), either detected by IVUS or OCT, are associated with a higher risk of distal embolization and periprocedural myocardial infarction.[20-24]

In order to facilitate plaque characterization, spectral analysis of ultrasound signal has been incorporated into IVUS

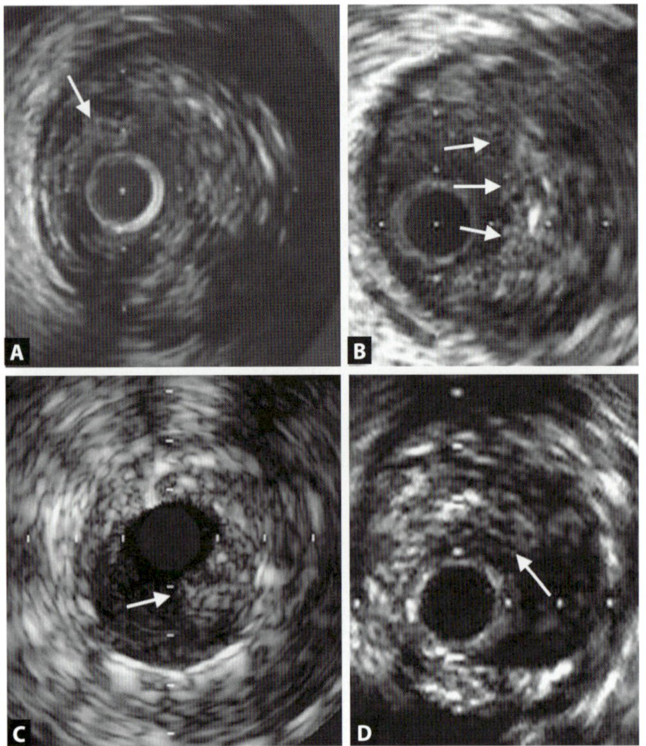

Figs 8.13A to D Examples of intracoronary thrombosis detected on IVUS. Fresh thrombus (A and B) is less bright than organized thrombus (C and D)

technology in order to provide virtual histology (VH), which can discriminate four types of tissue: calcium is represented in white, lipid-rich necrotic core in red, fibro-fatty plaque in light green and fibrous tissue in dark green.[25] However, compared to standard IVUS, VH has a lower resolution.

IVUS can also identify positive and negative vessel remodelling, defined as enlargement or narrowing of the EEM cross-sectional area at the site of lesion; beyond its role in appropriate stent sizing, positive remodelling has been linked to the presence of inflammation and vulnerable plaque.[26]

Lesion Severity Assessment

Both imaging methods are very precise in assessing the minimal lumen area (MLA) at the level of the plaque. However, unlike fractional flow reserve (FFR), there is not a universally accepted threshold for intervening. Broadly speaking, when trying to define the critical threshold for intravascular imaging data, two approaches have been applied in clinical studies:

1. Comparing intravascular imaging to FFR or to non-invasive functional tests, trying to identify a threshold for ischemia
2. Analyzing events in treated and untreated patients based on severity and morphology of baseline intravascular imaging assessment: in this regard, not only MLA is considered, but also plaque burden (which is better defined with IVUS) and histological features of the

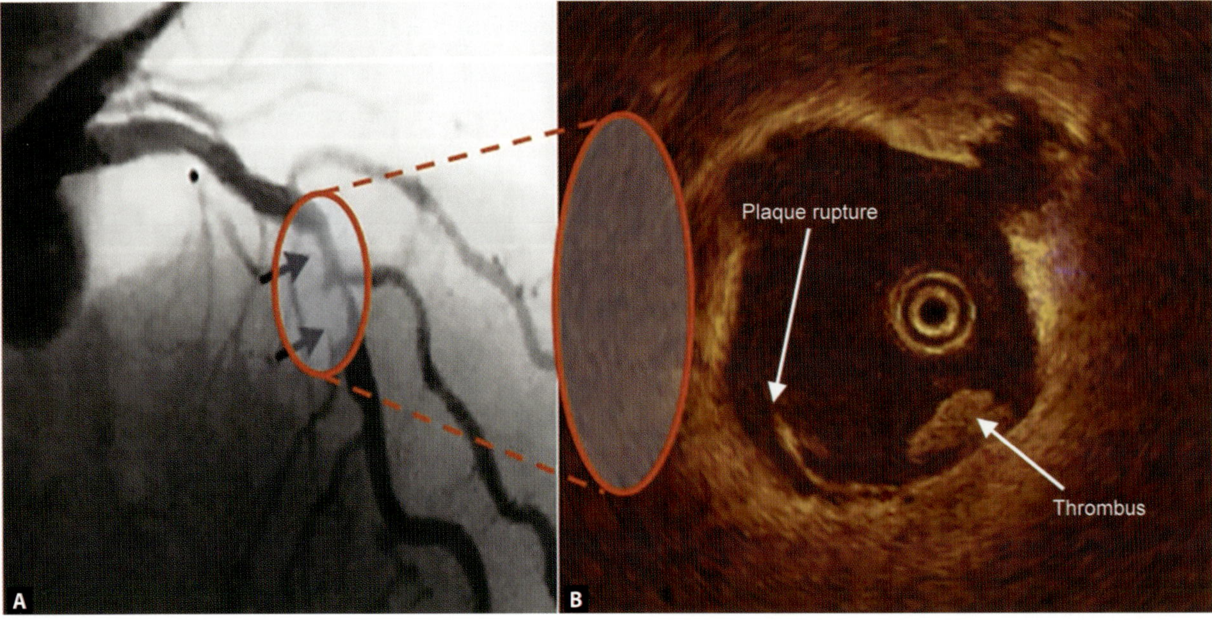

Figs 8.14A and B Angiography performed in a patient with acute coronary syndrome, showing severe stenosis at mid LAD; OCT performed at the same site showed a ruptured plaque with overlapped thrombus. These details are obtained with OCT (and not IVUS) and can be very useful for a more appropriate strategy selection

plaque (e.g. the presence of TCFA, which is instead better identified by OCT) have been taken into account by some Authors, in the hypothesis that PCI may "passivate" a lesion at risk.[27]

Although this latter hypothesis is fascinating, it has never been demonstrated that treating a plaque based on its vulnerable appearance can improve clinical outcomes. Therefore, provided that today the presence of an ischemia-generating lesion represents the most accepted indication for revascularization, IVUS and OCT have often been compared to FFR. In this regard, it is clear that the critical MLA value depends on reference vessel size; moreover, plaque length and features (e.g. smooth vs. uneven surface) may have a role in determining the pressure gradient across the lesion.

Naganuma et al. correlated IVUS with FFR in 132 non-LM intermediate lesions; in the overall cohort, a MLA value <2.70 mm^2 predicted an FFR <0.80 with 79.5% sensitivity and 76.3% specificity; the accuracy of IVUS could be incremented by considering a cutoff of 2.84 mm^2 in vessels ≥3 mm and 2.59 mm^2 for vessels with a reference diameter <3 mm.[28] However, the correlation with FFR and MLA was only moderate; plaque morphology in this study did not significantly affect FFR measurements.

D'Ascenzo et al., in a recently published metanalysis on >2500 patients investigated with both FFR and intravascular imaging, confirmed the modest predictive value of MLA (either defined by IVUS or OCT) in determining the functional significance of non-LM lesions.[29] On the other hand, a MLA value >4 mm^2 (except for LM lesions—see below) can rule out ischemia with a high negative predictive value.

In order to improve the predictive value of IVUS, Cho and colleagues tried to combine two different parameters, i.e. MLA and plaque burden: in their cohort of 945 lesions, they identified as optimal thresholds a MLA <3 mm^2 and a plaque burden >75%. However, combining these two parameters did not add to the diagnostic accuracy of IVUS in predicting FFR value; MLA retained a higher predictive value compared to plaque burden.[30]

IVUS in Assessment of Severity of LM Lesions

While the diagnostic accuracy for ischemia in non-LM lesions is only modest, IVUS has an established value in assessing severity of left main lesions;[29] due to the above-mentioned technical issues, limited data are available about the use of OCT in LM lesions.

Jasti et al., in a cohort of 55 ambiguous LM stenosis, found that an IVUS MLA of 5.9 mm^2 or an MLD of 2.8 mm were predictive of FFR < 0.75 with 93% sensitivity and 95% specificity.[31] Importantly, prognosis was excellent in patients with FFR ≥ 0.75 who were treated medically. These results were prospectively validated in the LITRO study, which enrolled 354 patients with intermediate LM lesions: in patients with a LM MLA >6 mm revascularization was deferred and the prognosis in medical therapy was excellent.[32]

According to Kang et al., an IVUS MLA of 4.8 and 4.1 mm^2 were predictive of an FFR value <0.80 and <0.75 respectively; however, no clinical follow-up was performed in this study.[33] All patients with a MLA >6 mm^2 had a negative FFR; 82% of patients with MLA <4.8 mm^2 had an FFR <0.80. The population examined in this study was Asian: it could therefore be hypothesized that the lower threshold identified in this paper may be linked to the lower body surface area of the study population. Interestingly, the authors found a high incidence of plaque rupture by IVUS (33%), and ruptured plaques had a lower FFR value than non-ruptured ones, even if average MLA was not significantly different.

Several IVUS studies have suggested that plaques with a different location in the LM may have different pathological features: lesions in the distal part or at the bifurcation often present a higher degree of plaque burden, are more frequently ruptured and calcified; ostial stenoses are instead frequently fibrotic, with a smaller plaque burden, and often show a recoil phenomenon after balloon angioplasty, reflecting the presence of elastic fibers.[34-36] Moreover, pre-PCI assessment of longitudinal vessel reconstruction may help in predicting the risk of carinal shifting after main vessel stenting.

Due to non-coaxial alignment, IVUS measurements may be falsely overestimated at the LCx ostium; sometimes, a pullback performed from the LCx will give different results also on the LM compared to a pullback performed from LAD: in these situations, it must be kept in mind that artefacts can lead to MLA overestimation (when the vessel lumen is imaged in a non-axial plane) but not to underestimation: the lower value should therefore be considered.

Procedure Optimization

After stent implantation, IVUS and OCT can identify stent underexpansion (i.e. an adequate minimal stent area (MSA) is not obtained based on the reference lumen diameter) and/or malapposition (presence of struts not in contact with the vessel wall—Figures 8.15A and B). Both situations can usually be corrected by postdilating the stent with adequately sized balloons at sufficient pressure (Figs 8.16 and 8.17); the pre-PCI use of intravascular imaging should minimize indeed the risk of stenting undilatable plaques, by suggesting appropriate lesion preparation in case of severe calcification. Both underexpansion and malapposition are linked to a higher incidence of stent thrombosis and restenosis. Maehara et al., in a post-hoc comparison of two prospective studies analysing IVUS- and OCT-guided PCI, found a comparable degree of stent expansion with the two methods.[37]

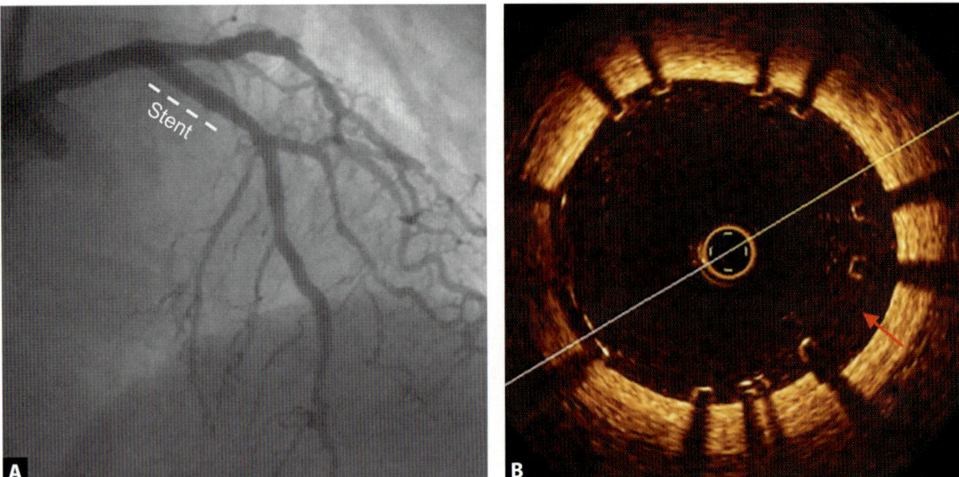

Figs 8.15A and B (A) Angio following stent deployment in proximal LAD, showing an excellent angiographic result; (B) OCT control at the same site, showing malapposition of the stent (arrows) not detected by angiography

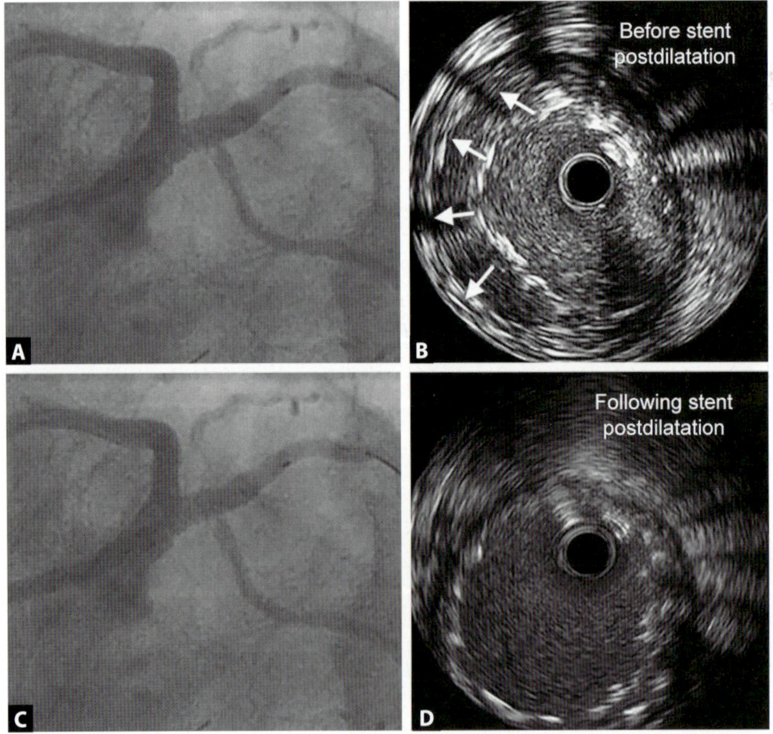

Figs 8.16A to D Optimization of PCI by IVUS guidance: (A) Angio following stent deployment in crossover from ostial LM to proximal LAD. Angiographic result seems optimal; (B) IVUS revealed a significant stent underexpansion and malapposition in LM; (C) Angio following postdilatation with larger, non-compliant balloon at high pressure, similar to the previous result in A; (D) IVUS check following postdilatation, showing full expansion and good apposition of the stent in LM

The AVIO (angiography Versus IVUS optimization) study proposed a minimal acceptable MSA based on stent size: a target area of at least 6 mm^2 should be obtained for a 3 mm stent; this target area is increased or decreased by 2 mm^2 for every 0.5 mm increase or decrease in stent size (e.g. 4 mm^2 for a 2.5 mm stent; 8 mm^2 for a 3.5 mm stent and so on).[38] This randomized trial showed a higher post-procedural lumen diameter for lesions assigned to IVUS-guided PCI, but—in contrast to the above-mentioned studies—failed to show a clinical benefit of IVUS in term of MACE reduction.

Both IVUS and OCT can easily assess completeness of lesion coverage, as well as the presence of gaps between

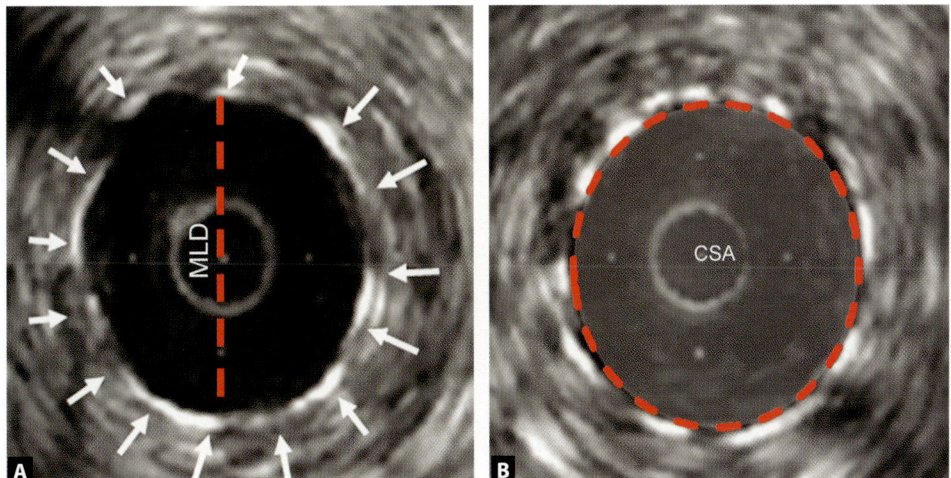

Figs 8.17A and B IVUS- guided stent expansion: optimal final MLD and final CSA (compared to reference MLD and CSA), full and circular expansion of the stent with homogeneous distribution of stent struts (arrows) and complete apposition of the stent to vessel wall

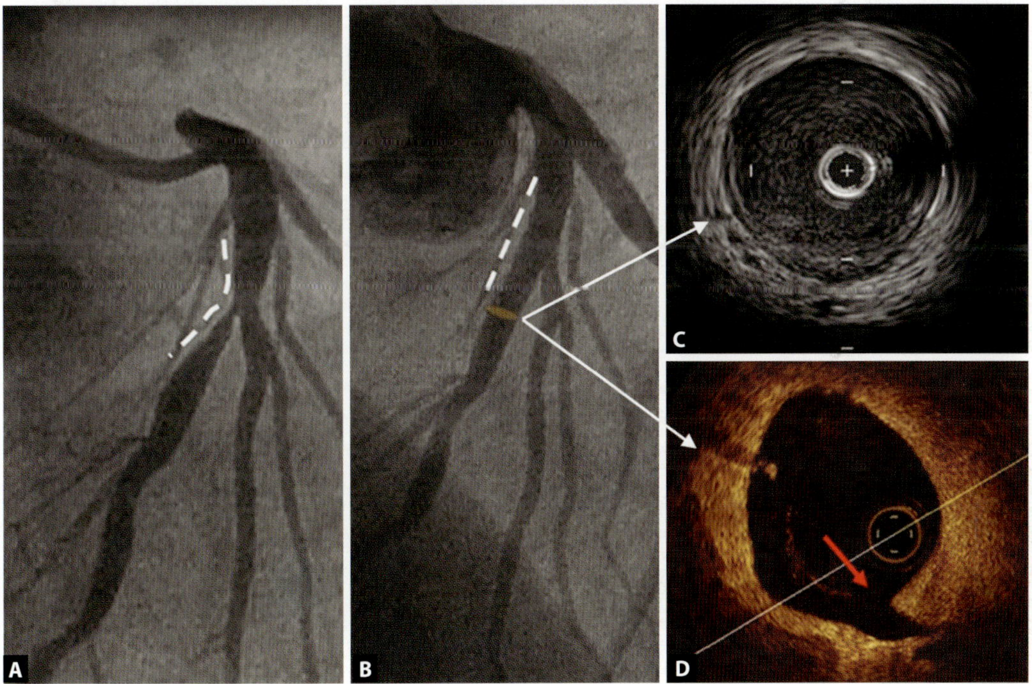

Figs 8.18A to D OCT and dissection: (A) Baseline angio in patients with LAD-I Diagonal bifurcation lesion (Medina 0,1,0); (B) Final angio after provisional T Stenting with single stent showing excellent final result; (C) Final IVUS at distal edge of the stent: no dissections are observed; (D) Final OCT at the same site (distal edge of the stent) showing a small dissection, missed by both angio and IVUS (arrow)

stents; the histological features of the plaque at stent edges could potentially have implications on the risk of subsequent target lesion failure.[39]

In a recently published paper on around 1'000 lesions treated with OCT-guided PCI, the Authors have identified signs of suboptimal stent implantation in nearly one third of cases; those signs included:

- Stent under expansion (MSA < 4.5 mm^2)
- Edge dissection (>200 μm in width)
- Reference lumen area <4.5 mm^2 at stent edges

- Malapposition >200 μm
- In-stent plaque prolapse/thrombus (defined as a mass >0.5 mm inside stent struts).

The presence of suboptimal stent deployment was an independent preditor of subsequent MACE at follow up.[40]

On the other hand, Chamié and colleagues identified stent edge dissections in nearly 40% of cases where OCT was used; the majority of these were not apparent at angiography, and only a minority of dissections detected by OCT were stented: untreated dissections had the same outcomes at 12 months compared to patients with no dissections, raising doubts about the clinical meaning of these findings (Figs 8.18A to D).[41]

IVUS also can detect angiographically silent edge dissections (Figs 8.19A and B) in around 10% of cases after stent implantation;[42,43] the natural history of these lesions appears however benign in most cases, provided that area of stenosis at the dissection site is <60%.[44]

Intravascular imaging is particularly useful in evaluating PCI at bifurcation sites (Figs 8.20A and B): indeed, in this setting (and particulary at side-branch ostium) malapposition and incomplete lesion coverage frequently occur; moreover, OCT and IVUS can detect and quantify jailing of the side-branch ostium, and OCT can provide high quality 3D reconstructions of bifurcation anatomy (Figs 8.21A and B). The use of IVUS for bifurcation stenting has been associated with better long-term survival and outcomes.[8]

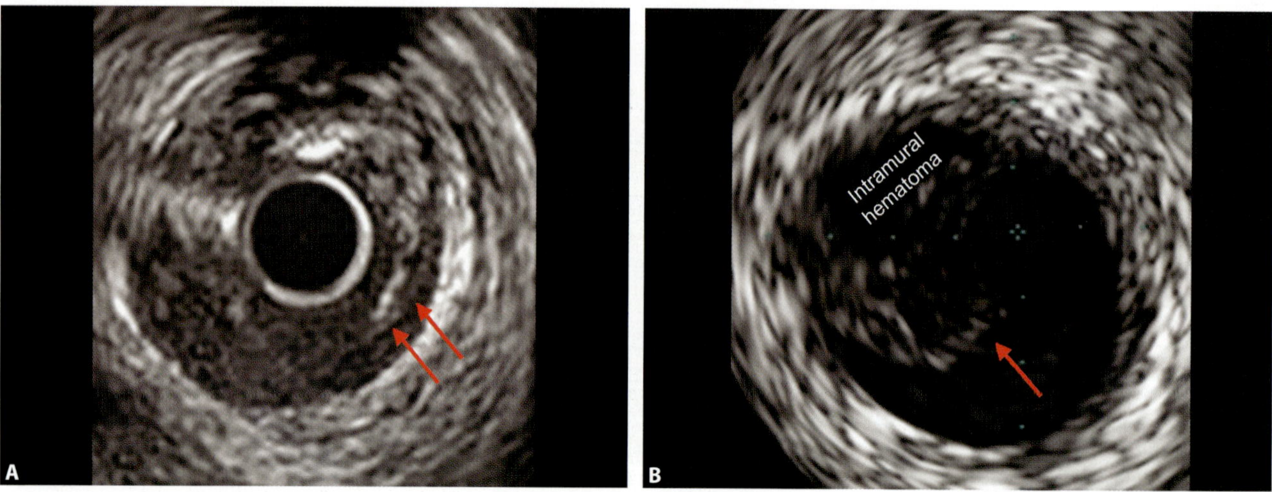

Figs 8.19A and B Coronary dissection: Dissecting intimal flap is well recognized (A—arrows), associated with intramural hematoma (B)

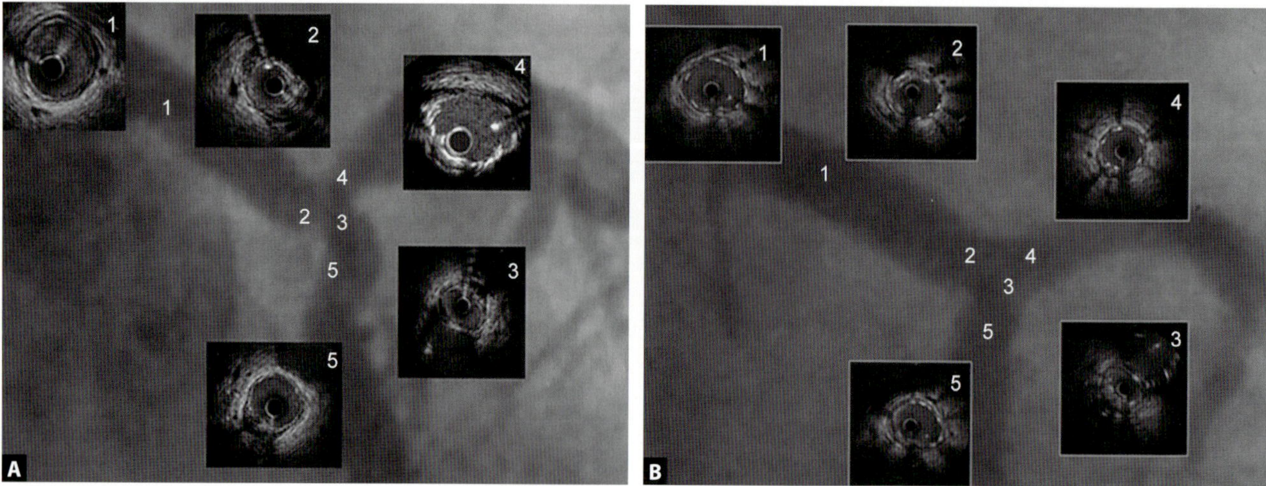

Figs 8.20A and B IVUS-guided left main bifurcation PCI: (A) Distal left main lesion defined by IVUS: IVUS images at LM shaft (1), distal LM (2), carina (3), ostial LAD (4) and ostial LCX (5), showing Medina 1,1,1 lesion; (B) Final IVUS check following PCI with two stent strategy (modified T approach) and post-dilatation at high pressure with appropriately sized NC balloons and final kissing, showing optimal ostial coverage and stent expansion and apposition at all checked sites: LM shaft (1), distal LM (2), carina (3), ostial LAD (4) and ostial LCX (5)

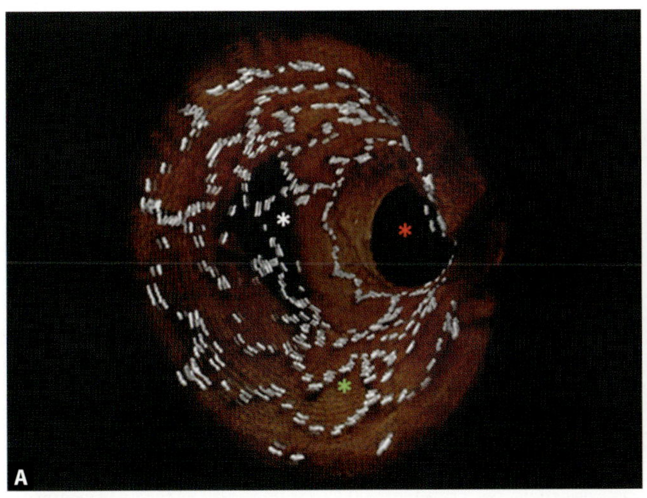

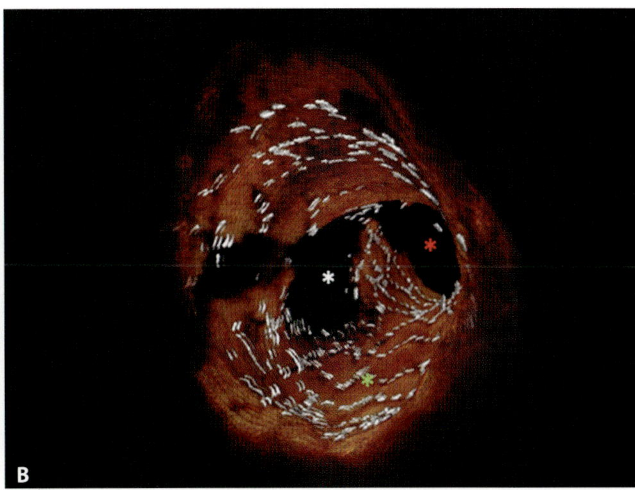

Figs 8.21A and B Peri-procedural use of OCT: 3D-OCT volume rendering provides a unique 3D imaging reconstruction of the stent, allowing the assessment of struts crossing by guide wires as well as stent deformation during complex bifurcation stenting procedures
Courtesy: Dr Y Fujino

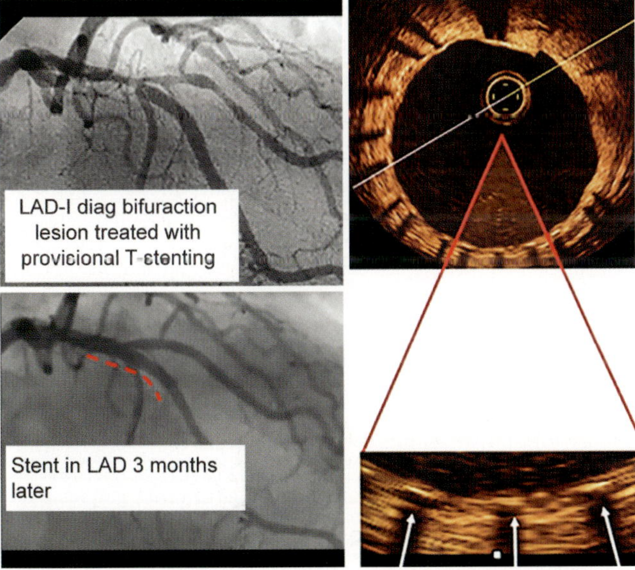

Fig. 8.22 OCT for the evaluation of vessel healing after stenting: OCT in LAD three months following II generation DES deployment, showing complete coverage of stent struts, which can be well observed on the magnified segment of the OCT image. The arrows indicate the covered struts

Long-term Post-PCI Assessment

OCT, due to its high resolution, is the method of choice for assessing stent struts coverage by endothelium (Fig. 8.22); this finding, beyond its usefulness in research, might guide the indication for dual antiplatelet therapy duration in selected patients.

Neointimal tissue is depicted in high detail by OCT, and different patterns of neointimal growth have been identified; however, the clinical significance of these findings is currently poorly understood. In particular, OCT can identify the presence of in-stent "neo-atherosclerosis", which is often implicated in restenosis manifesting late and/or with unstable angina, and probably reflects a totally different phenomenon from restenosis due to excessive intimal proliferation.[45]

A limitation of OCT in stented segment is instead represented by shadowing beyond struts, which hampers visualization of vessel wall behind the stent.

In analyzing stent failure, intravascular imaging can provide clues for its causes, such as underexpansion, malapposition (either early- or late-acquired), fracture, incomplete strut coverage, high residual plaque burden or dissection at stent edges: identification of these conditions is paramount in applying the most appropriate treatment in order to prevent further restenosis or thrombosis.

A particular role of intravascular imaging is represented by long-term assessment after bioresorbable scaffold (BRS) implantation, as it can identify struts degradation and assess vascular remodelling and motility after resolution of the "caging" effect.[46] BRS struts appear at IVUS as a double bright lign, while at OCT they are imaged as black boxes without backscattering.

REFERENCES

1. Ahn JM, Kang SJ, Yoon SH, Park HW, Kang SM, Lee JY, et al. Meta-analysis of outcomes after intravascular ultrasound-guided versus angiography-guided drug-eluting stent implantation in 26,503 patients enrolled in three randomized trials and 14 observational studies. The American Journal of Cardiology. 2014;113(8):1338-47.
2. Jang JS, Song YJ, Kang W, Jin HY, Seo JS, Yang TH, et al. Intravascular ultrasound-guided implantation of drug-eluting

stents to improve outcome: a meta-analysis. JACC Cardiovascular Interventions. 2014;7(3):233-43.

3. Zhang Y, Farooq V, Garcia-Garcia HM, Bourantas CV, Tian N, Dong S, et al. Comparison of intravascular ultrasound versus angiography-guided drug-eluting stent implantation: a meta-analysis of one randomised trial and ten observational studies involving 19,619 patients. EuroIntervention : journal of EuroPCR in collaboration with the Working Group on Interventional Cardiology of the European Society of Cardiology. 2012;8(7):855-65.
4. Singh V, Badheka AO, Arora S, Panaich SS, Patel NJ, Patel N, et al. Comparison of inhospital mortality, length of hospitalization, costs, and vascular complications of percutaneous coronary interventions guided by ultrasound versus angiography. The American Journal of Cardiology. 2015;115(10):1357-66.
5. Hong SJ, Kim BK, Shin DH, Kim JS, Hong MK, Gwon HC, et al. Usefulness of intravascular ultrasound guidance in percutaneous coronary intervention with second-generation drug-eluting stents for chronic total occlusions (from the Multicenter Korean-Chronic Total Occlusion Registry). The American Journal of Cardiology. 2014;114(4):534-40.
6. Patel Y, Depta JP, Patel JS, Masrani SK, Novak E, Zajarias A, et al. Impact of intravascular ultrasound on the long-term clinical outcomes in the treatment of coronary ostial lesions. Catheterization and cardiovascular interventions: official journal of the Society for Cardiac Angiography & Interventions. 2013.
7. Witzenbichler B, Maehara A, Weisz G, Neumann FJ, Rinaldi MJ, Metzger DC, et al. Relationship between intravascular ultrasound guidance and clinical outcomes after drug-eluting stents: the assessment of dual antiplatelet therapy with drug-eluting stents (ADAPT-DES) study. Circulation. 2014;129(4):463-70.
8. Kim SH, Kim YH, Kang SJ, Park DW, Lee SW, Lee CW, et al. Long-term outcomes of intravascular ultrasound-guided stenting in coronary bifurcation lesions. The American Journal of Cardiology. 2010;106(5):612-8.
9. Park SJ, Kim YH, Park DW, Lee SW, Kim WJ, Suh J, et al. Impact of intravascular ultrasound guidance on long-term mortality in stenting for unprotected left main coronary artery stenosis. Circulation Cardiovascular Interventions. 2009;2(3):167-77.
10. Paulo M, Sandoval J, Lennie V, Dutary J, Medina M, Gonzalo N, et al. Combined use of OCT and IVUS in spontaneous coronary artery dissection. JACC Cardiovascular Imaging. 2013;6(7):830-2.
11. Kume T, Okura H, Kawamoto T, Yamada R, Miyamoto Y, Hayashida A, et al. Assessment of the coronary calcification by optical coherence tomography. EuroIntervention : journal of EuroPCR in collaboration with the Working Group on Interventional Cardiology of the European Society of Cardiology. 2011;6(6):768-72.
12. Mudra H, Regar E, Klauss V, Werner F, Henneke KH, Sbarouni E, et al. Serial follow-up after optimized ultrasound-guided deployment of Palmaz-Schatz stents. In-stent neointimal proliferation without significant reference segment response. Circulation. 1997;95(2):363-70.
13. Fujino Y, Bezerra HG, Attizzani GF, Wang W, Yamamoto H, Chamie D, et al. Frequency-domain optical coherence tomography assessment of unprotected left main coronary artery disease-a comparison with intravascular ultrasound. Catheterization and cardiovascular interventions : official journal of the Society for Cardiac Angiography & Interventions. 2013;82(3):E173-83.
14. Moussa I, Di Mario C, Moses J, Reimers B, Di Francesco L, Martini G, et al. Coronary stenting after rotational atherectomy in calcified and complex lesions. Angiographic and clinical follow-up results. Circulation. 1997;96(1):128-36.
15. Lindsay AC, Paulo M, Kadriye K, Tejeiro R, Alegria-Barrero E, Chan PH, et al. Predictors of stent strut malapposition in calcified vessels using frequency-domain optical coherence tomography. The Journal of Invasive Cardiology. 2013;25(9):429-34.
16. Low AF, Kawase Y, Chan YH, Tearney GJ, Bouma BE, Jang IK. In vivo characterisation of coronary plaques with conventional grey-scale intravascular ultrasound: correlation with optical coherence tomography. EuroIntervention: Journal of EuroPCR in Collaboration with the Working Group on Interventional Cardiology of the European Society of Cardiology. 2009;4(5):626-32.
17. Tearney GJ, Yabushita H, Houser SL, Aretz HT, Jang IK, Schlendorf KH, et al. Quantification of macrophage content in atherosclerotic plaques by optical coherence tomography. Circulation. 2003;107(1):113-9.
18. Moreno PR, Falk E, Palacios IF, Newell JB, Fuster V, Fallon JT. Macrophage infiltration in acute coronary syndromes. Implications for plaque rupture. Circulation. 1994;90(2):775-8.
19. Kume T, Akasaka T, Kawamoto T, Ogasawara Y, Watanabe N, Toyota E, et al. Assessment of coronary arterial thrombus by optical coherence tomography. The American Journal of Cardiology. 2006;97(12):1713-7.
20. Jang JS, Jin HY, Seo JS, Yang TH, Kim DK, Park YA, et al. Meta-analysis of plaque composition by intravascular ultrasound and its relation to distal embolization after percutaneous coronary intervention. The American Journal of Cardiology. 2013;111(7):968-72.
21. Uetani T, Amano T, Ando H, Yokoi K, Arai K, Kato M, et al. The correlation between lipid volume in the target lesion, measured by integrated backscatter intravascular ultrasound, and post-procedural myocardial infarction in patients with elective stent implantation. European Heart Journal. 2008;29(14):1714-20.
22. Shibuya M, Okamura A, Hao H, Date M, Higuchi Y, Nagai H, et al. Prediction of distal embolization during percutaneous coronary intervention for unstable plaques with grayscale and integrated backscatter intravascular ultrasound. Catheterization and cardiovascular interventions : official Journal of the Society for Cardiac Angiography & Interventions. 2013;81(3):E165-72.
23. Lee T, Yonetsu T, Koura K, Hishikari K, Murai T, Iwai T, et al. Impact of coronary plaque morphology assessed by optical coherence tomography on cardiac troponin elevation in patients with elective stent implantation. Circulation Cardiovascular interventions. 2011;4(4):378-86.
24. Tanaka A, Imanishi T, Kitabata H, Kubo T, Takarada S, Tanimoto T, et al. Lipid-rich plaque and myocardial perfusion after successful stenting in patients with non-ST-segment elevation acute coronary syndrome: an optical coherence tomography study. European Heart Journal. 2009;30(11):1348-55.
25. Garcia-Garcia HM, Gogas BD, Serruys PW, Bruining N. IVUS-based imaging modalities for tissue characterization: similarities and differences. The International Journal of Cardiovascular Imaging. 2011;27(2):215-24.
26. Pasterkamp G, Schoneveld AH, van der Wal AC, Haudenschild CC, Clarijs RJ, Becker AE, et al. Relation of arterial geometry

to luminal narrowing and histologic markers for plaque vulnerability: the remodeling paradox. Journal of the American College of Cardiology. 1998;32(3):655-62.

27. Bourantas CV, Serruys PW, Nakatani S, Zhang YJ, Farooq V, Diletti R, et al. Bioresorbable vascular scaffold treatment induces the formation of neointimal cap that seals the underlying plaque without compromising the luminal dimensions: a concept based on serial optical coherence tomography data. EuroIntervention : journal of EuroPCR in collaboration with the Working Group on Interventional Cardiology of the European Society of Cardiology. 2015;11(8):746-56.
28. Naganuma T, Latib A, Costopoulos C, Takagi K, Naim C, Sato K, et al. The role of intravascular ultrasound and quantitative angiography in the functional assessment of intermediate coronary lesions: correlation with fractional flow reserve. Cardiovascular revascularization medicine : including molecular interventions. 2014;15(1):3-7.
29. D'Ascenzo F, Barbero U, Cerrato E, Lipinski MJ, Omede P, Montefusco A, et al. Accuracy of intravascular ultrasound and optical coherence tomography in identifying functionally significant coronary stenosis according to vessel diameter: A meta-analysis of 2,581 patients and 2,807 lesions. American heart journal. 2015;169(5):663-73.
30. Cho YK, Nam CW, Han JK, Koo BK, Doh JH, Ben-Dor I, et al. Usefulness of combined intravascular ultrasound parameters to predict functional significance of coronary artery stenosis and determinants of mismatch. EuroIntervention : journal of EuroPCR in collaboration with the Working Group on Interventional Cardiology of the European Society of Cardiology. 2015;11(2):163-70.
31. Jasti V, Ivan E, Yalamanchili V, Wongpraparut N, Leesar MA. Correlations between fractional flow reserve and intravascular ultrasound in patients with an ambiguous left main coronary artery stenosis. Circulation. 2004;110(18):2831-6.
32. de la Torre Hernandez JM, Hernandez Hernandez F, Alfonso F, Rumoroso JR, Lopez-Palop R, Sadaba M, et al. Prospective application of pre-defined intravascular ultrasound criteria for assessment of intermediate left main coronary artery lesions results from the multicenter LITRO study. Journal of the American College of Cardiology. 2011;58(4):351-8.
33. Kang SJ, Lee JY, Ahn JM, Song HG, Kim WJ, Park DW, et al. Intravascular ultrasound-derived predictors for fractional flow reserve in intermediate left main disease. JACC Cardiovascular Interventions. 2011;4(11):1168-74.
34. Sano K, Mintz GS, Carlier SG, de Ribamar Costa J, Jr., Qian J, Missel E, et al. Assessing intermediate left main coronary lesions using intravascular ultrasound. American heart journal. 2007;154(5):983-8.
35. Maehara A, Mintz GS, Castagna MT, Pichard AD, Satler LF, Waksman R, et al. Intravascular ultrasound assessment of the stenoses location and morphology in the left main coronary artery in relation to anatomic left main length. The American journal of cardiology. 2001;88(1):1-4.
36. Tyczynski P, Pregowski J, Mintz GS, Witkowski A, Kim SW, Waksman R, et al. Intravascular ultrasound assessment of ruptured atherosclerotic plaques in left main coronary arteries. The American journal of cardiology. 2005;96(6):794-8.
37. Maehara A, Ben-Yehuda O, Ali Z, Wijns W, Bezerra HG, Shite J, et al. Comparison of Stent Expansion Guided by Optical Coherence Tomography Versus Intravascular Ultrasound: The ILUMIEN II Study (Observational Study of Optical Coherence Tomography [OCT] in Patients Undergoing Fractional Flow Reserve [FFR] and Percutaneous Coronary Intervention). JACC Cardiovascular interventions. 2015;8(13):1704-14.
38. Chieffo A, Latib A, Caussin C, Presbitero P, Galli S, Menozzi A, et al. A prospective, randomized trial of intravascular-ultrasound guided compared to angiography guided stent implantation in complex coronary lesions: the AVIO trial. American Heart Journal. 2013;165(1):65-72.
39. Gonzalo N, Serruys PW, Okamura T, Shen ZJ, Garcia-Garcia HM, Onuma Y, et al. Relation between plaque type and dissections at the edges after stent implantation: an optical coherence tomography study. International Journal of Cardiology. 2011;150(2):151-5.
40. Prati F, Romagnoli E, Burzotta F, Limbruno U, Gatto L, La Manna A, et al. Clinical Impact of OCT Findings During PCI: The CLI-OPCI II Study. JACC Cardiovascular Imaging. 2015;8(11): 1297-305.
41. Chamie D, Bezerra HG, Attizzani GF, Yamamoto H, Kanaya T, Stefano GT, et al. Incidence, predictors, morphological characteristics, and clinical outcomes of stent edge dissections detected by optical coherence tomography. JACC Cardiovascular interventions. 2013;6(8):800-13.
42. Sheris SJ, Canos MR, Weissman NJ. Natural history of intravascular ultrasound-detected edge dissections from coronary stent deployment. American Heart Journal. 2000;139(1 Pt 1):59-63.
43. Liu X, Tsujita K, Maehara A, Mintz GS, Weisz G, Dangas GD, et al. Intravascular ultrasound assessment of the incidence and predictors of edge dissections after drug-eluting stent implantation. JACC Cardiovascular Interventions. 2009;2(10): 997-1004.
44. Nishida T, Colombo A, Briguori C, Stankovic G, Albiero R, Corvaja N, et al. Outcome of nonobstructive residual dissections detected by intravascular ultrasound following percutaneous coronary intervention. The American Journal of Cardiology. 2002;89(11):1257-62.
45. Kang SJ, Mintz GS, Akasaka T, Park DW, Lee JY, Kim WJ, et al. Optical coherence tomographic analysis of in-stent neoatherosclerosis after drug-eluting stent implantation. Circulation. 2011;123(25):2954-63.
46. Serruys PW, Ormiston JA, Onuma Y, Regar E, Gonzalo N, Garcia-Garcia HM, et al. A bioabsorbable everolimus-eluting coronary stent system (ABSORB): 2-year outcomes and results from multiple imaging methods. Lancet. 2009;373(9667): 897-910.

CHAPTER

9 Difficult Situations of Angioplasty: Ectasia/Aneurysm and Thrombus

Anish Chandarana

INTRODUCTION

Coronary artery ectasia (CAE) represents a form of atherosclerotic coronary artery disease (CAD) in majority and it is seen in 3–8% of patients undergoing coronary angiography. The presence of ectatic segments produces sluggish blood flow and clinically presents as exercise-induced angina or myocardial infarction (MI), regardless of the severity of coexisting stenotic coronary disease. Though, some understanding about the pathophysiology and natural history of this disease has developed over last 2–3 decades, many uncertainties related to diagnosis, methods of follow-up and application of various management strategies for these patients still prevail due to lack of robust clinical data. Patients of CAE with or without associated atherosclerotic CAD present extra challenges when they have to undergo percutaneous coronary intervention (PCI) due to uneven geometry, endothelial dysfunction (ED) and thromboembolism (TE). Special efforts are required to deal with large burden of intracoronary (IC) thrombus, which is present in most such cases. Deciding the need, timing and type of stent becomes a more serious consideration in a patient who has CAE than one who does not. Intravascular ultrasound (IVUS) and optical coherence tomography (OCT) have great potential to help in optimizing results of PCI in such patients with varied coronary anatomy and physiology.

DEFINITION AND PREVALENCE

Coronary artery ectasia, or aneurysmal CAD, is defined as dilatation of an arterial segment to a diameter at least 1.5 times that of the adjacent normal coronary artery or the largest segment of any coronary artery of the same individual in case if the same coronary artery has no normal segment.[1-3] CAE can be found in up to 4.9% of angiographic and in 0.2–1.4% of autopsy series. The largest study carried out in the context was Coronary Artery Surgery Study (CASS), in which 20,087 patients were studied, among whom 978 (4.9%) were found to have coronary ectasia.[4-7] A very high incidence of 10–12% has been found in Indian population with diverse demographic characteristics.[8] The CAE can be either diffuse, affecting the entire or most of the length of a coronary artery (ectasia), or localized (saccular or fusiform). It may be limited to one vessel or may involve multiple vessels, and based on extent of involvement Markis has suggested a classification of this disease. CAE is attributed to atherosclerosis in almost 50% of cases, whereas rest 50% cases can be attributed to congenital or other wide variety of acquired causes. In the great majority of these patients, ectasia coexists with atherosclerotic coronary artery disease.[2,9,10] Atherosclerotic CAE should also be differentiated from coronary aneurysms following coronary interventions. These include true or pseudo-aneurysms during coronary balloon angioplasty, following coronary stent placement, atherectomy and brachytherapy.[11,12] Occasionally, large ulcerated coronary plaques can be misinterpreted angiographically as coronary aneurysms.[13-15] Studies have documented the association of CAE with the presence of aneurysms in other vascular beds as well, probably owing to a common underlying pathogenetic mechanism. CAE has been seen more frequently in patients with aneurysms of the abdominal and ascending aorta. In one retrospective study, 8% of patients operated for abdominal aortic aneurysm had CAE, compared with 2.9% of patients who were operated for occlusive peripheral vascular disease.[16-18]

PATHOGENESIS

Studies of coronary arterial wall pathology highlighted the lack of uniformity in CAE. In patients with mixed CAE, Swanton et al. reported similar histological appearance to that of atherosclerosis with marked destruction and reduction of the medial elastic fibers with disruption of the internal and external elastic laminae.[3] On the other hand, the pure form of CAE showed smooth muscle hyalinization of the coronary fibromuscular media leaving the intima intact.[19] The hyalinization process has been linked to excessive nitric oxide (NO) production.[20,21] It has also been postulated that it represents a generalized deficit of the wall of the entire arterial system.[22,23] A theory of remodeling as pathological process has also been suggested based on the finding that early compensatory enlargement of human atherosclerotic coronary arteries occurs even before noticeable luminal narrowing, simulating CAE appearance.[24] The literature data failed to provide a pathognomonic biomarker for CAE; the ones quoted are known to be already abnormal in atherosclerosis and consequently would explain the same inflammatory response, with some markers quite higher in CAE than in atherosclerosis. Conventional inflammatory markers like cytokines, tumor necrosis factor (TNF) and interleukin 6 (IL-6) have been found to be elevated in 50% of CAE patients, particularly in those with evidence for atherosclerosis but have failed to differentiate between the two conditions.[25] Markers like inflammatory cells, e.g. leukocytes count; monocyte count and C-reactive protein are closely linked to the presence of CAE, although not specific.[26] Soluble adhesion molecules (e.g. intereclectar adhesion maleule (ICAM) and vascular cell adhesion molecule (VCAM) were also found to be higher in isolated CAE as well as in CAE with occlusive CAD compared with occlusive coronaries without CAE. These findings suggest that more severe coronary wall inflammation may play a role in CAE pathogenesis.[27]

CLINICAL COURSE AND NATURAL HISTORY

Although this entity has been the subject of many studies, a complete and comprehensive clinical picture has not emerged. CAE is considered an accompaniment or a variant of coronary atherosclerosis in many cases.[7] It has been suggested that the presence of the aneurysmal segments produces sluggish or turbulent blood flow, with an increased incidence of ischemic manifestations or occurrence of an acute MI as a result, regardless of the actual severity of the coexisting stenotic coronary lesions.[3,5,8] It has been postulated that patients with coronary ectasia but without significant coexistent CAD have a higher incidence of adverse events than individuals with normal coronary arteries. And similarly, it has been postulated that patients having significant stenotic CAD with ectasia do worse than patients having significant stenotic CAD without ectasia. Presence of ectasia has been historically considered to incur additional risk to the patients.[5,10]

Discrete aneurysms are much less common than diffuse ectasia and they are almost never found in arteries without severe stenosis. The underlying disease is more severe in patients with discrete aneurysms than in those with diffuse ectasia. Discrete aneurysms are more common in the left anterior descending coronary artery (LAD) while diffuse ectatic disease is more common in the right coronary artery (RCA).[28,29] Male sex predominates in CAE.[4,30] A positive family history and hypertension have been cited.[5] Hypercholesterolemia seems to be a predisposing factor; in one report, familial hypercholesterolemia was accompanied by coronary ectasia in 15% of patients, as compared with 2–5% of an age and sex matched control group.[31] Age seems to have no additional influence according to most investigators.[8]

Coronary artery disease (CAD) seems to be the main underlying etiology for CAE,[32] since 84.7% in the study by Vissilios et al.[29] 90.8% in CASS,[8] and 82.5% in the series of Farto-e-Abreu et al.[33] had coexisting stenotic CAD. Findings by Vissilios et al. indicated that, with a similar number of significant obstructive coronary lesions, exercise tolerance, incidence of angina pectoris or a previous Q-wave or non-Q-wave MI, and events at follow-up are comparable in patients of CAD with and without coronary ectasia. Patients with ectasia and insignificant CAD present with a definitely more benign picture. These patients with coronary ectasia and without significant CAD had a lower incidence of a previous MI, a higher exercise time and left ventricular ejection fraction, and significantly better follow-up results than patients with coexisting CAD. The CASS study also showed almost similar results. Patients with aneurysmal CAD were compared with patients with similar degree of stenotic CAD but without ectasia. In these two groups, no significant differences were noted when adjustment for arteriographic and ventriculographic findings was carried out, except for the fact that patients with aneurysmal disease had a higher incidence of documented MI. Patients with aneurysmal disease but with insignificant or no CAD were compared with those with no significant obstructive or aneurysmal disease. They found no difference between these two groups.[29]

Thus, it can be concluded that patients with coronary ectasia and coronary obstructive disease are almost similar in every respect to those with similar coronary obstructive disease but without ectasia. And though, pure ectasia is comparatively a quite benign disease, it is not completely innocuous, since there is a conspicuous difference in incidence of a previous MI and angina. This supports the notion that slow flow (SF), *in situ* thrombosis and distal embolization from mural thrombus within the ectatic segment may occur even in the absence of atherosclerotic lesions.

CLINICAL PRESENTATIONS AND DIAGNOSIS

Coronary artery ectasia (CAE) may be detected in the absence of symptoms; however, patients sometimes present with exercise-induced angina pectoris due to myocardial ischemia without coincident significant coronary artery stenosis, acute MI, or sudden death. Complications such as thrombus formation, distal embolization, shunt formation and rupture can occur, but the absolute risk is not known.[34-37] MI may also occur in the absence of significant coronary artery stenosis and is usually attributed to distal microembolization or thrombotic occlusion of an ectatic segment. Even though volumetric coronary blood flow is significantly higher in CAE, microvascular dysfunction that is reflected as reduced coronary flow reserve may be the underlying cause of myocardial ischemia, especially during exercise in patients with CAE.[38,39]

Cornary artery ectasia (CAE) may be detected noninvasively using echocardiography, computed tomography (CT), and magnetic resonance imaging (MRI).[34] Rare cases of giant coronary aneurysms can cause a pronounced bulge of the heart counter on chest X-rays.[40] The standard of reference for diagnosis of coronary aneurysm is coronary angiography (CAG), which provides information about the size, shape, location, and number of aneurysms.[41] Even CAG may be false negative, if the native vessel occludes.[35] Some aneurysms are detected calcified during angiography evaluation.[42,43] IVUS examination allows for distinguishing true from false aneurysms. In the former, the aneurysmal wall contains the medial tissue that shows continuity with the media of the adjacent normal coronary segment; in the latter, the aneurysm is limited only by adventitial tissue or even just by the visceral pericardium.[44] CAE may also break through to the right atrium, right ventricle, or coronary sinus, creating left to-right shunts.[34,35] If a rupture into a heart chamber occurs, a continuous murmur may be present and cardiac decompensation may ensue,[34] while a rupture into pericardium produces massive hemopericardium and cardiac tamponade.[45] Rapid enlargement of coronary aneurysms has also been reported.[46]

MEDICAL MANAGEMENT

Optimizing medications is of paramount importance in CAE patients, irrespective of the fact whether additional PCI or surgery is to be performed.

Risk Factors Modification

It has been strongly advocated that all patients with angiographic evidence of CAE should receive aggressive modification of coronary risk factors whether or not obstructive CAD is present.[47] This is to be achieved through therapeutic lifestyle changes and guideline based medicines as and when required.

Antiplatelet and Anticoagulation Treatment

To avoid thromboembolism, antiplatelet and anticoagulation therapies are reasonable and probably beneficial despite lack of evidence-based medicine.[35]

Aspirin has been the gold standard single agent used for this entity. Role of addition of the second antiplatelet agent (clopidogrel or prasugrel or ticagrelor) for primary prevention, in asymptomatic or symptomatic patients without history of intervention has not been well documented.

Since the follow-up course of the patients of CAE with or without coexisting stenotic disease is favorable, the recommendation for systemic anticoagulation instead of aspirin may need to be reconsidered.[3] This recommendation is based on case studies or at the most, study of a very small number of patients with ectasia and that has been reiterated since then without any controlled, randomized trials.[48] Anticoagulation carries a certain risk of hemorrhage. The expected ischemic benefits of anticoagulation must far outweigh the dangers of hemorrhage to make a routine use of oral anticoagulant drug.[49] With no infarcts or death in two years in the series of Vissilios P et al. and in five years in the series of Farto-e-Abreu,.[33] it would be difficult to justify classically defined anticoagulant treatment, unless mini-dose anticoagulation was employed. However, very large numbers of patients would be required for such a study.

Renin-angiotensin Aldosterone System (RAAS) Inhibitors

Based on the association of angiotensin converting enzyme (ACE) gene polymorphism and CAE, ACE inhibitors could be useful in the suppression of CAE progression, but this has yet to be proven.[50] Obviously, multiple trials have suggested positive role of these agents in preventing adverse cardio and cerebrovascular events in high-risk patients.

Statin Therapy

Because elevated matrix metalloproteinase (MMP)-3 levels likely contribute to the development of coronary aneurysms, some statins could be beneficial by inhibiting MMP-3 activity.[40] Though no such dedicated large trial has been done, it is reasonable to believe that statins due to their pleiotropic actions can help reduce symptoms and events in CAE patients with or without obstructive CAD.

Vasodilator and Antianginal Treatment

Trimetazidine can also improve coronary flow in CAE by increasing plasma adenosine levels. However, administration of nitroglycerin and nitrate derivates may induce angina pectoris in patients with CAE and should be avoided.[36] Beta-blockers and calcium channel blockers would be preferable agents to help angina.

PERCUTANEOUS INTERVENTION IN CORONARY ARTERY ECTASIA

coronary artery ectasia (CAE) produces a serious challenge to the interventional world. Indications for intervention are generally the same as they are for patients without CAE. Mainly they include (1) effort angina not well controlled with medicines or with high-risk features during stress test; (2) acute coronary syndrome (ACS) with ST-segment elevation MI (STEMI), as primary or rescue PCI or as a part of pharmacoinvasive approach and (3) ACS without ST-segment elevation when there are features of high risk; in the presence of significant obstruction to coronary blood flow risking sizable part of myocardium. Uneven geometry with variable internal dimensions, frequent presence of thrombus with high chance of distal embolization, inherent endothelial dysfunction and the presentation, which is ACS, more often than not, make decision process and procedure itself very complex.

IMAGING TO HELP CORONARY ANGIOGRAPHY

Coronary Angiography

It is the gold standard tool to help in diagnosing CAE, assessing the need of intervention, planning the revascularization strategy and confirming the adequacy of the procedure. Inherent limitations of CAG to depict the precise anatomy and its functional significance are well known to the interventional world. These limitations are further exaggerated in a patient with CAE due to many reasons.

Though we get basic information like presence, severity and length of lesions; diameter of the vessel wall at the site of the lesion and in normal segments; thrombolysis in myocardial infarction (TIMI) blood flow and tissue myocardial perfusion (TMP) blush grade in the concerned artery and its supply territory; presence of thrombus, calcium and spontaneous coronary artery dissection (SCAD); stent expansion and edge dissection, etc. CAG by itself is rarely sufficient to comprehensively help the interventionalist to make a decision regarding need of intervening and performance measures to optimize the acute and long-term results.

Three other technologies can be of great additional help in selected patients with CAE. For reasons already discussed, these technologies could be of much more importance in patients with CAE than in patients who have significant CAD without CAE.

Intravascular Ultrasound

Intravascular ultrasound (IVUS) provides valuable information regarding cross-sectional coronary vascular structure. It plays a key role in percutaneous coronary intervention (PCI) by accurately assessing coronary anatomy, assisting in selection of treatment strategy, and defining optimal stenting outcomes.[51-53] IVUS-guided PCI with bare metal stent (BMS) has been shown to be associated with a lower risk of angiographic restenosis and target vessel revascularization (TVR) than PCI guided by angiography alone.[54,55] A meta-analysis reported the benefit of IVUS-guided drug eluting stent (DES) implantation compared with angiography-guided implantation in reducing the risk of death, MI, stent thrombosis (ST) and repeat revascularization.[56]

The major use for IVUS is to plan interventional strategy and optimize stent deployment. IVUS accurately assesses reference lumen dimensions and lesion length for appropriate stent sizing. IVUS findings such as severe superficial calcium, or thrombus, can alter the mechanical or pharmacological strategy, including rotational atherectomy for plaque modification, more potent antiplatelet and anticoagulation therapies, or mechanical thrombectomy. Poststent IVUS assessment may detect complications of PCI and suboptimal results of the procedure including stent deployment. This helps to decide and execute further interventions for optimal stent implantation, thereby minimizing stent-related immediate and long-term adverse clinical outcomes.[57,63]

Intravascular ultrasound (IVUS) cannot directly estimate the functional significance of coronary stenosis and therefore, IVUS-derived minimal lumen area (MLA) cannot replace the role of noninvasive or invasive functional studies in making clinical decisions about whether to dilate a coronary lesion that does not involve left main coronary artery (LMCA).[58,59]

Visual estimation or quantitative angio-graphic analyses of vessel dimension for stent deployment seem inaccurate, more so when stenosis exists with ectasia. Angiographic success cannot always be linked with optimal stent expansion, even with high pressure balloon inflation during the stenting procedure.[60-62] This is of much greater significance while doing PCI for CAD with ectasia. Adequate post deployment stent evaluation by IVUS is very important to achieve optimal stent expansion.

There is no large scale, randomized, controlled trial comparing IVUS-guided PCI with conventional angiography-guided PCI in patients having CAD with ectasia. A meta-analysis is recently performed by Ahn and colleagues to evaluate the clinical impact of IVUS-guided PCI with DES implantation compared with conventional angiography-guided PCI. In this analysis of more than 26,000 patients, IVUS-guided PCI was associated with a significantly reduced risk of TLR and MI, as well as a lower risk of death, ST and composite of death, MI or repeat revascularization over a follow-up period of 12–48 months.[56,63] Overall IVUS-guided PCI strategy led to more frequent post dilatations, higher balloon inflation pressures, larger balloon sizes, larger stent dimensions, larger minimum lumen diameter and more, longer and wider dimension stenting.

Intravascular ultrasound (IVUS) is useful to confirm the presence of intramural hematoma (IMH) and a double lumen, identify the true lumen and severity of luminal compression. IVUS with its higher tissue penetration strength of 10 mm, enables the evaluation of external elastic lamina and the entire extent of dissected segments, even in patients with large caliber coronary vessels or intraluminal red thrombus. It provides complete thickness vessel visualization with the assessment of significantly longer diseased segment and larger false lumen areas. However, optical coherence tomography (OCT) with its superior tissue resolution can better visualize intimal ruptures and intraluminal thrombi, due to its insufficient tissue penetration it does not provide detailed assessment of full thickness of the arterial wall. This becomes clinically very relevant in ectatic vessels.[64-67]

Optical Coherence Tomography

With its superior resolution, which is 10-fold higher than IVUS, OCT provides good amount of qualitative and quantitative information regarding vessel lumen diameter, plaque morphology, lesion length and lesion characteristics. It is a wonderful tool to guide PCI strategy.[68] It can provide highly accurate and reproducible lumen area measurements.[69] The relationship between OCT-derived MLA, IVUS derived MLA and fractional flow reserve (FFR) have been examined.[70] But the safety and efficacy of a strategy of performing or deferring PCI based on OCT-derived MLA has not been determined. And based on the presence of robust clinical evidence for physiologic lesion assessment with FFR, use of OCT-derived anatomic criteria as a surrogate for functional significance cannot be a standard approach.[71-73] Excellent spatial resolution of OCT makes it an ideally suited imaging tool to guide PCI of nonostial lesions. The advantages include, reproducible and accurate lesion length and reference vessel luminal measurements to guide stent selection, the ability to characterize plaque components to determine the risk of periprocedural MI,[74-76] the potential ability to identify and avoid "geographic miss" related to partial coverage of higher-risk lipid plaque lesions, and optimizing stent results by identifying stent underexpansion, malapposition, and edge dissection.[77-79]

Optical coherence tomography (OCT) helps to visualize clearly the surface and subsurface of the coronary vessel with high tissue contrast, providing superb clarity of plaque composition with much easier interpretation compared to IVUS.[80] It can identify thin cap fibroatheroma, intraluminal thrombus and differentiate plaque erosion/rupture with a high level of accuracy.[77,81-84] By providing a longitudinal view, it promptly identifies the lesion site and severity with automatic detection of MLA and the extension of the atherosclerotic disease. After stent implantation, it is more accurate than IVUS in detecting the morphologic details of suboptimal stent implantation, including underexpansion, malapposition, residual thrombus, plaque prolapse, and edge dissections.[85,86]

To date there are no prospective, randomized trials assessing the role of OCT for guiding PCI. However, several reports have shown the potential of OCT to support clinical decision making in PCI.[79,87-90] Prati and colleagues compared the 1-year clinical outcomes in 335 patients with OCT guidance with a matched control group undergoing PCI with angiographic guidance alone.[79] The protocol provided several treatment recommendations based on OCT findings: (a) edge dissections (width > 200 micrometer) with reference lumen narrowing (lumen area < 4 mm^3) were treated with additional stenting; (b) stent underexpansion (in-stent MLA ≤ 90% of the average reference lumen area, or MLA ≤ 100% of the lowest lumen area of the reference segment) had further dilatation with a non-compliant balloon of the same size at 18 atmosphere or greater, or with a semicompliant balloon with a diameter 0.25 mm larger, at 14 atmosphere or greater; (c) stent malapposition at a distance of greater than 200 micrometer required further dilatation of the implanted stent with a noncompliant or semicompliant balloon; and (d) residual intraluminal thrombus after stenting was further dilated with a noncompliant or semicompliant balloon of the same diameter, for 60 seconds. OCT identifies suboptimal features requiring additional interventions in 35% of cases. On unadjusted analysis, the OCT group had a significantly lower 1-year risk of cardiac death, cardiac death or MI, and the composite of cardiac death, MI or repeat revascularization compared with angiographic guidance alone. After adjustments by multivariate and propensity score-adjusted analysis, OCT-guided PCI was associated with a lower risk of cardiac death or MI. At a technical level, the difference between the treatment groups was driven mainly by the elimination of all potential adverse OCT features.[90] Thus, this and few other studies suggest that OCT has potential clinical benefit in planning and mapping PCI procedures to optimize the results of stent implantation.[79,87-90]

Optical coherence tomography (OCT) can map the vessel pathology (lesion type, extension, geometry, and branch relationship).[91] The accurate identification of plaque components and normal segments helps to decide how to treat the lesion and where to land the stent to avoid immediate ischemic complications. Imperfect stent placement (landing a stent over a thin cap fibroatheroma) has been linked with higher risk of periprocedural MI, edge dissections, no-reflow, and may lead to increased risk of neoatherosclerosis and late ST.[76,92,93] OCT helps to differentiate between thrombus, calcium and tissue protrusion very easily. However, in a setting of ACS with complete thrombotic occlusion of the vessel (TIMI 0-1 flow), restoration of vessel patency with thrombectomy needs to be achieved before the OCT performance to ensure adequate clearing of the vessel lumen during contrast injection so that adequate images can be obtained. The effectiveness of thrombus removal and any further need for thrombus aspiration can be easily identified. Relationship between the remaining thrombus and the location of major side branches can be visualized. It has been documented that remaining thrombus may increase the risk of subsequent stent failure (e.g. ST, acquired incomplete stent apposition owing to clot reabsorption, and neoatherosclerosis). In such settings, enhanced vessel constriction makes it difficult to select the appropriate stent diameter and length. OCT greatly helps to assess the lumen and select the stent size accordingly. Stent underexpansion, malapposition, edge dissection, and complete coverage of the culprit lesion should be evaluated and corrected to optimize the results in ACS.[94-98]

Fractional Flow Reserve

Fractional flow reserve (FFR) is considered nowadays as the gold standard for invasive assessment of physiologic stenosis significance and an indispensable tool for decision making in coronary revascularization. Use of FFR in the catheterization laboratory accurately identifies which lesions should be stented and improves the outcome in most elective clinical and angiographic conditions. Functionally, significant stenosis should be revascularized, if technically possible.[99-101] On the other hand, if a stenosis has no functional significance, the outcome of medical treatment is excellent with an MI and a mortality rate of approximately 1% per year.[101,102] FFR is an accurate and lesion-specific index to indicate whether a particular stenosis or coronary segment can be held responsible for ischemia.[103,104] It has been shown that deferring stenting in an FFR-negative stenosis (i.e. in the nonischemic zone) is safe and associated with excellent long-term outcome. It has also been shown that revascularization of an FFR-positive stenosis (i.e. in the ischemic zone) is associated with significant decrease in ischemia and an improved outcome.[99,102,103]

Fractional flow reserve has been a safe, rapid, easy and extremely relevant clinical tool to define the functional significance of a given coronary lesion in different settings like intermediate severity stenosis, diffuse disease, ACS, and in multivessel disease. In the acute phase of MI, FFR is neither reliable nor useful to assess the culprit lesions. From 5 days after the MI, FFR can be used as usual to indicate residual ischemia of the infarct-related or remote arteries.[105,106] In CAD with ectasia, stenotic lesions are of intermediate severity more often than not, and FFR would be of a great relevance.

INTERVENTIONAL PHARMACOLOGY

Various medications are used either orally, parenterally or intracoronary to achieve adequate antiplatelet, anticoagulation and vasodilatation effects before, during and after PCI. These medicines aim at minimizing ischemic risks, produced by the disease itself and by mechanical intervention. They optimize the outcomes by helping establish optimum flow in the coronary arteries and achieve myocardial perfusion. In the absence of separate studies for patients of CAE, all medicines which are used generally for all other patients may be used even for these patients.

Vasodilators

They are administered for various indications: to facilitate standardized and accurate vessel size measurements, for prevention and treatment of slow-flow or no-reflow phenomenon after PCI and to treat arterial spasm during PCI. Most of the agents are given intracoronary as multiple boluses, diluted with saline and at short intervals to achieve desired rapid effects with small dose. Saline flush after each bolus is mandatory.

Nitroglycerin

It releases nitric oxide (NO) through an enzymatic reaction.[107] It causes vasodilatation without hypotension up to doses of 200 μg.

Nitroprusside

It is a direct NO donor. It does cause transient hypotension. It is given as 50–100 μg boluses.[108]

Nicorandil

It can be given as a slow intravenous infusion at a rate of 2–4 mg/hour or can be given as intracoronary boluses of 2–4 mg each.

In patients with CAE who present with stable angina, oral nitrates have been found to negatively affect the symptoms. Relevance of this fact to intracoronary use of nitrates is not assessed.

Verapamil

It dilates smooth muscles in the coronary arteries to achieve vasodilatation.[109] Due to different mechanism of actions, nitroglycerin and verapamil are frequently combined as "cocktail". Due to its negative inotropic and chronotropic effects, it is contraindicated in patients with left ventricular dysfunction and severe bradycardia. Diltiazem also can be used.[110]

Adenosine

It causes coronary dilatation by blocking adenosine type 2a receptors and L-type calcium channels in vascular smooth muscle cells. It can be given as a continuous high dose intravenous infusion or small dose intracoronary boluses of 15–50 μg. Important side effects are bradycardia, hypotension and bronchospasm. These all effects are transient and rapidly reversible.

Vasodilators in the Treatment of No-flow or Slow-flow

This phenomenon may describe vasospasm and downstream embolization of debris during PCI or suboptimal reperfusion of an infarct artery attributed to endothelial injury in addition to embolization and vasospasm.[111] Most studies investigating the utility of vasoactive agents to prevent or treat no-reflow have been conducted in the setting of PCI for ACS wherein there is highest risk of no-reflow. Greater effectiveness is achieved if these drugs are administered in the culprit distal vascular bed through an infusion microcatheter rather than when they are given intravenously or intracoronary through the guiding catheter, which is placed at the mouth of the coronary artery. A meta-analysis of 3821 patients from 10 randomized controlled trials, undergoing PCI for ACS showed adjunct therapy with adenosine was associated with a reduction in no-reflow and subsequently improved clinical outcomes.[112] Compared with placebo, adenosine significantly reduced postprocedural no-reflow with an odds ratio of 0.25 (95% confidence interval 0.08–0.73, p = 0.01). But adenosine failed to reduce ST-segment resolution, symptoms of heart failure, reinfarction and mortality. Nitroprusside and nicorandil also have been shown to improve coronary flow without hard clinical endpoint benefit.[113-115]

Keeping the pathophysiology of CAE in mind, use of intracoronary vasodilator agents is intuitively appealing; there is no scientific data available for this subgroup of patients.

Antiplatelet and Anticoagulation Treatment

Choice of various antiplatelet and anticoagulation agents depends on many variables like, age, clinical presentation, comorbidities (mainly diabetes, impaired renal and liver function), coadministration of other medicines (mainly steroids or nonsteroidal anti-inflammatory drugs), overall bleeding versus ischemic risk of the patient and vascular/lesion characteristics once it is known. It is well-documented that both–major bleeding and ischemic events–have adverse effects on short and long-term prognosis including mortality. Careful selection of right agents and right doses is very crucial to optimize PCI outcome.

Aspirin

It is a must component of dual antiplatelet treatment (DAPT) unless a patient has severe allergy to it.[116] Small maintenance dose (75–150 mg/day) and coadmistering proton pump inhibitor when there is a clinical indication, helps reducing bleeding events.[117,118]

Clopidogrel

It is one of the three currently used adenosine diphosphate (ADP) P2Y12 receptor inhibitors used during PCI. The pivotal Clopidogrel in Unstable Angina to Prevent Recurrent Events (CURE) trial, by showing 20% reduction in the composite endpoint of cardiovascular death, MI or stroke compared with placebo in medically and invasively managed patients with non-ST elevation (NSTE) ACS, established a firm role for use and continuation of clopidogrel for 12 months after NSTEACS.[119-121] Though clopidogrel has not been evaluated against placebo in any large outcome study in the setting of primary PCI, based on extrapolation of data from PCI-CURE, it has become a part of DAPT in all patients undergoing primary PCI (PPCI) also. A 600-mg loading dose is preferred over 300-mg loading dose, given the enhanced and more rapid platelet inhibition achieved with the higher dose as well as the reported beneficial effects in STEMI patients.[122-126]

There are few issues with clopidogrel including, late onset and offset of action, significant inpatient variability in the response to it (explained in part by genetic polymorphism of the *CYP2C19* gene), potential interactions with many drugs and food and resistance to its action as suggested by high on-treatment platelet reactivity. In worst scenario, this has shown to increase risk of MI and stent thrombosis.[121,127]

Prasugrel

This third generation thienopyridine has been shown to have more rapid, enhanced and consistent antiplatelet effects than clopidogrel, even compared with higher clopidogrel doses in a non-STEMI setting.[126] The clinical efficacy and safety of prasugrel (60-mg loading dose followed by 10-mg/day maintenance dose) compared with clopidogrel (300-mg loading dose followed by 75-mg/day maintenance dose) has been evaluated in a large-scale, multicenter, randomized Trial to Assess Improvement in Therapeutic Outcomes by Optimizing Platelet Inhibition with Prasugrel–Thrombolysis in Myocardial Infarction (TRITON–TIMI) 38, which enrolled 13,608 moderate to high-risk patients of ACS undergoing planned PCI.[128] In the overall population, over a follow-up period of 14.5 months, a significant 19% relative reduction of the primary efficacy endpoint (composite of cardiovascular death, nonfatal MI, or nonfatal stroke) was seen with prasugrel compared to clopidogrel. But there was a 32% increased risk of non-coronary artery bypass grafting (CABG) surgery related TIMI major bleeding. There was no net clinical benefits in patients aging >75 years and in those weighing <60 kg, and a net clinical harm in patients with prior cerebrovascular events. In STEMI patients or patients with diabetes, prasugrel provided ischemic benefits without increasing bleeding.[129]

Ticagrelor

This direct and reversible inhibitor of platelet has more rapid onset and offset of action, and provides a greater and more consistent platelet inhibition than the standard clopidogrel dosing.[130] The clinical efficacy and safety of ticagrelor (180 mg loading dose followed by 90 mg twice a day maintenance dose) compared with clopidogrel (300 mg to 600 mg loading dose followed by 75 mg/day maintenance dose) has been evaluated in a large-scale, multicenter, randomized PLATelet Inhibition and patient Outcomes (PLATO) trial enrolling 18,624 moderate to high risk patients of ACS (NSTEACS invasively or medically managed or STEMI managed with PPCI).[131] In the overall population, over a follow-up period of 12 months, a significant 16% relative reduction of the primary efficacy endpoint (composite of cardiovascular death, nonfatal MI, or nonfatal stroke) was seen with ticagrelor compared to clopidogrel. A significant lowered rate of cardiovascular death and overall death was also observed in ticagrelor arm. Overall, bleeding risk was similar in two arms, but ticagrelor was associated with 31% relative increased risk of non-CABG related TIMI major bleeding. In the prespecified STEMI subgroup with 7544 patients, ticagrelor was associated with lower rates of primary composite endpoints, all cause mortality and MI, and higher rates of stroke, with similar bleeding risk.[132]

Cangrelor

This reversible ADP P2Y12 receptor inhibitor is available in intravenous form with a short half-life of 3–6 minutes. Randomized, controlled trials comparing this agent with clopidogrel during PCI have shown mixed results. Cangrelor versus Standard Therapy to Achieve Optimal Management of Platelet Inhibition (CHAMPION PHOENIX) trial showed a consistent benefit of cangrelor given as intravenous infusion during PCI, in preventing ischemic complications like death, MI, and stent thrombosis, compared with clopidogrel given just before or after PCI.[133]

In PCI of patients having CAE, due to more thrombotic milieu, prasugrel or ticagrelor would be considered preferred second antiplatelet agent over clopidogrel, whenever there is need of DAPT.

Glycoprotein Receptor Inhibitors (GPI) and Parenteral Anticoagulation

It has been documented that addition of platelet glycoprotein IIb/IIIa receptor inhibitors (GPI) reduced the short-term ischemic risk and long-term mortality in patients undergoing PCI in the setting of ACS or angiographically visible thrombus.[134,135] Intense platelet inhibition produced by these agents (abciximab, tirofiban, integrilin), however, resulted in increased rates of bleeding complications,[136,137] associated with prolonged hospitalizations, increased costs, and late mortality.[138]

Interventional practice and pharmacotherapy continued to evolve, with development of refined, thinner-strut stent designs associated with less thrombogenicity,[139] early administration of platelet ADP P2Y12 receptor antagonists to patients with ACS or undergoing PCI,[140] and introduction of the more potent P2Y12 inhibitors ticagrelor and prasugrel.[128,131] In this context, the balance of benefit versus risk with GPI became less clear. In a randomized trial among patients who had received clopidogrel before elective PCI, GPI did not reduce ischemic complications but did increase bleeding.[141] Subsequent trials in higher-risk patients with ACS showed efficacy of GPI in reducing ischemic complications of PCI,[142] but also showed that these agents could be reserved for selective use in those patients with substantial thrombus burden, high-risk anatomy, or intraprocedural complications.[136] With a view to have faster onset of effect and to be able to get desired effects at a smaller dose, intracoronary administration of GPI has been tested for all of the three agents with variable success. A series of trials were then carried out among patients undergoing PCI for elective indications or ACS, demonstrating that substitution of the direct thrombin inhibitor bivalirudin for the combination of heparin plus a GPI consistently reduced bleeding complications by as much as 40%.[143-145] Neither ischemic events nor long-term mortality was increased with bivalirudin in those trials, and this agent eventually supplanted heparin and GPI during PCI for many patients.

Further, the role of GPI in combination with ticagrelor or prasugrel for ACS remains to be defined. Both of these newer oral antiplatelet agents have superior ischemic benefits in ACS patients at a cost of increased bleeding risk.

In the modern era of PCI, there may still be a role for judicious use of GPI in patients who have high ischemic risk like those with substantial thrombus burden, high-risk anatomy, or intraprocedural complications, particularly in the settings of ACS and/or when newer oral antiplatelet agent is not given due to one or other reasons. When GPI is used, all possible efforts to minimize bleeding risk, e.g. obtaining radial arterial access for PCI, adjusting GPI dose as per age and kidney function, giving only loading dose of GPI, avoiding concurrent use of NSAIDs, administration of PPI, etc. should be implemented.[146,147]

Intracoronary Thrombolytic Therapy

Although administration of fibrinolytic agents is intuitively appealing as a means to reduce pre-existing thrombus burden and prevent new thrombus formation within a treated coronary vessel, the potential of these agents for thrombin generation, platelet activation and bleeding complications appear to limit their effectiveness. Though many case reports have been published and discussed, no large-scale randomized trials have been performed to assess the efficacy of thrombolytic therapy during coronary interventions. Synthesis of data from small prospective trails or retrospective series does not demonstrate a benefit of thrombolysis in reducing acute or chronic ischemic complications. Boscareli D et al. presented one such data of local fibrinolysis with low dose (one-third of systemic) tenecteplase or alteplase, which was administered via a 6F-infusion catheter in 30 STEMI patients with a large thrombus burden. A thrombus was qualified as large when its maximal dimension was ≥2 vessels (TIMI thrombus grade 4 and 5). TIMI flow grade improved from 0/1 at baseline (93%) to ≥2 in most patients (97%). Blush grade 2–3 was observed in 85% and more than 50% ST-segment resolution was seen in 82%.[148] The largest study, Thrombolysis and Angioplasty in Unstable Angina (TAUSA) trial showed no benefit of intracoronary urokinase used before angioplasty as an adjunct. No difference in the incidence of intracoronary thrombus formation was observed between the two groups, but patients receiving urokinase paradoxically had higher rates of abrupt vessel closure.[149]

Statin Therapy

The inflammatory response of distal embolization and platelet aggregate interaction with leukocytes contributes to the degree of myonecrosis that is frequently seen after PCI. In ARMYDA and ARMYDA-2 trials, statin showed significant reduction in periprocedural MI as measured by serum CK-MB or troponin I levels. Anti-inflammatory effects of statin were evidenced through attenuated rise of various inflammatory markers after PCI in patients who received statin.[150]

Long-term Oral Anticoagulation Treatment

In patients with ACS, irrespective of the management strategy, 12-month DAPT has been found to be very effective in reducing ischemic endpoints at an acceptable bleeding risk. Triple antithrombotic therapy for variable period with aspirin, clopidogrel and oral vitamin K antagonist (VKA) warfarin have been used for ACS patients who have an additional indication for the later, like atrial fibrillation, deep vein thrombosis or those with mechanical valve prosthesis. Balancing between ischemic benefits versus bleeding risk is crucially important for optimizing long- term prognosis. A randomized, multicenter, open-label Triple Therapy in Patients on Oral Anticoagulation after Drug Eluting Stent Implantation (ISAR-TRIPLE) trial did show that 6 weeks of triple therapy is as effective as and has less bleeding risk as compared to 6 months of triple therapy.[151] On the basis of the ISAR-TRIPLE study, 6 weeks certainly seems like a reasonable starting point, titrating the duration and intensity of triple antithrombotic therapy upward or downward, depending on patient and lesion characteristics. In another trial—**W**hat is the **O**ptimal antiplat**E**let and anticoagulant therapy in patients with oral anticoagulation and coronary **S**ten**T**ing (WOEST), combination of clopidogrel and VKA showed equal efficacy in preventing thrombotic complications with less bleeding risk as compared to triple combination including aspirin in addition.[152] Newer anticoagulation agents including rivaroxaban, apixaban and debigatran have been tested as a part of dual or triple therapy in patients with recent ACS with or without specific indication for oral anticoagulation agent. As expected, most of these trials have shown modest reduction in ischemic events with substantial increase in bleeding, specifically when triple therapy was used. Newer antiplatelet agents, prasugrel and ticagrelor have not been well tested in randomized controlled trial with any oral anticoagulation agent either alone or with aspirin.[153]

DEALING WITH THE THROMBUS

Thrombus in Coronary Artery and Its Impact

Data from observational studies.[154] and randomized trials,[155] have clearly indicated that the presence of thrombus on the angiogram is an independent predictor of major adverse clinical events due to an increased risk of abrupt closure, distal embolization, and procedural failure.[156-159] Among the

7917 patients in a pooled analysis of eight clinical trials, those with angiographically visible thrombus more frequently suffered abrupt closure and in-hospital death or MI.[160] Angiographically, thrombus is defined as an intraluminal filling defect with contrast on 3 sides or an area of contrast staining noted within the stenosis and not having the angiographic characteristics of dissection. IVUS and OCT are quite useful imaging tools to confirm the angiographic finding.

Evidences have suggested that bleeding and blood transfusions following PCI may be independent determinants of long-term adverse outcomes.[161,162] Various efforts to reduce risk of bleeding includes obtaining transradial rather than transfemoral access, smaller sheaths, shorter sheath dwell time, reduced intensity of intraprocedural anticoagulation, and the avoiding post-procedure use of heparins. However, this represents a challenge as novel and more potent antithrombotic agents developed for ACS patient population invariably appear to be associated with a greater risk of bleeding.[128,162] This highlights the ground for mechanical adjunctive antithrombotic devices.

Distal Embolization

Distal embolization is a universal phenomenon during PCI for MI or for lesions with significant thrombus burden, occurring predominantly at the time of first balloon inflation and stent deployment. Moreover, thrombus burden is an independent predictor of adverse outcomes. Thus, there is a need to develop novel strategies to remove thrombus during PCI, preventing macro- and micro-embolization and the resulting microvascular dysfunction in patients with thrombotic lesions with the goal of improving outcomes.[163]

The concept of embolic protection device (EPD) use during PCI for acute MI or for lesions with significant amount of thrombus is attractive and intuitive. However, the larger randomized trials did not confirm the initial favorable impression regarding EPD use in primary PCI during acute MI. The Enhanced Myocardial Efficacy and Removal by Aspiration of Liberated Debris (EMERALD) trial, which compared PCI with PercuSurge GuardWire distal protection to PCI without EPD, failed to show benefit of EPD use for ST-segment resolution, infarct size between days 5 and 14, and major adverse cardiac events at 6 months. Similar disappointing results were seen with the use of FilterWire distal protection in the setting of PCI for acute MI. Delay caused in restoring epicardial flow, further embolization caused while crossing the lesion with the device, incomplete aspiration of liberated debris, leaking of vasoactive substances released from the ruptured plaques, lack of protection to side branches and reperfusion injury could be the most probable reasons of such negative results of EPD.[164-166] Contrary to this, PCI for vein graft is greatly helped by use of PercuSurge GuardWire system and other distal embolic protection filter devices. Primary endpoint of composite of death, Q-wave MI, non-Q-wave MI, emergent bypass surgery, or target vessel revascularization at 30 days were improved, mainly driven by reduction in non-Q-wave MI. There was significant and drastic reduction in no-reflow.[167,168] There have been no dedicated trials for EPD use in patients with CAE undergoing PCI, but selecting the size of and the site for parking the device, maneuvering the device down the artery, etc. can be important issues due to uneven geometry.

Aspiration Thrombectomy (AT)

After documented failure of rheolytic mechanical thrombectomy, the utility of AT in primary PCI has been studied extensively. It is quite understandable, that removal of some or possibly most of the offending thrombus at the culprit lesion site may prevent distal embolization, improve epicardial coronary flow, and reduce microvascular obstruction and the no-reflow phenomenon. On the other hand, the thrombectomy catheter itself is one more device that may cause distal thrombus embolization, and its insertion adds to cost and procedure time prior to definitive balloon angioplasty and/or stenting. Many trials and meta-analyses did show improvement in immediate and short-term surrogate endpoints like TIMI flow and TMP blush grade suggesting better microvascular perfusion, reduced occurrence of slow-flow or no-reflow phenomenon, reduced infarct size, and better left ventricular performance.[169] The most important question, whether these immediate positive effects are leading to improvement in long-term clinical outcomes and mortality, has been answered by many trials.

The TAPAS (Thrombus Aspiration During Percutaneous coronary Intervention in Acute Myocardial Infarction Study) was a single center trial involving 1,071 patients, which demonstrated not only a significant improvement in the primary outcome of myocardial blush grade but a nearly 50% reduction in mortality at 1 year.[170] Subsequently, the TASTE (Thrombus Aspiration during ST-Segment Elevation Myocardial Infarction) trial, which randomized over 7,000 patients to thrombus aspiration or PCI alone, suggested that routine aspiration does not reduce either 30-day or 1-year mortality in patients undergoing PPCI.[171] The TOTAL (Trial of Routine Aspiration Thrombectomy With PCI versus PCI Alone in Patients With STEMI) trial randomized 10,063 patients with STEMI referred for primary PCI within 12 hours of onset to either AT (Export catheter) followed by PCI or conventional PCI. The primary composite outcome, cardiovascular death, MI, cardiogenic shock, or New York Heart Association (NYHA) class IV chronic heart failure at 180 days was not different between the two arms. Similarly, primary composite outcomes and incidences of cardiovascular death, recurrent MI, cardiogenic shock, TLR and stent thrombosis were unchanged at the end of one year by routine additional use of AT. Additional routine thrombectomy did improve periprocedural reperfusion markers; there was reduced risk of distal embolization and incomplete ST-segment resolution. But 30-day stroke risk was increased, and that was a worrisome finding. It is noteworthy that 7.1% patients from PCI only group needed bailout AT.[172] Thus, three large, randomized trials (TASTE, TOTAL and INFUSE-AMI [Intracoronary Abciximab and Aspiration Thrombectomy in Patients with Large Anterior Myocardial Infarction]) did not observe a benefit in clinical outcomes with routine AT compared with conventional PCI during acute MI revascularization. These findings have made ACC/AHA revise the STEMI guideline recommendation for AT use, from class IIa to class III.

A meta-analysis of many trials which included TAPAS and INFUSE-AMI trials, on the role of AT during PCI in acute MI, reported a significantly better TIMI blush grade and ST-segment resolution in the manual AT group compared with the conventional PCI group. Consistently, they also reported a lower incidence of major adverse cardiovascular events and lower mortality in the AT group.[173] The meta-regression analysis performed on the same studies by De Rossa et al. showed that the beneficial effect of AT over PCI alone is higher for longer ischemic times, and this effect is evident for both mortality and the rate of major adverse cardiovascular events. This phenomenon can easily be explained because of the fact that the efficacy of PCI rapidly decreases over time, as for all treatments of AMI, whereas AT seemingly holds its efficacy over time.[174] De Vita et al. also reported that increasing time to treatment was associated with a significantly decreased reperfusion rate in patients treated with PCI alone, but no such trend was observed in patients treated with AT and PCI. Although no mechanism has been identified for this phenomenon, it is tempting to speculate that distal embolization may became more relevant in later stages when the thrombus is increasingly organized and more apt to disrupt in insoluble fragments. It is conceivable that AT will have a U-shaped relationship with ischemic time; with very longer ischemic times, the thrombus becomes more organized and is subsequently harder to retrieve with manual aspiration catheters.[175] Thiele et al. performed a multicenter, randomized trial to compare the adjunctive AT with conventional PCI in patients with NSTEMI presenting within 72 hours after symptom onset and with thrombus over culprit lesion demonstrated by angiography. The investigators conclude that adjunctive AT did not lead to an improvement of myocardial reperfusion (microvascular obstruction assessed by magnetic resonance imaging within 4 days) and infarct size in patients with NSTEMI.[176] The changes in thrombus composition-thrombus getting more organized and difficult to be aspirated, and loss of salvageable myocardium as time lapsed might have contributed to failure of AT as an adjunctive tool.[177]

Though, there are no dedicated trials for AT in patients with CAE, it is intuitively appealing and can scientifically be backed that many patients with this anatomical variation would benefit by use of aspiration thrombectomy, especially when they present with STEMI or angiographically visible large thrombus burden.

STENT? NOT TO STENT? DEFERRED STENTING?

Uneven geometry with variable diameters of normal, stenotic and ectatic areas in the coronary artery to be intervened presents a serious decision dilemma while performing PCI in most of the patients with CAE. A significant thrombus burden with endothelial dysfunction may be found even when a patient has presented with stable coronary disease. Primary PCI with stenting or early PCI immediately after coronary reperfusion with fibrinolytic, for a significant residual stenosis, reduces myocardium at risk, improves prognosis, and is the current standard of care for acute STEMI.[178-179] No-reflow, an acute reduction in myocardial blood flow despite a patent epicardial coronary artery involves microvascular obstruction secondary to distal embolization of clot, microvascular spasm, and thrombosis.[180] No-reflow occurs in approximately 10% of cases of primary PCI and is associated with patient characteristics such as advanced age and delayed presentation and coronary characteristics such as a completely occluded culprit artery and heavy thrombus burden.[180-184] No therapies have been shown to prevent no-reflow with consistency, and when it occurs, treatment by administration of vasodilator drugs,[185] and intra-aortic balloon counterpulsation therapy is empirical.[179,180,185,186]

Two different approaches have been used by many operators for selected patients:

No Stent Implantation

This strategy can be adopted when there is complete restoration of epicardial blood flow with no residual significant lesion or flow-limiting dissection with plaque rupture after balloon angioplasty or aspiration thrombectomy or combination of both. Earlier studies have shown that elective patients with residual stenosis ≤30%[187,188] or ≤35% and FFR ≥ 0.9[189] after balloon angioplasty had favorable clinical outcomes at long-term follow-up. Good intermediate-term results with only balloon angioplasty have been reported in few cases with stable or unstable CAD with ectasia.[190] Because of the relatively larger reference vessel size of the CAE patient, recurrence causing real ischemia by functional study using a pressure wire would be less even if the visual angiographic restenosis appears to be significant compared with recurrence in the usual native coronary arteries. This suggests that balloon angioplasty alone can potentially be a good treatment option in selected CAE patients with significant stenosis. In the era of drug eluting balloon, "parallel ballooning" using two drug-eluting balloons has also been proposed and tried by some operators.

Furthermore, as only thrombus aspiration is nontraumatic to the vessel wall, event-free outcomes after thrombus aspiration without additional angioplasty may be related to diminished vessel injury. During balloon angioplasty and stenting, platelet aggregation, inflammation and intimal proliferation are induced and these mechanisms may result in restenosis or occlusion.[191,192] The case for no stenting under such circumstances is made stronger by the fact that the heterogeneity of the coronary artery morphology and relatively larger vessel size complicates decision to determine stent type, size, and complete expansion with the usual coronary devices. Underexpansion and malapposition due to thrombus are worrisome issues with potentially serious short and long-term consequences.

Deferred Stent Implantation

Stenting after few hours of primary procedure of either balloon dilatation only or aspiration thrombectomy only or both, might allow time for reduction in coronary thrombus burden and recovery of microvascular function. After initial coronary reperfusion and normalization of coronary blood flow, brief deferral of stenting might reduce the occurrence of no-reflow compared with usual care with immediate stenting and thus, may help increase myocardial salvage.

Carrick D et al.[193] did a prospective, randomized, controlled, parallel group, single center trial of Deferred Stenting Versus Immediate Stenting to Prevent No- or Slow-Reflow in Acute ST-Segment Elevation Myocardial Infarction (DEFER-STEMI They selected STEMI patients at high risk of no-reflow if radial artery access was used and one or more of the following inclusion criteria were met: (a) clinical history that included MI, increased age (i.e. 65 years of age or older), duration of symptoms >6 h; (b) culprit coronary artery abnormalities including an occluded artery (TIMI flow grade 0/1 at initial angiography), heavy thrombus burden (TIMI grade 2 or higher), long lesion length (≥24 mm), small vessel diameter (i.e.≤2.5 mm); (c) clinical signs of acute microvascular injury after initial reperfusion with persistent ST-segment elevation >50%. Patients with the absence of normal (TIMI flow grade 3) coronary blood flow after initial reperfusion with aspiration thrombectomy with or without balloon angioplasty and patients with cardiogenic shock were excluded. The residual severity of the culprit stenosis was not relevant to participation provided TIMI flow grade 3 was evident. The deferred PCI strategy involved an intention-to-stent 4 to 16 h after initial coronary reperfusion. This time interval was based on a balance between competing benefits and risks. The treatment protocol for deferred patients included transfer to the coronary care unit, continuous intravenous infusion of GPI therapy (tirofiban 0.15 mg/kg/min) and administration of subcutaneous low molecular weight heparin [(LMWH) enoxaparin 1 mg/kg every 12 h] for up to 16 hours. The radial artery sheath used for PCI was retained or removed according to operator and patient preference. The usual care PCI strategy included immediate stenting in the catheter laboratory and intravenous GPI therapy for 12 h (tirofiban 0.15 mg/kg/min). In this trial they observed that significantly fewer patients in the deferred stenting group had no-/slow-reflow, no reflow and intraprocedural thrombotic events and TIMI flow grades at the end of PCI were higher in the deferred stenting group. Myocardial salvage index at 6 months was greater in the deferred stenting group. This was achieved at a small cost of recurrent STEMI in a few patients in the deferred stenting group before the second procedure.

Many other clinical trials including MIMI (Minimal Invasive Procedure for Myocardial Infarction), PRIMACY (Primary Reperfusion Secondary Stenting Trial), and DANAMI-3 (DANish Study of Optimal Acute Treatment of Patients with ST-elevation Myocardial Infarction) have assessed different approaches to deferred stenting in primary PCI. Recent studies, including 3 nonrandomized case series,[194-196] and a systematic review,[197] support the notion that deferred stenting may be safe in appropriately selected STEMI patients.

Overall, for this simple, pragmatic, and potentially widely applicable strategy, the balance of the benefit of reduced no-reflow versus the risk of recurrent myocardial infarction needs to be tested in a large multicenter, randomized, controlled trial.

PRIMARY PERCUTANEOUS CORONARY INTERVENTION IN CORONARY ARTERY ECTASIA

Yip HK et al. retrospectively analyzed 924 consecutive patients with AMI who underwent emergency primary PCI. Of these 924 patients, only 24 patients (2.6%) had an infarct-related artery (IRA) with aneurysmal dilation. Coronary angiography revealed high thrombus burden with subsequent high occurrence of no-reflow phenomenon and distal embolization after primary PCI in these patients. The incidence of cardiogenic shock and the 30-day mortality rate were also higher. In spite of this, survival rate was 90.9% during a mean follow-up of 19 ± 30 months.[198]

Similarly, Erden I et al. retrospectively analyzed 643 consecutive patients with AMI who underwent emergency primary PCI. Of these 643 patients, only 31 patients (4.8%) had an ectatic IRA. Impaired epicardial arterial flow, thrombus burden score of IRA, impaired TMP blush grade, and distal embolization were significantly higher, whereas ST-segment resolution and collateral vascular development were significantly lower in patients with ectatic IRA. They concluded that IRA ectasia was an independent predictor of adverse outcome.[199]

WHICH STENT?

Because of the heterogeneity of the coronary artery morphology and relatively larger vessel size, it is difficult to determine stent type, size, and to achieve complete expansion with the usual coronary devices. There have been very limited data regarding revascularization of stenotic ectatic coronary arteries and there are, in fact, no specific guidelines for selecting or preferring one stent over the other. Because of the variable size and morphology of the coronary arteries with CAE, various stents have been utilized during PCI.

Bare Metal Stent (BMS) versus Drug-eluting Stent (DES) versus Bioresorbable Scaffold

There are no randomized controlled data for superiority of one over the other in patients with CAD and ectasia. However, looking to the data of current second and third generation DES in overall spectrum of CAD, it is quite practical to believe that DES could potentially be a better choice in this subset of patients also. Very likely, due to larger lumen and stent diameter in many such cases, restenosis rate may not be very high even with BMS. And if it is true, cost-effectiveness calculations for DES versus BMS may be different. Similarly, there is no data about use of BVS in CAE. Whichever stent is used, more critical issue is to size it properly and once done, to expand it properly to avoid malapposition.

Successful implantation of two DESs (3.5 × 180-mm sirolimus-eluting stents) parallel to each other in an ectatic artery has also been reported with IVUS guidance.[200] Though, like many other approaches adopted for intervention in CAE, long-term safety and efficacy of this technique remains to be established.

Covered Stent

Idea of using a covered stent in the segment harboring a saccular aneurysm is quite old and many operators have tried it. In most of such cases proximal and distal landing zones for the stent are near normal coronary segments, helping to exclude the aneurysm.[201] The Jostent® polytetrafluoroethylene (PTFE)-covered, balloon-expandable stent (Abbott Vascular instruments Deutschland GmbH, Rangendingen, Germany) has been shown to be an effective device for the percutaneous management and exclusion of coronary aneurysms.[202-205] Stefanadis et al. reported the successful deployment of an autologous venous graft-covered stent to a coronary aneurysm.[206] Interestingly, the MASTER (MGUARD for Acute ST Elevation Reperfusion) trial showed that the use of a mashed stent, designed to trap and exclude a thrombus, helped maintaining the efficacy of PCI over time in patients with ST-segment elevation myocardial infarction.[207] This stent can be another option for use in CAE.

Peripheral Stent

Using peripheral balloon and stent devices for the management of huge coronary ectasia may be a more proper option for the coronary interventionist because of experience, familiarity and accessibility. Although, some extra resistance and friction during device positioning owing to the relatively larger profile compared with the usual coronary device is expected, many successful cases without immediate mechanical complications or subsequent cardiovascular events have been reported with the balloon and stent designed for peripheral artery disease.

Agirbasli et al. reported 3 cases of coronary angioplasty with intratherapeutic peripheral biliary stents for CAE.[208] This was, perhaps, the first report of using a peripheral biliary stent in a coronary vascular structure. Subsequently, many operators have used balloon expandable renal stents for this purpose. High pressure inflation is the most risky step while using these relatively bulky and large devices.

Self-expanding Stents

The use of this type of stent helps to avoid high pressure inflations as needed in case of balloon expandable stent, provides continued self expansion as opposed to tubular stent, and facilitates improved 'fit' in difficult anatomy by confirming to vessel wall with reduced malapposition. It would mimic the shape and diameter of the vessel to achieve perfect apposition with no risk of vessel wall-stent diameter mismatch and so would help reduce stent thrombosis and restenosis. Not only it adapts to anatomic changes during the post-AMI phase to maintain apposition but also, it can grow up to almost 6.0 mm, a diameter which is difficult to be achieved with balloon expandable stents. Adequate lesion site preparation and a quick post-dilatation are strongly recommended in self-expandable stents even if the stent is looking nice immediately post-deployment.

Newer generation of self-expandable STENTYS stent has been described to treat ectatic aneurysmal coronary lesions.[209] STENTYS stent is made from nitinol with nickel-titanium alloy and would self-expand and conform to the vessel lumen over time. However, the longer and bigger sized STENTYS stent has lower profile. Using 7F guide catheter for better support and careful deployment of the stent to avoid a forward jump complication of the device are necessary interventional arts. Even use of two overlapping STENTYS stents with the aid of platinum radio-opaque end markers under fluoroscopic guidance has also been reported. Despite its self-apposing characteristic, it is still prudent to perform postdilatation to ensure optimal stent strut apposition.[210-213]

Self-expandable PTFE stents (Symbiot®, Boston Scientific, Natick, Mass, USA) may be preferable in aneurysms of great longitude that are located in vessels with angulations or in those with larger diameters; however, only limited experience is available.[214]

Whatever stent is used, meticulous care to size it properly with the use of OCT or IVUS is almost a must in all cases of CAD with ectasia.

SURGICAL TREATMENT OF CORONARY ARTERY ECTASIA

In the symptomatic patient not suitable for stent insertion, surgical excision or ligation of the aneurysm with bypass graft of the affected coronary arteries may be the procedure of choice. Coronary artery ectasia that presents with life-threatening complications such as heart chamber compression or fistula formation with severe shunts require prompt surgical intervention. Coronary artery aneurysm of at least three to four times, the size of the original vessel diameter is considered as an absolute indication for surgical intervention by many, because of the propensity for complications such as compression, rupture, or thrombosis. Coronary bypass graft with ligation of the aneurysm is an alternative surgical treatment for aneurysms of the LMCA. In some patients with LMCA aneurysm, ligation of the aneurysm may be difficult. Surgical therapy is reserved for those with large thrombotic aneurysms or with myocardial ischemia and significant associated CAD.[41, 215-218]

REFERENCES

1. Seabra-Gomes R, Somerville J, Ross DN, Emanuel R, Parker DJ, Wong M. Congenital coronary artery aneurysms. Br Heart J. 1974;36:329-35.
2. Falsetti HL, Carroll RJ. Coronary artery aneurysm: A review of the literature with a report of 11 new cases. Chest. 1976:69;630-6.
3. Swanton RH, Thomas ML, Coltart DJ, Jenkins BS, Webb-Peploe MM, Williams BT. Coronary artery ectasia variant of occlusive coronary arteriosclerosis. Br Heart J. 1978;40:393-400.
4. Hartnell GG, Parnell BM, Pridie RB. Coronary artery ectasia, its prevalence and clinical significance in 4993 patients. Br Heart J. 1985;54:392-95.
5. Markis JE, Joffe CD, Cohn PF, Feen DJ, Herman MV, Gorlin R. Clinical significance of coronary arterial ectasia. Am J Cardiol. 1976;37:217-22.
6. Oliveros RA, Falsetti HL, Carroll RJ, Heinle RA, Ryan GF. Atherosclerotic coronary artery aneurysm. Report of five cases and review of literature. Arch Intern Med. 1974;134:1072-6.
7. Swaye PS, Fisher LD, Litwin P, et al. Aneurysmal coronary artery disease. Circulation. 1983;67:134-8.
8. Sharma SN, Kaul U, Sharma S, Wasiv HS, Manchanda SC, Bahl VK, et al. Coronary arteriographic profile in young and old Indian patients with ischemic heart disease: a comparative study. Indian Heart J. 1990;42:365-9.
9. Sophie Mavrogeni. Coronary artery ectasia: from diagnosis to treatment, a review article. Hellenic J Cardiol. 2010;51:158-63.
10. Befeler B, Aranda MJ, Embi A, Mullin FL, El-Sherif N, Lazzara R. Coronary artery aneurysms: study of the etiology, clinical course and effect on left ventricular function and prognosis. Am J Med. 1977;62:597-607.
11. Cohen P, O'Gara PT. Coronary artery aneurysms: a review of the natural history, pathophysiology, and management. Cardiol Rev. 2008;16:301-4.
12. Bell MR, Garratt KN, Bresnahan JF, Edwards WD, Holmes DR. Relation of deep arterial resection and coronary artery aneurysms after directional coronary atherectomy. J Am Coll Cardiol. 1992;20:1474-81.
13. Pavlakis GP, Stella PR. Coronary aneurysm formation after primary coronary angioplasty. Hellenic J Cardiol. 2008;49:106-10.
14. Condado JA, Waksman R, Gurdiel O, et al. Long-term angiographic and clinical outcome after percutaneous transluminal coronary angioplasty and intracoronary radiation therapy in humans. Circulation. 1997;96:727-32.
15. Sanidas EA, Vavuranakis M, Papaioannou TG, et al. Study of atheromatous plaque using intravascular ultrasound. Hellenic J Cardiol. 2008;49:415-21.
16. Stajduhar KC, Laird JR, Rogan KM, Wortham DC. Coronary arterial ectasia: increased prevalence in patients with abdominal aortic aneurysm as compared to occlusive atherosclerotic peripheral vascular disease. Am Heart J. 1993;125:86-92.
17. Daoud AS, Pankin D, Tulgan H, Florentin RA. Aneurysms of the coronary artery. Report of ten cases and review of literature. Am J Cardiol. 1963;11:228-37.
18. al-Harthi SS, Nouh MS, Arafa M, al-Nozha M. Aneurysmal dilatation of the coronary arteries: diagnostic patterns and clinical significance. Int J Cardiol. 1991;30:191-4.
19. Condado JA, Waksman R, Gurdiel O, et al. Long-term angiographic and clinical outcome after percutaneous transluminal coronary angioplasty and intracoronary radiation therapy in humans. Circulation. 1997;96:727-32.

20. Fukuda S, Hashimoto N, Naritomi H, Nagata I, Nozaki K, Kondo S, et al. Prevention of rat cerebral aneurysm formation by inhibition of nitric oxide synthase. Circulation. 2000;101:2532-8.
21. Johanning JM, Franklin DP, Han DC, Carey DJ, Elmore JR. Inhibition of inducible nitric oxide synthase limits nitric oxide production and experimental aneurysm expansion. J Vasc Surg. 2001;33:579-86.
22. Usama Boles, Roby Rakhit, Man Fi Shiu, et al. Coronary artery ectasia as a culprit for acute myocardial infarction: review of pathophysiology and management. Available on-line at *www.anakarder.com* doi:10.5152/akd.2013.227
23. England JF. Herbicides and coronary ectasia. Med J Aust. 1981;2:260.13.
24. Glagov S, Weisenberg E, Zarins CK, Stankunavicius R, Kolettis GJ. Compensatory enlargement of human atherosclerotic coronary arteries. N Engl J Med. 1987;316:1371-5.
25. Adiloğlu AK, Can R, Nazlı C, Ocal A, Ergene O, Tınaz G, et al. Ectasia and severe atherosclerosis: relationships with Chlamydia pneumonia, helicobacter pylori, and inflammatory markers. Tex Heart Inst J. 2005;32:21-7.
26. Li JJ, Nie SP, Qian XW, Zeng HS, Zhang CY. Chronic inflammatory status in patients with coronary artery ectasia. Cytokine. 2009;46:61-4.
27. Turhan H, Erbay AR, Yaşar AS, Aksoy Y, Bicer A, Yetkin G, et al. Plasma soluble adhesion molecules;intercellular adhesion molecule-1, vascular cell adhesion molecule-1 and E-selectin levels in patients with isolated coronary artery ectasia. Coron Artery Dis. 2005;16:45-50.
28. Tunick PA, Slater J, Kronzon I, Glassman E. Discrete atherosclerotic coronary artery aneurysm:a study of 20 patients. JAm Coil Cardiol. 1990;15:279-82.
29. Demopoulos VP, Olympios CD, Fakiolas CN, et al. The natural history of aneurysmal coronary artery disease. Heart. 1997;78:136-41.
30. Holsinger DR, Osmundson PJ, Edwards JE. The heart in periarteritis nodosa. Circulation 1962;25:610-29.
31. Sudhir K, Ports TA, Amidon TM, Goldberger JJ, Kane JP, Yock P, et al. Increased prevalence of coronary ectasia in heterozygous familial hypercholesterolemia. Circulation. 1995;91: 1375-80.
32. Starc R, Janezic AS, Cijan A. Angiographic evidence of coronary artery ectasia: our experience. Cor Vasa. 1991;33:288-93.
33. Farto-e-Abreu P, Mesquita A, Silva JA, Seabra Comez R. Coronary artery ectasia: clinical and angiographic characteristics and prognosis. Rev Port Cardiol. 1993;12:305-10.
34. Chia HM, Tan KH, Jackson G. Non-atherosclerotic coronary artery aneurysms: Two case reports. Heart. 1997;78(6):613-6.
35. Anfinsen OG, Aaberge L, Geiran O, Smith HJ, Aakhaus S. Coronary artery aneurysms mimicking cardiac tumor. Eur J Echocardiogr. 2004;5(4):308-12.
36. Dogan A, Ozaydin M, Gedikli O, Altinbas A, Ergene O. Effect of trimetazidine on exercise performance in patients with coronary artery ectasia. Jpn Heart J. 2003;44(4):463-70.
37. Desai MY, Biederman RW, Mankad S. Incidental echocardiographic detection of coronary artery aneurysm in a patient with multiple vascular aneurysms. Echocardiography. 2004;21(3): 265-7.
38. Akyurek O, Berkalp B, Sayin T, Kumbasar D, Kervancioglu C, Oral D. Altered coronary flow properties in diffuse coronary artery ectasia. Am Heart J. 2003;145(1):66-72.
39. Payam SP, Niroomand F. Coronary artery aneurysm: A review. Clin. Cardiol. 2006;29;439-43.
40. Tanabe M, Onishi K, Hiraoka N, Kitamura T, Okinaka T, Ito M, Isaka N, Nakano T. Bilateral giant coronary aneurysms diagnosed non-invasively by dynamic magnetic resonance imaging. Int J Cardiol. 2004;94(2-3):341-2.
41. Tengiz I, Ercan E, Aliyev E, Sekuri C, Duman C, Altuglu I. Elevated levels of matrix metalloprotein-3 in patients with coronary aneurysm: A case control study. Curr Control Trials Cardiovasc Med. 2004;5(1):doi:10.1186/1468-6708-5-10.
42. Abbate A, Patti G, Dambrosio A, Di Sciascio G. Left main coronary artery aneurysm: A case report and review of the literature. Ital Heart J. 2001;2(9):711-4.
43. Sarkar DA, Smith EE, Brecker SJ. Giant coronary aneurysms. Lancet. 2004;363(9402):37.
44. Rubartelli P, Terzi G, Borgo L, Giachero C. Coronary artery aneurysm after stent implantation: Acute and long-term results after percutaneous treatment with a stent graft. Ital Heart J. 2002;3(3):202-5.
45. Oe H, Ehara S, Yoshikawa J. Crab claw-like appearance on coronary angiography. Heart. 2005;91(4):437.
46. Aqel RA, Zoghbi GJ, Iskandrian A. Spontaneous coronary artery dissection, aneurysms, and pseudoaneurysms: A review. Echocardiography. 2004;21(2):175-82.
47. Baman TS, Cole JH, Devireddy CM, Sperling LS. Risk factors and outcomes in patients with coronary artery aneurysms. Am J Cardiol. 2004;93:1549-51.
48. Ebert PA, Peter RH, Gunnells JC, Sabiston DC. Resecting and grafting of coronary artery aneurysm. Circulation. 1971;43:593-8.
49. Kitamura S, Kawashima Y, Miyamoto K, Kobayashi T, Matsuda H, Ohgitani N, et al. Multiple coronary artery aneurysms resulting in myocardial infarction in a young man. J Thorac Cardiovasc Surg. 1975;70:290-7.
50. Gulec S, Aras O, Atmaca Y, Akyurek O, Hanson NQ, Sayin T, Tsai MY, Akar N, Oral D. Deletion polymorphism of the angiotensin I converting enzyme gene is a potent risk factor for coronary artery ectasia. Heart. 2003;89(2):213-4.
51. Mintz GS, Nissen SE, Anderson WD, et al. American College of Cardiology Clinical Expert Consensus Document on Standards for Acquisition, Measurement and Reporting of Intravascular Ultrasound Studies (IVUS). A report of the American College of Cardiology Task Force on Clinical Expert Consensus Documents. J Am Coll Cardiol. 2001;37:1478-92.
52. Mintz GS. Clinical utility of intravascular imaging and physiology in coronary artery disease. J Am Coll Cardiol. 2014;64:207-22.
53. Mintz GS, Weissman NJ. Intravascular ultrasound in the drug-eluting stent era. J Am Coll Cardiol. 2006;48:421-9.
54. Casella G, Klauss V, Ottani F, et al. Impact of intravascular ultrasound-guided stenting on long-term clinical outcome: a meta-analysis of available studies comparing intravascular ultrasound-guided and angiographically-guided stenting. Catheter Cardiovasc Interv. 2003;59:314-21.
55. Parise H, Maehara A, Stone GW, et al. Meta-analysis of randomized studies comparing intravascular ultrasound versus angiographic guidance of percutaneous coronary intervention in pre-drug-eluting stent era. Am J Cardiol. 2011;107:374-82.
56. Ahn JM, Kang SJ, Yoon SH, et al. Meta-analysis of outcomes after intravascular ultrasound-guided versus angiographically-

guided drug-eluting stent implantation in 26503 patients enrolled in three randomized trials and 14 observational studies. Am J Cardiol. 2014;113:1338-47.
57. McDaniel MC, Eshtehardi P, Sawaya FJ, et al. Contemporary clinical applications of coronary intravascular ultrasound. JACC Cardiovasc Interv. 2011;4:1155-67.
58. Kang SJ, Lee JY, Ahn JM et al. Validation of intravascular ultrasound-derived parameters with fractional flow reserve for assessment of coronary stenosis severity. Circ Cardiovasc Interv. 2011;4:65-71.
59. Nishioka T, Amanullah AM, Luo H, et al. Clinical validation of intravascular ultrasound imaging for assessment of coronary stenosis severity: comparison with stress myocardial perfusion imaging. J Am Coll Cardiol. 1999;33:1870-8.
60. Nakamura S, Colombom A, Gaglione A, et al. Intracoronary ultrasound observations during stent implantation. Circulation 1994;89:2026-34.
61. Brodie BR, Cooper C, Jones M, et al. Post-dilatation clinical comparative study. Is adjunctive balloon post dilatation necessary after coronary stent deployment? Final results from POSTIT trial. Catheter Cardiovasc Interv. 2003;59:184-92.
62. de Ribamar Costa J Jr, Mintz GS, Carlier SG, et al. Intravascular ultrasound assessment of drug-eluting stent expansion. Am Heart J. 2007;153:297-303.
63. Seung-Jung Park, Jung-Min Ahn. Intravascular ultrasound for the assessment of coronary lesion severity and optimization of percutaneous coronary intervention. Clinics Review articles, Intravascular Imaging: OCT and IVUS, Interventional Cardiology Clinics. 2015;4,3: 383-95.
64. Christopher F, Jacqueline S. Optical coherence tomography in the diagnosis and management of spontaneous coronary artery dissection. Clinics Review articles, Intravascular Imaging: OCT and IVUS, Interventional Cardiology Clinics. 2015;4,3:309-20.
65. Alfonso F, Paulo M, Dutary J. Endovascular imaging of angiographically invisible spontaneous coronary artery dissection. JACC Cardiovasc Interv. 2012;5:452-3.
66. Paulo M, Sandoval J, Lennie V, et al. Combined use of OCT and IVUS in spontaneous coronary artery dissection. JACC Cardiovasc Imaging. 2013;6:830-2.
67. Poon K, Bell B, Raffel OC, et al. Spontaneous coronary artery dissection: utility of intravascular ultrasound and optical coherence tomography during percutaneous coronary intervention. Circ Cardiovasc Interv. 2011;4:e5-7.
68. Bezerra HG, Costa MA, Guagliumi G, eta al. Intracorornary optical coherence tomography: a comprehensive review clinical and research applications. JACC Cardiovasc Interv. 2009;2(11):1035-46.
69. Arabindra B, Lopez JJ. Technical considerations and practical guidance for intracoronary optical coherence tomography, Intravascular Imaging: OCT and IVUS. Interventional Cardiology Clinics. 2015;4(3):239-49.
70. Gonzalo N, Escaned J, Alfonso F, et al. Morphometric assessment of coronary stenosis relevance with optical coherence tomography: a comparison with fractional flow reserve and intravascular ultrasound. J Am Col Cardiol. 2012;59:1080-9.
71. Briguari C, Anzuini A, Aeroldi F, et al. Intravascular ultrasound criteria for assessment of the functional significance of intermediate coronary artery stenoses and comparison with fractional flow reserve. Am J Cardiol. 2001;87:136-41.
72. Koo BK, Yang HM, Doh JH, et al. Optimal intravascular ultrasound criteria and their accuracy for defining the functional significance of intermediate coronary stenoses of different locations. JACC Cardiovasc Interv. 2011;4:803-11.
73. Waksman R, Legutko J, Singh J, et al. First: Fractional flow reserve and intravascular ultrasound relationship study. J Am Col Cardiol. 2013;61:917-23.
74. Lee T, Kakuta T, Yonestu T, et al. Assessment of echo-attenuated plaque by optical coherence tomography and its impact on post-procedural creatinine kinase-myocardial band elevation in elective stent implantation. JACC Cardiovasc Interv. 2011;4:483-91.
75. Lee T, Yonetsu T, Koura K, et al. Impact of coronary plaque morphology assessed by optical coherence tomography on cardiac troponin elevation in patients with elective stent implantation. Circ Cardiovasc Interv. 2011;4:378-86.
76. Port I, D Vito L, Burzotta F, et al. Predictors of periprocedural (type IVa) myocardial infarction, as assessed by frequency-domain optical coherence tomography. Circ Cardiovasc Interv. 2012;5:89-96. S 1-6.
77. Bouma BE, Tearney GJ, Yabushita H, et al. Evaluation of intracoronary stenting by intravascular optical coherence tomography. Heart. 2003;89:317-20.
78. Guagliumi G, Sirbu V, Musumeci G, et al. Examination of the in-vivo mechanisms of late drug-eluting stent thrombosis: findings from optical coherence tomography and intravascular ultrasound imaging. JACC Cardiovasc Interv. 2012;5: 12-20.
79. Prati F, D Vito L, Biondi-Zoccai G, et al. Angiography alone versus angiography plus optical coherence tomography to guide decision-making during percutaneous coronary interventions: the Centro per la Lotta contro l'Infarto-optimization of percutaneous coronary intervention (CLI OPCI) study. Euro Intervention. 2012;8:823-9.
80. Gutierrez H, Arnold R, Gimeno F, et al. Optical coherence tomography. Initial experience in patients undergoing percutaneous coronary intervention. Rev Esp Cardiol. 2008;61:976-9.
81. MacNeil BD, Lowe HC, Takano M, et al. Intravascular modalities for detection of vulnerable plauque: Current status. Arterioscler Thromb Vasc Biol. 2004;23:1333-42.
82. Jang IK, Bouma BE, Kang DH, et al. Visualization of coronary atherosclerotic plaques in patients using optical coherence tomography: comparison with intravascular ultrasound. J Am Coll Cardiol. 2002;39:604-9.
83. Tearney GJ, Yabushita H, Houser SL, et al. Quantification of macrophage content in atherosclerotic plaques by optical coherence tomography. Circulation. 2003;107:113-9.
84. Barlis P, Schmitt JM, Current and future developments in intracoronary optical coherence tomography imaging. Eurointervention. 2009;4: 529-33.
85. Prati F, Guagliumi G, Mintz GS, et al. Expert review document part 2: methodology, terminology and clinical applications of optical coherence tomography for the assessment of interventional procedures. Eur Heart J. 2012;33:2513-20.
86. Radu MD, Raber L, Heo J, et al. Natural history of optical coherence tomography-detected non-flow-limiting edge dissections following drug eluting stent implantation. Euro Intervention. 2014;9(9):1085-94.

87. Imola F, Mallus MT, Rammazotti V, et al. Safety and feasibility of frequency domain optical coherence tomography to guide decision making in percutaneous coronary intervention. Euro Intervention. 2010;6:575-81.
88. Stefano GT, Bezerra HG, Mehanna E, et al. Unrestricted utilization of frequency domain optical coherence tomography in coronary interventions. Int J Cardiovasc Imaging. 2013;29(4):741-52.
89. Viceconte N, Chan PH, Barrero EA, et al. Frequency domain optical coherence tomography for guidance of coronary stenting. Int J Cardiol. 2013;1(166):722-8.
90. Riber L, Radu MD, Optimising cardiovascular outcomes using optical coherence tomography-guided percutaneous coronary interventions. Euro Intervention. 2012;22(8):765-71.
91. Stefano GT, Bezerra HG, Attizzani G, et al. Utilization of frequency domain optical coherence tomography and fractional flow reserve to assesss intermediate coronary stenosis: conciliating anatomic and physiologic information. Int J Cardiovasc Imaging. 2011;27:299-308.
92. Joner M, Finn AV, Farb A, et al. Pathology of drug-eluting stents in humans: delayed healing and late thrombotic risks. J Am Coll Cardiol. 2006;48:193-202.
93. Chamie D, Bezerra HG, Attizzani GF, et al. Incidence, predictors, morphological characteristics and clinical outcomes of stent edge dissection detected by optical coherence tomography. JACC Cardiovasc Interv. 2013;6:800-13.
94. Onuma Y, Thussen L, van genus RJ, et al. TROFI Investigators. Randomized study to assess the effects of thrombus aspiration on flow area in patients with ST-segment elevation myocardial infarction: an optical frequency domain imaging study-TROFI trial. Eur Heart J. 2013;34:1050-60.
95. Magro M, Regar E, Gutierrez-Chico JL, et al. Residual atherothrombotic material after stenting in acute myocardial infarction-an optical coherence tomographic evaluation. Int J Cardiol. 2013;167:656-63.
96. Nakazawa G, Finn AV, Joner M, et al. Delayed arterial healing and increased late stent thrombosis at culprit sites after drug-eluting stent placement for acute myocardial infarction patients: an autopsy study. Circulation. 2008; 118:1138-45.
97. Gonzalo N, Barlis P, Serruys PW, et al. Incomplete stent apposition and delayed tissue coverage are more frequent in drug-eluting stents implanted during primary percutaneous coronary intervention for ST-segment elevation myocardial infarction than in drug-eluting stents implanted for stable/ unstable angina: insights from optical coherence tomography. JACC Cardiovasc Interv. 2009;2:445-52.
98. Bernelli C, Sirbu V, Guagliumi G. Percutaneous coronary intervention planning and optimization with optical coherence tomography. Intravascular Imaging: OCT and IVUS, Interventional Cardiology Clinics. 2015;4(3):251-84.
99. Davies RF, Goldberg AD, Forman S. Asymptomatic Cardiac Ischemia Pilot (ACIP) study two-year follow-up;outcomes of patients randomized to initial strategies of medical therapy versus revascularization. Circulation 1997;95:2037-43.
100. Shaw LJ, Heller GV, Casperson P, et al. Gated myocardial perfusion single photon emission computed tomography in the Clinical Outcomes Utilizing Revascularization and Aggressive drug Evaluation (COURAGE) trial, Veterans Administration Cooperative study no. 424. J Nucl Cardiol. 2006;13: 685-98.
101. Pijls NH, Fearon WF, Tonino PA, et al. Fractional flow reserve versus angiography for guiding percutaneous coronary intervention in patients with multivessel coronary artery disease: 2-year follow-up of the FAME (Fractional Flow Reserve Versus Angiography for Multivessel Evaluation) study. J Am Coll Cardiol. 2010;56:177-84.
102. Pijls NHJ, van Schaardenburgh P, Manoharan G, et al. Percutaneous coronary intervention of functionally non-significant stenosis: 5-year follow-up of the DEFER study. J Am Coll Cardiol. 2007;49:2105-11.
103. Pijls NH, van Son JA, Kirkeeide RL, De Bruyne B, Gould KL. Experimental basis of determining maximum coronary, myocardial, and collateral blood flow by pressure measurements for assessing functional stenosis severity before and after percutaneous transluminal coronary angioplasty. Circulation. 1993;87:1354-67.
104. De Bruyne B, Baudhuin T, Melin JA, et al. Coronary flow reserve calculated from pressure measurements in humans. Validation with positron emission tomography. Circulation 1994;89:1013-22.
105. Wijns W, De Bruyne B, Vanhoenacker P. What does the clinical cardiologist need from non-invasive cardiac imaging: Is it time to adjust practices to meet evolving demands? J Nucl Cardiol. 2007;14:366-70.
106. Main: Nico HJ, Jan-Willem EM. Functional Measurement of Coronary Stenosis. J Am Coll Cardiol. 2012;59(12).
107. Mayer B, Beretta M. The enigma of nitroglycerine bioactivation and nitrate tolerance: news, views and troubles. Br J Pharmacol. 2008;155:170-84.
108. Ignarro LJ, Lipton H, Edwards JC, et al. Mechanism of vascular smooth muscle relaxation by organic nitrate, nitrites, nitroprusside and nitric oxide: evidence for the involvement of s-nitrothiols as active intermediates. J Pharmacol Exp Ther. 1981;218:739-49.
109. Braun LT. Calcium channel blockers for the treatment of coronary artery spasm: rationale, effects and nursing responsibilities. Heart Lung 1983;12:226-32.
110. Fugit MD, Rubal BJ, Donovan DJ. Effects of intracoronary nicardipine, diltiazem and verapamil on coronary blood flow. J Invasive Cardiol. 2000;12:80-5.
111. Levine GN, Bates ER, Blakenship JC, et al. 2011 ACCF/AHA/ SCAI Guidelines for Percutaneous Intervention. A report of the American College of Cardiology Foundation/American Heart Association Task Force on Practice Guidelines and the Society for Cardiovascular Angiography and Interventions. J Am Coll Cardiol. 2011;58:e44-122.
112. Navarase EP, Buffon A, Andeatti F, et al. Adenosine improves post-procedural coronary flow but not clinical outcomes in patients with acute coronary syndrome: a meta-analysis of randomized trials. Atherosclerosis. 2012;222: 1-7.
113. Ito H, Taniyama Y, Iwakura K, et al. Intravenous nicorandil can preserve microvascular integrity and myocardial viability in patients with reperfused anterior wall myocardial infarction. J Am Coll Cardiol. 1999;33:654-60.
114. Amit G, Cafri C, Yaroslavtsev S, et al. Intracoronary nitroprusside for the prevention of the no-reflow phenomenon after primary percutaneous coronary intervention in acute myocardial infarction. A randomized, double-blind, placebo-controlled clinical trial. Am Heart J. 2006;152:887.e1-14.

115. Claessen B, Henriques J PS. Vasoactive and antiarrhythic drugs during percutaneous coronary intervention. Interventional Cardiology Clinics, Interventional Pharmacology. 2013;2(4): 665-70.
116. Antithrombotic Trialists' Collaboration. Collaborative meta-analysis of randomized trials of antiplatelet therapy for prevention of death, myocardial infarction, and stroke in high risk patients, BMJ. 2002;324:71-86.
117. Weil J, Colin-Jones D, Langman M, et al. Prophylactic aspirin and risk of peptic ulcer bleeding. BMJ. 1995;310:827-30.
118. Kunadian V, Sinclair H, Sutton A, Dangas D. Aspirin, platelet P2Y12 receptor inhibitors, and other oral antiplatelet: Comparative Pharmacology and role in elective PCI. Interventional Cardiology Clinics, Interventional Pharmacology. 2013;2(4):527-36.
119. Yusuf S, Zhao F, Mehta SR, et al. Effects of clopidogrel in addition to aspirin in patients with acute coronary syndromes without ST-segmentation elevation. N Engl J Med. 2001;345:494-502.
120. Mehta SR, Yusuf S, Peters RJ, et al. Effects of pre-treatment with clopidogrel and aspirin followed by long-term therapy in patients undergoing percutaneous coronary intervention: the PCI_CURE study. Lancet. 2001;358:527-33.
121. Bagai J, Banerjee S, Brilakis E. Combination antithrombotic management for non-ST segment elevation acute coronary syndromes. Interventional Cardiology Clinics, Interventional Pharmacology. 2013;2(4):553-72.
122. Wijns W, Kohl P, Danchin N, et al. Task Force on Myocardial Revascularization of the European Society of Cardiology (ESC) and the European Association of Cardio-Thoracic Surgery (EACTS), European Association for Percutaneous Cardiovascular Interventions (EAPCI). Guidelines on myocardial revascularization. Eur Heart J. 2010;31:2501-55.
123. Levine GN, Bates ER, Blakenship JC et al. 2011 ACCF/AHA/SCAI Guidelines for Percutaneous Intervention. A report of the American College of Cardiology Foundation/American Heart Association Task Force on Practice Guidelines and the Society for Cardiovascular Angiography and Interventions. J Am Coll Cardiol. 2011;58:e44-122.
124. Dangas D, Mehran R, Guagliumi G, et al. HORIZONS-AMI Trial investigators. Role of clopidogrel loading dose in patients with ST-segment elevation myocardial infarction undergoing primary angioplasty: results from the HORIZONS-AMI (harmonizing outcomes with revascularization and stents in acute myocardial infarction) trial. J Am Coll Cardiol. 2009;54: 1438-46.
125. CURRENT-OASIS 7 Investigators, Mehta SR, Bassand JP, Chrolavicius S, et al. Dose comparison of clopidogrel and aspirin in acute coronary syndromes. N Engl J Med. 2010;363:930-42.
126. Capranzano P, Tamburino C, Dangas G. combination antithrombotic management of STEMI with pharmacoinvasive strategy, primary PCI, or Rescue PCI. Interventional Cardiology Clinics, Interventional Pharmacology. 2013;2(4): 573-84.
127. Holmes DR Jr, Dehmer GJ, Kaul S, et al. ACCF/AHA clopidogrel clinical alert: approaches to the FDA "boxed warnings": a report of the American College of Cardiology Task Force on Clinical Expert Consensus Documents and the American Heart Association endorsed by the Society for Cardiovascular Angiography and Interventions and the Society of Thoracic Surgeons. J Am Coll Cardiol. 2010;56:321-41.
128. Wiviott SD, Braunwald E, MacCabe CH, et al. Prasugrel versus clopidogrel in atients with acute coronary syndromes. N Engl J Med. 2007;357:2001-15.
129. Montalescot G, Wiviott SD, Braunwald E, et al. TRITON-TIMI 38 investigators. Prasugrel compared with clopidogrel in patients undergoing percutaneous coronary intervention for ST-elevation myocardial infarction (TRITON-TIMI 38): double blind randomized controlled trial. Lancet. 2009;373:723-31.
130. Gurbel MPA, Bliden KP, Butler K, et al. Randomized double-blind assessment of the ONSET and OFFSET of the antiplatelet effects of ticagrelor versus clopidogrel in patients with stable coronary artery disease: the ONSET/OFFSET study. Circulation. 2009;120:2577-85.
131. Wallentin L, Backer RC, Budaj A, et al. Ticagrelor versus clopidogrel in patients with acute coronary syndromes. N Engl J Med. 2009;361:1045-57.
132. Steg PG, James S, Harrington RA, et al. PLATO study group. Ticagrelor versus clopidogrel in patients with ST-elevation acute coronary syndromes intended for reperfusion with primary percutaneous coronary intervention: a Platelet Inhibition and Patient Outcomes (PLATO) trial subgroup analysis. Circulation. 2010;122:2131-41.
133. Bhatt GD, Stone GJ, Mahaffey KW et al. Effects of platelet inhibition with cangrelor during PCI on ischemic events. N Engl J Med. 2013;368:1303-13.
134. EPISTENT Investigators. Randomized placebo controlled and balloon-angioplasty-controlled trial to assess safety of coronary stenting with use of platelet glycoprotein-IIb/IIIa blockade. Lancet. 1998;352:87-92.
135. Topol EJ, Lincoff AM, Kereiakes DJ, et al. Multi-year follow-up of abciximab therapy in three randomized, placebo-controlled trials of percutaneous coronary revascularization. Am J Med. 2002;113:1-6.
136. Giugliano R, White J, Bode C, et al. Early versus delayed, provisional eptifibatide in acute coronary syndromes. N Engl J Med. 2009;360:2176-90.
137. Horwitz PA, Berlin JA, Sauer WH, Laskey WK, Krone RJ, Kimmel SE. Bleeding risk of platelet glycoprotein IIb/IIIa receptor antagonists in broad-based practice (results from the Society for Cardiac Angiography and Interventions Registry). Am J Cardiol. 2003;91:803-6.
138. Mehran R, Pocock S, Nikolsky E, et al. Impact of bleeding on mortality after percutaneous coronary intervention. J Am Coll Cardiol Intv. 2011;4:654-64.
139. Palmerini T, Biondi-Zoccai G, Della Riva D, et al. Stent thrombosis with drug-eluting stents. J Am Coll Cardiol. 2013;62:1915-21.
140. Bellemain-Appaix A, O'Connor S, Silvain J, et al. Association of clopidogrel pretreatment with mortality, cardiovascular events, and major bleeding among patients undergoing percutaneous coronary intervention. A systematic review and meta-analysis. JAMA. 2012;308:2507-16.
141. Kastrati A, Mehilli J, Schulhlen H, et al. A clinical trial of abciximab in elective percutaneous coronary intervention after pretreatment with clopidogrel. N Engl J Med. 2004;350:232-8.
142. Kastrati A, Mehilli J, Neumann F, et al. Abciximab in patients with acute coronary syndromes undergoing percutaneous coronary intervention after clopidogrel pretreatment. JAMA. 2006;295:1531-8.

143. Lincoff AM, Bittl JA, Harrington RA, et al. Bivalirudin and provisional glycoprotein IIb/IIIa blockade compared with heparin and planned glycoprotein IIb/IIIa blockade during percutaneous coronary intervention. The REPLACE-2 trial. JAMA. 2003;289:853-63.
144. Stone G, McLaurin BT, Cox DA, et al. Bivalirudin for patients with acute coronary syndromes. N Engl J Med. 2006;355:2203-16.
145. Stone G, Witzenbichler B, Guagliumi G, et al. Bivalirudin during primary PCI in acute myocardial infarction. N Engl J Med. 2008;358:2218-30.
146. Safley DM, Venkitachalam L, Kennedy KF, Cohen DJ. Impact of glycoprotein IIb/IIIa inhibition in contemporary percutaneous coronary intervention for acute coronary syndromes: insights from the National Cardiovascular Data Registry. J Am Coll Cardiol Intv. 2015;8:1574-82.
147. Lincoff AM. What Role for Glycoprotein IIb/IIIa Inhibition in Contemporary Coronary Intervention? JA CC: Cardiovasc Interv. 2015;8(12):1583-5.
148. Boscareli D, Vaquerizo B, Faustin MG, et al. Intracoronary thrombolysis in patients presenting with ST-segment elevation myocardial infarction presenting with massive intraluminal thrombus and failed aspiration. Eur Heart J: Acute Cardiovascular Care. 2014;3(3):229-36.
149. Topol E. Textbook of Interventional Cardiology, Abrupt Vessel Closure. pp.475-89.
150. Patti G, Colonna G, Pasceri V, et al. Randomized trial of high loading dose of clopidogrel for reduction of periprocedural myocardial infarction in patients undergoing coronary interventions: Results from the ARMYDA-2 (Antiplatelet therapy for Reduction of Myocardial Damage during Angioplasty) study. Circulation. 2005;111:2099-2.
151. Fiedler K, Meing M, Mehilli J, et al. Triple Therapy in Patients on Oral Anticoagulation after Drug Eluting Stent Implantation (ISAR-TRIPLE). J Am Coll Cardiol. 2015;65(16):1619-29.
152. Willem JM Dewilde et al. Use of clopidogrel with or without aspirin in patients taking oral anticoagulant therapy and undergoing percutaneous coronary intervention: an open-label, randomized, controlled trial. Lancet. 2013;381(9872):1107-15.
153. Jonas O, Lars W, John H, et al. New oral anticoagulants in addition to single or dual antiplatelet treatment after an cute coronary syndrome: a systemic review and meta-analysis. Eur Heart J. 2013:34:1670-80.
154. Singh M, Berger PB, Ting HH, et al. Influence of coronary thrombus on outcome of percutaneous coronary angioplasty in the current era (the Mayo Clinic experience). Am J Cardiol. 2001;88:1091-6.
155. Blankenship JC, Tasissa G, O'Shea JC, et al. on behalf of ESPRIT Investigators. Effect of glycoprotein IIb/IIIa receptor inhibition on angiographic complications during percutaneous coronary intervention in the ESPRIT trial. J Am Coll Cardiol. 2001;38:653-8.
156. Khan MM, Ellis SG, Aguirre FV, et al. Does intracoronary thrombus influence the outcome of high risk percutaneous transluminal coronary angioplasty? Clinical and angiographic outcomes in a large multicenter trial. EPIC Investigators. Evaluation of IIb/IIIa Platelet Receptor Antagonist 7E3 in Preventing Ischemic Complications. J Am Coll Cardiol. 1998;31:31-6.
157. de Feyter PJ, van den Brand M, Laarman GJ, van Domburg R, Serruys PW, Suryapranata H. Acute coronary artery occlusion during and after percutaneous transluminal coronary angioplasty. Frequency, prediction, clinical course, management, and follow-up. Circulation. 1991;83:927-36.
158. Detre KM, Holmes DR Jr, Holubkov R, et al. Incidence and consequences of periprocedural occlusion. The 1985-1986 National Heart, Lung, and Blood Institute Percutaneous Transluminal Coronary Angioplasty Registry. Circulation 1990;82:739-50.
159. Ellis SG, Roubin GS, King SB III, et al. Angiographic and clinical predictors of acute closure after native vessel coronary angioplasty. Circulation. 1988;77:372-9.
160. Singh M, Reeder GS, Ohman EM, et al. Does the presence of thrombus seen on coronary angiogram affect outcome after percutaneous coronary angioplasty? An angiographic trials pool data experience. J Am COLL Cardiol. 2001;38:624-30.
161. Ndrepepa G, Berger PB, Mehilli J, et al. Periprocedural bleeding and 1-year outcome after percutaneous coronary interventions: appropriateness of including bleeding as a component of a quadruple end point. J Am Coll Cardiol. 2008;51:690-7.
162. Lennon RJ, Holmes DR, Prasad A, et al. Percutaneous coronary intervention in native vessels with angiographically visible thrombus temporal trends and impact of drug-eluting Stents. JACC: Cardiovasc Interv. 2010;3(9):937-46.
163. Jaffe R, Dick A, Strauss BH, et al. Prevention and treatment of microvascular obstruction-related myocardial injury and coronary no-reflow following percutaneous coronary intervention, A Systematic Approach. JACC Cardiovasc Interv. 2010;3(7):695-704.
164. Stone GW, Webb J, Cox DA, et al. Distal microcirculatory protection during percutaneous coronary intervention in acute ST-segmentation elevation myocardial infarction: A randomized controlled trail. JAMA. 2005;293:1063-72.
165. Glick M, Jander N, Bestehorn HP, et al. Randomized evaluation of the effects of filter-based distal protection on myocardial perfusion and infact size after primary percutaneous catheter intervention in myocardial infarction with and without ST-segment elevation. Circulation. 2005;112:1462-69.
166. Ali OA, Bhindi R, McMohan AC, et al. Distal protection in cardiovascular medicine: Current status. Am Heart J. 2006;152:207-16.
167. Baim DS, Wahr D, George B, et al. Randomized trial of distal embolic protection device during percutaneous intervention of saphenous vein aorto-coronary bypass grafts. Circulation. 2002;105:1285-90.
167. Mauri L, Rogers C, Baim DS, et al. Devices for distal protection during percutaneous revascularization. Circulation. 2016;113:2651-56.
169. Bavry AA, Kumbhani DJ, Bhatt DL. Role of adjunctive thrombectomy and embolic protection devices in acute myocardial infarction: a comprehensive meta-analysis of randomized trials. Eur Heart J. 2008;29:2989-3
170. Vlaar PJ, Svilaas T, van der Horst IC, et al. Cardiac death and reinfarction after 1 year in the Thrombus Aspiration during Percutaneous coronary intervention in Acute myocardial infarction Study (TAPAS): a 1-year follow-up study. Lancet. 2008;371:1915-20.

171. Lagerqvist B, Fröbert O, Olivecrona GK, et al. Outcomes 1 year after thrombus aspiration for myocardial infarction. N Engl J Med. 2014;371:1111-20.
172. Jolly SS, Cairns JA, Yusuf S, et al. On behalf of the TOTAL Investigators. Outcomes after thrombus aspiration for ST elevation myocardial infarction: 1-year follow-up of the prospective randomised TOTAL trial. Lancet. 2016;387(10014): 127-35.
173. Kumbhani DJ, Bavry AA, Desai MY, Bangalore S, Bhatt DL. Role of aspiration and mechanical thrombectomy in patients with acute myocardial infarction undergoing primary angioplasty: an updated meta-analysis of randomized trials. J Am Coll Cardiol. 2013;62:1409-18.
174. De Rosa S, Caiazzo G, Torella D, Indolfi C. Intracoronary versus intravenous abciximab bolus administration (letter). J Am Coll Cardiol. 2014;63:1340-1.
175. De Vita M, Burzotta F, Porto I, et al. Thrombus aspiration in ST elevation myocardial infarction: comparative efficacy in patients treated early and late after onset of symptoms. Heart. 2010;96:1287-90.
176. Thiele H, de Waha S, Zeymer U, et al. Effect of aspiration thrombectomy on microvascular obstruction in NSTEMI patients: the TATORT-NSTEMI trial. J Am Coll Cardiol. 2014;64: 1117-24.
177. Hung C, et al. Aspiration thrombectomy: Time should be considered. J Am Coll Cardiol. 2015;65:55-62.
178. Keeley EC, Boura JA, Grines CL. Primary angioplasty versus intravenous thrombolytic therapy for acute myocardial infarction: a quantitative review of 23 randomized trials. Lancet. 2003;361:13-20.
179. O'Gara PT, Kushner FG, Ascheim DD, et al. 2013 ACCF/AHA guideline for the management of ST-elevation myocardial infarction: a report of the American College of Cardiology Foundation/American Heart Association Task Force on Practice Guidelines. J Am Coll Cardiol. 2013;61:485-510.
180. Jaffe R, Charron T, Puley G, Dick A, Strauss BH. Microvascular obstruction and the no-reflow phenomenon after percutaneous coronary intervention. Circulation. 2008;117:3152-6.
181. Morishima I, Sone T, Okumura K, et al. Angiographic no-reflow phenomenon as a predictor of adverse long-term outcome in patients treated with percutaneous transluminal coronary angioplasty for first acute myocardial infarction. J Am Coll Cardiol. 2000;36:1202-9.
182. Antoniucci D, Valenti R, Migliorini A, et al. Direct infarct artery stenting without predilation and no-reflow in patients with acute myocardial infarction. Am Heart J. 2001;142:684-90.
183. Ndrepepa G, Tiroch K, Keta D, et al. Predictive factors and impact of no reflow after primary percutaneous coronary intervention in patients with acute myocardial infarction. Circ Cardiovasc Interv. 2010;3:27-33.
184. Harrison RW, Aggarwal A, Ou FS, et al. American College of Cardiology National Cardiovascular Data Registry. Incidence and outcomes of no-reflow phenomenon during percutaneous coronary intervention among patients with acute myocardial infarction. Am J Cardiol. 2013;111:178-84.
185. Vijayalakshmi K, Whittaker VJ, Kunadian B, et al. Prospective, randomized, controlled trial to study the effect of intracoronary injection of verapamil and adenosine on coronary blood flow during percutaneous coronary intervention in patients with acute coronary syndromes. Heart. 2006;92: 1278-84.
186. Levine GN, Bates ER, Blankenship JC, et al. 2011 ACCF/AHA/SCAI guideline for percutaneous coronary intervention: a report of the American College of Cardiology Foundation/American Heart Association Task Force on Practice Guidelines and the Society for Cardiovascular Angiography and Interventions. J Am Coll Cardiol. 2011;58:e44-122.
187. Rodriguez A, Ayala F, Bernardi V, et al. Optimal coronary balloon angioplasty with provisional stenting versus primary stent (OCBAS): Immediate and long-term follow-up results. J Am Coll Cardiol,1998;32:1351-57.
188. Foley DP, Serruys PW. Provisional stenting — stent-like balloon angioplasty: Evidence to define the continuing role of balloon angioplasty for percutaneous coronary revascularization. Semin Interv Cardiol 1996;1:269-73.
189. Bech GJ, Pijls NH, de Bruyne B, et al. Usefulness of fractional flow reserve to predict clinical outcome after balloon angioplasty. Circulation. 1999;99:883-8.
190. Suk-Kyu Oh, Seung-Woon Rha, Hyungdon Kook, et al. Two different successful angioplasty methods in patients with stenotic coronary artery ectasia. Chonnam Med J. 2012;48(3):185-9.
191. Fokkema ML, Vlaar PJ, Svilaas T. Thrombus aspiration as definitive mechanical intervention for ST-Elevation myocardial infarction: A report of five cases. Cathlab Digest. 2008;16(6).
192. Welt FGP, Rogers C. Inflammation and restenosis in the stent era. Arterioscler Thromb Vasc Biol. 2002;22:1769-76.
193. Carrick D, Oldroyd KG, McEntegart M, et al. A randomized trial of deferred stenting versus immediate stenting to prevent no-or slow-reflow in acute ST-segment elevation myocardial infarction (DEFER-STEMI). J Am Coll Cardiol. 2014;63:2088-98.
194. Isaaz K, Robin C, Cerisier A, et al. A new approach of primary angioplasty for ST-elevation acute myocardial infarction based on minimalist immediate mechanical intervention. Coron Artery Dis. 2006;17:261-9.
195. Kelbæk H, Engstrøm T, Ahtarovski KA, et al. Deferred stent implantation in patients with ST-segment elevation myocardial infarction: a pilot study. Euro Intervention. 2013;8:1126-33.
196. Escaned J, Echavarría-Pinto M, Gorgadze T, et al. Safety of lone thrombus aspiration without concomitant coronary stenting in selected patients with acute myocardial infarction. Euro Intervention. 2013;8:1149-56.
197. Freixa X, Belle L, Joseph L, et al. Immediate vs. delayed stenting in acute myocardial infarction: a systematic review and meta-analysis. Euro Intervention. 2013;8:1207-16.
198. Yip HK. Chen MC, Wu CJ. Clinical features and outcome of coronary artery aneurysm in patients with acute myocardial infarction undergoing a primary percutaneous coronary intervention. Cardiology. 2002;98:132-40.
199. Erden I, Erden EC, Özhan H, et al. Outcome of primary percutaneous intervention in patients with infarct-related coronary artery ectasia. Angiology. 2010;61(6):574-79.
200. Rha SW, Wani SP, Oh DJ. Parallel stenting using two sirolimus-eluting stents in an ectatic coronary artery stenosis. Heart. 2007;93:976.
201. Stefanadis C, Toutouzas K, Tsiamis E, Toutouzas P. New stent design for autologous venous graft-covered stent preparation: first human application for sealing of a coronary aneurysm.

Catheterization and Cardiovascular Interventions. 2002;55: 222-7.
202. Fineschi M, Gori T, Sinicropi G, Bravi A: Polytetrafluoroethylene (PTFE) covered stents for the treatment of coronary artery aneurysms. Heart. 2004;90(5):490.
203. Burzotta F, Trani C, Romagnoli E, Mazzari MA, Savino M, Schiavoni G, Crea F. Percutaneous treatment of a large coronary aneurysm using the selfexpandable Symbiot PTFE-covered stent. Chest. 2004;126(2):644-5.
204. Briguori C, Sarais C, Sivieri G, Takagi T, DiMario C, Colombo A. Polytetrafluoroethylene-covered stent and coronary artery aneurysms. Cathet Cardiovasc Interv. 2002;55(3): 326-30.
205. Erol MK, Bozkurt E, Arslan S. Percutaneous sealing of coronary aneurysm by grafted stent implantation. Heart. 2004;90(11):1309.
206. Stefanadis C, Toutouzas K, Tsiamis E. Toutouzas P. New stent design for autologous venous graft-covered stent preparation: first human application for sealing of a coronary aneurysm. Catheter Cardiovasc Interv. 2002;55:222-7.
207. Dudek D, Abizaid A, Silber S, et al. One-year results from the MASTER trial, a prospective, randomized, multicenter evaluation of an embolic protection stent (MGuard) in patients with STEMI undergoing primary PCI. J Am Coll Cardiol. 2013;62 Suppl 1:B14.
208. Agirbasli M, Morris DC, Marshall JJ. The use of intrastent peripheral stent in large coronary arteries: report of three cases. Catheter Cardiovasc Interv. 2000;50:498-501.
209. Yew KL. Novel use of absorb bioresorbable vascular scaffold and STENTYS self-apposing coronary stent for complex saphenous vein grafts intervention, Int J Cardiol. 2014;18663:e1-e2.
210. Moretti C, Omedè P, Presutti DG, et al. Shaping an ectatic coronary artery: Stentys implantation. Int J Cardiol. 2014;171(3):459-61.
211. Laborde JC, Borenstein N, Behr L, Ramcharitar S. Stentys coronary bifurcation stent. Euro Intervention. 2007;3(1):162-5.
212. La Manna A, Geraci S, Tamburino C. A self-expandable coronary stent system to treat complex coronary stenosis complicated by poststenotic aneurysm: an optical coherence tomographic evidence-based case report. J Invasive Cardiol. 2011;23(12):E277-80.
213. Giordano A, Corcione N, Polimeno M, et al. No surprising forward jump when deploying a self-expandable stent: two cases exploiting the combination of Emboshield Nav6 BareWire and Stentys devices. Int J Cardiol. 2013;168(3):3079-81.
214. Burzotta F, Trani C, Romagnoli E, Mazzari MA, Savino M, Schiavoni G, et al. Percutaneous treatment of a large coronary aneurysm using the self-expandable Symbiot PTFE-covered stent. Chest. 2004;126:644-5.
215. Elahi MM, Dhannapuneni RV, Keal R. Giant left main coronary artery aneurysm with mitral regurgitation. Heart. 2004;90(12):1430.
216. Badmanaban B, Mallon P, Campbell N, Sarsam MA. Repair of left coronary artery aneurysm, recurrent ascending aortic aneurysm, and mitral valve prolapsed 19 years after Bentall's procedure in a patient with Marfan syndrome. J Card Surg. 2004;19(1):59-61.
217. Turkay C, Golbasi I, Sahin N, Kabukcu M, Bayezid O. Surgical management of an atherosclerotic aneurysm of the left main coronary artery. J Thorac Cardiovasc Surg. 2001;122(3):626-7.
218. Ebert PA, Peter RH, Gunnells JC, Sabiston DC. Resecting and grafting of coronary artery aneurysm. Circulation. 1971;43:593-8.

CHAPTER

10

Multivessel Percutaneous Coronary Intervention: Interventional Cardiologist's Perspective

K Sarat Chandra, S Nagendra Boopathy

INTRODUCTION

Coronary artery disease (CAD) remains one of the leading causes of morality all over the world. India, with its high prevalence of diabetes, has been experiencing a high incidence of CAD. The last three decades have found significant improvement in the management of CAD especially in the field of coronary interventions. Though percutaneous coronary intervention (PCI) is the treatment of choice in single and most of the double vessel disease cases, there is continuing debate about the choice of revascularization in patients with triple vessel disease. In this review, we discuss about the choice of revascularization in the management of patients with multivessel disease.

MULTIVESSEL DISEASE

More than half the patients with stable ischemic heart disease will have multivessel disease while the incidence of the same is higher in the setting of acute coronary syndromes and diabetes mellitus (DM).[1] Revascularization in such patients depends on various factors that include DM, coronary anatomy (syntax score), clinical presentation of the patient, comorbid conditions associated with the patient, cost of therapy (Pharmacoeconomics) and patient's choice. Though western literature deals with almost all the above factors, pharmacoeconomics of therapy is often missed while considering the therapy for a patient In our approach, we classify the patients based on their clinical presentation into patients with acute coronary syndrome and those with stable ischemic heart disease (Flow chart 10.1).

Multivessel Intervention in Patients with Stable Ischemic Heart Disease

Though many studies comparing the efficacy of balloon angioplasty and bare metal stents with coronary artery bypass graft surgery (CABG) are available, they are not contemporary and are not appropriate in this era of drug eluting stents (DES) and latest generation dual antiplatelet therapy.[2-6] Hence, we intend to limit our discussion to leading and relatively recent trials comparing the efficacy of DES vs CABG. Best evidence comparing DES to CABG comes from two studies. They are SYNTAX [Percutaneous Coronary Intervention versus Coronary-Artery Bypass Grafting for Severe Coronary Artery Disease][4,5] and BEST TRIAL (Trial of Everolimus-Eluting Stents or Bypass Surgery for Coronary Disease).[6]

SYNTAX

SYNTAX trial compared CABG with first generation DES, paclitaxel eluting stent (Taxus) in patients with left main and multivessel disease. 1800 patients were randomly assigned to CABG (n = 897) or PCI (n = 903). As the five year results are now available, we would like to emphasize them rather than the 12 month results. After 5 years of follow-up, major adverse cardiac and cerebral events (MACCE) were 26.9% in the CABG group and 37.3% in the PCI group ($p < 0{\cdot}0001$). Incidence of myocardial infarction and repeat revascularization in the CABG vs PCI were 3.8% vs 9.7% [$p < 0.0001$] and 13.7% vs 25.9% [$p < 0.0001$] respectively. Though the 12 months results showed significantly increased incidence of stroke in the CABG arm, 5 year results showed only a trend towards increased incidence of stroke with CABG (3.7% vs 2.4%; $p = 0.09$). All cause mortality was similar between the groups (11.4% in the CABG group vs 13.9% in the PCI group; $p = 0.10$). In the sub group analysis based on the SYNTAX score, it was reconfirmed that patients with lower syntax score (<23) did equally well in both PCI and CABG arms [28.6% in the CABG vs 32.1% in the PCI group ($p = 0.43$)]. It was found that MACCE was significantly increased with PCI in intermediate (23–32) and higher SYNTAX (>32) groups (25.8% in CABG group vs 36.0% in the PCI intermediate score group; $p = 0.008$; 26.8% vs 44.0% in the high SYNTAX score group; $p < 0.0001$).

Flow chart 10.1 Approach to multivessel PCI

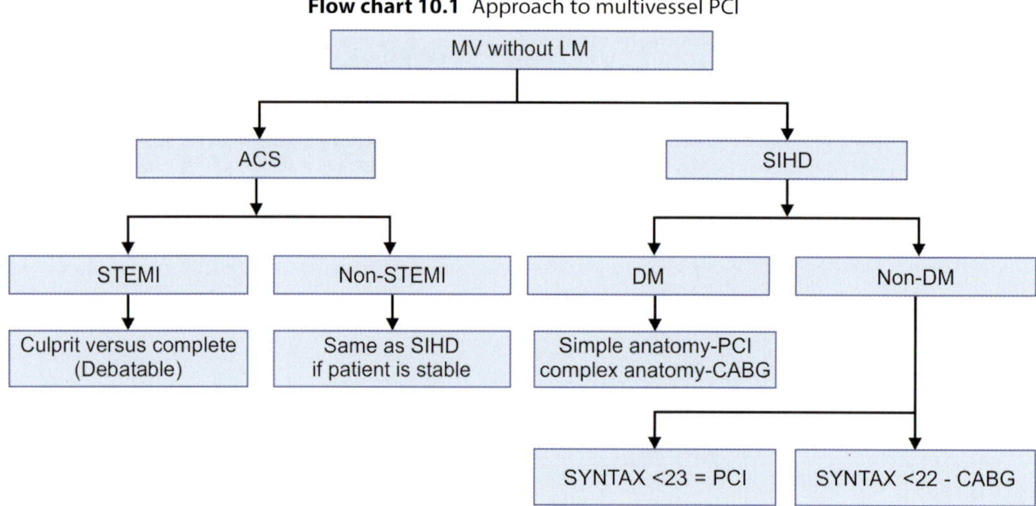

Abbreviations, MV, multivessel; LM, left main; ACS, acute coronary syndrome; SIHD, stable ischemic heart disease; STEMI, ST elevation myocardial infarction; Non-STEMI, Non-ST elevation myocardial infarction; DM, diabetes mellitus; PCI, percutaneous coronary intervention; CABG, coronary artery bypass graft surgery

It was also observed that overall MACCE were similar between PCI and CABG arms in the sub group analysis for left main disease which was predefined and powered [31.0% in the CABG group vs 36.9% in the PCI group (p = 0.12)]. MACCE was similar between arms in patients with low/intermediate SYNTAX scores but significantly increased in PCI patients with high scores.[7] With few limitations in its design, SYNTAX study plays a significant role in decision making in managing patients with CAD at present. One of the presumed limitations of SYNTAX was the use of first generation stent, Taxus in the PCI arm. This question was addressed in the second study BEST.

BEST STUDY

BEST is a multicenter, randomized study which was terminated prematurely after recruiting 880 patients due to slow enrollment before it reached its proposed recruitment of 1776. Out of 880 patients with two and three vessel CAD randomized to PCI with EES or CABG, those with left main disease were excluded. It was observed that MACE (a composite of death, MI, or target-vessel revascularization at two years) in the PCI group was higher than that of CABG at 4.6 years (15.2 vs 10.6%; hazard ratio [HR] 1.47, 95% CI 1.01–2.13), p = 0.04). Though there was no difference in the composite safety end point of death, MI, or stroke, the rates of any repeat revascularization and spontaneous MI were found to be increased significantly after PCI. It needs to emphasized that more patients in CABG arm had complete revascularization as compared to the PCI arm.

It is prudent to consider a large sized observational study[8] addressing the issue of multivessel PCI. Out of 34,819 patients with two and three vessel CAD (left main disease patients were excluded), propensity matching was done. 9223 patients who underwent multivessel PCI with everolimus eluting stent and 9223 patients who received CABG were studied. At a mean follow-up of 2.9 years, risk of death was similar between both the arms (3.1% per year and 2.9% per year, respectively; hazard ratio, 1.04; 95% confidence interval [CI], 0.93–1.17; p = 0.50). It was observed that patients who underwent PCI had higher risks of myocardial infarction (1.9% per year vs 1.1% per year; hazard ratio, 1.51; 95% CI, 1.29–1.77; $p < 0.001$) and repeat revascularization (7.2% per year vs 3.1% per year; hazard ratio, 2.35; 95% CI, 2.14–2.58; $p < 0.001$), and a lower risk of stroke (0.7% per year vs 1.0% per year; hazard ratio, 0.62; 95% CI, 0.50–0.76; $p < 0.001$). The higher risk of myocardial infarction with PCI compared to CABG was not significant among patients with complete revascularization but was significant among those with incomplete revascularization. All this evidence makes it clear that we should try to provide near complete revascularization if PCI is selected as a strategy of revascularization.

Multivessel Intervention in Patients with Acute Coronary Syndromes

Incidence of multivessel disease is more common in patients with ACS than those with SIHD.[1] Till a couple of years ago, only culprit vessel PCI was done during primary PCI in patients with ST-segment elevation myocardial infarction (STEMI).

Three recently published studies have questioned this approach. They are PRAMI [>50% nonculprit vessel was intervened,[9] CvLPRIT [>70% nonculprit vessel was intervened,[10] and DANAMI-PRIMULTI [Used FFR for the assessment of nonculprit lesion.[11] Results of these trials has made ACC/AHA to change their recommendations for nonculprit vessel interventions during STEMI as Class IIb from Class III. It is too premature to come to a conclusion regarding non culprit vessel PCI during STEMI at present. We need to wait for the results of a larger trial named COMPLETE which is expected to enroll 3900 patients. Revascularization of patients with NSTEACS who are electrically and hemodynamically stable is same as patients with SIHD.

Multivessel PCI in Patients with Diabetes

Till recently, no large RCT was available directly answering the issue of revascularization in patients with DM. FREEDOM is a global, multicentric, randomized controlled trial that compared CABG vs multivessel PCI in patients with diabetes mellitus.[12] Patients with left main disease were excluded from the study. 1900 patients were studied. Median follow-up period was 3.0 years. It was found that primary composite outcome (all-cause mortality, nonfatal MI and nonfatal stroke) occurred more frequently in PCI arm (26.6% vs 18.7%) irrespective of the syntax score. As known before, MI was more often seen after PCI while stroke was more common after CABG. In addition to it, FREEDOM also found that patients in PCI arm had higher mortality which was not seen in other studies like sub group analysis of SYNTAX and CARDIA trials.[13] Major guidelines updated themselves after the results of FREEDOM were published making CABG as the first line of revascularization in patients with diabetes mellitus. It needs to be stressed that all of patients received first generation DES in FREEDOM.

The effect of first generation DES (Paclitaxel eluting stent, Taxus, Boston Scientific, USA) versus second generation DES (Everolimus eluting DES-Xience, Abbott, USA) was studied by U Kaul et al.[14] They found that first generation stents are inferior to second generation stents. In TUXEDO trial, 1830 patients with DM and CAD were randomly assigned to receive either paclitaxel eluting stent or everolimus eluting stent. PES failed to meet the noninferiority criterion for the primary end point which was target-vessel failure, defined as a composite of cardiac death, target-vessel myocardial infarction, or ischemia-driven target-vessel revascularization at the 1-year follow-up [5.6% vs 2.9%; risk difference, 2.7 percentage points [95% confidence interval, 0.8–4.5]. Significantly higher 1-year target vessel failure rate was observed in the paclitaxel-eluting stent group than in the everolimus-eluting stent group (p = 0.005), spontaneous myocardial infarction (3.2% vs. 1.2%, p = 0.004), stent thrombosis (2.1% vs. 0.4%, p = 0.002), target-vessel revascularization (3.4% vs 1.2%, p = 0.002), and target-lesion revascularization (3.4% vs. 1.2%, p = 0.002). Could the exclusive use of everolimus eluting stent have changed the results in FREEDOM trial is a matter of debate. It should be emphasized that most of these trials excluded sicker patients which include patients with LV dysfunction, low eGFR, prior stroke, frail individuals and higher Euroscore. The choice of revascularization in such patients remains unclear and need to tailored for each individual.

There are some points to remember. Modern antiplatelet agents like prasugrel or ticagrelor were not used in FREEDOM trial. We are now aware that prasugrel has a particular advantage for diabetics in that it reduces stent thrombosis. Compared to the clopidogrel group in the TRITON TIMI 38 study, the prasugrel group had a 52% relative reduction for stent thrombosis.[15]

With regard to ticagrelor, the pivotal PLATO trial has shown that at 12 months, the primary end point [a composite of death from vascular cause, myocardial infarction, or stroke] occurred in 9.8% of patients receiving ticagrelor as compared with 11.7% in those receiving clopidogrel. Myocardial infarction has also been shown to be reduced in the ticagrelor arm (5.8% in the ticagrelor group vs 6.9% in the clopidogrel group, p ¼ 0.005).[16]

Thus the use of modern generation P2 Y12 inhibitors if used in FREEDOM trial might have made a difference to the outcomes.

We made an attempt to compare the 2 year results of FREEDOM surgical arm with 2 year results of latest generation Everolimus and zotarolimus eluting stents as shown in (Table 10.1).[17] Although these are different trials with different endpoints, one can draw some idea from this table and it appears that the results are reasonably comparable. Is it possible that if one of these modern drug eluting stents were used in FREEDOM trial the results could have been different?

FAME 3[18] will answer the role of FFR in the treatment of multivessel disease which will lead to revascularization of physiologically significant lesions rather than anatomically significant lesions. It is very clear to us that 2nd generation DES outperforms first generation DES. Similarly it is very clear that FFR guided PCI is superior to angiography guided PCI. It is also found that functional syntax score not only converts patients from higher syntax to lower syntax score but also a better tool in assessing the risk of death and MI. This may create paradigm shift in the management of multi-vessel PCI.

RECOMMENDATIONS

- In patients with single vessel disease, double vessel disease (RCA and LCX), triple vessel disease with low syntax

Table 10.1 Comparison of FREEDOM surgical arm with outcomes of Xience V trials and RESOLUTE All Comers trial

Clinical endpoints	*FREEDOM trial [CABG arm]*	*Meta-analysis of Xience V trials*	*RESOLUTE all corners trial*	
	2 years after randomization	*Clinical outcomes at 2 years data in diabetic patients*	*Clinical outcomes at 2 years*	
			Resolute	*Xience V*
Primary composite outcome	11.9%	10.1%	12.5%	12.9%
Myocardial infarction	4.7%	4.2%	5.5%	5.0%
Cardiovascular death	1.3%	2.1%	2.6%	2.2%

score and without diabetes (Flow chart 10.1), we strongly suggest PCI as the initial strategy of revascularization.

- In patients with diabetes and triple vessel disease with low SYNTAX score, the option of CABG should be given as first line treatment. PCI is reasonable alternative provided all the lesions are anatomically simple.
- In patients with intermediate and high SYNTAX score irrespective of their diabetic status, CABG is the choice of revascularization.

REFERENCES

1. Dangas G, Mehran R, Wallenstein S. Correlation of angiographic morphology and clinical presentation in unstable angina. J Am Coll Cardiol. 1997;29(3):519-25.
2. van Domburg RT, Foley DP, Breeman A, et al. Coronary artery bypass graft surgery and percutaneous transluminal coronary angioplasty. Twenty-year clinical outcome. Eur Heart J. 2002;23:543.
3. Daemen J, Boersma E, Flather M, et al. Long-term safety and efficacy of percutaneous coronary intervention with stenting and coronary artery bypass surgery for multivessel coronary artery disease: a meta-analysis with 5-year patient-level data from the ARTS, ERACI-II, MASS-II, and SoS trials. Circulation. 2008;118:1146.
4. Serruys PW, Morice MC, Kappetein AP, et al. Percutaneous coronary intervention versus coronary-artery bypass grafting for severe coronary artery disease. N Engl J Med. 2009;360:961.
5. Mohr FW, Morice MC, Kappetein AP, et al. Coronary artery bypass graft surgery versus percutaneous coronary intervention in patients with three-vessel disease and left main coronary disease: 5-year follow-up of the randomised, clinical SYNTAX trial. Lancet. 2013;381(9867):629-38.
6. Park SJ, Ahn JM, Kim YH, et al. Trial of everolimus-eluting stents or bypass surgery for coronary disease. N Engl J Med. 2015; 372:1204.
7. Morice MC, Serruys PW, Kappetein AP, et al. Five-year outcomes in patients with left main disease treated with either percutaneous coronary intervention or coronary artery bypass grafting in the synergy between percutaneous coronary intervention with taxus and cardiac surgery trial. Circulation. 2014;129(23):2388-94.
8. Bangalore S, Guo Y, Samadashvili Z, Blecker S, et al. Everolimus-eluting stents or bypass surgery for multivessel coronary disease. N Engl J Med. 2015;372(13):1213.
9. Wald DS, Morris JK, Wald NJ, et al. Randomized trial of preventive angioplasty in myocardial infarction. N Engl J Med. 2013;369(12):1115-23.
10. Gershlick AH, Khan JN, Kelly DJ, et al. Randomized trial of complete versus lesion-only revascularization in patients undergoing primary percutaneous coronary intervention for STEMI and multivessel disease: the CvLPRIT trial. J Am Coll Cardiol. 2015;65(10):963-72.
11. Engstrøm T, Kelbæk H, Helqvist S, et al. Complete revascularisation versus treatment of the culprit lesion only in patients with ST-segment elevation myocardial infarction and multivessel disease (DANAMI-3—PRIMULTI): an open-label, randomised controlled trial. Lancet. 2015;386(9994):665-71.
12. Farkouh ME, Domanski M, Sleeper LA, et al. Strategies for multivessel revascularization in patients with diabetes. N Engl J Med. 2012;367:2375.
13. Kapur A, Hall RJ, Malik IS, et al. Randomized comparison of percutaneous coronary intervention with coronary artery bypass grafting in diabetic patients. 1-year results of the CARDia (Coronary Artery Revascularization in Diabetes) trial. J Am Coll Cardiol. 2010;55:432.
14. Kaul U, Bangalore S, Seth A, et al. Paclitaxel-eluting versus everolimus-eluting coronary stents in diabetes. N Engl J Med. 2015;373(18):1709-19.
15. Wiviott SD, Braunwald E, McCabe CH, et al. TRITON-TIMI 38 Investigators. Prasugrel versus clopidogrel in patients with acute coronary syndromes. N Engl J Med. 2007;357:2001-15.
16. Wallentin L, Becker R. Ticagrelor versus clopidogrel in patients with acute coronary syndromes. N Engl J Med [Internet]. 2009;361:1045-57 [cited 2013 Jan 7].
17. Jariwala P, Chandra S. 'FREEDOM' trial: Have the interventional cardiologists lost their freedom? Indian Heart J. 2013;65(1): 114-6.
18. Zimmermann FM, Bruyne De, Pijls NH, et al. Rationale and design of the Fractional Flow Reserve versus Angiography for Multivessel Evaluation (FAME) 3Trial: a comparison of fractional flow reserve guided percutaneous coronary intervention and coronary artery bypass graft surgery in patients with multivessel coronary artery disease. Am Heart J. 2015;170(4):619-26.

CHAPTER

11 Multivessel Coronary Angioplasty: Cardiac Surgeons' Viewpoint

Kaushal Pandey

INTRODUCTION

Coronary artery disease and its complications are the single largest cause of death and morbidity in the world; more so in the developed world. This disease is also enjoying the same status in India; though the causes are different. While there is evidence that the incidence of this disease is declining in the North American continent, mainly attributable to decline in smoking and the population becoming health conscious; the incidence in our country has assumed epidemic proportions. The incidence of this disease is still rising in our country, mainly because of increase of diabetes mellitus in our population. The society still continues with use of tobacco in various forms and a large population remaining ignorant and is still not health conscious. The medical records keeping in India has not evolved, even though we have many institutions of international class. It is difficult for me to give exact numbers of coronary artery bypass graft (CABG) or percutaneous transluminal coronary angioplasty (PTCA) being performed in the country. An educated guess estimates CABG numbers to be around 1,25,000 for the year 2015 and over 3,00,000 PTCA patients. These numbers may not tell us the whole story.

A large segment of our population is still unserviced or simply not capable of affording these procedures in either public or private hospitals. We have reasons to believe that these numbers can rise at a rate of 15% per year in the next decade.

The standard modalities of treatment for coronary artery disease are:

- Medical management with beta-blockers, statins and antiplatelet drugs
- PTCA
- CABG

In this chapter, we will discuss the role of PTCA and CABG in patients with multivessel coronary artery disease. There will be emphasis on advantages and disadvantages of each of these procedures. Short and long term results with specific reference to stent and graft patency will be discussed. We shall also analyze which patients will do better with PTCA or CABG. We will conclude by giving a surgeon's view point on this complex and difficult decision making and provide a scientific basis to our recommendation on PTCA and/or CABG in patients with multivessel coronary artery disease. It is a fortunate situation that patients with multivessel coronary artery disease can have treatment from two different specialties. The same disease can be treated by cardiologist using stents of different types which continue to evolve. The same patient can also be treated by a coronary artery bypass surgery either on pump or an off pump CABG. While the two procedures are radically different to each other, they still treat the same disease and the treatment remains palliation.

Coronary angioplasty is a percutaneous intervention performed either through femoral artery approach or radial artery approach. It tackles the coronary stenosis right where the stenosis is by implantation of a stent. One or more stents can be implanted in the same artery. The procedure is performed under local anesthesia. It usually requires a short hospitalization and early return to work.

Coronary bypass surgery is a surgical procedure performed through sternotomy or a thoracotomy. It makes use of cardiopulmonary bypass or it can be performed on beating heart. Bypass surgery is done using arterial or vein grafts. These grafts are usually anastomosed to healthy distal segments of coronary artery, well away from the diseased segment. It requires general anesthesia, frequently postoperative ventilation, two or more days of intensive care unit (ICU) management and almost a week in hospital stay. Return to work is delayed and frequently be around four to six weeks.

HISTORY

The scientific basis for treatment of coronary artery disease was established by the works of F Mason Sones and other cardiologists working at the Clevelend Clinic. Between the years 1951 and 1960, over 2,00,000 coronary angiography procedures were performed by Sones and his colleagues. Sones published his landmark article in the year 1961. In this article, he described artherosclerotic anatomy of the coronary arteries. He showed that coronary stenosis usually occur in the proximal part of the coronary arteries leaving the distal vessel free of disease. He also demonstrated that these lesions also affect the bifurcation of coronary arteries. He further showed that if the vessel was chronically occluded, it was collateralized by the other arteries. In this very article, Sones talks about how this information can be used in future for the treatment of coronary artery disease. The mid 1960s saw performance of first coronary artery bypass procedures. Renee Favaloro performed the first CABG at Clevelend Clinic, using saphenous vein grafts. Vasilii Kolesov, a Russian Surgeon performed the first left internal mammary artery (LIMA) to left anterior descending (LAD) bypass, which was done off pump. The era of 1970s saw further refinements in CABG, with emphasis on reducing mortality. 1970s and 1980s also saw development of standard techniques worldwide in CABG, especially with use of LIMA, radial artery and vein grafts. The era of 1990s established the superiority of arterial grafts, especially bilateral internal mammary (BIMA) and radial artery. The new millennium established off pump coronary artery bypass (OPCAB), minimally invasive coronary artery surgery (MICAS) and other less invasive procedures. This happened more as a means by the surgeon to thwart the rapid increase in PTCA worldwide. To date coronary artery surgery study (CASS) remains the single largest study of any surgical procedure in the world. In fact CABG is the most widely researched surgical procedure in the world.

While advances in CABG were taking place, it was always believed by the cardiologists and their patients that the procedure was very invasive. It had a mortality which was on the decline, but there was a fair bit of morbidity. We were all concerned about the occasional mediastinitis, neurocognitive disorder and delayed return to work. There was always a problem of early graft failure and sometimes Redo CABG. Patients with graft failure and Redo CABG somehow did not do well. The biggest problem with the procedure was that it was operator dependent. Top surgeons and some institutions gave out outstanding results, both short term and long term. The average and less than average surgeons and institutions could never match them.

In the mid 1970s, the early results of CASS study started to come out. Frequently the outcomes were not good and there were too many complications. Cardiologists started to look at developing alternative procedures to CABG. Andreaz Gruentzig performed the first balloon angioplasty in the year 1977. Rightfully, he is called the Father of PTCA. Balloon angioplasty continued to evolve and evolve rapidly. It became a frequently performed procedure in the late 1980s. Early half of the 1990s established balloon angioplasty as the standard treatment for single vessel coronary artery disease. 1990s also saw the use of bare metal stents. The new millennium ushered in newer and newer stents; each better than the previous one. Drug eluting stents created a major revolution in the development of PTCA. Stent thrombosis and stent stenosis became uncommon. Soon they became the standard of practice for management of patients with multivessel coronary artery disease. Stents continued to evolve in many directions, making PTCA even more attractive.

The medical industry behind stents has ensured standardization of the procedure. As a result, cardiologists worldwide are able to perform complex PTCA and give out uniformly good outcomes. The individual skill element has definitely been diluted. There is no unpredictability in PTCA outcomes today. Surgery continues to remain skill dependent. As a result, there is major discrepancy in results and outcome following CABG. CABG may not evolve further. PTCA continues to evolve and its numbers continue to rise worldwide; at the expense of CABG. PTCA has indeed become an alternative, and that too an attractive one over the CABG.

PERCUTANEOUS CORONARY INTERVENTION VERSUS CORONARY ARTERY BYPASS GRAFT IN LOW RISK MULTIVESSEL CORONARY ARTERY DISEASE

Low risk multivessel coronary artery disease patients include patients with no diabetes, no renal failure, no hyperlipidemia, ejection fraction > 35% and low syntax score.

Meta-analysis of 15 randomized clinical trial (RCT) of PCI vs CABG in multivessel disease (Table 11.1). It demonstrates that only 5% of screened patients were actually randomized to the two therapies. Importantly, all patients studied have ejection fractions of 50%. The incidence of triple vessel disease in these trials is only 35%. It should not be surprising to find that CABG and PCI are similar in outcomes as these trials exclude all the high-risk patients which may benefit from CABG over multivessel intervention (i.e. diabetics, low LV function and triple vessel disease or left main). However, one might argue these trials reflect the natural proportion of multivessel disease in the population, and an appropriate ratio to be representative of 'all comers' with CAD; but then we should be very cautious in generalizing these results to all CAD patients.[1]

Hoffman et al. reported a meta-analysis of thirteen RCT of CABG vs. PCI involving 7,964 patients followed up to eight years. In the overall analysis, neither strategy provided a statistically significant survival advantage at one, three, or

Table 11.1 Summary of 15 RCT of PCI vs CABG in multivessel disease

Trial	*No. of screened*	*Randomized (%)*	*Stent*	*3-vessel disease (%)*	*Proximal LAD*	*EF>50%*	*Diabetes (%)*
ERACI	127	9	–	45	–	100	11
EAST	392	4	–	40	70	100	25
GABI	359	4	–	18	–	–	10
CABRI	1054	3	–	40	–	100	12
MASS	142	69	–	–	100	100	21
BARI	1829	12	–	41	36	100	24
SIMA	121	–	–	–	100	100	11
LAUSANNE	134	3	–	0	100	–	12
RITA	1011	4	–	12	–	–	6
TOULOSE	152	3		29	–	–	14
AWESOME	454	–	+	45	–	–	–
ERACI–II	450	2	+	56	–	–	17
ARTS	1205	5	+	32	–	100	19
SOS	988	5	+	38	45	100	14
MASS–II	408	2	+	41	–	–	–
Summary	8826	5		35	41	100	16

Abbreviations: RCT, randomized clinical trials; PCI, percutaneous coronary interventions; CABG, coronary artery bypass graft; LAD, left anterior descending artery; EF, ejection fraction

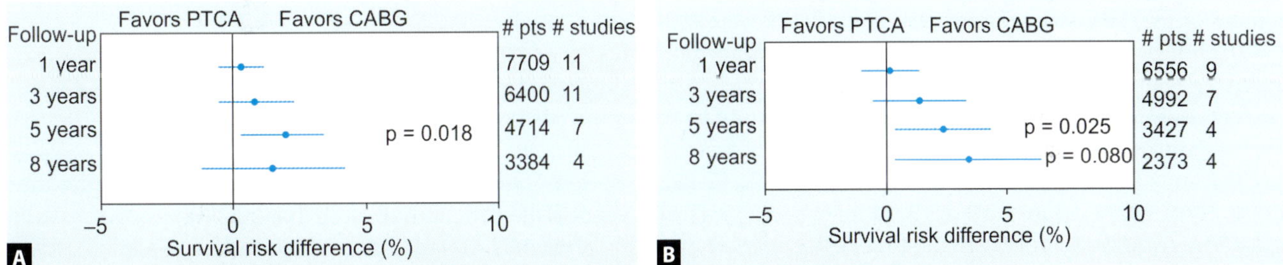

Figs 11.1A and B Risk difference for all-cause mortality for years 1, 3, 5, and 8 post-initial revascularization. All trials (A) and multivessel coronary artery disease (B). The lines represent 95% confidence intervals. Event rates for the coronary bypass arm at 1, 3, 5, and 8 years for all trials (A) were 3.0%, 4.7%, 7.1%, and 13.7%; for multivessel trials (B) were 3.4%, 5.3%, 8.9%, and 15.8%
Abbreviations: CABG, coronary artery bypass graft; PTCA, percutaneous transluminal coronary angioplasty

eight years. At 5 years, there was a statistically significant 1.9% RD advantage favoring CABG (Fig. 11.1A). Subgroup analysis of multivessel trials showed a similar survival advantage for CABG at years 5 and 8 (Fig. 11.1B). The long-term survival advantage for CABG is consistent with observational studies suggesting greater benefit from CABG over PTCA for patients with CAD.

However, it must be noted that all data at 5 and 8 years are from earlier studies that did not employ stents in the initial revascularization procedure. The trend favoring CABG for survival at 3 years in prestent trials was no longer present in the stent era, despite a decrease in absolute mortality following CABG. Whether the introduction of stents and improvements in CABG will affect long-term results remains to be seen.[2]

Mercado et al. published the results of a meta-analysis on CABG vs PCI (with stents) for multivessel disease in 2005. Investigators included four RCT (Arterial Revascularization Therapies Study, Stent or Surgery Trial, Argentine Randomized Trial of Percutaneous Transluminal Coronary Angioplasty vs CABG in Multivessel Disease 2, and Medicine, Angioplasty, or Surgery Study 2) that compared PCI with multivessel stenting (n = 1518) vs CABG (n = 1533). One year after the initial procedure, PCI with multiple stenting and CABG provided a similar degree of protection against death, myocardial infarction, or stroke in patients with microvascular disease (MVD). Repeat revascularization procedures occurred more frequently in patients in the PCI group compared to CABG (18% vs 4.4%; hazard ratio 4.4 and 95% confidence interval 3.3–5.9).[3]

RESULTS OF ARTERIAL REVASCULARIZATION THERAPIES STUDY II TRIAL

Between April 1997 and June 1998, a total of 1,205 patients were randomly assigned to PCI with bare metal stent (BMS) (n = 600) or CABG (n = 605) in 67 participating centers in the arterial revascularization therapies study (ARTS) I trial. Between February 2003 and November 2003, 607 patients at 45 participating centers were treated by PCI using sirolimus-eluting stent (SES) and entered into the ARTS II study. Table 11.2 presents their baseline demographic and angiographic characteristics. The percentage of percutaneous triple-vessel treatment was 46.6% in SES versus 18.0% in BMS ($p < 0.001$). The mean number of significant lesions per patient was 3.6 ± 1.3 in SES versus 2.8 ± 1.0 in CABG ($p < 0.001$) and 2.8 ± 1.0 in BMS. SES patients received 3.7 ± 1.5 stents with an average total stented length of 72 ± 32 mm compared with 2.8 ± 1.3 stents and 48 ± 22 mm in BMS patients ($p < 0.001$). In the SES population, SYNTAX score and logistic euroSCORE were 20.8 ± 9.51 and 2.16 ± 15.2, respectively. Clinical follow-up at 5 years was available in 97.6% of ARTS II population. The 5-year event rates are depicted in Table 11.3 and Figures 11.2A to D. The survival rate in ARTS II was comparable to the historical, surgical, and PCI groups from ARTS I (SES: 94.5%, CABG: 92.6%, BMS: 92.0%). The death/CVA/MI event-free survival was 87.1% in ARTS II, versus 86.0% (log-rank $p = 0.42$) and the 81.9% (log-rank $p = 0.008$) in the CABG and BMS cohorts, respectively. At 5-years follow-up, the major adverse cardiac and cerebral events (MACCE)-free survival rate in ARTS II (72.5%), which had been comparable to the surgical cohort of ARTS I at 3 years, was significantly lower than CABG (78.9%, $p = 0.02$), and significantly higher than BMS (58.5%, log-rank $p < 0.001$). At 5 years, SES had a safety record comparable to CABG and superior to BMS, and a MACCE rate that was higher than in patients treated with CABG, and lower than in those treated with BMS. Approximately one-third of the events seen with SES could be prevented through the elimination of early, late, and very late stent thrombosis.[4]

In summary, it would be safe to conclude that CABG and PCI are both reasonable options in patients with multivessel CAD with normal LV function. There may be a slight mortality benefit long-term of CABG over balloon angioplasty plain old balloon angioplasty (POBA) which is nullified with the use of stents. However, there is approximately four times more repeat procedures in patients treated initially with PCI compared to CABG which is about half of what is seen with balloon angioplasty.[2]

PERCUTANEOUS CORONARY INTERVENTION VERSUS CORONARY ARTERY BYPASS GRAFT IN HIGH-RISK MULTIVESSEL CORONARY ARTERY DISEASE

Diabetes is predicted to be major health burden in India in coming years. CAD in diabetics has been shown to be more aggressive and to be associated with an impaired event-free survival after both CABG and PCI because of smaller vessel sizes, longer lesion length, greater plaque burden, and a possibly differently acting restenotic cascade than in nondiabetics.[5,6]

CABG was considered to be choice of treatment for complicated coronary lesion but due to recent advances and standardization in PCI in this subset of patient increasingly PTCA is offered.

CABG has been regarded by some as a preferred revascularization method because of its ability to bypass this large amount of plaque burden and to achieve more complete revascularization rates, making the need for repeat revascularizations less likely. New York registry of 37,212 CABG and 22,102 PCI patients with more than double vessel disease showed that after three years, CABG significantly reduced the risk of death. If the patients had more than double vessel disease and proximal LAD surgery, patients were 35% more likely than the others to be alive after three years. If the patients had more than double vessel disease but no proximal LAD lesion then surgery patients were 24% more likely than the others to be alive after three years.[7]

Van Domburgh et al. reported the results of a single-center matched-propensity controlled cohort study which revealed the late outcome after stenting or CABG for treatment of multivessel disease. In this matched cohort study with an 8-year follow-up, survival was better and less repeat revascularizations were needed among patients undergoing elective CABG for the treatment of multivessel disease as compared with the stent group.[8]

Pell et al. compared the survival following CABG vs PCI in diabetic and nondiabetic patients. Results showed that PCI had 3.6 times higher mortality rates at two-year follow-up in patients with diabetes.[9]

A propensity analysis of long-term survival after surgical or percutaneous revascularization in 6033 patients with MVD and high-risk features (diabetes or left ventricular dysfunction) showed that PCI had 2.3 times higher mortality rate than CABG at five-year follow-up.[10]

Table 11.2 Baseline and procedural characteristics of ARTS II and I population

	SES (n = 607)	*CABG (n = 605)*	*BMS (n = 600)*	*SES/CABG difference (95% CI)*	*SES/BMS difference (95% CI)*
Baseline characteristics					
Male sex	77	76	77	0.6% (–4.2% to 5.4%)	–0.4% (–5.2% to 4.4%)
Age (yrs)	63 ± 10	61 ± 9	61 ± 10	1.5 (0.4–2.6)	2.1 (1.0–3.2)
Body mass index (kg/m²)	27.5 ± 4.1	27.4 ± 3.7	27.2 ± 3.7	0.2 (–0.3 to 0.6)	0.3 (–0.1 to 0.8)
Risk factors					
Myocardial infarction	34	42	44	–7.6% (–13.0% to –2.1%)	–9.9% (–15.4% to –4.4%)
Diabetes	26	16	19	10.3% (5.8%–14.9%)	7.5% (2.8%–12.2%)
Hypertension	67	45	45	22.3% (16.8%–27.7%)	22.5% (17.1%–28.0%)
Hypercholesterolemia	74	58	58	16.4% (11.2%–21.7%)	16.1% (10.8%–21.4%)
Family history of MI or sudden death at age <55 yrs	36	42	39	–6.0% (–11.5% to –0.5%)	–3.2% (–8.7% to 2.2%)
Current smoker	19	26	28	–6.5% (–11.2% to –1.8%)	–8.7% (–13.4% to –3.9%)
Peripheral vascular disease	7	5	6	1.8% (–0.9% to 4.5%)	1.4% (–1.3% to 4.2%)
Indication for treatment					
Stable angina	53	58	56	–4.8% (–10.4% to –0.8%)	–3.1% (–8.7% to 2.5%)
Unstable angina	36	37	38	–0.8% (–6.2% to 4.6%)	–1.3% (–6.7% to 4.2%)
Silent ischemia	10	5	6	5.6% (2.6%–8.5%)	4.4% (1.3%–7.5%)
Angiographic characteristics					
Ejection fraction	60 ± 12	60 ± 13	61 ± 12	–0.2 (–1.6 to 1.3)	–0.8 (–2.2 to 0.7)
No. of lesions with stenosis >50%	3.6 ± 1.3	2.8 ± 1.0	2.8 ± 1.0	0.8 (0.6–0.9)	0.8 (0.6–0.9)
No. of diseased vessels					
1	0	4	4	–3.4% (–5.0% to –1.8%)	–3.6% (–5.3% to –2.0%)
2	46	66	69	–20.1% (–25.6% to –14.6%)	–22.4% (–27.9% to –17.0%)
3	54	30	27	23.5% (18.1%–28.9%)	26.1% (20.7%–31.4%)
Vessel territory with stenosis (% of lesions)					
Right coronary artery	29	29	31	–0.4% (–3.3% to 2.5%)	–2.1% (–5.0% to 0.9%)
Left main	0	0	0	–0.1% (–0.2% to 0.1%)	–0.1% (–0.2% to 0.1%)
Left anterior descending	42	41	39	0.4% (–2.7% to 3.6%)	2.1% (–1.1% to 5.3%)
Left circumflex artery	29	29	29	0.0% (–2.9% to 3.0%)	0.0% (–2.9% to 3.0%)
Lesion length (visual) (% of lesions)					
Discreet (<10 mm)	61	68	66	–7.3% (–10.4% to –4.2%)	–4.7% (–7.9% to –1.5%)
Tubular (10–20 mm)	27	25	27	2.0% (–0.9% to 4.9%)	–0.1% (–3.0% to 2.8%)
Diffuse (>20 mm)	12	7	7	5.3% (3.4%–7.2%)	4.8% (2.9%–6.7%)
Lesion classification (% of lesions)					
Type A	7	7	6	0.0% (–1.6% to 1.6%)	0.9% (–0.7% to 2.5%)
Type B1	23	31	26	–7.9% (–10.8% to –5.1%)	–3.0% (–5.8% to –0.2%)
Type B2	56	54	60	1.9% (–1.3% to 5.1%)	–3.7% (–6.9% to –0.5%)
Type C	14	8	8	6.0% (4.0%–8.0%)	5.9% (3.9%–7.8%)

Contd...

Contd...

	SES (n = 607)	*CABG (n = 605)*	*BMS (n = 600)*	*SES/CABG difference (95% CI)*	*SES/BMS difference (95% CI)*
Procedural characteristics					
Bifurcation requiring double wiring	34	32	35	2.2% (–0.9% to 5.3%)	–0.6% (–3.7% to 2.6%)
Number of stents implanted	3.7 ± 1.5	–	2.8 ± 1.3	–	0.9 (0.7–1.0)
Total stent length (mm)	72.5 ± 32.1	–	47.6 ± 21.7	–	24.9 (21.8–28.1)
Maximum dilatation pressure (atm)	16.4 ± 2.9	–	14.6 ± 2.8	–	1.7 (1.4–2.1)
Direct stenting (% of lesions)	34.6	–	3.3	–	31.3% (29.1%–33.6%)
Duration of procedure (min)	85 ± 43	193 ± 67	99 ± 50	–108.2 (–114.6 to –101.8)	–13.6 (–18.9 to –8.3)
Postprocedural hospital stay (days)	3.4 ± 2.7	9.6 ± 4.9	3.9 ± 3.7	–6.2 (–6.6 to –5.8)	–0.5 (–0.9 to –0.2)

Values are % or mean ± SD. Data are expressed per patient unless stated otherwise.

Abbreviations: BMS, bare-metal stent; CABG, coronary artery bypass graft; CI, confidence interval; MI, myocardial infarction; PCI, percutaneous coronary intervention; SES, sirolimus-eluting stent(s)

In a recent study of patients with multivesel disease and ≥5 years of follow-up, CABG was found to have a significant survival advantage over patients undergoing stent implantation.[11] This advantage was maintained among most subgroups, including males, those >65 years of age, patients without a history of PCI, CABG, or myocardial infarction (MI), nondiabetics, diabetics, patients with an ejection fraction (EF) >40%, patients with either 2- or 3-vessel disease, and for both complete and incomplete PCI. The only subgroups in which the survival advantage trended toward stent implantation were those with a previous history of coronary revascularization (either previous CABG or PCI). CABG patients also experienced fewer repeat revascularizations (CABG or PCI) and MI, and 41% fewer events for the composite end point of major adverse cardiac events (MACE).

These results are consistent with the reports of other observational studies.[8,10] However, at one year, as in the SOS trial, there was no significant difference in the outcome of mortality.[12]

However, it should be noted that most of the prior trials of CABG vs PCI included outdated technology and techniques for both procedures.

Most of the randomized clinical trials report similar 5-year mortality rates for both CABG and PCI.

The trials which have been mentioned above do not represent the ground realty. The surgical patients in the above study have had left internal mammary artery (LIMA) + saphenous venous graft (SVG) as the standard surgical procedure. Emphasis on complete revascularization was not adhered to. Today the surgical patients have multiple arterial grafts, complete revascularization and frequently multiple grafts on the same artery. Similarly, the stents have also advanced in technology. Today, the patients are getting fourth generation drug eluting stents (DES) and even bifurcation stents.

Two of the largest trials of CABG vs PCI ever performed, FREEDOM (Future Revascularization Evaluation in Patients with Diabetes Mellitus: Optimal Management of Multivessel Disease) and SYNTAX trials (The Synergy between PCI with TAXUS and Cardiac Surgery), both using DES and minimally invasive surgery results are available. The most important trial of CABG versus PCI is the SYNTAX Trial, whose 5-year outcomes have recently been published[13] (Table 11.4).

Highlights of SYNTAX Trial-in contrast to all the previous randomized trials of CABG versus PCI, which had enrolled only highly selected patient groups, SYNTAX was a relative 'all comer' trial in patients with multivessel and/or left main stem disease. And also SYNTAX maintained parallel registry that looked at outcomes in 1,078 patients who were ineligible for randomization.

Overall, at five-years, 26.9% of CABG and 37.3% of PCI patients reached the composite endpoint ($p < 0.001$) of death (11.4% vs 13.9%; $p = 0.10$), MI (3.8% vs 9.7%; $p < 0.001$), CVA (3.7% vs 2.4%; $p = 0.09$), or repeat revascularization (13.7% vs 25.9%; $p < 0.001$).[13]

After five years patients who underwent coronary artery bypass grafting continued to have better outcomes than with

Table 11.3 Clinical end points at 5 years (hierarchical and nonhierarchical MACCE up to 1,800 days, per patient) counted since date of procedure

	SES (n = 607)	*CABG (n = 602)**	*BMS (n = 600)*	*SES/CABG difference (95% CI)*	*SES/BMS difference (95% CI)*
Hierarchical					
Death	33 (5.4)	43 (7.1)	47 (7.8)	−1.7 (−4.4 to 1.0)	−2.4 (−5.2 to 0.4)
CVA	17 (2.8)	16 (2.7)	19 (3.2)		
MI	27 (4.4)	24 (4.0)	41 (6.8)		
Death/CVA/MI	77 (12.7)	83 (13.8)	107 (17.8)	−1.1 (−4.9 to 2.7)	−5.1 (−9.2 to −1.1)
Revascularization	88 (14.5)	42 (7.0)	140 (23.3)		
(re) CABG	15 (2.5)	5 (0.8)	47 (7.8)		
(re) PTCA	73 (12)	37 (6.1)	93 (15.5)		
Any MACCE	165 (27.2)	125 (20.8)	247 (41.2)	6.4 (1.6–11.2)	−14 (−19.3 to −8.7)
Nonhierarchical					
CVA	22 (3.6)	20 (3.3)	23 (3.8)	0.3 (−1.8 to 2.4)	−0.2 (−2.3 to 1.9)
MI	35 (5.8)	34 (5.6)	49 (8.2)	0.1 (−2.5 to 2.7)	−2.4 (−5.3 to 0.5)
Revascularization	123 (20.3)	52 (8.6)	181 (30.2)	11.6 (7.7–15.5)	−9.9 (−14.8 to −5.0)
(re) CABG	17 (2.8)	7 (1.2)	63 (10.5)	1.6 (0.1–3.2)	−7.7 (−10.5 to −4.9)
(re) PTCA	108 (17.8)	49 (8.1)	138 (23.0)	9.7 (5.9–13.4)	−5.2 (−9.7 to −0.7)

*Three patients on the waiting list died.

Values are n (%).

Abbreviations: CVA, cardiovascular accident; MACCE, major adverse cardiac and cerebrovascular event; PTCA, percutaneous transluminal coronary angioplasty

PCI. This was especially evident in patients with three-vessel disease. In triple vessel disease, patients CABG outcomes were superior to PCI ($p < 0.001$). After 4 years CABG vs PCI stroke rates equalized in triple vessel disease.

In the PCI group, almost five stents/patient were used for a total length of about 9 cm. Despite this, only a little over 50% were completely revascularized. In the CABG group, about three grafts/patient were placed for a revascularization of 63.2%, only marginally better than in the PCI. Despite this, during the five-year follow-up PCI patients underwent repeat revascularization at more than double the rate in triple vessel disease (12.6 vs 25.4; $p < 0.001$), LMD (15.5 vs 27.7; $p < 0.001$).

Four-year results suggest that CABG remains the standard of care for patients with complex lesions (intermediate or high SYNTAX score). With less complex disease (low SYNTAX scores), PCI is an acceptable revascularization alternative.[13]

Multivessel CAD, the optimal revascularization strategy in patients with diabetes had also been controversial but has recently been settled by the freedom trial.[14]

This trial randomized 1900 patients with diabetes and multivessel CAD already receiving aggressive medical therapy, to CABG or DES. The 5-year primary composite outcome occurred in 26.6% of the PCI group and 18.7% of the CABG group ($p = 0.005$). These findings were true for all the risk factors examined, but especially for patients with poor heart function (LVEF <40%) (Table 11.5 and Figures 11.3A and B).

Crucially, the benefit of CABG was driven by highly significant absolute reductions in both death (5.4%; $p = 0.049$) and myocardial infarction (7.9%; $p < 0.001$), but with a higher risk of stroke in the CABG group (5.2% vs 2.4%; $p = 0.03$). In long-term follow-up, the rate of myocardial infarction was significantly higher in the PCI group than in the CABG group, whereas the rate of stroke was significantly higher in the CABG group. However, the higher relative risk of stroke among patients undergoing CABG was evident only early in the postprocedural period.

Syntax and freedom trials are the main studies available for scientific evaluation of CABG vs PTCA. Both these trials are actually applicable to the clinical scenario prevailing in our own country. Diabetes and its sequelae, especially the diffuse nature of coronary artery disease is well represented in both these studies. CABG outcomes, especially at long term clearly supersede PTCA outcomes.

QUALITY OF LIFE AFTER PERCUTANEOUS CORONARY INTERVENTION VERSUS CORONARY ARTERY BYPASS GRAFT

Quantification of quality of life is a difficult task as it has to take many factors into consideration most importantly freedom from angina or heart failure, freedom from need for medication,

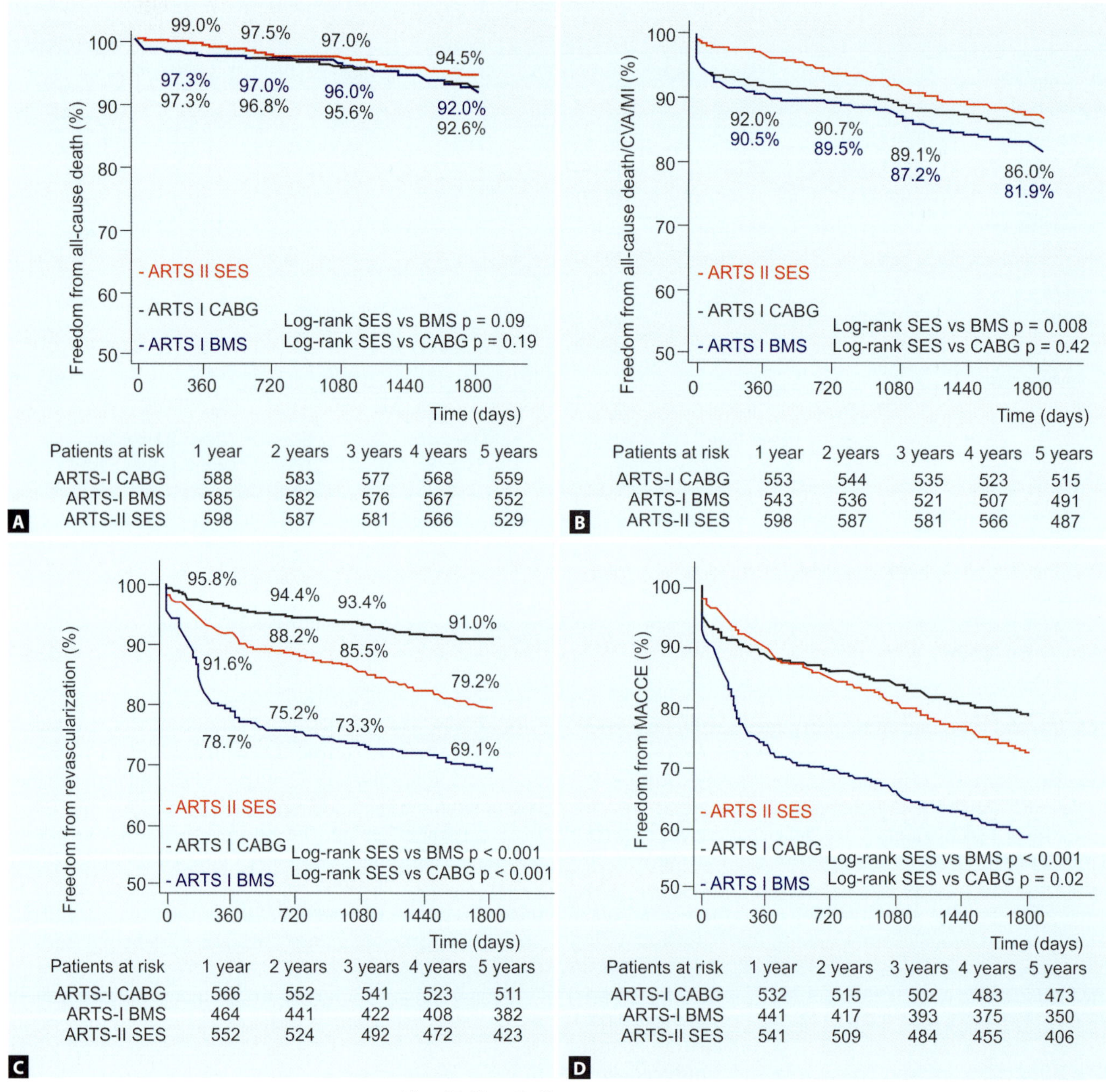

Figs 11.2A to D Five years event rates

Table 11.4 SYNTAX 5-year results for patients with three-vessel disease

Outcome	*CABG, n = 549 (%)*	*PCI, n = 546 (%)*	*p*
Primary end point: MACCE	24.2	37.5	<0.001
All-cause death	9.2	14.6	0.006
Cardiac death	4.0	9.2	<0.001
MI	3.3	10.6	<0.001
Cerebrovascular accident	3.4	3.0	0.66
Repeat revascularization	12.6	25.4	<0.001
Safety end point: All-cause death/cerebrovascular accident/MI	14.0	22.0	<0.001

Table 11.5 5-year primary composite outcome

Outcome	*2 years after randomization*		*5 years after randomization*		*Patients with event*		*p value**
	PCI	*CABG*	*PCI*	*CABG*	*PCI*	*CABG*	
	Number (percent)				*Number*		
• Primary composite††	121 (13.0)	108 (11.9)	200 (26.6)	146 (18.7)	205	147	0.005‡
– Death from any cause	62 (6.7)	57 (6.3)	114 (16.3)	83 (10.9)	118	86	0.049
– Myocardial infarction	62 (6.7)	42 (47)	98 (13.9)	48 (6.0)	99	48	<0.001
– Stroke	14 (1.5)	24 (2.7)	20 (2.4)	37 (5.2)	22	37	0.03§
• Cardiovascular death	9 (0.9)	12 (1.3)	73 (10.9)	52 (6.8)	75	55	0.12

* P values were cakulated with the use of the log-rank test on the basis of all available follow-up data (i.e. more than 5 years).

† The primary composite outcome was the rate of death from any cause. myocardial infarction, or stroke.

‡ p = 0.006 in the as-treated (nonintention-to-treat) analysis.

§ p = 0.16 by the Wald test of the Cox regression estimate for study-group assignment in 1712 patients after adjustment for the average glucose level after the procedure.

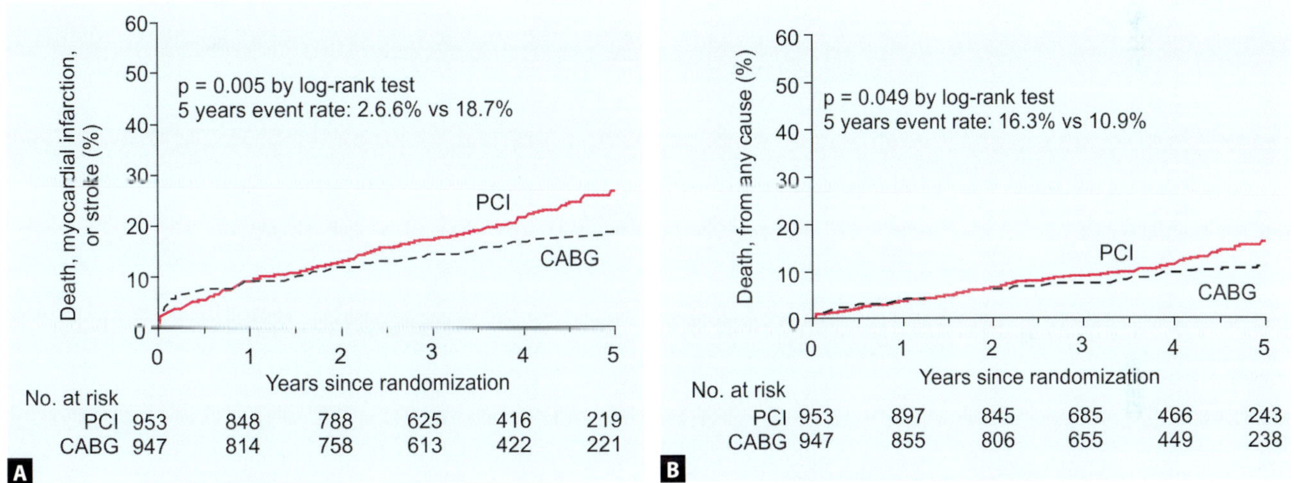

Figs 11.3A and B Percentage of death with (A) and without (B) cardiovascular disease during 5 years

rehospitalization, and reintervention; and patients exercise capacity. Most surviving patients have a satisfactory quality of life early after CABG, but the probability of retaining this gradually begins to decline after about 5 years.[15]

In 2013, Abdallah et al. compared health status outcomes after PCI vs CABG by analyzing the FREEDOM trial. More than 80% of the population had 3-vessel CAD, and more than 90% had LAD involvement. At baseline, both groups of patients reported significant health status limitations attributable to CAD.

The overall questionnaire response rate was >80% for eligible patients during the first 3 years of follow-up and >70% in years 4 and 5. Compared with baseline, both groups demonstrated substantial improvement in the Seattle angina questionnaire-angina frequency (SAQ-AF) subscale that was apparent by 1 month and sustained throughout the 5-year follow-up period (Fig. 11.4A). Between group comparisons demonstrated that CABG resulted in slightly higher scores than DES-PCI on the SAQ-AF subscale at the 1-year and 2-year follow-up time points (mean difference 1.0 and 1.3 points, respectively (Table 11.6). By 3 years, however, there was no significant difference in angina relief between the DES-PCI and CABG groups. When analyzed as a categorical variable, the proportion of angina free patients tended to be slightly greater with CABG than with DES-PCI at 6 months (83.7% vs 78.1%), 12 months (83.5% vs 79.5), and 24 months (83.3% vs 81.0%), although the differences were only statistically significant at 6 and 12 months.

The results for the SAQ physical limitation and Seattle angina questionnaire-quality of life (SAQ-QoL) subscales

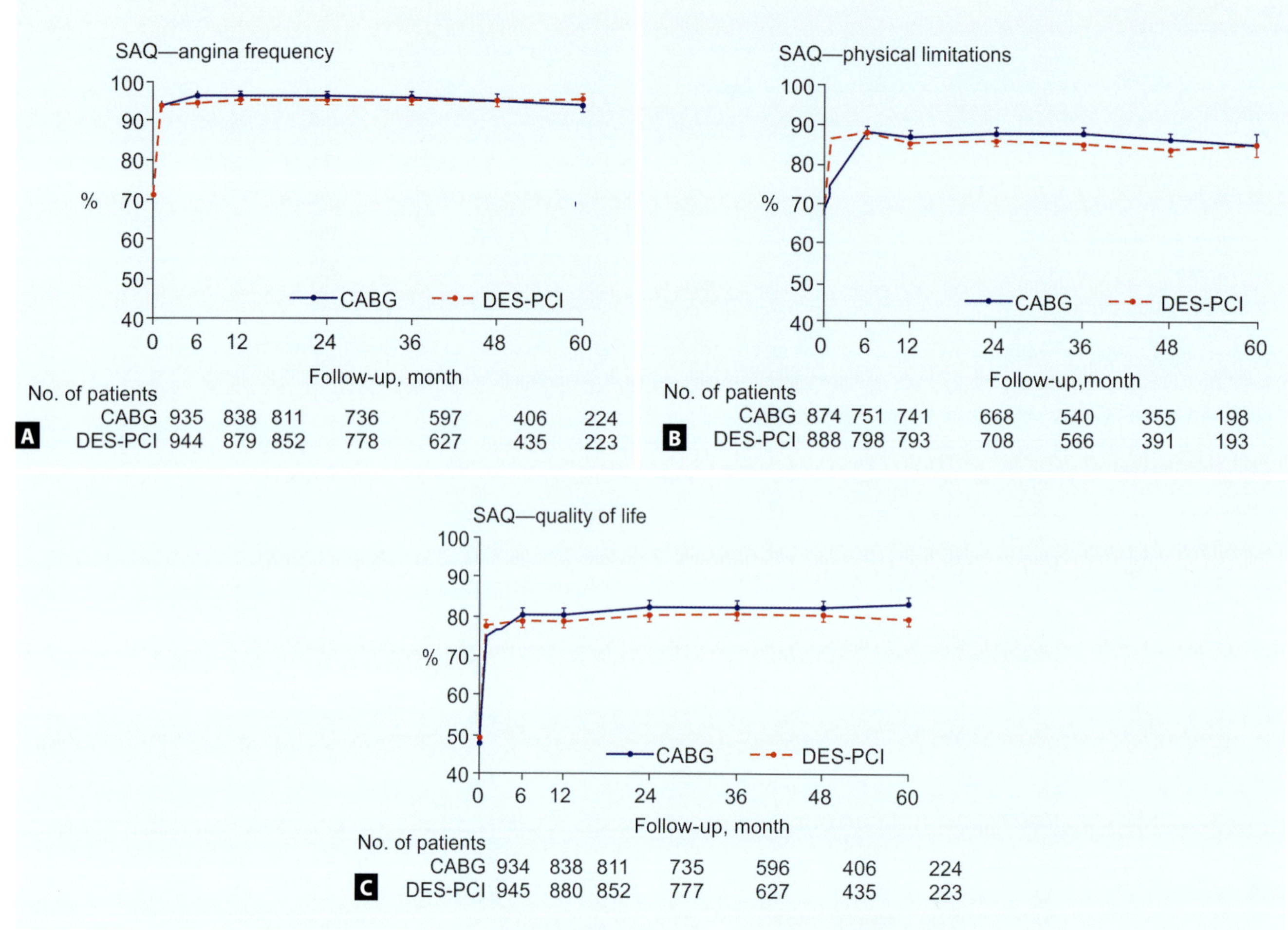

Figs 11.4A to C Seattle Angina questionnaire results. Mean scores (with 95% CI error bars) for the angina frequency (A), physical limitation (B), and quality of life (C) subscales of the Seattle Angina questionnaire (SAQ). Scores for each subscale range from 0 to 100, with higher scores representing better health status or quality of life

are summarized in Figures 11.4B and C, respectively. At 1 month, DES-PCI resulted in greater improvement compared with CABG for both the physical limitations (mean difference 8.1 points, 95% CI –9.9 to –6.3, $p < 0.001$) and QoL (mean difference 1.9 points, 95% CI –3.6 to –0.2, $p = 0.03$) subscales. By six months, scores for the SAQ QoL subscale were similar for the two treatment groups but remained modestly higher with DES-PCI for the physical limitations subscale (mean difference 2.3 points, 95% CI –3.8 to –0.9, $p = 0.002$). By 1 year, however, scores for both the physical limitations and QoL subscales were higher with CABG [mean differences 2.0 (95% CI 0.4 to 3.6, $p = 0.01$) and 1.9 points (95% CI 0.4 to 3.4, $p = 0.01$), respectively]. CABG continued to demonstrate better outcomes with respect to these two SAQ subscales through two and three years of follow-up. Beyond year 3, there were no consistent between-group differences for any of the SAQ subscales (although there were significant differences in favor of CABG at 5 years for the physical limitations and QoL subscales).

Results for the RDS are summarized in Figure 11.5. Both DES-PCI and CABG resulted in substantial reductions in the level of dyspnea over time, but the rate of improvement was more rapid with DES-PCI. At one month, DES-PCI patients were more likely to be free of limitations due to dyspnea than patients randomized to CABG (RDS 0: 67.6% vs 58.0%, $p < 0.001$). These between group differences were no longer apparent by 6 months (65.2% vs. 66.9%, $p = 0.99$).[16]

Bypass Angioplasty Revascularization Investigation two Diabetes (BARI-2D) Trial in which an indirect comparison demonstrated a slightly greater benefit of CABG than PCI on the duke activity status index (a measure of functional status) when compared with medical therapy.[17]

Table 11.6 Mean effect of CABG and PCI on disease specific health status according to longitudinal models, adjusted for baseline

Scale/Time point	*Treatment difference (CARG – PCI)*	*95% CI*	*P value*
SAQ—Angina frequency			
1 month	0.3	–0.7 to 1.4	0.54
6 months	0.7	–0.2 to 1.6	0.12
12 months	1.0	0.2–1.9	0.02
24 months	13	0.3–2.2	0.01
36 months	1.0	–0.1 to 2.0	0.07
48 months	0.2	–1.1 to 1.5	0.79
60 months	–1.2	–3.3 to 0.9	0.28
SAQ—Physical limitation			
1 month	–8.1	–9.9 to –6.3	<0.001
6 months	–2.3	–3.8 to –0.9	0.002
12 months	2.0	0.4–3.6	0.01
24 months	4.4	23–6.1	<0.001
36 months	2.5	0.5–4.5	0.01
48 months	1.0	–1.4 to 3.4	0.42
60 months	4.6	0.8–8.3	0.02
SAQ—Quality of life			
I month	–1.9	–3.6 to –0.2	0.03
6 months	0.4	–1.1 to 1.8	0.62
12 months	1.9	0.4–3.4	0.01
24 months	2.2	03–3.8	0.003
36 months	1.0	–0.7 to 2.7	0.25
48 months	0.6	–1.4 to 2.6	0.57
60 months	3.4	0.1 1–6.8	0.04

Abbreviations: CI, confidence interval; SAQ, Seattle angina questionnaire

Positive values indicate better quality of life with CARG.

Scores on the SAQ range from 0 to 100 with higher scores indicating better QoL. A score of 0 indicates daily angina or nitroglycerin use, severely limited physical activity due to cardiac disease and severely impacted quality of life for the SAQ–AF, SAQ–PL and SAQ–QoL respectively while a score of 100 indicates no angina or nitroglycerin use, no cardiac limitation on physical activity and no cardiac impact on Q0L on the same scales.

COST EFFECTIVENESS OF PERCUTANEOUS CORONARY INTERVENTION VERSUS CORONARY ARTERY BYPASS GRAFT

In a cost-effectiveness analysis of 1720 patients who were allocated to PCI, CABG or either therapy were followed for seven years. It was concluded that while the medical therapy and CABG were cost-effective at a conventional quality-adjusted life year of $60,000, PCI was not cost effective, and the additional benefit of stenting over best medical therapy was 'too small to justify the additional cost'. These findings are consistent with a previous report by the UK Health Technology Assessment Group, who also questioned whether the additional costs of DES were justifiable, warning that the widespread use of DES might reduce the gain in quality and possibly the duration of life arising from CABG in the long term.[18,19]

The second medicine, angioplasty, or surgery study (MASS II) analyzed the cost-effectiveness of medical therapy (MT), PCI and CABG by adjusting the cumulative costs for

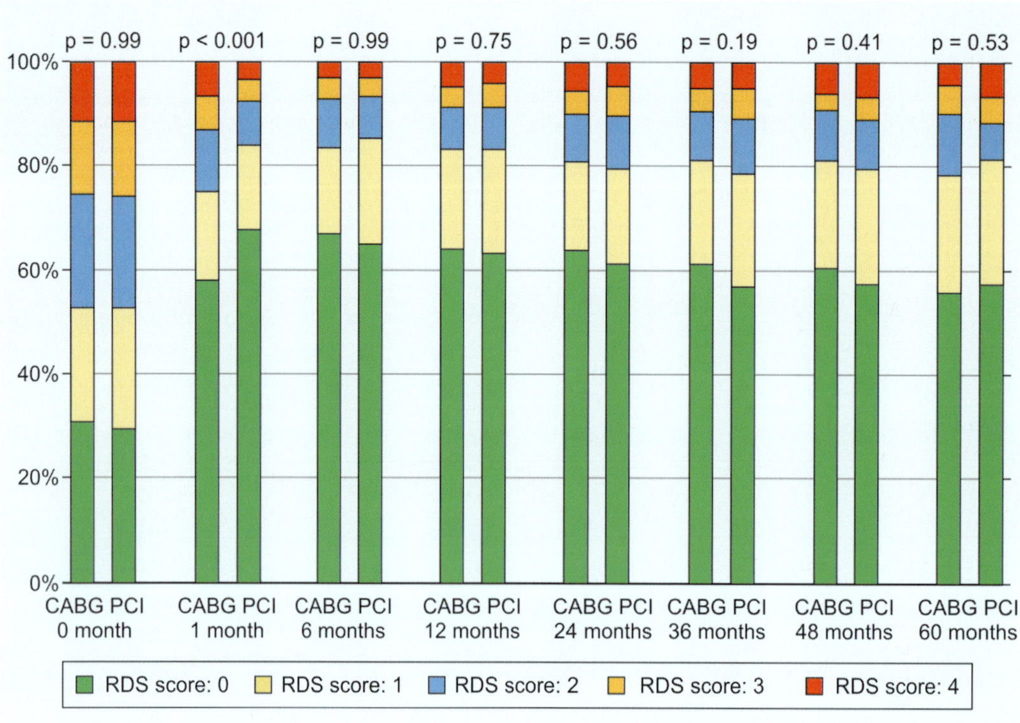

Fig. 11.5 Frequency of dyspnea-related limitation in physical activity according to the Rose Dyspnea Scale (RDS; range 0-4; higher scores represent more dyspnea)

average event-free time and angina-free proportion. The event-free costs were $9071.00 for MT; $19 967.00 for PCI; and $18 263.00 for CABG. Comparison of the event-free costs showed that there was a significant difference favoring MT versus PCI ($p = 0.01$) and versus CABG ($p = 0.01$) and CABG versus PCI ($p = 0.01$). The event-free plus angina-free costs were $16, 553.00, $25, 831.00, and $24, 614.00, respectively. The paired comparison of the event-free plus angina-free costs showed that there was a significant difference favoring MT versus PCI ($p = 0.04$), and versus CABG ($p = 0.001$); there was no difference between CABG and PCI ($p = 0.05$).

They concluded that in the long-term economic analysis, for the prevention of a composite primary end point, MT was more cost effective than CABG, and CABG was more cost-effective than PCI.[20]

The above issue has a slightly different inner meaning when applied to our own country. Our patients pay from their own pocket. Less than 20% of the patents are sponsored by employer or through insurance. Moreover, our patients need to return back to work earlier. Most of these patients are the sole earning members in their family.

CONCLUSION

Good Candidate for Percutaneous Transluminal Coronary Angioplasty

- Patients with good caliber coronary arteries and discrete lesions
- Patients with no comorbid condition
- Patients with good LV function
- Low syntax score patients.

Good Candidate for Coronary Artery Bypass Graft

- Patients with diffusely diseased coronary arteries, multiple lesions in LAD
- Patients with comorbid conditions including diabetes mellitus (DM), chronic renal failure (CRF) and other systemic diseases
- Patients with poor LV function and occluded arteries including chronic total occulsion (CTO)
- High syntax score.

Final Remark

- PTCA and CABG are complementary procedures. Both are palliative.
- Heart care team needs to evolve in the Indian set-up.
- Increased and judicious use of FFR will make both the practices scientific.

REFERENCES

1. Sorana O, Manchandab A, Schuelerc S. Percutaneous coronary intervention versus coronary artery bypass surgery in multivessel disease: a current perspective. Interactive Cardiovascular and Thoracic Surgery. 2009;8: 666-72.
2. Hoffman SN, TenBrook JA, Wolf MP, Pauker SG, Salem DN, Wong JB. A meta-analysis of randomized controlled trials comparing coronary artery bypass graft with percutaneous transluminal coronary angioplasty one- to eight-year outcomes. J Am Coll Cardiol. 2003;41:1293-304.
3. Mercado N, Wijns W, Serruys PW, Sigwart U, Flather MD, Stables RH, O'Neill WW, Rodriguez A, Lemos PA, Hueb WA, Gersh BJ, Booth J, Boersma E. One-year outcomes of coronary artery bypass graft surgery versus percutaneous coronary intervention with multiple stenting for multisystem disease: a meta-analysis of individual patient data from randomized clinical trials. J Thorac Cardiovasc Surg. 2005;130:512-9.
4. Patrick W Serruys, et al. 5-year clinical outcomes of the ARTS II (Arterial Revascularization Therapies Study II) of the sirolimus-eluting stent in the treatment of patients with multivessel de novo coronary artery lesions. J Am Coll Cardiol. 2010;55(11):1093-1101. doi:10.1016/j.jacc.2009. 11.049.
5. Lincoff AM. Important triad in cardiovascular medicine: diabetes, coronary intervention, and platelet glycoprotein IIbyIIIa receptor blockade. Circulation. 2003;107:1556-9.
6. Aronson D, Bloomgarden Z, Rayfield EJ. Potential mechanisms promoting restenosis in diabetic patients. J Am Coll Cardiol. 1996;27:528-35.
7. Hannan EL, Racz MJ, Walford G, Jones RH, Ryan TJ, Bennett E, Culliford AT, Isom OW, Gold JP, Rose EA. Long-term outcomes of coronary-artery bypass grafting versus stent implantation. N Engl J Med. 2005;352:2174-83.
8. Van Domburg RT, Takkenberg JJ, Noordzij LJ, Saia F, van Herwerden LA, Serruys PW, Bogers AJ. Late outcome after stenting or coronary artery bypass surgery for the treatment of multivessel disease: a single centermatched-propensity controlled cohort study. Ann Thorac Surg. 2005;79:1563-9.
9. Pell JP, Pell AC, Jeffrey RR, Jennings K, Oldroyd K, Eteiba H, Hogg KJ, Murday A, Faichney A, Colquhoun I, Berg G, Starkey IR, Flapan A, Mankad P. Comparison of survival following coronary artery bypass grafting vs percutaneous coronary intervention in diabetic and nondiabetic patients: retrospective cohort study of 6320 procedures. Diabet Med. 2004;21:790-2.
10. Brener SJ, Lytle BW, Casserly IP, Schneider JP, Topol EJ, Lauer MS. Propensity analysis of long-term survival after surgical or percutaneous revascularization in patients with multivessel coronary artery disease and high-risk features. Circulation. 2004;109:2290-5.
11. Bair TL, Muhlestein JB, May HT, Meredith KG, Horne BD, Pearson RR, LiQ, Jensen KR, Anderson JL, Lappe DL. Surgical revascularization is associated with improved long-term outcomes compared with percutaneous stenting in most subgroups of patients with multivessel coronaryartery disease: results from the intermountain heart registry. Circulation. 2007;116(11 Suppl):I226-31.
12. Coronary artery bypass surgery versus percutaneous coronary interventionwith stent implantation in patients with multivessel coronary artery disease (the stent or surgery trial): a randomised controlled trial. Lancet. 2002;360:965-70.
13. Mohr FW, Morice MC, Kappetein AP, et al. Coronary artery bypass graft surgery versus percutaneous coronary intervention in patients with three-vessel disease and left main coronary disease: 5-year follow-up of the randomised, clinical SYNTAX trial. Lancet. 2013;381:629-38.
14. Farkouh ME, Domanski M, Sleeper LA, et al. Strategies for multivessel revascularization in patients with diabetes. N Engl J Med. 2012;367:2375-84.
15. Booth DC, Deupree RH, Hultgren HN, DeMaria AN, Scott SM, Luchi RJ. Quality of life after bypass surgery for unstable angina. 5-year follow-up results of a veterans affairs cooperative study. Circulation. 1991;83:87.
16. Abdallah MS, et al. Quality of life after PCI vs. CABG among patients with diabetes and multivessel CAD: Results from the FREEDOM trial JAMA. 2013;310(15):1581-90. doi:10.1001/jama.2013.279208.
17. Brooks MM, Chung SC, Helmy T, et al. Health status after treatment for coronary artery disease and type 2 diabetes mellitus in the bypass angioplasty revascularization investigation 2 diabetes trial. Circulation. 2010;122(17):1690-9. [PubMed: 20937978].
18. Griffin SC, Barber JA, Manca A, Sculpher MJ, Thompson SG, Buxton MJ, Hemingway H. Cost effectiveness of clinically appropriate decisions on alternative treatments for angina pectoris: prospective observationalstudy. Br Med J. 2007;334:624–7.
19. Taggart DP. Coronary artery bypass graft vs percutaneous coronary angioplasty: CABG on the rebound? Current Opinion in Cardiology. 2007;22:517–23.
20. D'Oliveira Vieira R, et al. Cost-effectiveness analysis for surgical, angioplasty, or medical therapeutics for coronary artery disease 5-year follow-up of medicine, angioplasty, or surgery study (MASS) II trial. Circulation. 2012;126[Suppl 1]:S145–S50. doi: 10.1161/CIRCULATIONAHA.111.084442.

CHAPTER

12

Left Main Stenting

Shirish (MS) Hiremath, Omkar Thopte

INTRODUCTION

A critical lesion in the left main coronary artery (LMCA) has been observed in 3–5% of all the patients undergoing coronary angiography and in 10–30% undergoing coronary artery bypass grafting (CABG).[1]

Coronary artery bypass grofting (CABG) has been considered the standard care for such patients. However, since the introduction of percutaneous coronary intervention (PCI), the accumulation of experience, coupled with improved technology and pharmacology, has led to this approach being rapidly evolved and broadly adopted in LMCA stenosis. Several studies demonstrated that PCI and CABG show comparable long-term incidences of death, myocardial infarction (MI), but revascularization occurs less frequently in patients undergoing surgery.

The *LE MANS* (Study of Unprotected Left Main Stenting Versus Bypass Surgery) enrolled 105 patients with >50% left main narrowing, with or without multivessel coronary artery disease, who were equally suitable for PCI or CABG. At 1 year follow-up, the primary endpoint of mean ejection fraction increased with PCI compared with CABG (3.3 ± 6.7% after PCI vs 0.5 ± 0.8% after CABG; p = 0.047). The risk of major adverse cardiac and cardiovascular events (MACCE) at 1 year was similar (31% vs 25%; relative risk: 1.09 [95% CI: 0.85–1.38]), primarily due to the need for repeat revascularization in the PCI group.[2]

The *SYNTAX* (Synergy Between Percutaneous Coronary Intervention with TAXUS and Cardiac Surgery) trial provides the largest randomized dataset from which to assess the early and longer term safety and efficacy of PCI for left main disease. The trial used a novel method to calculate angiographic complexity, called the SYNTAX score and a higher SYNTAX score reflects greater anatomic complexity. Among the 750 patients in the unprotected left main cohort, 1 year major adverse cardiovascular and cerebrovascular events (MACCE) rates were similar for PCI and CABG (15.8% vs 13.7%, p = 0.48), with significantly lower rates of repeat revascularization in the patients randomly assigned to CABG (11.8% vs 6.5%, p = 0.02) at the cost of more strokes (0.3% vs 2.7%, p = 0.009).[3] In patients with low and intermediate SYNTAX scores (0–22 and 23–32), 1 year MACCE rates were numerically lower with PCI (7% vs 13% [p = 0.19]; 12.6% vs 15.5% [p = 0.54]), whereas in those with SYNTAX scores >32, MACCE rates after CABG were significantly better (25.3% vs 12.9%, p = 0.008). At the 3 years follow-up, there continued to be no significant difference within the overall left main cohort in the rate of MACCE between treatment strategies (26.8% vs 22.3%, p = 0.20); repeat revascularization was still more frequent with PCI (20.0% vs 11.7%, p = 0.004), whereas the risk of stroke after PCI remained lower (1.2% vs 4.0%, p = 0.02).[4] At the 5 year-follow-up, there continued to be no significant difference within the overall left main cohort in the rate of MACCE between treatment strategies (36.9% in PCI patients and 31.0% in CABG patients (hazard ratio (HR) 1.23 [0.95, 1.59]; p = 0.12). Stroke was significantly increased in the CABG group (PCI 1.5% vs CABG 4.3%, HR 0.33 [0.12, 0.92], p = 0.03) and repeat revascularization in the PCI arm (26.7% vs 15.5%, HR 1.82 [1.28, 2.57], p < 0.01). MACCE was similar between arms in patients with low/intermediate SYNTAX Scores but significantly increased in PCI patients with high scores (>33).[5]

In the recently published 5 years results of PRECOMBAT (Premier of Randomized Comparison of Bypass Surgery versus Angioplasty Using Sirolimus-Eluting Stent in Patients with Left Main Coronary Artery Disease) trial, 5 years-risk of death, myocardial infarction, or stroke was similar (8.4% and 9.6%; HR, 0.89; 95% CI, 0.52–1.52; p = 0.66) in patients with unprotected left main disease managed with PCI using DES (N = 300) and coronary artery bypass grafting (N = 300), but revascularizations were more common in patients undergoing PCI (hazard ratio: 2.18; 95% CI, 1.10–4.32; p = 0.02).[6]

A recent meta-analysis of 14,203 patients from 24 studies comparing PCI with coronary artery bypass grafting for unprotected left main lesions found no significant difference for all-cause mortality between PCI or CABG at 5 years. The need for target vessel revascularization (TVR) was significantly higher in patients undergoing PCI at all time points. However, occurrence of stroke was significantly less frequent in patients treated with PCI. There was no significant difference in combined MACCE between the 2 groups.[7]

Therefore, LMCA, PCI may be a potential alternative to CABG in selected situations.

In this chapter we will discuss the percutaneous treatment of LMCA disease using stepwise approach. The following is an overview of its management, highlighting specific technical issues.

Patients with LMCA are classified into two subgroups:

1. Protected (a previous CABG surgery to one or more branches of left coronary artery),
2. Unprotected LMCA (ULMCA, without such bypasses),

The LMCA is usually divided into three anatomical segments: ostium, shaft, and distal bifurcation. Distal bifurcation is exposed to a greater shear stress and is more prone to developing an atherosclerotic lesion. Clinical outcomes after revascularization may vary according to lesion location (nondistal vs distal) and LMCA complexity (simple Vs complex distal bifurcation).

ASSESSMENT OF LMCA LESION

Coronary angiography has been gold standard to define the severity of CAD. The cut-off for significant stenosis is a diameter stenosis >/ = 50%. The clue suggesting a significant LMCA disease is a drop of 'systolic and diastolic pressure' (pressure damping) at the time of catheter engagement. Another clue is the absence of contrast backflow into aorta (reflux of contrast into aorta) (Figs 12.1A and B).

ANGIOGRAPHIC EVALUATION OF LMCA

Left main length, lesion length, plaque burden, anatomic relationship between aorta and ostial segment, and side branches (SB) and LMCA disease in case of distal involvement (bifurcation angle), diameters, calcifications.

However, the coronary angiogram has several limitations. There is large intra and inter-observer variability in evaluation of its severity. Also due to its short-length, the presence of overlapping daughter branches, the lack of a reference segment, the concealment of diffuse atherosclerosis and issues of catheter placement and contrast 'streaming' for assessing the presence of ostial disease make the accurate assessment of the LMCA segment difficult even by the most experienced of clinicians. Therefore, additional tools such as fractional flow reserve (FFR) or intravascular ultrasound (IVUS) are often needed in order to assess intermediate LMCA stenosis.

FRACTIONAL FLOW RESERVE IN LMCA STENOSIS

Fractional flow reserve (FFR) is a validated, lesion-specific index that accurately reflects the functional significance of a coronary stenosis. FFR provides a precise estimation of the coronary blood supply for a specific myocardial territory, independent of hemodynamic parameters, such as heart rate, blood pressure or changes in myocardial contractility.[8]

Hamilos et al were the first to demonstrate the considerable discrepancy between coronary angiography and fractional flow reserve (FFR) in the evaluation of intermediate LMCA stenosis. Among the 213 patients in their study, 62 patients (29.1%) showed a 'visual functional

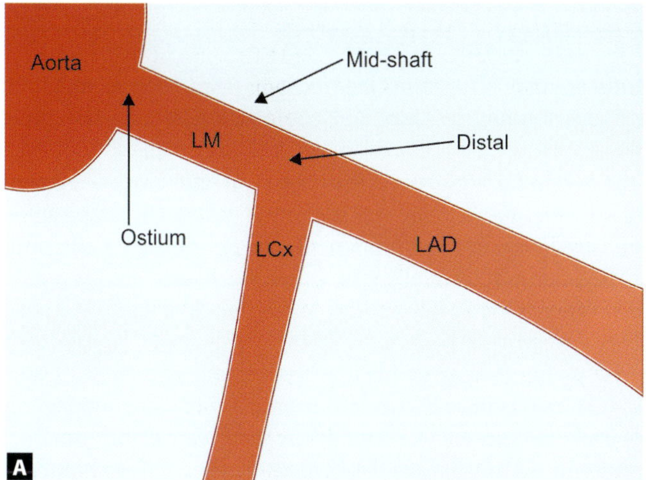

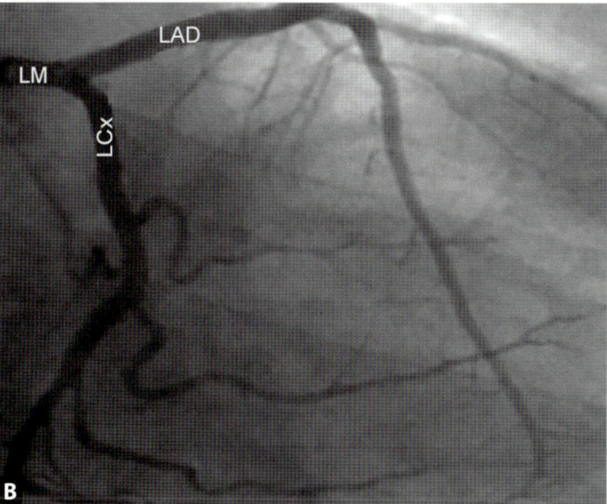

Figs 12.1A and B Schematic representation of left main coronary artery segments
Abbreviations: LAD, left anterior descending; LCx, left circumflex artery; LM, left main

mismatch' between angiographic significance and functional significance, 13 patients had a diameter stenosis >50% while the FFR was >0.80, and 49 patients had a diameter stenosis <50% while the FFR was <0.80. It is interesting to note that the prevalence of 'reverse mismatch,' which refers to angiographically insignificant but functionally significant stenosis, was dominant and as high as 79.0% among the mismatched patients. Figures 12.2A and B demonstrates the discrepancy between coronary angiography and FFR. The patients had an equivocal LMCA stenosis on angiography, and coronary artery bypass grafting (CABG) was performed only on patients with an FFR <0.80 across the LMCA stenosis. Mortality was surprisingly low for patients who were deferred CABG, based on FFR measurements.[9]

The main caveat when measuring FFR in the LMCA is that lesions are rarely isolated, making evaluation more complicated. Coexisting stenoses in the left anterior descending (LAD) or in the left circumflex artery (LCx) will tend to increase the FFR measured across an LMCA stenosis. The influence of downstream lesions on the FFR measurement in the LMCA depends on the severity of those lesions and on the size of the vascular territory supplied by the vessels. And hence, pullback curve should always be obtained in the case of lesions in left anterior descending (LAD) or left circumflex (LCx) artery in order to allow complete functional mapping of the epicardial coronary vasculature.

The guiding catheter should be disengaged from the ostium when performing measurements and intravenous adenosine 140 µg/kg/min is preferred over intracoronary adenosine.

IVUS TO GUIDE LMCA INTERVENTIONS

IVUS in Intermediate Lesions

There is a good correlation between IVUS measurement with FFR for assessing LMCA lesion significance. Abizaid et al were the first to report the importance of LMCA lumen dimensions by IVUS and they found that LMCA minimum lumen diameter (MLD) on IVUS was the strongest predictor of the rate of MACE. There was a progressive relationship between the degree of MLD compromise and subsequent MACE rates.[10]

Jasti et al performed FFR and IVUS measurements across angiographically indeterminate LMCA lesions. Compared with the FFR of <0.75 as being the 'gold-standard' measure of functional significance, an MLD of 2.8 mm on IVUS was found to have the highest sensitivity and specificity (93% and 95%, respectively) for identifying significant LMCA stenosis. This was followed by minimum lumen area (MLA) on IVUS of 5.9 mm^2 (93% sensitivity, and 95% specificity).[11]

Kang et al. investigated 55 patients with isolated UMLCA stenoses (30–80% diameter stenosis severity) that underwent IVUS and FFR before intervention. An MLA on IVUS of 4.8 mm^2 was found to best predict an FFR 0.80 (89% sensitivity, 83% specificity).[12]

From 121 patients with angiographically normal ULMCA lesions, Fassa et al. identified lower range of normal unprotected left main coronary artery (ULMCA) MLA to be 7.5 mm^2. After this, 214 patients with angiographically intermediate ULMCA lesions underwent IVUS. Of the patients with a ULMCA segment IVUS MLA >7.5 mm^2 were treated medically, whereas patients with an MLA <7.5 mm^2 were revascularized. At mean period of 3.3 years follow-up, they did not find any statistical difference in outcomes between these 2 patient groups.[13]

A recently multicenter *LITRO* study evaluated the safety of a lower predefined IVUS MLA threshold of 6 mm^2 to guide LMCA revascularization. A total of 354 patients were enrolled in 22 centers. In 179 patients with a ULMCA segment MLA of >6 mm^2, revascularization was deferred (although permitted for non-ULMCA lesions), whereas the remaining 152 patients with an MLA <6 mm^2 were revascularized (45% with PCI and 55% with CABG). The 2 years event-free survival of cardiac death and myocardial infarction (MI) was 97.7% in those patients who had no ULMCA revascularization, compared with 94.5% in the revascularized group (p = 0.5). Therefore, they suggested an MLA ≥6 mm^2 was a safe value for deferring revascularization of the LMCA. The results of this study provide further support for the utility of IVUS in angiographically indeterminate LMCA stenosis (Table 12.1).[14]

The 2011 American College and Cardiology Foundation (ACCF)/American Heart Association (AHA)/Society for Cardivascular Angiography and Interventions (SCAI) guidelines for PCI state that IVUS is reasonable for the assessment of angiographically indeterminate left main coronary artery disease (class IIa, Level of Evidence: B).

PERIPROCEDURAL IVUS

Intravascular ultrasound has recently been used to highlight the distribution, burden, and composition of atherosclerotic plaque within the LMCA segment and may help to determine interventional strategies. The length of the LMCA segment has been found to be an important factor in determining the predominant distribution of plaque. Shorter (<10 mm) LMCA harbour a slightly greater preponderance for plaque to distribute at the LMCA ostium. While, longer length (>10 mm) LMCA segments have been shown to harbour significantly more plaque burden within the distal bifurcation region.[15] Ostial LMCA lesions have less overall plaque burden, greater degrees of negative (constrictive remodeling) and less calcification than nonostial LMCA lesions. IVUS identified the diffuse nature of atherosclerosis involving not only the LMCA segment but also LAD and LCx (90% and 62% respectively) (Fig. 12.3).[16]

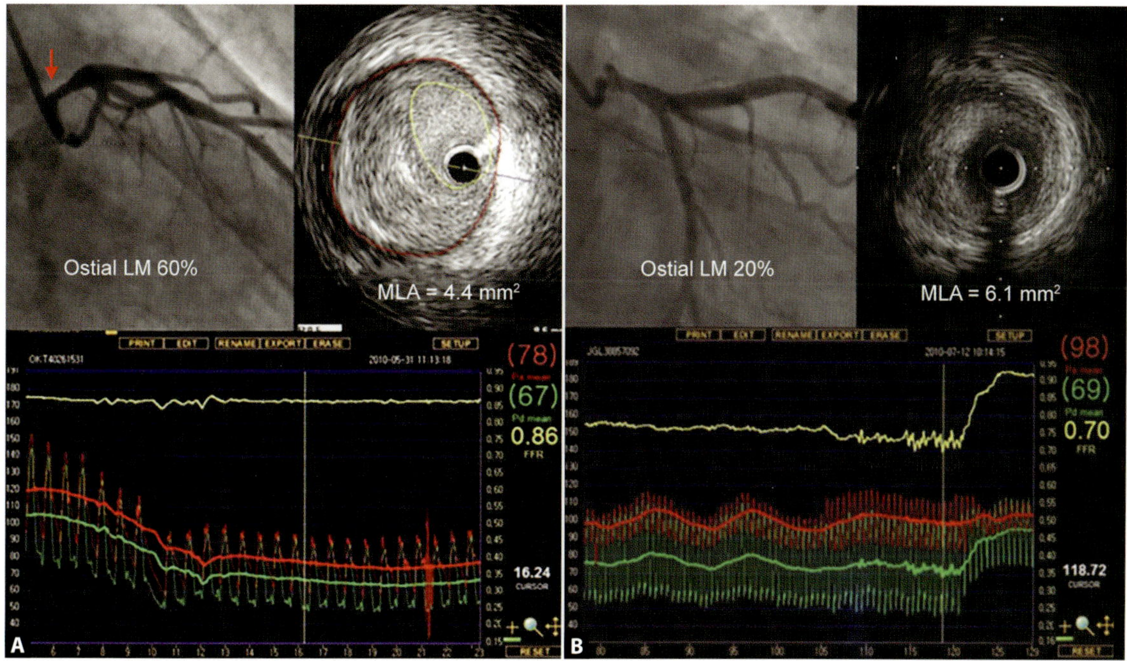

Figs 12.2A and B Representative case of visual–functional mismatch in LMCA stenosis: (A) Visually estimated percentage diameter stenosis was ≈60%, but FFR was 0.86; (B) Visually estimated percentage diameter stenosis was ≈20%, but FFR was 0.70

Abbreviations: FFR, fractional flow reserve; LM, left main; LMCA, left main coronary artery; MLA, minimal lumen area

Table 12.1 Use of IVUS to determine the significance of LMCA disease

Author	*IVUS criteria*	*Comment*
Abizaid et al.[10]	MLD	No specific cut off suggested. Progressive relationship between the degree of MLD compromise and subsequent MACE rates
Jasti et al.[11]	MLA, MLD	MLA <5.9 mm² and MLD <2.8 mm. FFR of 0.75 used as gold-standard reference
Kang et al.[12]	MLA	MLA of <4.8 mm² correlated with FFR <0.80.
Fassa et al.[13]	MLA	MLA 7.5 mm²
de la Torre Hernandez et al.[14]	MLA	MLA 6.0 mm²

Abbreviations: FFR; fractional flow reserve; IVUS, intravascular ultrasound; LMCA, left main coronary artery; MACE; major adverse cardiovascular events; MLA, minimum lumen area; MLD, minimum lumen diameter

In order to optimize the final procedure result (i.e. optimal stent expansion and apposition) and to assess any procedure-related complications (i.e. edge dissections, intramural hematomas, assessing plaque shift) IVUS plays a pivotal role.

The IVUS is critical for the optimization of postprocedural MLA after PCI to reduce restenosis rates. The most common site of restenosis invariably occurs at the ostium of the side-branch (i.e. LCx). In patients who had undergone a single stent strategy for LMCA, a postintervention ostial LCx MLA of >4 mm² was associated with a restenosis rate of 6% compared with 50% in those whose ostial LCx MLA was <4 mm² ($p = 0.04$). Similarly in those who received 2 stents, a postintervention ostial LCX MLA of >5.5 mm² was associated with a restenosis rate of 15% compared with 67% in those whose ostial LCX MLA was <5.5 mm² ($p = 0.03$).[17]

Suboptimal stent implantation (stent underexpansion) is important risk factor not only for DES restenosis but also for the more serious and rare event of ST.[18] IVUS is useful after stent implantation to determine the need for post-dilatation with appropriately sized noncompliant balloons based on average media-media diameters and to detect edge dissections which is known to associated with the occurrence of ST.[19]

Kang et al. investigated, the relationship between underexpansion in left main PCI with DES and adverse events. In the study, IVUS measurements were made at 4 locations: proximal left main, at the polygon of confluence, ostial left anterior descending, and ostial left circumflex in order to determine the stent area cut-off values associated with optimal outcomes. Investigators found that the best IVUS predictors of angiographic restenosis were minimal

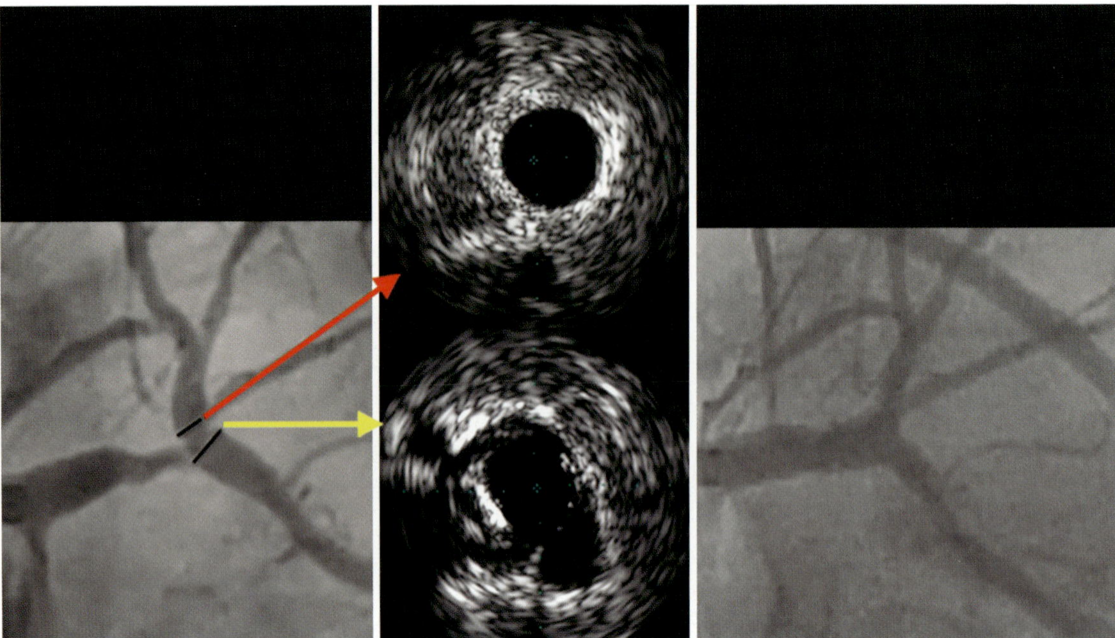

Fig. 12.3 Pre percutaneous coronary intervention (PCI) use of intravascular ultrasound (IVUS)

stent areas (MSA) of <8.2 mm^2 in the proximal left main, <7.2 mm^2 in the polygon of confluence, <6.3 mm^2 in the ostial left anterior descending, and <5.0 mm^2 in the ostial left circumflex.[20]

In *MAIN-COMPARE* (revascularization for unprotected left main coronary artery stenosis: comparison of percutaneous coronary angioplasty vs surgical revascularization) registry, 3-year outcomes revealed a significant low cumulative mortality rate within the IVUS-guided ULMCA PCI group receiving DES compared with the angiography guided group (4.7% vs 16%, p = 0.048).

Park et al showed that IVUS guidance was associated with a significantly lower risk of three-year mortality compared with angiography guidance.[21]

Similarly, in a multicenter registry evaluating 731 LMCA lesions (76.5% involving the distal left main) undergoing DES implantation, IVUS guidance was associated with reduced cardiac death.[22] However, in both the studies it did not modify the risk of MI or repeat revascularization.

The 2011 ACCF/AHA/SCAI guidelines for PCI state that IVUS may be considered for guidance of coronary stent implantation, particularly in cases of left main coronary artery stenting. (class IIb, Level of Evidence: B).

LESION PREPARATION (ROTATIONAL ATHERECTOMY)

Lesion preparation should be used:

- In presence of diffuse and severe calcification (Figs 12.4A to K)
- When balloon for predilation does not yield the lesion fully
- When it is difficult to cross the lesion with stent.

The 2011 ACCF/AHA/SCAI guidelines for PCI state that rotational atherectomy is reasonable for fibrotic or heavily calcified lesions that might not be crossed by a balloon catheter or adequately dilated before stent implantation. (Class IIa, Level of Evidence C).

We generally use IVUS information on the plaque morphology to determine lesion debulking strategy in the following way:

- Superficial calcium extending more than 180° may demand lesion preparation with rotational atherectomy (Rotablator),
- Severe fibrosis (particularly at the SB ostium) or moderate calcifications may demand noncompliant balloons sized to the media-to-media diameter.

INTRA-AORTIC BALLOON PUMP

A lower threshold for using an intra-aortic balloon pump (IABP) is suggested, particularly if the right coronary artery (RCA) is occluded, left ventricular function is severely reduced, or the LM, LAD, and/or LCx is significantly calcified.

AORTO-OSTIAL UNPROTECTED LEFT MAIN PCI

In approximately 5–35% of patients undergoing PCI for LMCA, the atherosclerotic plaque is limited only at the ostium

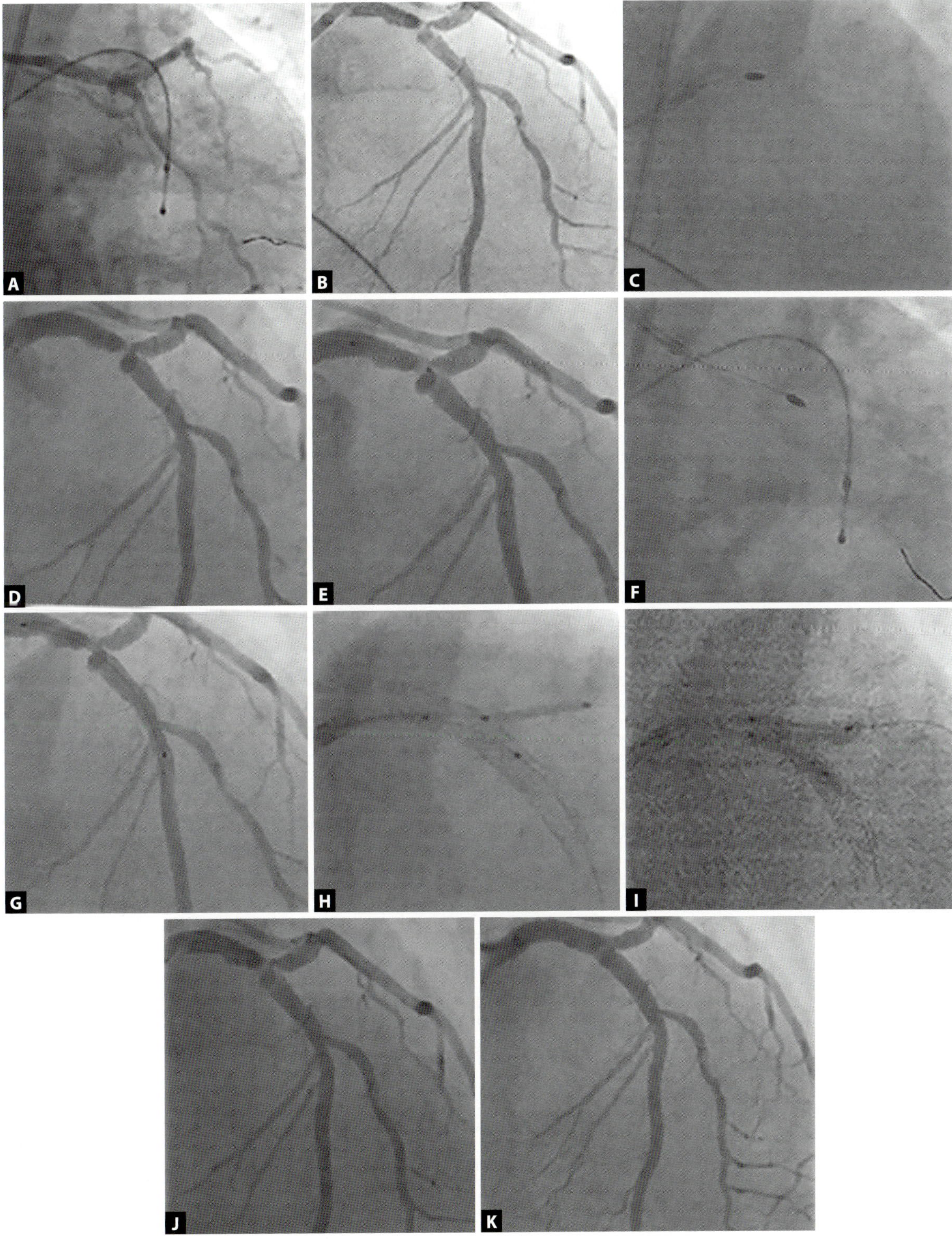

Figs 12.4A to K Lesion preparation with rotational atherectomy in LMCA stenting with T and protrusion (TAP) technique: (A and B) LCA engaged with 3.5 × 7 Fr EBU showing distal left main heavily calcific with 80% stenosis and ostial LAD and LCx heavy calcium with 90% stenosis; (C to F) Rotablation to LAD followed by to LCx done; (G and H) Stenting to LAD done (4.0 × 32 mm) and then across stent strut LCx stent (3.5 x 15) was placed (T and protrusion stenting technique); (I to K) Final kissing balloon inflation done with 3.5 x 8 NC balloon in LCx and 3.0 × 15 semicompliant balloon in LAD

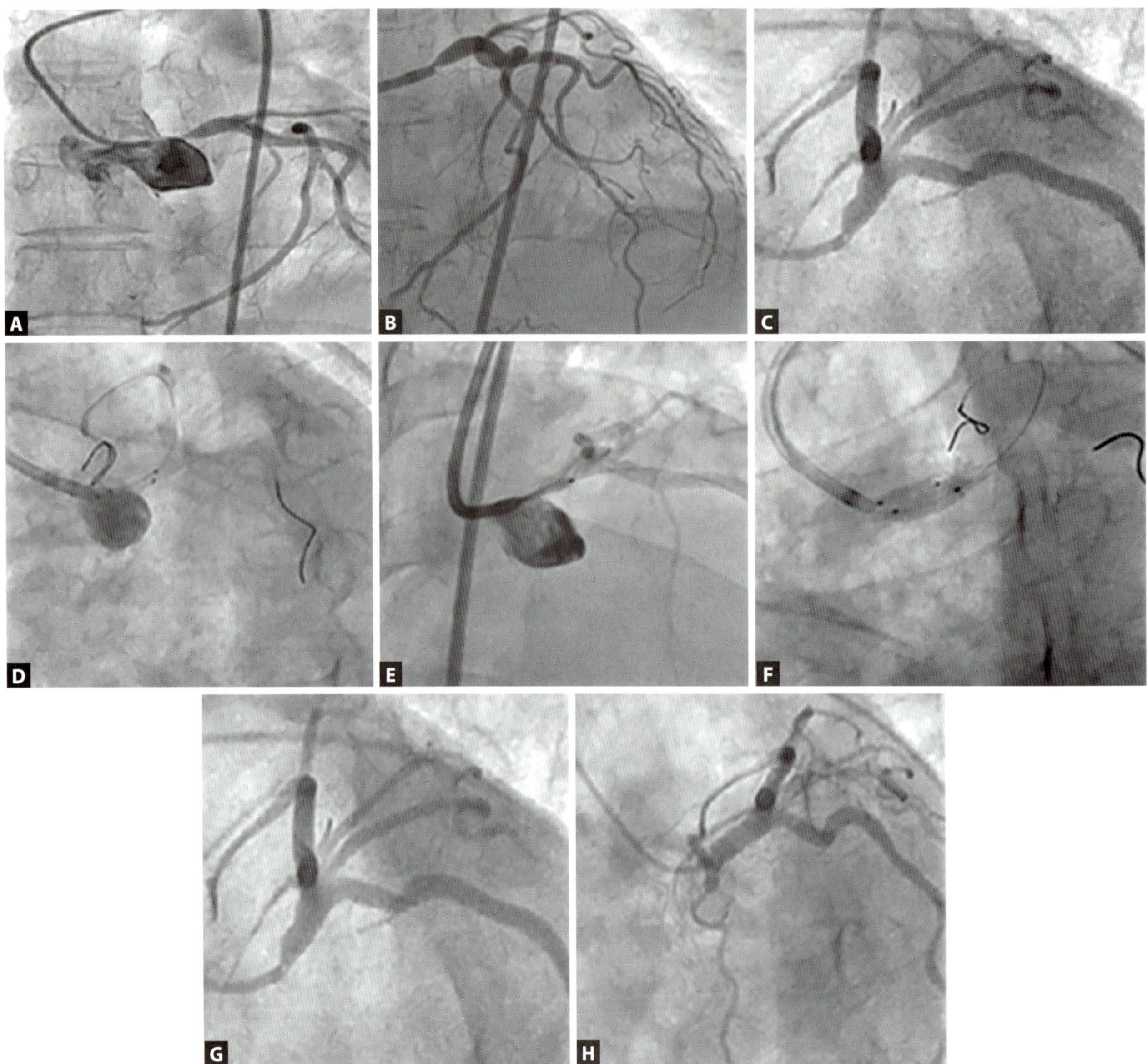

Figs 12.5A to H Aorto-ostial LMCA stenting. (A to C) LCA injections taken with JL 3.5 × 6F diagnostic catheter showing critical ostial left main stenosis; (D) LCA engaged with 3.5 × 7F EBU SH and LAD, LCx wiring done. Later predilation with 3.0 × 9 cutting balloon and 3.0 × 8 NC balloon done; (E) 4.0 x 8 DES deployed in left main ostium; (F) Postdilation done with two 3.0 × 8 NC balloons simultaneously (G and H) LCA injection shows excellent final result

or mid-shaft segment. PCI of nondistal lesions is well known to be associated with favorable angiographic and clinical outcomes.[23]

General principles PCI for an ostial ULMCA lesion are:

- Check for full predilatation
- Minimal usage of direct stenting

One specific feature of an ostial ULMCA lesion is the size of the reference vessel frequently more than 4.0 mm. It is important to allow the stent to protrude into the aorta for about 1–2 mm (Figs 12.5A to H) and to check for positioning in different views (i.e. cranial right anterior oblique and the caudal left anterior oblique). It is important to use a short stent to avoid fully covering the distal bifurcation. In contrast, the operator should be careful not to implant a stent too short in order to avoid dislodgement during postdilatation or while maneuvering the guiding catheter. We recommend the use of DES in ostial LMCA lesions, because aorto-ostial lesions are associated with a high restenosis rate, even if the reference vessel size is large.

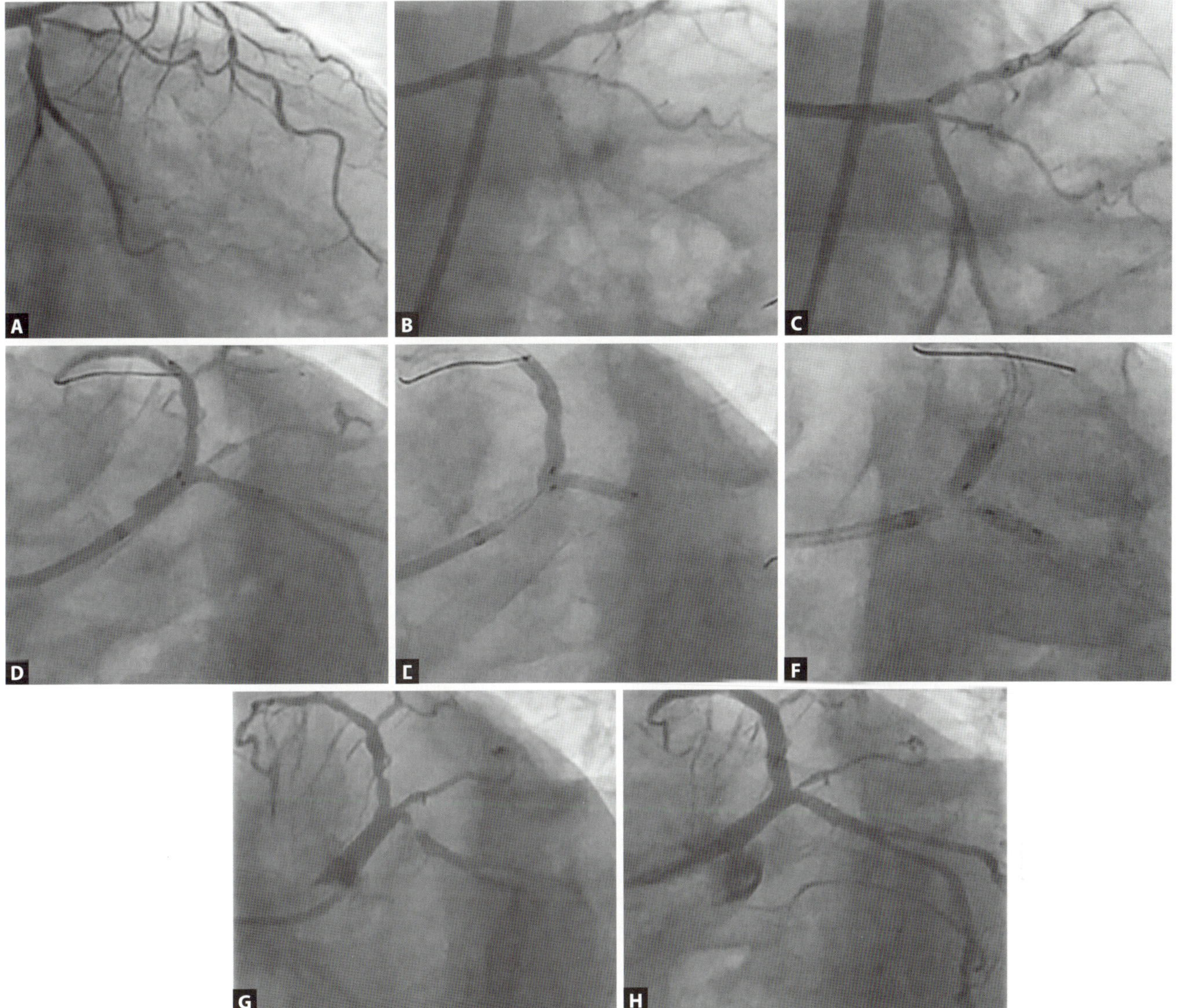

Figs 12.6A to H V Stent technique. (A) LCA engaged with 3.57 F EBU and showing ostioproximal LAD and ostioproximal LCx critical lesions, distal LMCA is normal; (B and C) LAD and LCx lesions were sequentially predilated with 2.5 × 12 semicompliant balloon followed by 3.0 × 8 NC balloon; (D and E) Later on 3.5 × 28 and 3.5 × 14 DES simultaneously deployed into LAD and LCx respectively; (F) Postdilation was done with 3.5 × 12 NC balloons simultaneously (G and H) Excellent end result

MID-SHAFT LEFT MAIN PCI

Lesions located at the body of the LMCA should be treated as ostial lesions. When lesion extends very close to the bifurcation and there is any doubt about possibility of plaque shift, then it is reasonable strategy is to extend the stent into the LAD. Also it may be necessary to wire the LCx in order to protect it and to facilitate rewiring. The final stent sizes are usually ≥4 mm. When target size is 4 mm, it is possible to utilize a 3.5 mm stent and to postdilate with a 4 mm noncompliant balloon.

LEFT MAIN BIFURCATION PCI

Distal bifurcation is involved in 60–90% of lesions involving LMCA.[1] PCI for distal LMCA has been shown to be associated with worse clinical outcome compared with nondistal LMCA PCI.[24] The results of distal LMCA PCI are highly dependent on the selection of the strategy and the optimal performance of the procedure.

The LMCA bifurcation varies not only in anatomy (plaque location and burden, diameter of branches and

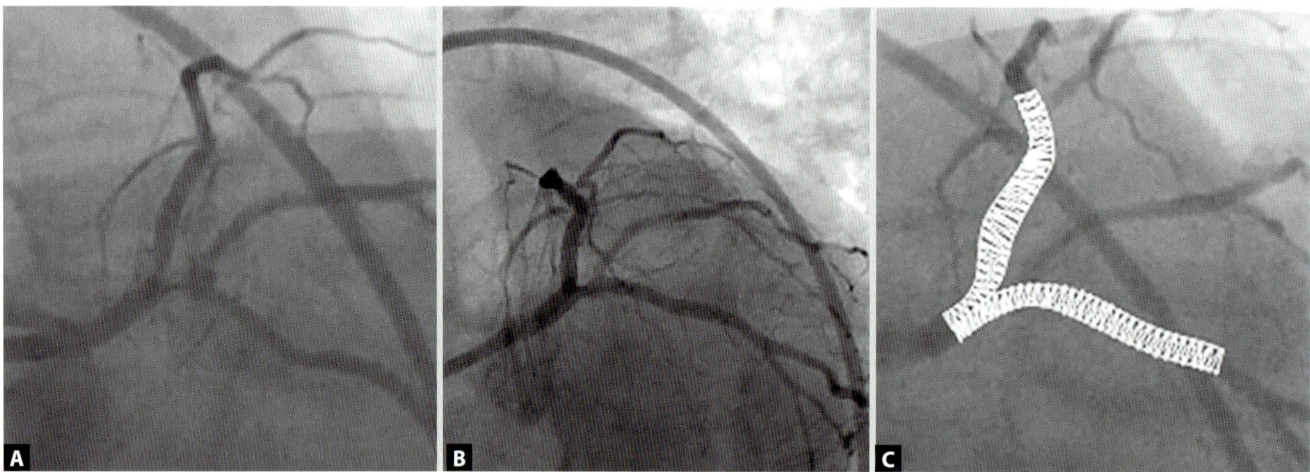

Figs 12.7A to C Simultaneous kissing stent (SKS) technique: (A) LCA engaged with lesions 3.5 7F EBU showing ostial LAD and LCx having 80% critical stenosis, both the were predialted with NC balloon; (B and C) 3.0 × 33 and 3.0 × 33 mm DES are positioned side by side creating a double barrel configuration and deployed simultaneously with excellent result

angle between branches) but also in the dynamic changes during PCI (plaque shift), and hence there is no single strategy that can be applied to every bifurcation (one-stent vs two-stent).

Current approaches may require two stents in about 50% of true (i.e. Medina 1, 1, 1/1, 0, 1/0, 1, 1) LMCA bifurcations.[25] In LMCA bifurcation the side branch may be as important as the main branch in terms of size and territory of distribution. We usually define the LAD as the MB and the LCx or RI as the SB. The most important factors to take into account when the operator is deciding between provisional stenting and two stent strategies are: plaque distribution, size of the SB, severity and length of the SB lesion, and angle of branch.

An ULMCA bifurcation lesion when is plaque located in the MB alone (Medina 1, 1, 0/1, 0, 0), it should be treated by implanting a stent from the ULMCA into the MB with a provisional approach to the SB. And after performing a FKBI, decision to implant a second stent should be taken in case of dissection or residual stenosis (≥50%).

Conversely, when the disease at the bifurcation involves both MB and SB (or three branches when RI is present), and if the SB is sufficiently large in diameter (i.e. ≥2.5 mm), or if the disease extends beyond the ostium (≥ 5 mm) then elective two stent strategy should be considered.

Next important variable to be considered LMCA bifurcation PCI is the angle between the branches. Bifurcations are classified according to the internal angle between MB and SB in V-shaped (angle <70°) and T-shaped (≥70°) lesions. Invariably in most of the cases LMCA bifurcation is T-shaped with an average angle of 80°. This is an important point to consider, because a T-shaped angle does not allow easy wire access to the SB and may not allow re-crossing into the SB with a wire, balloon or stent after MB stenting while, V-Shaped (angle <70°) is associated with the risk of plaque shift and compromise of the ostium, and SB occlusion.

Currently there are insufficient data to recommend which of the two-stent techniques is superior with regard to procedural and follow-up events. Based on the LMCA bifurcation anatomy preferred two stent strategies are summarized in Figures 12.6A to H. The V and the simultaneous kissing stent techniques are shown in Figures 12.6A to H and 12.7A to C, the T-technique in Figures 12.8A to J, the crush/mini-crush technique in Figures 12.9A to K, and the culotte technique in Figures 12.10A to F.

SUMMARY AND AUTHOR RECOMMENDATIONS

Evidence from RCTs involving more than 1,600 patients with left main disease who are suitable candidates for either CABG or PCI in the setting of less complex coronary anatomy (SYNTAX score <32) suggests that PCI may provide at least equivalent results to CABG in the setting of less complex coronary anatomy. Clinical outcomes after PCI appear worse in patients with more complex coronary anatomy, in particular those with SYNTAX scores >32.

Intravascular imaging and/or functional assessment before and after intervention may optimize clinical outcomes, although robust data supporting these approaches are lacking. The most important factors to take into account when the operator is deciding between provisional stenting and elective two stent strategy are: plaque distribution, size of the SB, severity and length of the SB lesion, and angle of branch. Currently there is insufficient data to determine which of the two-stent strategy is superior with regard to procedural and follow-up events.

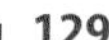

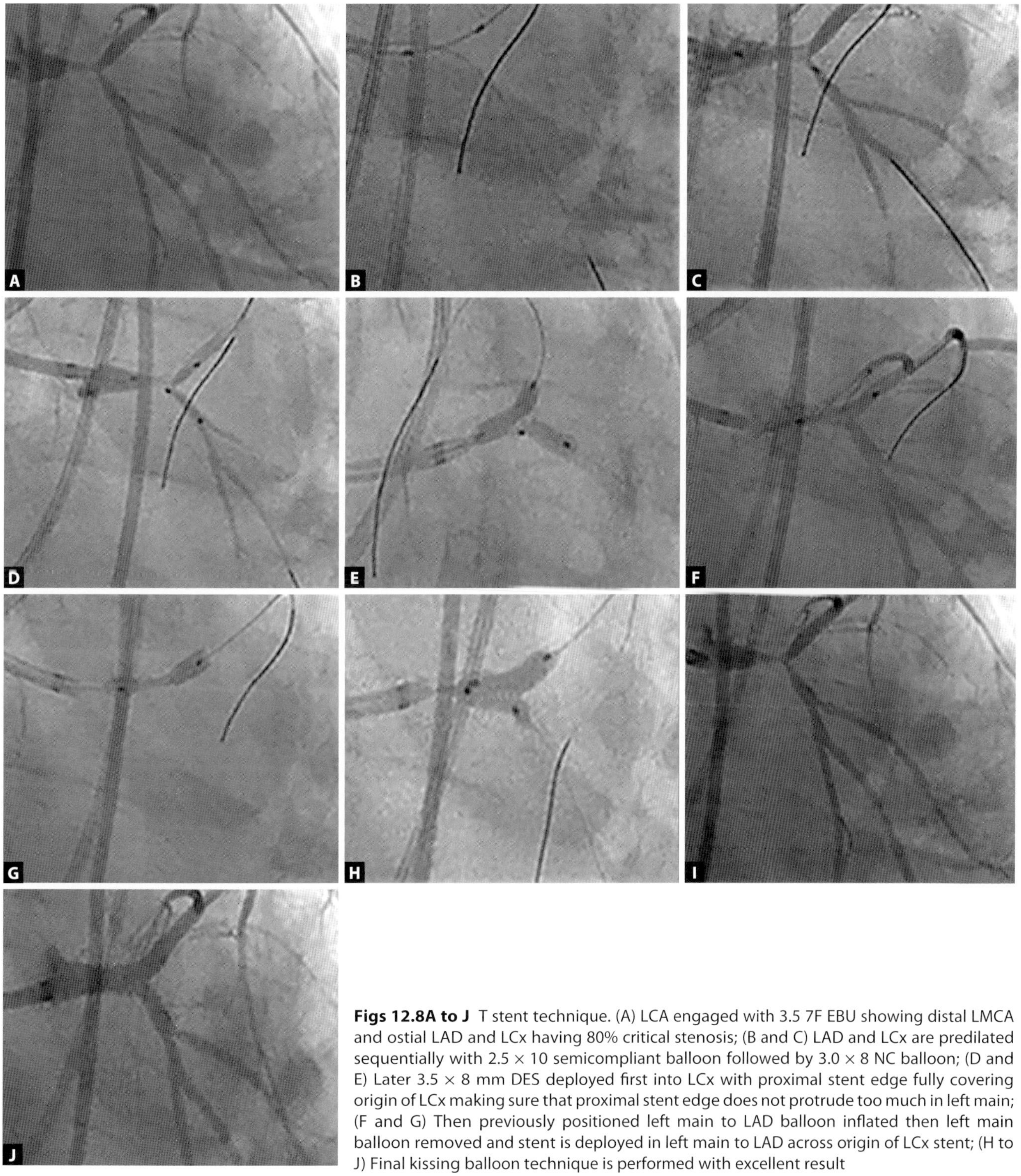

Figs 12.8A to J T stent technique. (A) LCA engaged with 3.5 7F EBU showing distal LMCA and ostial LAD and LCx having 80% critical stenosis; (B and C) LAD and LCx are predilated sequentially with 2.5 × 10 semicompliant balloon followed by 3.0 × 8 NC balloon; (D and E) Later 3.5 × 8 mm DES deployed first into LCx with proximal stent edge fully covering origin of LCx making sure that proximal stent edge does not protrude too much in left main; (F and G) Then previously positioned left main to LAD balloon inflated then left main balloon removed and stent is deployed in left main to LAD across origin of LCx stent; (H to J) Final kissing balloon technique is performed with excellent result

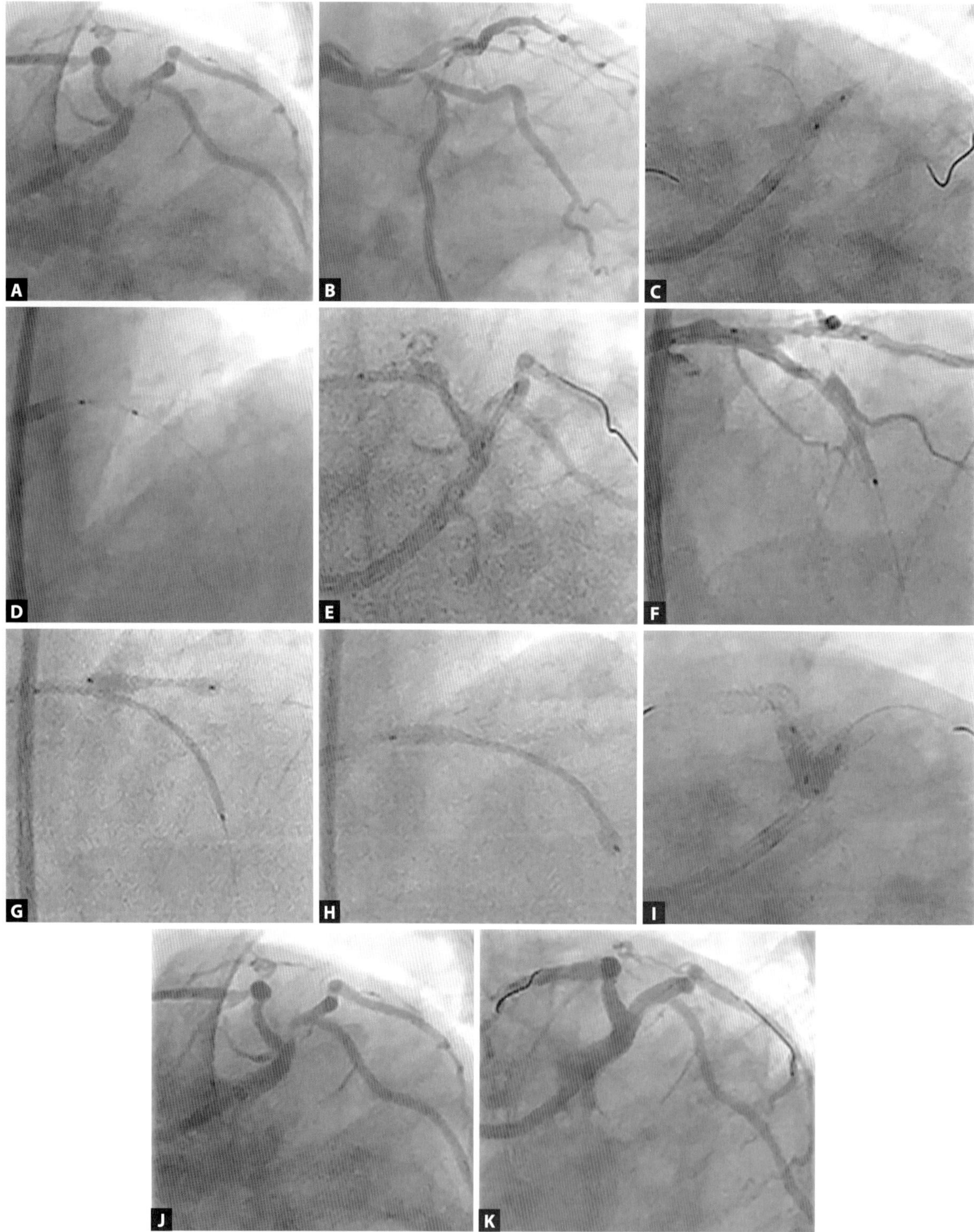

Figs 12.9A to K Mini crush technique. LCA injection shows distal left main tapering with 40% stenosis. Ostio-proximal LAD has 40–50% plaque and ostioproximal LCx has 90% stenosis. Both the lesions predilated with 2.5 × 10 NC and 3.0 × 8 NC balloons sequentially. Then 4.00 × 32 mm stent placed from LMCA to lad and and 3.5 × 15 mm stent placed in ostium of LCx so as to protrude by 3 mm in LMCA. LCx stent is deployed first and the balloon and wire are then removed. Prepositioned stent in the main LM LAD is deployed to completely cover and crush the protruding segment of the LCx stent against the vessel wall. A wire is then recrossed through the LM stent into the LCx, balloon dilation done across stent strut. Then kissing balloon inflation is done to finish the procedure

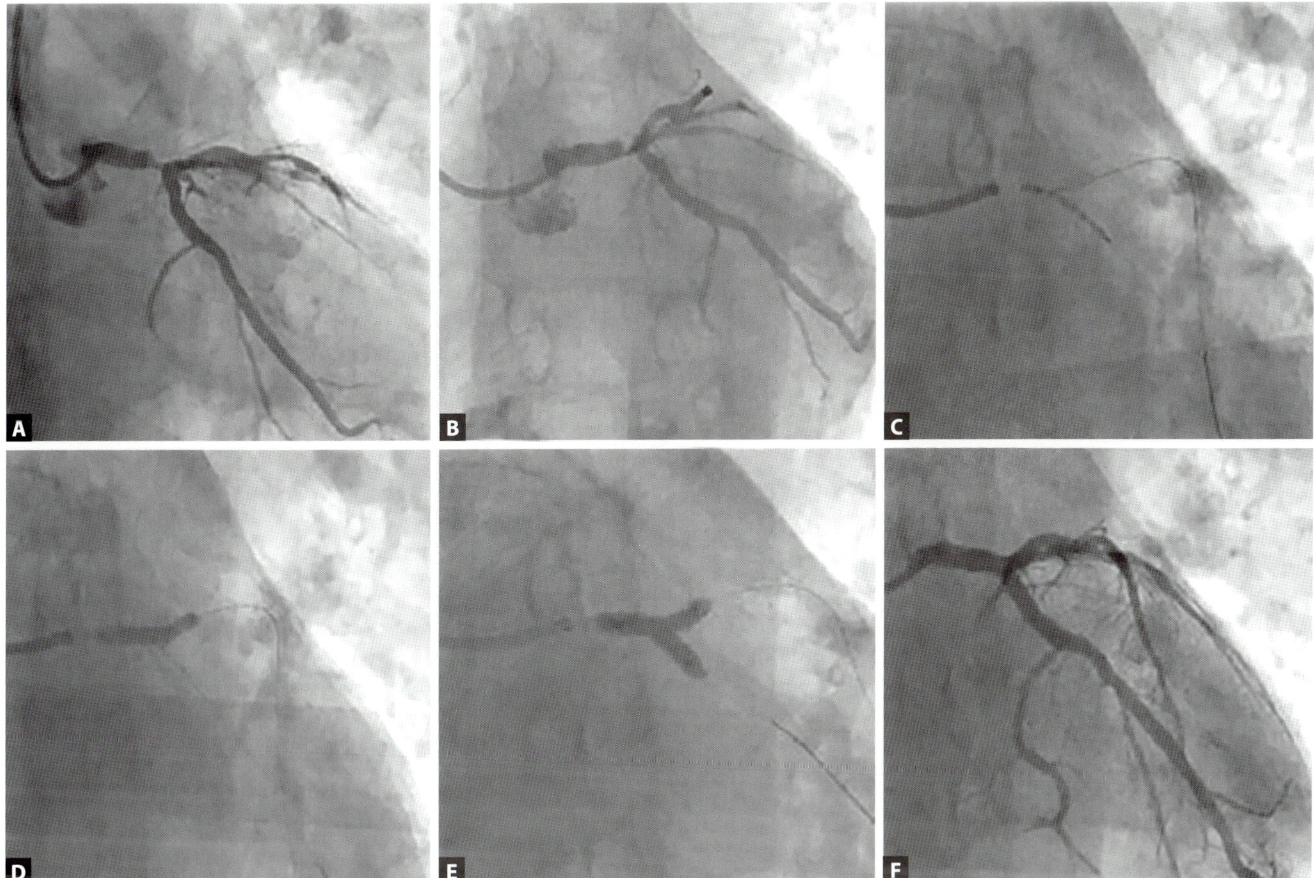

Figs 12.10A to F Culotte technique. (A to C) LCA injection showing distal left main 90% stenosis with LAD and LCx ostial 80% and 70% involvement. Both LAD and LCx are of equal size (3.5 mm). LMCA to LCx predilated with 3.0 × 10 mm NC balloon. Stent (3.5 x 18 mm) deployed across LMCA to LCx. Then through stent strut across LMCA to LAD balloon dilation done with 3.0 × 10 mm NC balloon; (D) 3.5 × 15 mm stent deployed across LMCA to LAD through stent struts; (E) Final Kissing balloon inflation done; (F) LCA injection showing excellent final result

The current ACCF/AHA/SCAI guideline recommends a Heart Team approach to revascularization is recommended in patients with unprotected left main (Class I, Level of evidence C). Also ACCF/AHA/SCAI guideline states that a calculation of the Society of Thoracic Surgeons (STS) and SYNTAX scores is reasonable in patients with unprotected left main. (Class IIa, Level of evidence B). Left main PCI is a reasonable alternative to CABG in patients who have anatomic conditions associated with good procedural and longer-term outcomes and who are at increased risk for surgery. (Class IIa, Level of Evidence B).

The EXCEL trial will provide more definitive data regarding the safety and efficacy of left main PCI compared with CABG in patients suitable for either treatment strategy.

REFERENCES

1. Park SJ, Park DW. Percutaneous coronary intervention with stent implantation versus coronary artery bypass surgery for treatment of left main coronary artery disease: is it time to change guidelines? Circ Cardiovasc Interv. 2009;2(1):59-68.
2. Buszman PE, Buszman PP, Kiesz RS, Bochenek A, Trela B, Konkolewska M, et al. Early and long-term results of unprotected left main coronary artery stenting: the LE MANS (Left Main Coronary Artery Stenting) registry. J Am Coll Cardiol. 2009;54(16):1500-11.
3. Morice MC, Serruys PW, Kappetein AP, Feldman TE, Stahle E, Colombo A, et al. Outcomes in patients with de novo left main disease treated with either percutaneous coronary intervention using paclitaxel-eluting stents or coronary artery bypass graft treatment in the Synergy Between Percutaneous Coronary Intervention with TAXUS and Cardiac Surgery (SYNTAX) trial. Circulation. 2010;121(24):2645-53.
4. Kappetein AP, Feldman TE, Mack MJ, Morice MC, Holmes DR, Stahle E, et al. Comparison of coronary bypass surgery with drug-eluting stenting for the treatment of left main and/or three-vessel disease: 3-year follow-up of the SYNTAX trial. Eur Heart J. 2011;32(17):2125-34.
5. Morice MC, Serruys PW, Kappetein AP, Feldman TE, Stahle E, Colombo A, et al. Five-year outcomes in patients with left main

disease treated with either percutaneous coronary intervention or coronary artery bypass grafting in the synergy between percutaneous coronary intervention with TAXUS and cardiac surgery trial. Circulation. 2014;129(23):2388-94.

6. Ahn JM, Roh JH, Kim YH, Park DW, Yun SC, Lee PH, et al. Randomized Trial of Stents Versus Bypass Surgery for Left Main Coronary Artery Disease: 5-Year Outcomes of the PRECOMBAT Study. J Am Coll Cardiol. 2015;65(20):2198-206.
7. Athappan G, Patvardhan E, Tuzcu ME, Ellis S, Whitlow P, Kapadia SR. Left main coronary artery stenosis: a meta-analysis of drug-eluting stents versus coronary artery bypass grafting. JACC Cardiovasc Interv. 2013;6(12):1219-30.
8. Pijls NH, De BB, Peels K, Van Der Voort PH, Bonnier HJ, Bartunek JKJ, et al. Measurement of fractional flow reserve to assess the functional severity of coronary-artery stenoses. N Engl J Med. 1996;334(26):1703-8.
9. Hamilos M, Muller O, Cuisset T, Ntalianis A, Chlouverakis G, Sarno G, et al. Long-term clinical outcome after fractional flow reserve-guided treatment in patients with angiographically equivocal left main coronary artery stenosis. Circulation. 2009;120(15):1505-12.
10. Abizaid AS, Mintz GS, Abizaid A, Mehran R, Lansky AJ, Pichard AD, et al. One-year follow-up after intravascular ultrasound assessment of moderate left main coronary artery disease in patients with ambiguous angiograms. J Am Coll Cardiol. 1999;34(3):707-15.
11. Jasti V, Ivan E, Yalamanchili V, Wongpraparut N, Leesar MA. Correlations between fractional flow reserve and intravascular ultrasound in patients with an ambiguous left main coronary artery stenosis. Circulation. 2004;110(18):2831-6.
12. Kang SJ, Lee JY, Ahn JM, Song HG, Kim WJ, Park DW, et al. Intravascular ultrasound-derived predictors for fractional flow reserve in intermediate left main disease. JACC Cardiovasc Interv. 2011;4(11):1168-74.
13. Fassa AA, Wagatsuma K, Higano ST, Mathew V, Barsness GW, Lennon RJ, et al. Intravascular ultrasound-guided treatment for angiographically indeterminate left main coronary artery disease: a long-term follow-up study. J Am Coll Cardiol. 2005;45(2):204-11.
14. de la Torre Hernandez JM, Hernandez HF, Alfonso F, Rumoroso JR, Lopez-Palop R, Sadaba M, et al. Prospective application of pre-defined intravascular ultrasound criteria for assessment of intermediate left main coronary artery lesions results from the multicenter LITRO study. J Am Coll Cardiol. 2011;58(4): 351-8.
15. Maehara A, Mintz GS, Castagna MT, Pichard AD, Satler LF, Waksman R, et al. Intravascular ultrasound assessment of the stenoses location and morphology in the left main coronary artery in relation to anatomic left main length. Am J Cardiol. 2001;88(1):1-4.
16. Oviedo C, Maehara A, Mintz GS, Araki H, Choi SY, Tsujita K, et al. Intravascular ultrasound classification of plaque distribution in left main coronary artery bifurcations: where is the plaque really located? Circ Cardiovasc Interv. 2010;3(2):105-12.
17. Kim YH, Park SW, Hong MK, Park DW, Park KM, Lee BK, et al. Comparison of simple and complex stenting techniques in the treatment of unprotected left main coronary artery bifurcation stenosis. Am J Cardiol. 2006;97(11):1597-601.
18. Cook S, Wenaweser P, Togni M, Billinger M, Morger C, Seiler C, et al. Incomplete stent apposition and very late stent thrombosis after drug-eluting stent implantation. Circulation. 2007;115(18):2426-34.
19. Dussaillant GR, Mintz GS, Pichard AD, Kent KM, Satler LF, Popma JJ, et al. Small stent size and intimal hyperplasia contribute to restenosis: a volumetric intravascular ultrasound analysis. J Am Coll Cardiol. 1995;26(3):720-4.
20. Kang SJ, Ahn JM, Song H, Kim WJ, Lee JY, Park DW, et al. Comprehensive intravascular ultrasound assessment of stent area and its impact on restenosis and adverse cardiac events in 403 patients with unprotected left main disease. Circ Cardiovasc Interv. 2011;4(6):562-9.
21. Park SJ, Kim YH, Park DW, Lee SW, Kim WJ, Suh J, et al. Impact of intravascular ultrasound guidance on long-term mortality in stenting for unprotected left main coronary artery stenosis. Circ Cardiovasc Interv. 2009;2(3):167-77.
22. Chieffo A, Park SJ, Meliga E, Sheiban I, Lee MS, Latib A, et al. Late and very late stent thrombosis following drug-eluting stent implantation in unprotected left main coronary artery: a multicentre registry. Eur Heart J. 2008;29(17):2108-15.
23. Chieffo A, Park SJ, Valgimigli M, Kim YH, Daemen J, Sheiban I, et al. Favorable long-term outcome after drug-eluting stent implantation in nonbifurcation lesions that involve unprotected left main coronary artery: a multicenter registry. Circulation. 2007;116(2):158-62.
24. Valgimigli M, Malagutti P, Rodriguez Granillo GA, Tsuchida K, Garcia-Garcia HM, van Mieghem CA, et al. Single-vessel versus bifurcation stenting for the treatment of distal left main coronary artery disease in the drug-eluting stenting era. Clinical and angiographic insights into the Rapamycin-Eluting Stent Evaluated at Rotterdam Cardiology Hospital (RESEARCH) and Taxus-Stent Evaluated at Rotterdam Cardiology Hospital (T-SEARCH) registries. Am Heart J. 2006;152(5):896-902.
25. Latib A, Colombo A, Sangiorgi GM. Bifurcation stenting: current strategies and new devices. Heart. 2009;95(6):495-504.

CHAPTER

13

Coronary Chronic Total Occlusion Intervention Technique

Masaki Tanabe, Jaskaran Singh Dugal, Ajit Mehta

INTRODUCTION

Coronary chronic total occlusion (CTO) is defined as 100% occlusion of the coronary arteries with thrombolysis in myocardial infarction (TIMI) 0 flow for at least 3 months, and is commonly found in patients undergoing coronary angiography. The duration of occlusion is often difficult to determine and is estimated based upon first onset of angina or dyspnea and/or prior history of myocardial infarction in the target vessel territory unless there is no prior angiography. However, it is important to implicate for the histopathological characteristics and the success rates associated with percutaneous coronary intervention (PCI).

Although no randomized controlled clinical trials comparing CTO-PCI with medical therapy have been published to date, there is a growing body of evidence suggesting clinical benefits of this field.[1] These benefits include improvement of anginal symptoms, decreased antianginal medication intake, improved exercise capacity, improved left ventricular systolic function, decreased risk of arrhythmia, improved tolerance of future coronary occlusion events, such as acute coronary syndrome, and improved survival among patients with successful versus failed CTO-PCI. Moreover, CTO is the most common reason for failing to achieve complete revascularization, and incomplete revascularization is associated with poorer clinical outcome compared with complete revascularization.

Application of drug-eluting stents (DES) has resulted in significant reduction of target vessel revascularization in non-CTO PCI, and has also led to a surge of interest in CTO-PCI. As a consequence, second-generation DES implantation is the current therapy of choice for percutaneous revascularization of CTO, because it is clear due to supporting clinical evidence in many meta-analyses that implantation of the second-generation DES improves long-term angiographic and clinical outcomes compared with first-generation DES, bare metal stents, and balloon angioplasty without using stents.[2]

Successful recanalization rates for CTO via the conventional antegrade approach remain suboptimal even today. The major reason for CTO-PCI failure is inability to cross the lesion with a guidewire. Many experienced centers have reported that contemporary crossing techniques and devices have significantly improved the likelihood of CTO-PCI success, as a retrograde approach to the CTO via a collateral channel has been developed for use in cases of complex CTO.[3]

This review will focus on current techniques for CTO-PCI with an emphasis on procedurally relevant histopathology and methodologies that have historically emerged from sites in Japan.[4,5]

HISTOPATHOLOGICAL CONSIDERATIONS

The CTO consists of a proximal and distal cap with an intervening occluded segment. The proximal cap is more likely to be fibrocalcific than the distal cap. This has implications for selection of a particular percutaneous approach and explains the rationale behind retrograde strategies.

In histopathological studies of CTO,[6] the intimal plaque of shorter-duration CTO was highly fibrotic plaque with noncalcified lesions, whereas the original lumen area mainly consisted of organized thrombi with microchannels defined as small lumen in CTO lesions with an average size of 200–300 µm (Figs 13.1 and 13.2). In contrast, longer-duration CTO consisted of harder intimal plaque and denser calcium formations without microchannels.[7]

The CTO has traditionally been divided into 'luminal' versus 'subintimal' spaces. The luminal space is defined as the space containing blood when the artery is patent and is encircled by the intimal (endothelial) layer. The subintimal space refers to the space external to the intimal layer but within the vessel architecture. This includes the media (smooth muscle) and adventitial layers. The internal elastic membrane (IEM) surrounds the intimal layer, while the external elastic

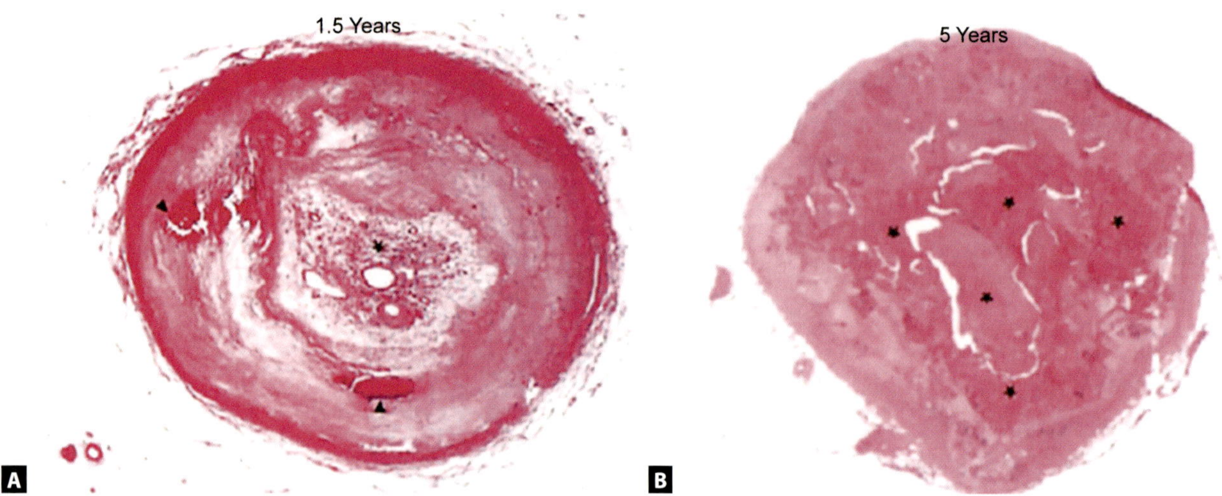

Figs 13.1A and B Histopathological images of chronic total occlusion. The cross-sectional histopathological images of angiographically occluded coronary artery in the different occluded period. (A) 1.5-year chronic total occlusion that has organized thrombus with microchannel in original lumen area (*) with some calcification (arrowheads) in dense fibrous tissue; (B) 5-year chronic total occlusion in which much calcium (*) was observed without microchannels. Image reproduced with permission from Dr Sumitsuji et al

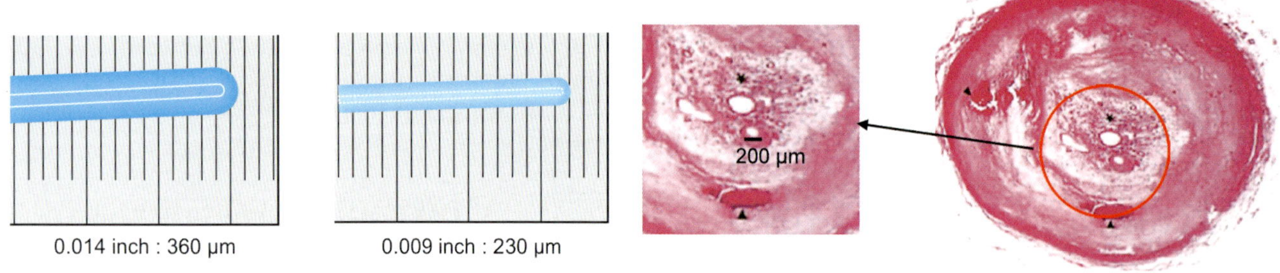

Fig. 13.2 What is the loose tissue tracking ? Some microchannels defined as small lumen in CTO lesion of the original lumen area with an average size of 200–300 μm were found. Loose tissue, histologically recanalized segments, was also found around microchannels. It may allow coronary guidewires to pass through the lumen of the CTO within endothelialized microchannels and across the occlusions. Image reproduced with permission from Dr Sumitsuji et al

membrane (EEM) surrounds the media and is bounded by adventitia. During CTO-PCI, subintimal wire passage is within the media between the IEM and the EEM following the path of least resistance. This theoretical distinction is relevant when discussing the various percutaneous interventional techniques against CTO.

Histologically recanalized segments (termed 'loose tissue') may allow coronary wires to pass through the lumen of the CTO within endothelialized microchannels and across the occlusions. On the other hand, nonrecanalized segments are predisposed to subintimal wire passage.[6] Angiographically, short occlusions with a tapered stump are more likely to have historically recanalized segments than longer occlusions or nontapered (ambiguous) entry.

CLINICAL CONSIDERATION AND PREPROCEDURAL PREPARATION

When revascularization with PCI is indicated, the procedure requires thorough planning. Procedural success depends on careful review of the angiogram including stump morphology, distribution and extent of calcification, and outline of collaterals (Figs 13.3A to E). Simultaneous double contrast injection is mandatory to make clear the morphology of the CTO segment, length of occlusion, presence and extent of collaterals, and the distal vascular bed beyond the CTO via the collateral-supplying side of the artery.

Predicting the difficulty of CTO crossing with a guidewire is important for case selection and procedural planning.

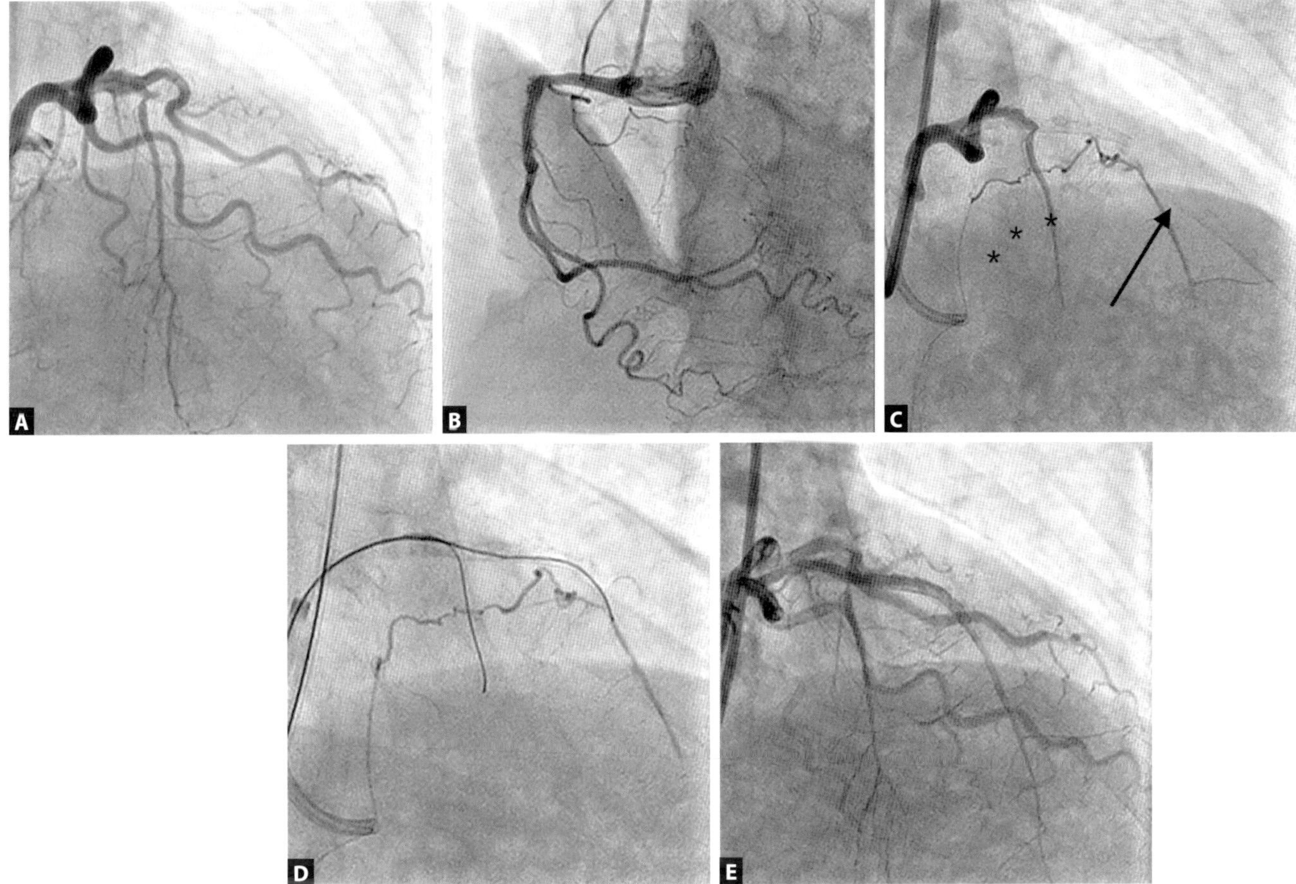

Figs 13.3A to E A case of being mandatory to detailed angiographic assessment using tip injection from a microcatheter for performance of CTO-PCI. (A and B) In the routine dual coronary angiography, it was unclear to visualize the exit of the left anterior descending-chronic total occlusion (LAD-CTO); (C) Under selective contrast injection from the tip of microcatheter in the conus branch (asterisks), the exit of the LAD-CTO (arrow) was visualized clearly; (D and E) Successful wire crossing and recanalization was achieved with the Gaia 3rd and a drug-eluting stent implantation, respectively

The multicenter CTO Registry of Japan (J-CTO) score,[8] which is determined by assigning one point to each of five variables (previously failed lesion, blunt type of entry, calcification, bending, and occlusion length), is currently widely used and is evolving to classify lesion complexity (Fig. 13.4). This score it has also been proposed as a predictor of procedural success as well as a numerical score with higher values indicating greater procedure complexity.

Chronic total coronary angiography can also assist in preplanning to build interventional strategies by providing additional data regarding morphological features of the CTO,[9] in particular vessel course and trajectory, tortuosity, occlusion length and location, and distribution of calcification (Figs 13.5 and 13.16).

Introduction of the procedure requires meticulous attention to arterial access. Bilateral femoral artery access is characteristic for CTO-PCI (in cases with no peripheral vascular disease) with side-hole guide catheters for each puncture site, one for visualization of the distal collaterals and for possible retrograde access, and the other for the antegrade approach. At least 7 Fr guiding catheters are proposed for CTO interventions. To obtain further support, long femoral sheaths (≥30 cm) are helpful, especially in cases of tortuous arteries. Backup support and side holes are essential elements in guide catheter selection: an extra backup type guide for the left coronary and an Amplatz type for the right. A shorter guide catheter (<90 cm) is also available for considering the retrograde approach, especially via a long collateral trajectory including epicardial collaterals and bypass grafts. Multiple simultaneous procedural steps, such as anchor balloon support and use of microcatheters, may be required with a 7 Fr system. When intravascular ultrasound (IVUS)-guided PCI is contemplated, it is better to use an 8F guide catheter to accommodate the two catheters (IVUS catheter and microcatheter).

Due to increased operator expertise and the development of modern devices, PCI for CTO is also feasible using radial access despite the lower backup force of the guiding catheter

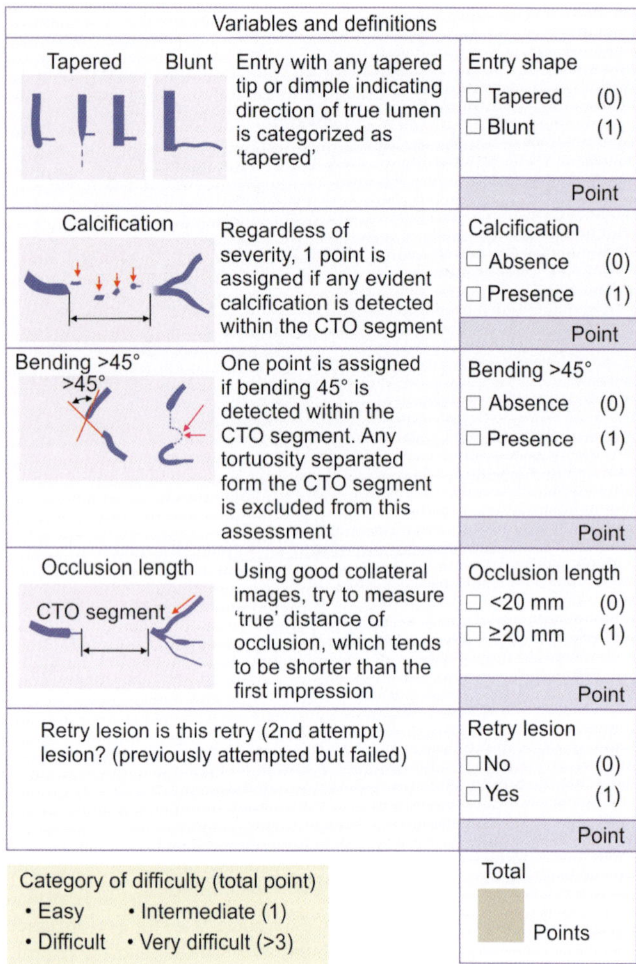

Variables and definitions		
Tapered / Blunt	Entry with any tapered tip or dimple indicating direction of true lumen is categorized as 'tapered'	Entry shape ☐ Tapered (0) ☐ Blunt (1) Point
Calcification	Regardless of severity, 1 point is assigned if any evident calcification is detected within the CTO segment	Calcification ☐ Absence (0) ☐ Presence (1) Point
Bending >45° >45°	One point is assigned if bending 45° is detected within the CTO segment. Any tortuosity separated form the CTO segment is excluded from this assessment	Bending >45° ☐ Absence (0) ☐ Presence (1) Point
Occlusion length CTO segment	Using good collateral images, try to measure 'true' distance of occlusion, which tends to be shorter than the first impression	Occlusion length ☐ <20 mm (0) ☐ ≥20 mm (1) Point
Retry lesion is this retry (2nd attempt) lesion? (previously attempted but failed)		Retry lesion ☐No (0) ☐Yes (1) Point
Category of difficulty (total point) • Easy • Intermediate (1) • Difficult • Very difficult (>3)		Total Points

Fig. 13.4 The J-CTO score is widely used to classify lesion complexity, which has also been proposed as a predictor of procedural success as well as a numeral score with higher values indicating greater procedure complexity. Reproduced with permission from Morino et al.

compared to transfemoral access.[10] A radial approach can be used for either interventional and/or guide catheter insertion of a donor artery. It may be increasing frequency of a combined femoral and radial access approach.

Procedural plans are then made based on the lesion angiographic characteristics, while maintaining flexibility in case the initially selected crossing approach fails to achieve progress.

ANTEGRADE APPROACH

Guidewire Tip Shape

The wire tip should be as short as possible (<1 mm), with an angle <45° initially (Figs 13.6A and B). A second, milder curve would be preferable to improve maneuverability of the wire. One exception to this rule is that a sharp (>60°) angle with a 1–2 mm bend, depending on the lumen size, is required to navigate the wire from the subintimal space back to the true lumen either as part of the parallel wire technique or IVUS-guided wiring. Stiff wires such as the Confianza Pro (9 g or 12 g; Asahi Intecc, Aichi, Japan) may be suitable in this situation.

Guidewire Manipulation

There are a number of different methods for guidewire manipulation, including controlled drilling and penetration strategies (Fig. 13.7) at the proximal cap, inside CTO, and distal cap. Each method has advantages and disadvantages, but overall either method works well for a short, focal, straight segment of a non-calcified CTO. For a long, tortuous, calcified occlusion, however, wiring should be tailored to the lesion characteristics. Hard plaques, such as calcifications and tortuosity inside the CTO segment, remain major obstacles for interventional revascularization. Even a tapered, stiff wire cannot penetrate calcification, but can minimize crossing deviation. However, the wire tends to dig deeper into the subintimal layer at a tortuous or angled CTO segment. Combination of penetration and controlled drilling strategies with microcatheter support may be preferable, with special attention paid to the wire tip in relation to the target lumen during practical procedures.

Microcatheters

Low profile, trackable, over-the-wire microcatheters are an indispensable tool for CTO-PCI, as they allow precise guidewire control and ease of wire exchange. It is crucial to advance the microcatheter close to the tip to enhance wire control. When wire exchange is necessary, saline is injected into the lumen to avoid introducing air. In addition, when a microcatheter must be exchanged over a guidewire, balloon dilation (e.g. 2.5 mm inside 7 F guide catheter) beyond the microcatheter can fix the wire and facilitate microcatheter exchange (balloon trapping). In Japan, the dedicated trapping balloon is commercially available (Kusabi catheter; Kaneka Medix, Osaka, Japan).

Among the available microcatheters, both Finecross (Terumo, Tokyo, Japan) and Caravel (Asahi Intecc) have the advantage of good trackability, while the latter also has a large lumen for selective injection, whereas Corsair (135 cm, and 150 cm; Asahi Intecc) has more support, even beyond a hard plaque or tortuous segment.

Antegrade Wire Escalation

A number of dedicated CTO guidewires are available, but key elements to recognize are: (a) tapered (0.009 inch) or not; (b) polymer jacket or not; (c) stiffness, and (d) trackability.

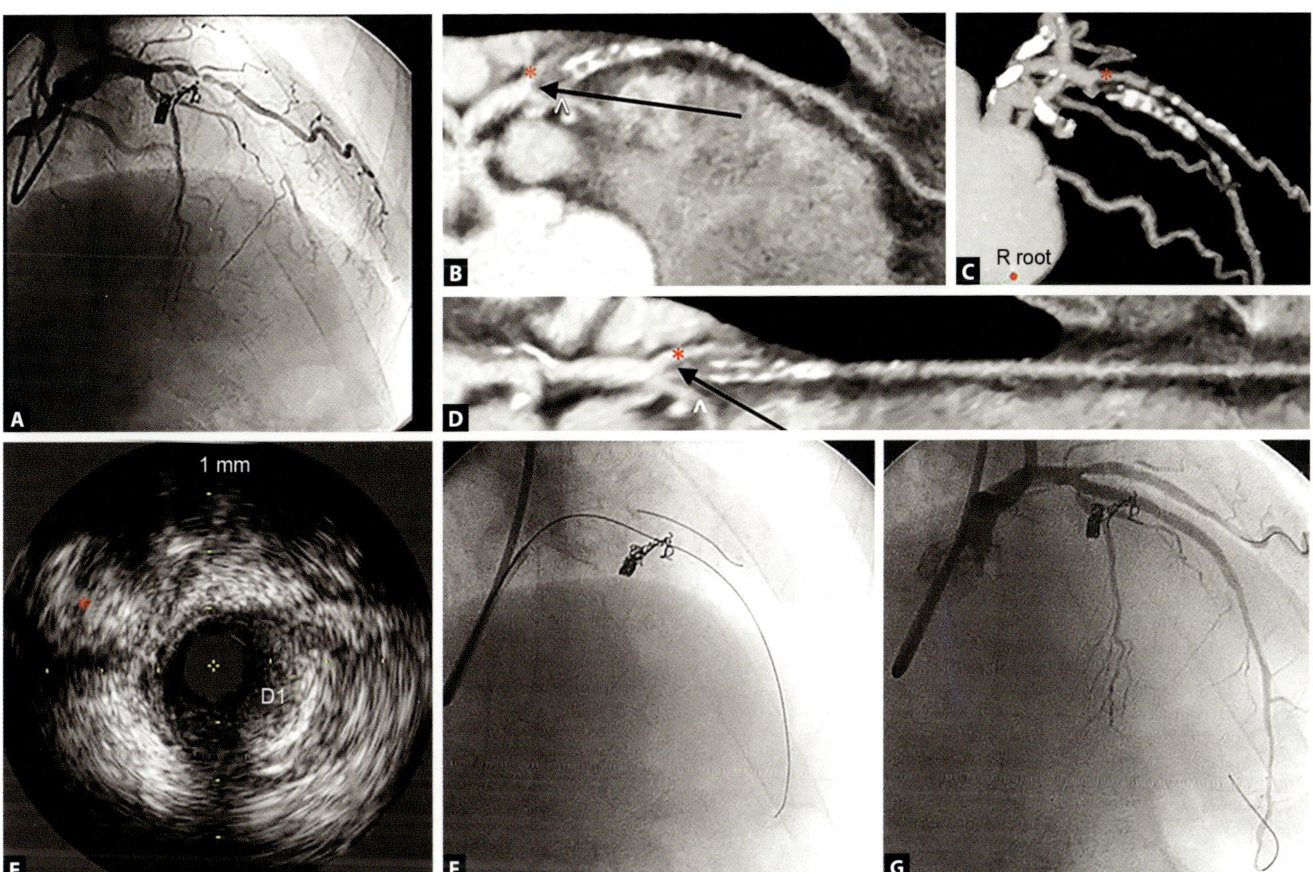

Figs 13.5A to G A case of proximal LAD-CTO. The CT coronary angiography had great contributed to the identification of the trajectory of the CTO. (A) In the baseline coronary angiography, The entry of the LAD-CTO was unclear. To Look for the precise position of the CTO entry using other imaging modalities seemed to be mandatory before coronary intervention; (B to D) The coronary CTA described the CTO entry of the LAD-CTO clearly. The CTO entry was shown by arrows. It was the center of the trifurcation that was sandwiched between the first diagonal branch (red asterisks) and the first septal branch (white arrowheads); (E)The online IVUS image guidance during the antegrade wiring was confirmed the position of the CTO entry (red asterisk). It was the opposite side to the ostium of the first diagonal branch (D1); (F) Antegrade wiring was successful in passing through the proximal LAD-CTO using the Confienza Pro under the IVUS guidance; (G) Successful revascularization was achieved with two drug-eluting stents implantation

As penetration force of a wire derives from tip load (stiffness), diameter, and lubricity, new operators can pick one or two work-force wires at the beginning to learn CTO-PCI.

Antegrade wire escalation is the most commonly used CTO crossing approach. Gradual escalation of wire tip load (wire escalation strategy) aims to traverse the CTO with the safest wire, reducing the risk of perforation, avoiding migrating into the subintimal space. A microcatheter is advanced to the proximal cap of the occlusion, followed by crossing attempts using various guidewires. Currently, the most common initial guidewire choice is a soft tip, polymer-jacketed tapered guidewire (such as the XT-R; Asahi Intecc) with the aim of seeking out microchannels to traverse the CTO in the intimal space. If this fails to cross, then either a stiff, polymer-jacketed wire (such as the ULTIMATE bros.3; Asahi Intecc) as needed in fibrous CTO segments for loose tissue tracking or intimal plaque tracking or a stiff, tapered wire (such as the Confianza Pro 12; Asahi Intecc) is used for penetration into hard or calcified plaque. The recent introduction of composite core stiff guidewires of the Gaia families (Gaia 1st, 2nd, and 3rd; Asahi Intecc), which theoretically allow greater directional control within the body of the CTO without compromising penetration power, could further improve antegrade wiring success due to good torque control, and active and intentional wire control. Consequently, early incorporation during wire escalation may be feasible for loose tissue and intimal plaque tracking, as well as retrograde distal cap penetration.

On the other hand, the theoretically useful and comprehensive method using the 'wire step down' approach involves performing wire exchange of a softer and more

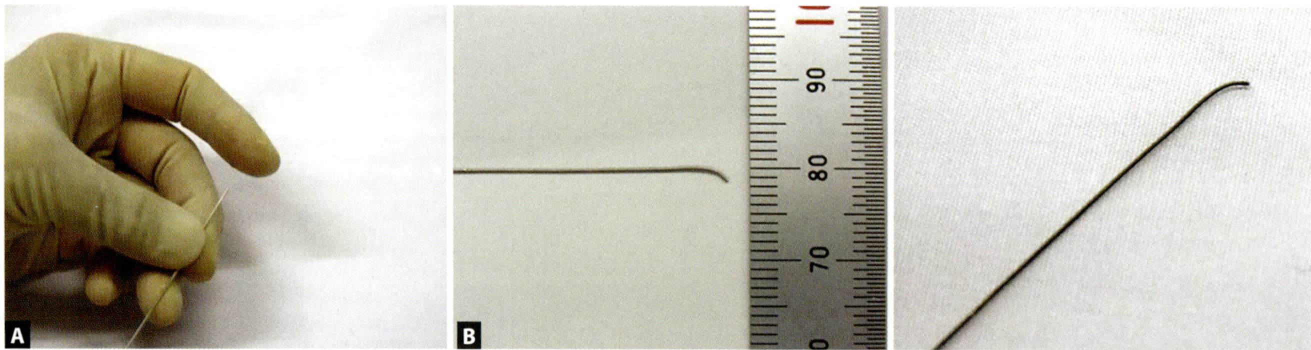

Figs 13.6A and B How to shape a guidewire tip curve for CTO-PCI? Coronary chronic total occlusion guide wire configuration. (A) It is preferable to shape a guidewire by inserting it through an introducer; (B) The very short (<1 mm), curved (<45°) tip of a wire is mandatory for initial coronary chronic total occlusion probing over a microcatheter

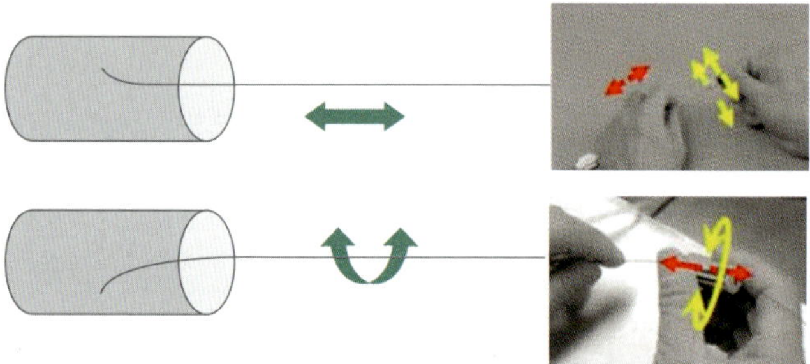

Fig. 13.7 Penetration versus controlled drill for intimal plaque tracking. Directional control of the wire tip is more precise in 'penetration'. Advancement of the wire tip is easier in 'controlled drill'. During practical procedures, combination of penetration and controlled drilling strategy with a microcatheter support can be required and preferable, paying special attention to the wire tip in relation to the target lumen. Image reproduced with permission from Dr Sumitsuji

trackable wire within the body of the CTO after successful penetration of the part in the hard plaque using a stiff wire. It is feasible for the step down wire to pass through the same hole made by the stiff wire tip even though microcatheters obstruct its advancement.

Wire escalation procedures are usually performed with microcatheter support. Over-the-wire (OTW) balloons are used in some cases, as they induce wire bias and have a profile that may make it difficult to cross the occluded segment after successful wiring. Clearly, the microcatheter offers several advantages for wire maneuvering. First, it provides added support to the wire and increases penetration force. Second, it allows maintenance of position once the lesion is crossed and for wire exchange or wire reshaping. Corsair is a dedicated catheter that has features of a microcatheter as well as a support catheter; it is becoming the initial microcatheter of choice for most CTO interventions, and is usually able to traverse occluded segments once wiring has occurred.

During antegrade wiring within the CTO segment, understanding the course of the guidewire is critical both for enhancing the likelihood of success and for minimizing the risk of complications. This can be accomplished in most cases using dual coronary injection. If the guidewire enters the distal true lumen (as confirmed in two orthogonal projections), the microcatheter is advanced past the occlusion, and the guidewire is exchanged for a workhorse guidewire, followed by balloon angioplasty and stent implantation.

If the guidewire tip exits with deviation of the vessel, it is withdrawn and may be redirected in cases without complications. If the guidewire crosses the occlusion but enters the subintimal space, true lumen reentry would be required using a 'parallel wire' technique.

Parallel Wire Technique

When the distal lumen fails to be visualized as the guidewire crosses, this suggests subintimal passage of the wire, expanding the area injured by the wire tip (the subintimal layer) and compromising the true lumen. The next step will be the parallel wire technique with a stiffer wire before losing sight of the distal lumen.[11]

In the setting of the parallel wire strategy, the first wire that enters the subintimal space is left in position to seal the tract, act as a marker, and minimize contrast injection. Continued advancement of this wire close to the distal cap should be avoided as it can cause collapse of the distal true lumen and make reentry difficult. A second penetrating guidewire is therefore introduced using a microcatheter and an attempt is made at redirection to aim the intimal wiring into the true lumen from the proximal portion within the occluded segment (Figs 13.8A and B).

The key points are:

- The second wire should be stiffer and more torquable, such as Confianza Pro

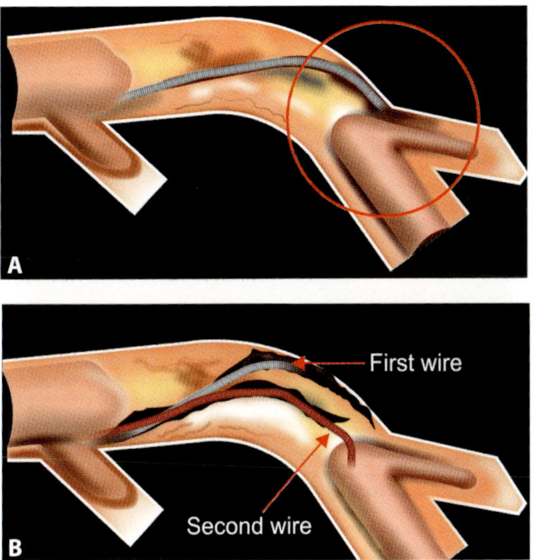

Figs 13.8A and B Schematic diagram of parallel wire technique. (A) The first wire migrated into the subintimal space and made a false lumen (red circle). It was left in position to seal that tract and act as a marker and minimize contrast injection as well; (B) The second penetrating guidewire was attempt to redirection for the aiming at intimal wiring into the true lumen from proximal portion within occluded segment. Image reproduced with permission from Dr NH Lee

- The wire should start from a different CTO entry point, using at least two different orthogonal views
- Penetration wiring will minimize expansion of the injured area
- Time for wiring will be limited due to potential expansion of the subintimal space, unless it may lead to eventual loss of distal vessel visualization.

The Crusade Catheter (Kaneka Medix, Osaka, Japan) is a double-lumen microcatheter that contains both a monorail and an OTW port. It is ideally suited to parallel wiring by allowing the introduction of multiple wires without removal of the catheter from an optimal position (Figs 13.9A to F). Moreover, it maintains a coaxial position toward the true lumen and it is considered that guidewire support is much stronger than the pushing force of other microcatheters due to its minimal shaft movement during second guidewire maneuvering.

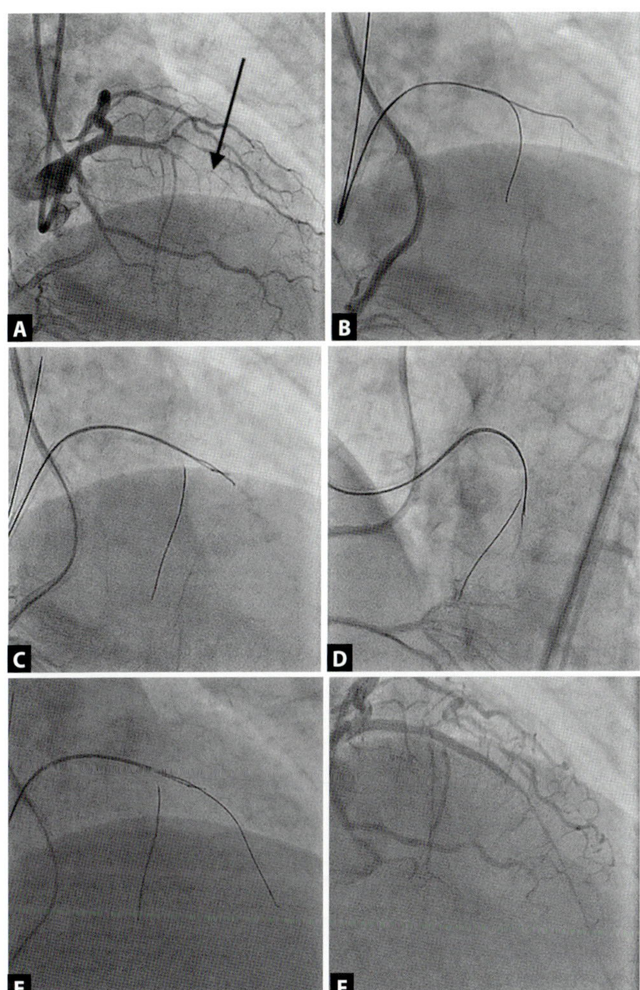

Figs 13.9A to F A case of parallel wire technique using the Crusade double lumen catheter: (A) The LAD-CTO had a tiny true lumen at the CTO exit and diffusely diseased of the distal true lumen beyond the CTO segment (black arrow); (B) The antegrade guidewire using the Gaia 2nd was migrated into the subintimal space at the CTO exit; (C and D) Attempting parallel wire technique; The second penetrating guidewire (Gaia 3rd) was introduced of the OTW lumen of the Crusade double lumen microcatheter which was reloaded on the RX lumen of it. The Gaia 3rd made at redirection for the aiming at intimal wiring into the true lumen from proximal portion within occluded segment under two different orthogonal views [C; right anterior oblique (RAO) cranial view, the 2nd wire was redirected downward. D; left anterior oblique (LAO) cranial view, the 2nd wire was redirected left side]; (E) The second penetrating guidewire (Gaia 3rd) was successful in re-routing within the intima of the CTO segment and passed through the distal true lumen; (F) Complete revascularization was achieved with a drug-eluting stent implantation

Anchor Techniques

Anchor techniques can be useful to increase guide catheter support. The anchor wire technique involves placement of a second support wire in a side branch proximal to the occlusion to increase support from the guide catheter as well as to stabilize its position. The side branch balloon anchoring technique (Figs 13.10A and B) involves inflating an appropriately sized balloon in the side branch for stabilization and to increase support of the guide catheters, (*See* Figs 13.16 and 13.34) such as when they are backing out or when more penetration power of the guidewires is required (Figs 13.11A to D).[12]

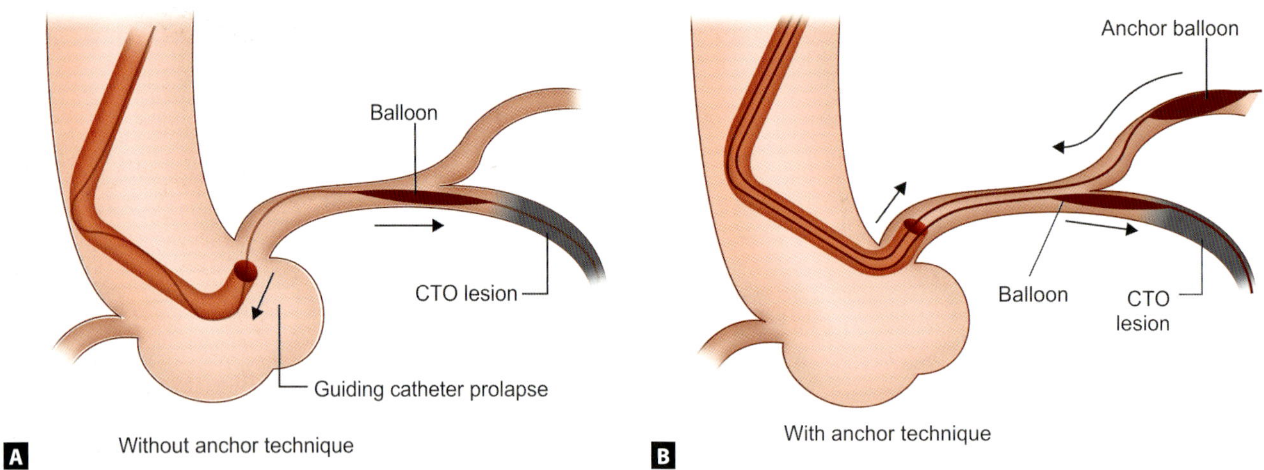

Figs 13.10A and B Schematic diagram of anchor technique. (A) Without anchor technique; (B) With anchor technique. Image reproduced with permission from Dr Fujita

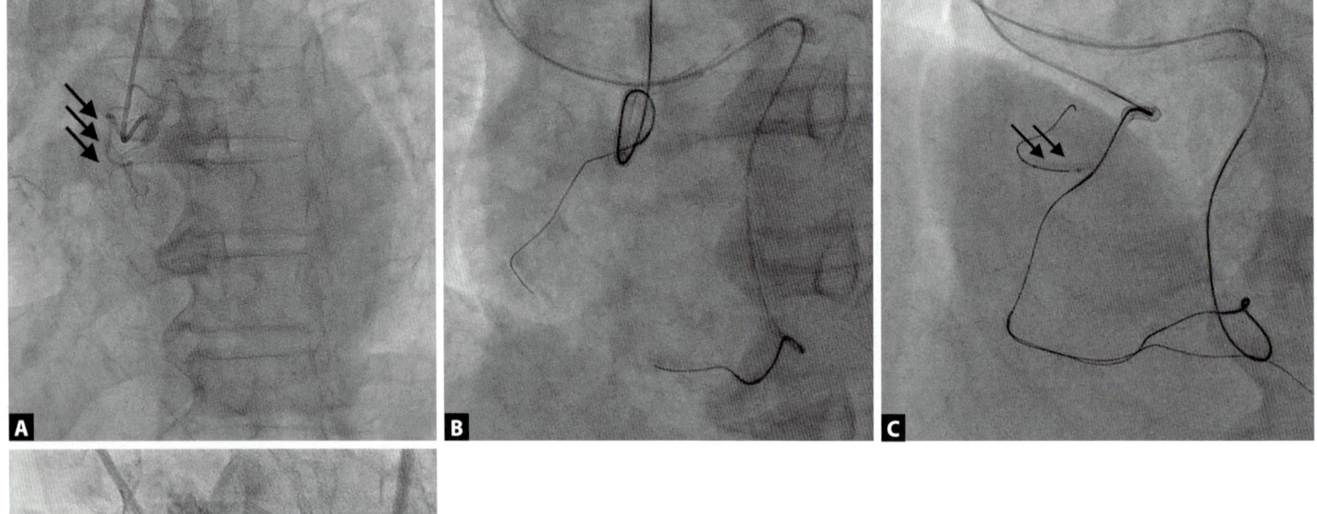

Figs 13.11A to D A case of side branch balloon anchoring technique. (A) In the baseline angiography, the RCA had an anomalous origin from the left coronary sinus of Valsalva, and it had a CTO at the proximal portion after branching the small branch (black arrows); (B) Considering anatomical problem, the CTO-PCI was started by retrograde approach first, before antegrade wire escalation. After that, antegrade wiring was continued using the Gaia 2nd with the Corsair microcatheter support. However, the antegrade guidewire did not work well because of poor backup guide catheter support; (C) For stabilization and increasing backup support of the antegtrade guide catheter, side branch balloon anchoring technique was performed using the 2.0 mm balloon dilatation (black arrows). After that, the antegrade Gaia 2nd was successful in passing through the CTO segment under kissing wire technique to the retrograde guidewire; (D) Complete revascularization was achieved with three drug-eluting stents implantation as a final result

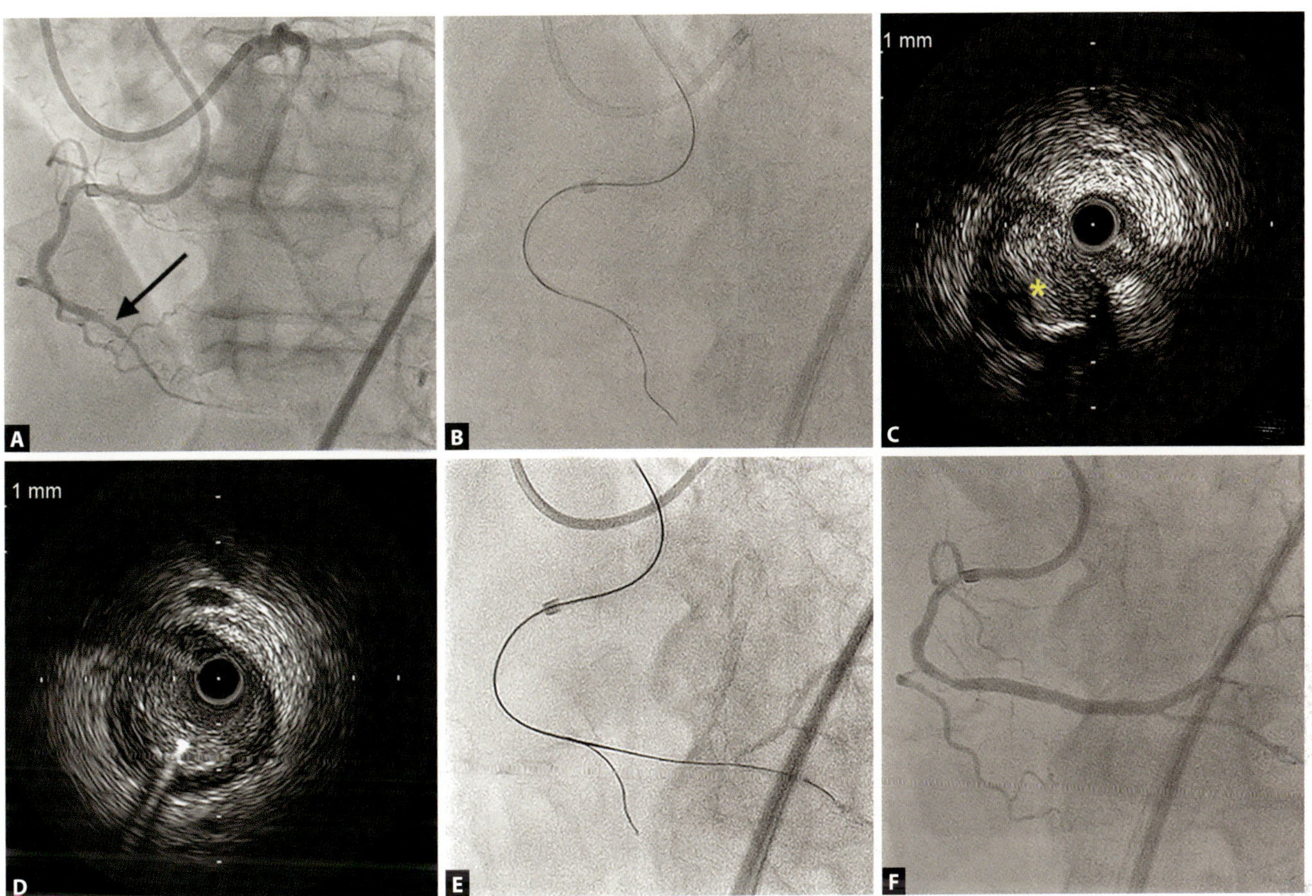

Figs 13.12A to F A case of IVUS guided wiring (side branch method): (A) The RCA-CTO entry had no stump at the bifurcation of the acute marginal branch (black arrow); (B) The IVUS catheter (Navifocus WR, Terumo, Tokyo, Japan) was placing in the proximal portion of the acute marginal branch and the second wire (Miracle Neo.3, Asahi Intecc, Aichi, Japan) was navigated with the Corsair microcatheter support; (C) An online IVUS image at the CTO entry: the true lumen of the CTO entry was shown by yellow asterisk; (D) The online IVUS image showed the second guidewire tip using the Miracle Neo.3 was successfully puncturing into the intima from the CTO entry; (E) Successful antegrade wire crossing was achieved with wire step down method using a Gaia 1st; (F) Successful interventional revascularization was achieved by two drug-eluting stents deployment

In the coaxial anchor balloon technique, a balloon (the OTW balloon is preferable in this situation) is inflated in the coronary artery proximal to the occlusion, enhancing the penetration capacity. The disadvantages of these methods include the risk of injury at the site of anchor balloon inflation, which is usually inconsequential in these side branches but may cause ischemia if the side branch supplies a large myocardial territory. The risk can be minimized by inflating the anchor balloon at relatively low pressure. They occasionally include modification of the proximal vessel anatomy and hinder antegrade wiring.

Intravascular Ultrasound-guided Wiring Technique

Intravascular ultrasound (IVUS) is an imaging modality used to depict a cross-sectional view of the coronary tree, which can focus upon the composition of the plaque, distribution of calcification, consistency at the CTO entry, reference vessel size, and side branch anatomy. Hence, IVUS is applicable in CTO-PCI in the setting of: (a) side branch method (Figs 13.12 and 13.5) involving navigating and penetrating the second guidewire into the true lumen from the proximal cap, while an IVUS catheter can be placed in the proximal side branch, and (b) true lumen reentry method (Figs 13.13 and 13.16) which is performed to assess a favorable reentry location from the proximal true lumen. Currently, IVUS-guided true lumen puncture is the last resort for getting a wire into the distal true lumen, as the method can be applied even after losing sight of the distal vascular bed on angiography due to subintimal space advance without limitation. An IVUS catheter is advanced into the presumed subintimal space and is monitored to orient the second wire to the true lumen. The key points are: (a) ability to translate cross-sectional images

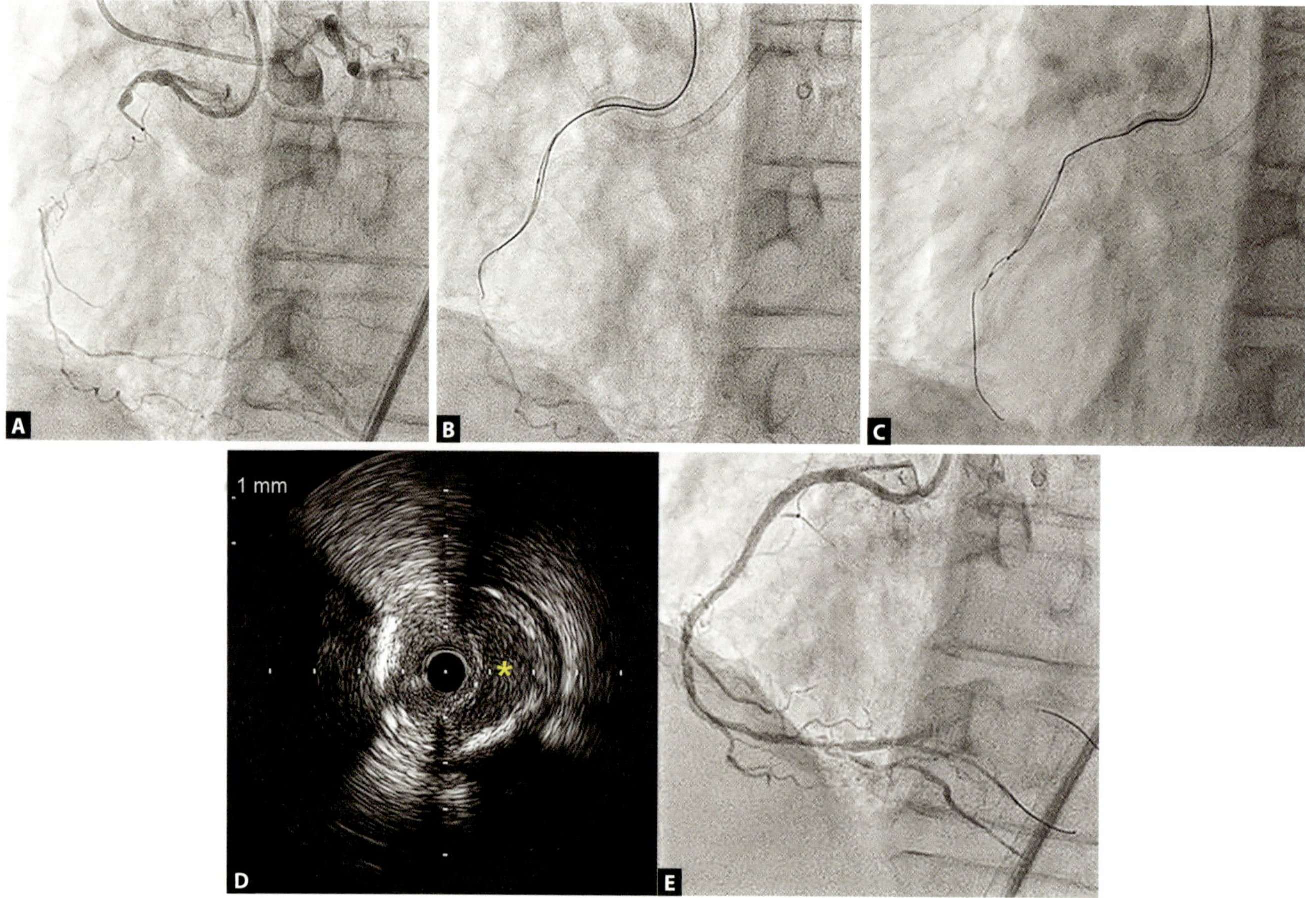

Figs 13.13A to E A case of IVUS guided wiring (reentry method). (A) The proximal RCA-CTO had no stump at the CTO entry and long occlusion segment up to the middle RCA; (B) Antegrade wires were migrated into subintimal space under parallel wire technique. Moreover, there were no fair interventional collaterals; (C) The IVUS catheter (Navifocus WR) was placing in the CTO segment on the wire which was migrated into the subintimal space and the second wire (Gaia 2nd) was navigated with the Corsair microcatheter support and penetrated to the favorable re-entry location from the proximal true lumen; (D) The IVUS image, which was after remounted on the successful passing guidewire, showed the false lumen (yellow asterisk) with semilunar shape that extended subintimal space at the right side; (E) Final result after drug-eluting stents implantation

of IVUS into three dimensions is needed; (b) the second wire should be a stiff, tapered wire over a microcatheter, and therefore, an 8 F guide is mandatory; (c) the reentry point should be closer to the proximal cap. Thus, the operator must understand the anatomy of coronary arteries in terms of IVUS interpretation.

It is preferable during CTO-PCI to use an IVUS catheter in which the imaging transducer is closer to its tip, such as the Eagle eye platinum (Volcano, San Diego), which has a short tip solid state, and the Navifocus WR (Terumo), which has better deliverability.

Antegrade Subintimal Tracking

Once the wire advances into the subintimal tissue, it is difficult to enter the true lumen without dedicated reentry techniques and technologies, because intimal plaque located between the true lumen and subintima is more resistant than the subintimal tissue. From the histopathological view, the subintimal tissue is weak longitudinally, and therefore enlargement of the subintimal space pushes the plaque toward the distal true lumen, resulting in its collapse. Both of these situations make guidewire crossing more difficult and increase the risk of ischemic myocardial injury.

There are a number of methods to manage antegrade subintimal tracking. The reentry technique with a stiff wire requires that the wire tip strength be directed from the subintima toward the true lumen as well as having the strength to penetrate the tissue located between true lumen and subintima. Although not easy to perform, selecting the reentry position in the bending part or the bifurcated part of the vessel affords a greater chance at successful reentry.

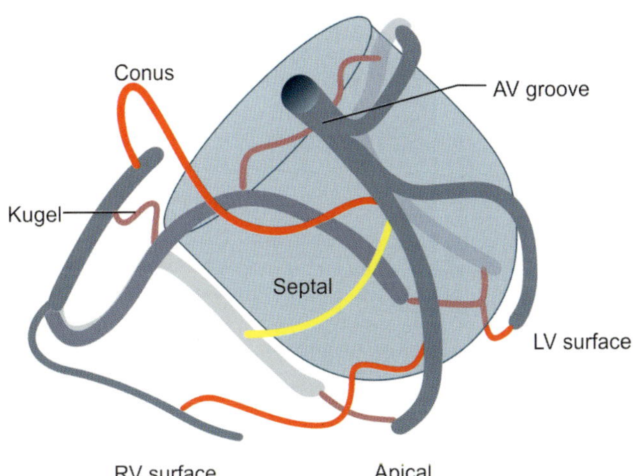

Fig. 13.14 Classification and terminology of collateral channels
Image reproduced with permission from Dr Sumit siji

- Septal channel
  - RCA PDA/PLA-(septal)-LAD
  - Septal to septal (Ipsilateral intraseptal)
- Epicardial channel
  - Conus branch-LAD
  - Kugel artery
  - RV surface
    - RV branch-LAD
    - AM branch-LAD
    - RV branch-RCA PDA
  - LV surface
    - RCA PDA-(apex)- LAD
    - RCA PLA-Diagonal
    - RCA PLA-LCX OM/PL branch
    - LCX OM branch-LCX PL branch
    - Diagonal-LCX OM/PL branch
    - Diagonal-distal LAD
    - Diagonal to Diagonal
  - AV groove
    - RCA PLA-LCX AC branch
    - LCX AC branch-LCX AC branch

Fig. 13.15 Collateral channels potentially applicable to retrograde approach

Abbreviations: AC, atrial circumflex; AM, acute marginal; PDA, posterior descending artery; PL, posterolateral; PLA, posterolateral artery; OM, obtuse marginal

The subintimal tracking and reentry (STAR) technique[13] or 'antegrade dissection and reentry' devices, such as the CrossBoss catheter (Boston Scientific, Boston, MA) and the Stingray balloon (Boston Scientific) (although these are not commercially available at present in Japan), have been reported previously as options for the reentry technique.

However, these subintimal wire tracking methods still pose a risk of side branch occlusion and subsequent myocardial injuries. If the wire reaches the distal true lumen through subintimal wire crossing in some segment without compromising many side branches, subintimal stenting with drug-eluting stents may be practical and long-term patency may also be excellent. On the other hand, when a guidewire is steered into the distal segment of a true lumen supplying a limited area of myocardium, stenting may result in suboptimal flow. The slow flow at the end will be associated with a high propensity of restenosis or even reocclusion. Therefore, CTO-PCI should be planned to minimize subintimal wiring and maximize a long-term benefit of stenting.

Retrograde Approach

The retrograde approach to CTO crossing can significantly increase success rates, particularly in challenging lesions. A guidewire is advanced into the artery distal to the occlusion through collateral channels (occasionally through bypass graft as a conduit) followed by CTO crossing against the original direction of blood flow. Currently, it is not only reserved as a second-line strategy for failed intimal antegrade crossing, but is also utilized as an initial strategy considering angiographic morphology, such as good candidates for interventional collaterals, ambiguous proximal cap, ostial CTO, and stumpless CTO or long trajectory of the CTO segment.

The retrograde approach has some advantages compared to the antegrade approach, because the distal cap of the CTO segment is easier to enter than the proximal cap as it is more frequently tapered and is often softer than the proximal cap, likely due to exposure to lower filling pressure, and is less frequently anatomically ambiguous.

Collateral crossing is facilitated by the use of dedicated microcatheters (such as Corsair and Caravel) and guidewires, such as the composite core Sion guidewire (Asahi Intecc), and soft polymer-jacketed guidewires (such as Sion black; Asahi Intecc), and XT-R. After confirmation of guidewire crossing into the distal true lumen, the microcatheter is advanced to the distal cap, followed by CTO crossing, which is usually done using wire escalation.

Angiographic collaterals can be divided into septal and epicardial channels, which have different characteristics. Detailed classification and terminology are shown in Figures 13.14 and 13.15. Trans-septal collaterals are preferred over epicardial collaterals because they are easier to cross with guidewires and carry a lower risk of tamponade in case of rupture. Successful guidewire crossing is not always predictable based on angiographic appearance. In addition, small side branches, tortuosity, such as corkscrew morphology, acute bends, tiny and unclear connections, are often obstacles to wire negotiation. Consequently, it may be mandatory to perform careful guidewire manipulation with repeat injections through the microcatheter, i.e. so-called

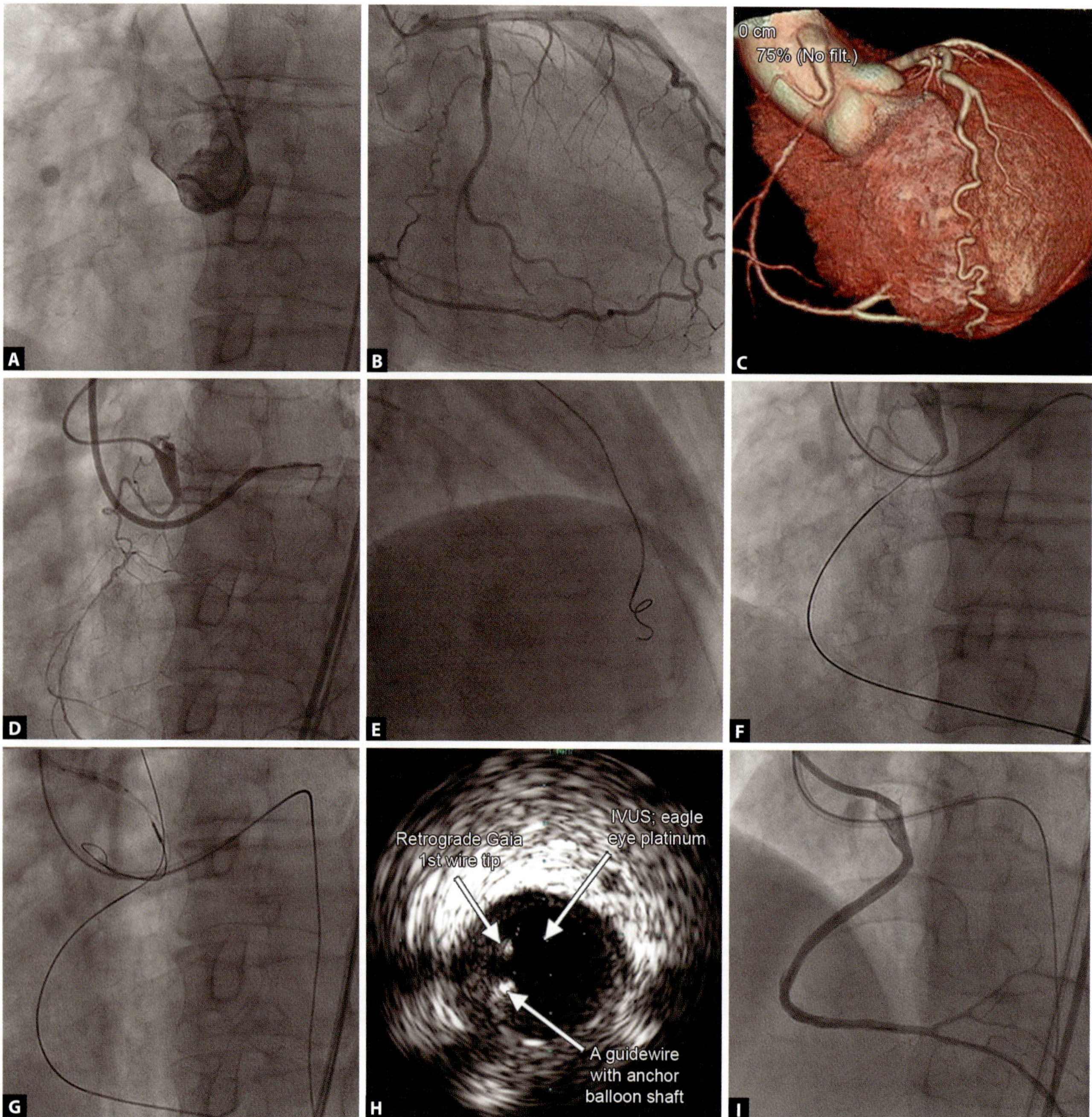

Figs 13.16A to I A case of retrograde wire direct cross under IVUS guidance. (A) The RCA ostium was unclear because diagnostic catheters were unable to engage despite trials using some kinds of catheters; (B) An epicardial collateral from the LAD distal to the RCA PD branch via the LV apex and an epicardial collateral via AV groove from LCX AC branch to RCA PL branch were shown; (C) In CT angiography, the RCA had a CTO at the proximal portion and anomalous origin. The RCA ostium was above the LCA ostium and originated from the anterior wall of the ascending aorta; (D) The angiographic feature of the CTO segment was clearly visible in bilateral injection due to successful cannulation to the RCA ostium using a AL3 diagnostic catheter. The entry of the CTO featured completely blunt shape just after branching the Conus branch, moreover, the exit of the CTO featured a little ambiguous shape; (E) The RCA CTO-PCI was performed by retrograde approach using the epicardial collateral via the LV apex using the SUOH (Asahi Intecc) with the combination of the Corsair microcatheter; (F) Subsequently, retrograde wiring within the CTO segment was attempted using the XT-R (Asahi Intecc), however, it was migrated into the subintimal space at the CTO entry; (G) Performance of retrograde wire direct cross was attempted using the Gaia 1st with side branch balloon (2.0 mm) anchor to the Conus branch and on-line IVUS (Eagle Eye Platinum) guidance simultaneously. Accordingly, the retrograde gaia 1st was successful in puncturing within the true lumen of the CTO entry and passing through the anomalous RCA ostium; (H) The on-line IVUS image during the procedure; (I) After construction wire externalization in the retrograde manner, three DESs were implanted from the proximal portion to the distal bifurcation of the RCA as a final result

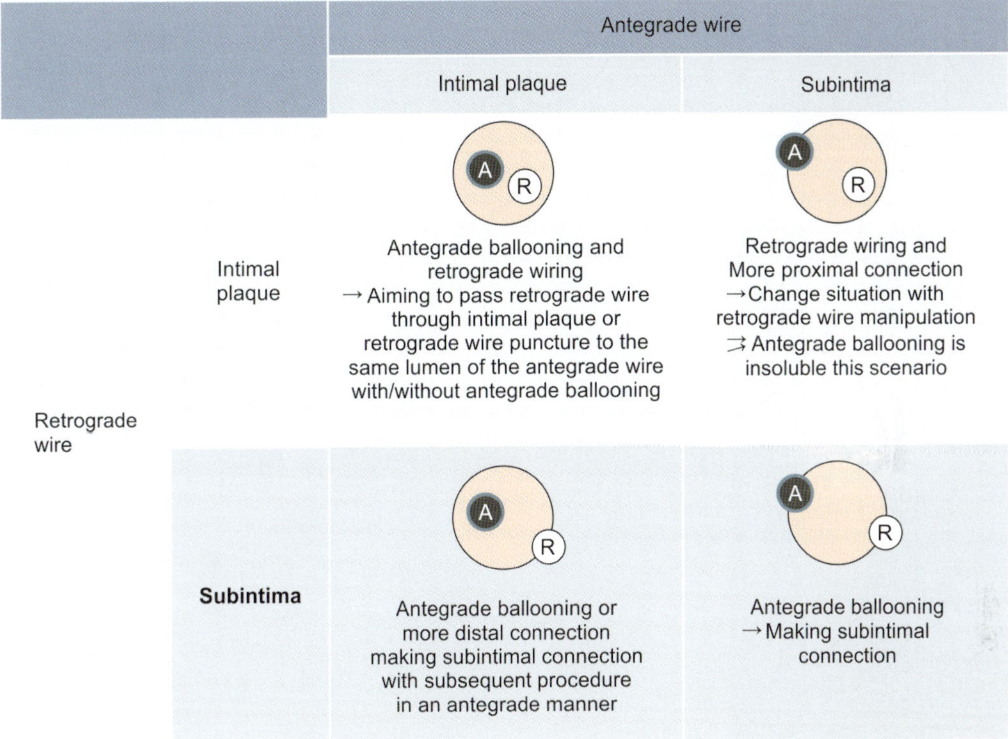

Fig. 13.17 Four possible scenarios for the antegrade and retrograde gidewire that require different strategies for successful retrograde CTO crossing

'tip injection', to confirm the position in the correct channel. If perforation occurs, bleeding is normally contained and rarely results in catastrophic outcomes. On the other hand, epicardial collaterals are fragile and associated with high mortality if rupture occurs and remains untreated (usually via cardiac tamponade).

Saphenous vein bypass grafts (SVG) are large and easy to cross with wires for the retrograde approach (*See* Fig. 13.26). Even degenerated or acutely occluded SVG[14] can serve as conduits for the retrograde approach to the distal arterial segment of chronically occluded native coronary arteries.

In contrast to the antegrade strategy, subintimal tracking is not considered a failure as it facilitates procedural success using various strategies, such as the reverse controlled antegrade and retrograde subintimal tracking (CART) technique.

The retrograde wire escalation strategy is usually performed with a microcatheter to advance the exit of the CTO. If the retrograde guidewire passes through the CTO segment in the intimal space, it is then externalized, which is termed retrograde wire direct crossing (Figs 13.16A to I). IVUS evaluation may be used over the antegrade wire to confirm that the retrograde wire is luminal prior to advancement through the proximal vessel.

Failure of luminal retrograde wire crossing, which means that the guidewire migrates within the subintimal space or fails to advance within the intima due to hard plaque, requires in additional complex procedural steps involving antegrade guidewire navigation within the CTO segment (if not already present), which is termed antegrade preparation. There are four possible scenarios for antegrade and retrograde guidewires that require different strategies for successful retrograde CTO crossing (Fig. 13.17).

First, both antegrade and retrograde wires are in the intimal space. In this case, the objective is either to advance the antegrade or retrograde guidewire with the opposing wire as a landmark toward the opposing channel, which is termed the kissing wire technique (Figs 13.18 and 13.11). Antegrade balloon dilatation is the next strategic procedural step. This expands the antegrade channel and shortens the CTO length to increase the chance of the retrograde guidewire advancing in the intima toward the antegrade guiding catheter. The next scenario is that both antegrade and retrograde wires are in the subintimal space. The two sides are usually connected when the antegrade space is enlarged via balloon dilatation. This is known as the reverse CART technique (Figs 13.19 to 13.22, 13.30 and 13.34).

The least favorable scenario occurs where the retrograde wire is subintimal and the antegrade wire lies in the true lumen. The difficulty arises because of a large layer of tissue between the two wires. Aggressive antegrade dilatation may disrupt the body of the CTO and open a passage into the

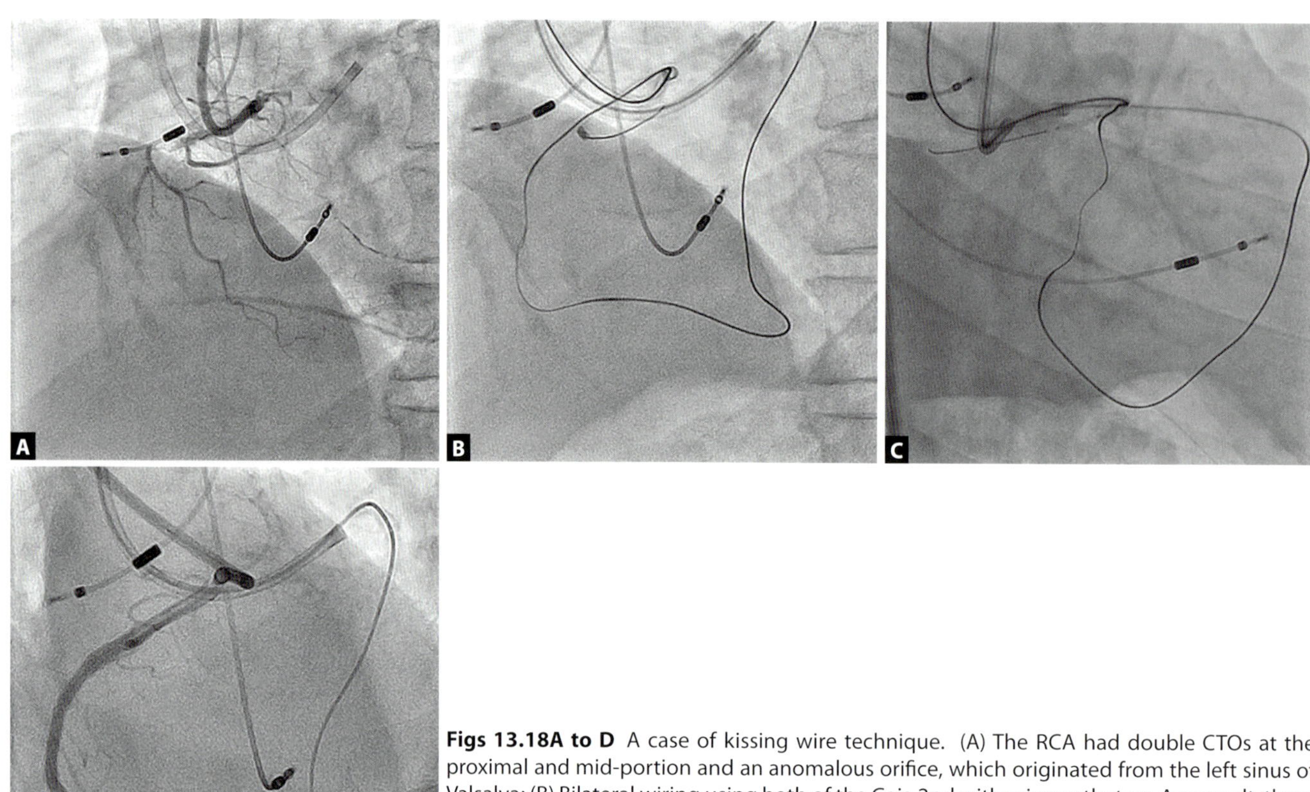

Figs 13.18A to D A case of kissing wire technique. (A) The RCA had double CTOs at the proximal and mid-portion and an anomalous orifice, which originated from the left sinus of Valsalva; (B) Bilateral wiring using both of the Gaia 2nd with microcatheters. As a result, these wire tip came close within intimal plaque of distal CTO segment in a left anterior oblique view; (C) Bilateral wire tip crossed exactly in the same lumen in a right oblique view with kissing wire technique; (D) Complete the CTO-PCI procedure after wire externalization in a retrograde manner and three drug-eluting stents deployment as a final procedural step

Make connection between antegrade and retrograde subintimal space utilizing behavior of subintimal dissection.

Antegrade wire automatically gets into distal true lumen.

Fig. 13.19 Concept of CART technique
Abbreviation: CART, controlled antegrade and retrograde subintimal tracking

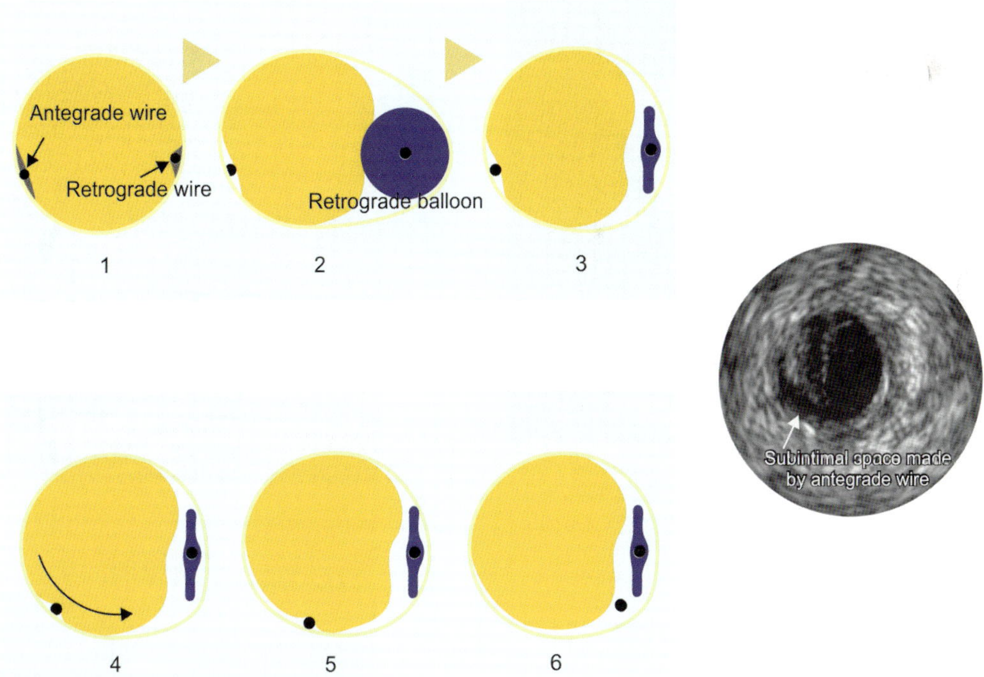

Fig. 13.20 Schematic diagram of CART (cross sectional view) technique. The antegrade wire was advanced into the CTO segment and migrated into the subintimal space. The retrograde wire introduced the CTO segment and finally into the subintimal space (1). After advancing a small balloon over the retrograde wire into the subintima, and the balloon was inflated inside the CTO segment (2). To keep this subintimal open, the deflated balloon was left in place (3). The two subintimal dissections provide a re-entry space for the antegrade wiring (4). Finally, the antegrade wire was navigated into the same lumen made by balloon inflation (black arrow of 4).
Abbreviation: CART, controlled antegrade and retrograde subintimal tracking

subintimal space. This will allow the retrograde wire to engage the newly created space and hence the antegrade true lumen. Finally, the retrograde wire is intimal and the antegrade wire is subintimal. Retrograde advancement of the wire until it reaches an adjacent subintimal space as the antegrade wire and finishing with reverse CART to connect the spaces is an efficient strategic procedural step.

During bilateral wire maneuvering, IVUS guidance (See Figs 13.16, 13.27 and 13.30) can contribute to the decision regarding the subsequent procedural step and confirm the positions of the antegrade and retrograde guidewires based on four possible scenarios.

The most commonly used retrograde crossing technique is the reverse CART technique (Figs 13.25 to 13.28, 13.30 and 13.34). In reference to latest advances in CTO techniques for both the antegrade approach and the retrograde approach, the next-generation guidewires of the wire families, Gaia 1st, Gaia 2nd, and Gaia 3rd (Asahi Intecc), enable precise wire direction control by efficient use of deflection mechanisms. In the retrograde approach, the Gaia families bring the 'contemporary reverse CART technique,' (Figs 13.23A to D) which is less traumatic and is a reasonable new wiring concept to facilitate the procedure. This method will likely be adopted as a standard retrograde procedure (Figs 13.25A to I).

After successful luminal connection due to these retrograde procedural steps, it is necessary to externalize the retrograde guidewire. Wiring the antegrade guide catheter with retrograde wire manipulation is the simplest technique to externalize a guidewire, and should be the first choice whenever possible. After the retrograde wire that crossed the CTO segment enters the antegrade guide, a trapping balloon is inflated within the antegrade guide next to the wire to facilitate advancement of the retrograde microcatheter into the antegrade guide catheter. However, wiring the antegrade guide may not always be possible, e.g. in cases of aorto-ostial CTO, noncoaxial guide positioning, and large vessel caliber. If wiring the antegrade guide catheter with the retrograde wire fails, then the snaring method can be performed (Figs 13.28 and 13.33). Therefore, CTO operators should fully comprehend the characteristics of various snaring catheters, snaring position, and manner of wire snaring.

For wire externalization, after advancement of the retrograde microcatheter into the antegrade guide catheter, the retrograde wire is removed and replaced with a dedicated

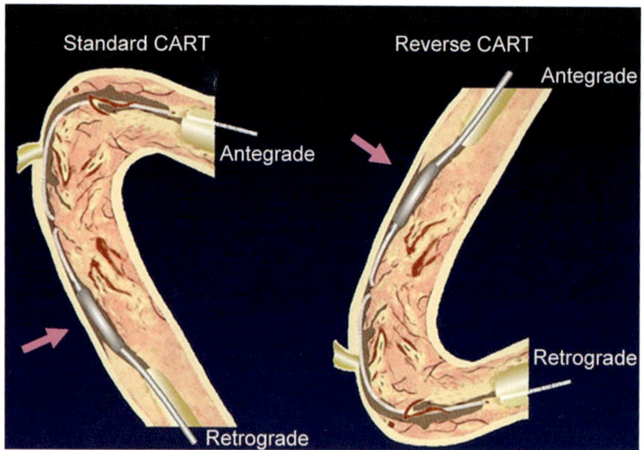

Fig. 13.21 Schematic diagram of contrast the standard CART with the reverse CART. The CART has major procedural limitations, which is required to deliver over-the-wire balloon retrogradely through a collateral channel. With the advent of dedicated soft wires and the Corsair microcatheter, more complex collaterals have been successfully crossed in a retrograde fashion. Accordingly, the retrograde wire with the microcatheter such as the Corsair cross CTO close to the proximal cap through a retrograde collateral, then, the appropriately sized balloon dilates antegradely the CTO to create an optimal re-entry space for the retrograde wire

long-shaft guidewire (>300 cm), such as the RG3 guidewire (Asahi Intecc) with a tapered 0.009-inch tip and length of 330 cm, which is threaded through the antegrade guide catheter hub. A rapid exchange balloon is then introduced on the distal tip of the externalized wire through the antegrade guide. The balloon usually crosses the occlusion easily, because completion of wire externalization provides excellent support for equipment delivery.

After retrograde crossing and during PCI, the retrograde microcatheter should remain in the distal portion of the native artery covering the collateral channel. Removal prior to PCI completion may result in wire-induced collateral transection with resulting rupture, as the externalized wire can exert significant shear stress or tension.

Once the balloon has opened the occlusion, two options are available, considering the correlation with the crossing collateral and the distal lumen of the target artery dependent on the specific case. The first involves continuing with ballooning and stenting the vessel over the externalized wire. This provides excellent support for passage of long stents. Alternatively, an antegrade workhorse wire can be advanced to the distal true lumen of the target artery through the newly opened space. In the setting of this procedure, the introduction of a double-lumen microcatheter over the externalized wire, such as the Crusade catheter, can prevent migration into the false lumen and pass through the newly opened space via the OTW lumen (Figs 13.26 and 13.34).

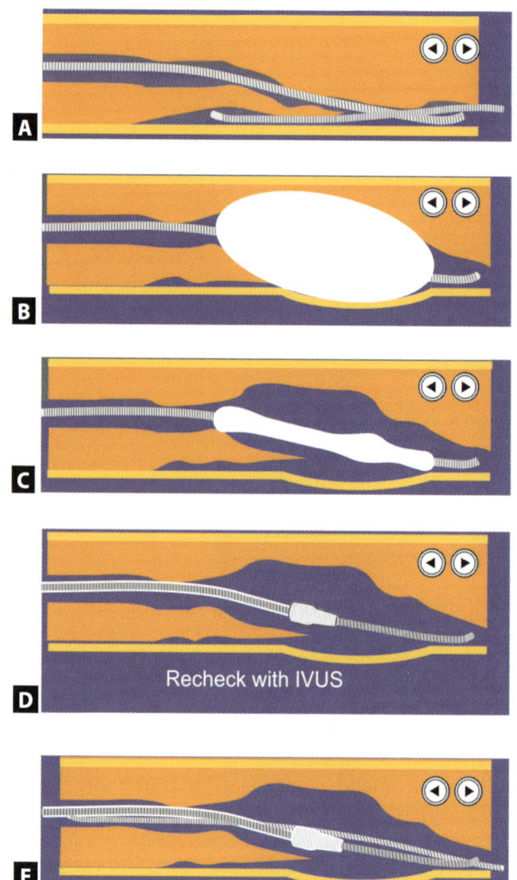

Figs 13.22A to E Schematic diagram of IVUS-guided reverse CART. (A) Showing both antegrade and retrograde wire in subintimal space; (B and C) Dilation of subintimal space with balloon on antegrade wire to make connection; (D) Checking with intravascular ultrasound (IVUS) for the location of subintimal space; (E) Retrograde wire passed from subintimal space into antegrade true lumen via connection made by antegrade balloon under IVUS guidance. Right arrowhead indicates distal lumen, and left arrowhead indicates proximal lumen

Abbreviation: CART, controlled antegrade and retrograde tracking

Image reproduced with permission from Rathore et al.

This is crucial to preserve large side branches, which exist at the CTO exit, to avoid compromise by the subsequent procedure involved plaque modification. On positioning the stent implantation, it is necessary to use contralateral injections to avoid propagation of antegrade hydraulic dissections.

As mentioned previously, CTO-PCI should be planned to minimize subintimal wiring and maximize the long-term benefit of stenting. However, it may be necessary to implant stents within the subintimal space to a certain degree, because the reverse CART technique became the mainstream of

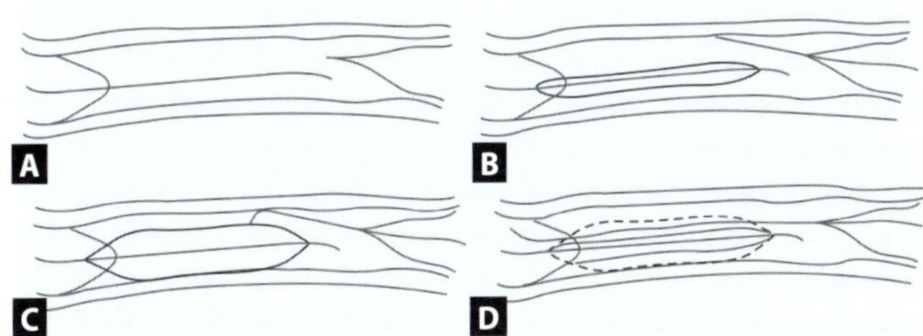

Figs 13.23A to D Contemporary reverse CART. (A) An antegrade guidewire is advanced within intima as distally as possible; (B) Small balloon is also advanced along with the antegrade guidewire and a retrograde guidewire (Gaia families may be preferable) is delivered; (C) At the suitable point, the antegrade inflated balloon should be targeted and the retrograde guidewire is manipulated for puncture to the center of the balloon using deflection mechanism; (D) The retrograde guidewire cross the CTO segment through the space which made by antegrade balloon inflation
This method will be popularized as a standard retrograde procedure which is less traumatic and reasonable according to CTO wire control mechanics although the next generation CTO wire is required for efficient use of deflection mechanism. Image reproduced with permission from Dr Y Uehara for presentation TCTAP 2015.

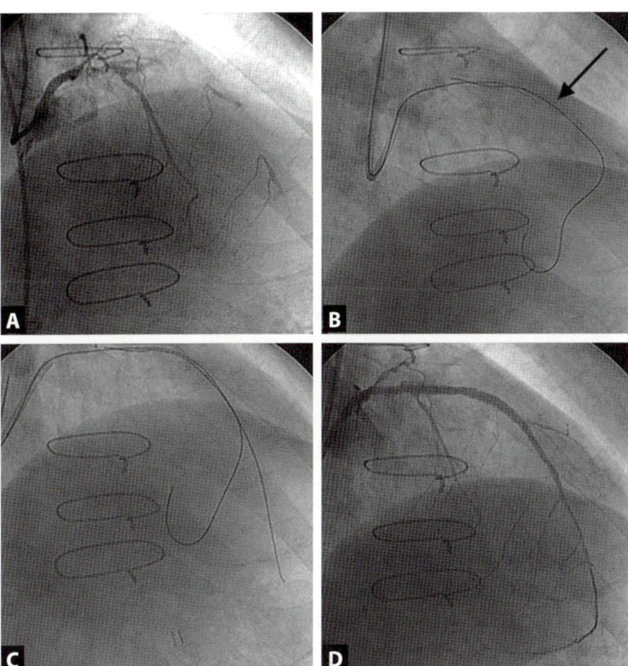

Figs 13.24A to D A case of standard CART technique. (A) The LAD-CTO from the proximal to the midportion, which had graft failure due to left internal thoracic artery (LITA) graft occlusion. There was a fair ipsilateral intraseptal collateral; (B) A small size (2.0 mm) of OTW balloon (black arrow) was retrogradely navigated via the ipsilateral collateral and it had provided the "space" for antegrade wire re-entry by dilatation; (C) The antegrade wire was successfully passed the CTO segment through the re-entry space by CART technique; (D) Complete revascularization against the LAD-CTO was achieved with two drug-eluting stents implantation as a final result

retrograde CTO-PCI methodology, and there are supporting data suggesting clinical benefits of 2nd generation DES implantation after reverse CART.

CART TECHNIQUE

Dr Kato developed a more comprehensive retrograde approach in 2005.[15] The CART technique (Fig. 13.19) consists of antegrade wiring through the CTO where retrograde balloon dilation creates local subintimal dissection to facilitate wire crossing to the distal true lumen. Figure 13.20 shows how retrograde balloon dilation contributes to mobilization of the two separate wires merging into the same lumen.

However, this technique has major procedural limitations, in that it is necessary to deliver the OTW balloon retrogradely through a collateral channel and estimate retrograde balloon size empirically (Figs 13.24A to D).

REVERSE CART® TECHNIQUE

With the advent of dedicated soft wires and novel microcatheters, more complex collaterals have been successfully crossed in a retrograde manner. By 2008, the concept of a channel dilator materialized as the Corsair microcatheter, which enables the wire to access the distal CTO through any collateral channel.[16]

When the retrograde wire with the microcatheters crosses CTO close to the proximal cap through a retrograde collateral, the appropriately sized balloon based on the reference vessel size can fully dilate the CTO to create an optimal reentry space for the retrograde wire. Once the retrograde guidewire enters the guide catheter, the microcatheter can also be advanced over the trapping wire to exchange the wires for 300 cm wire externalization. Over this long wire, additional 'antegrade' balloon dilation and stent delivery can be achieved. This is the beginning of the current predictable and reliable retrograde approach called reverse CART, (Figs 13.21, 13.25 to 13.28, 13.30 and 13.34) which was also developed by Kato.[16]

In this technique, once the antegrade balloon has been dilated for retrograde wire reentry, contrast injection should not be used until the last stent deployment. Otherwise, pressurized contrast agent is injected into the dilated segment, causing spiral dissection or hematoma (hydrostatic pressure-induced dissection).

Several modifications of the reverse CART technique have been developed. The 'IVUS-guided reverse CART technique'[17] (Figs 13.22A to E) allows more precise sizing of the balloon to maximize the space created for reentry without risking vessel perforation as well as visualization of the retrograde wire tip

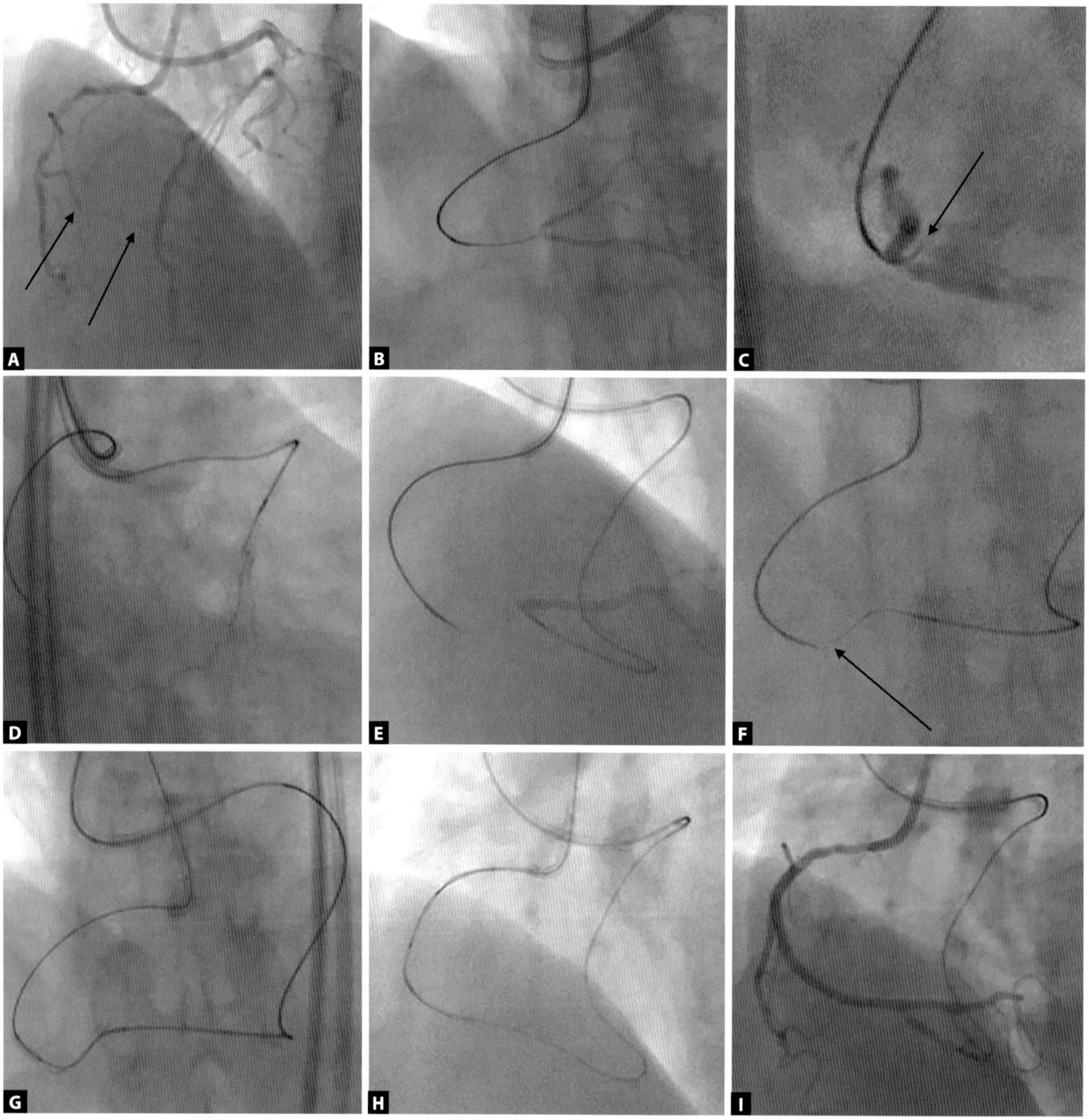

Figs 13.25A to I A typical case of (contemporary) reverse CART technique. (A) The RCA had a CTO from the midportion to the distal bifurcation (black arrow); (B and C) The antegrade wiring using the Gaia 2nd with the Corsair was performed, but migrated into the subintimal space at the CTO exit. It was not clear in a left cranial view, but in a right oblique (black arrow). However, the "antegrade preparation" had been completed at that point; (D) Subsequently, the procedure has changed to retrograde approach. The fair connection to the RCA distal was described in a tip injection from the Corsair via the trans-septal collateral; (E) Tip injection from the retrograde Corsair after successful negotiation to the septal channel using the Sion (Asahi Intecc.); (F) The retrograde wiring using the Gaia 2nd . It was successfully penetrated within the CTO exit and advanced toward the antegrade wire tip (black arrow); (G) Performance of (contemporary) reverse CART technique. A small sized balloon (2.0 mm) was advanced antegradely at the suitable point of the CTO segment and inflated. The retrograde Gaia 2nd punctured the antegrade balloon to cross the CTO retrogradely; (H) The retrograde Gaia 2nd easily entered the same space (into intimal plaque) which was made by the antegrade balloon inflation and successfully passed through the CTO segment; (I) After construction wire externalization in the retrograde manner, two long DESs were implanted at the CTO segment of the RCA as a final result

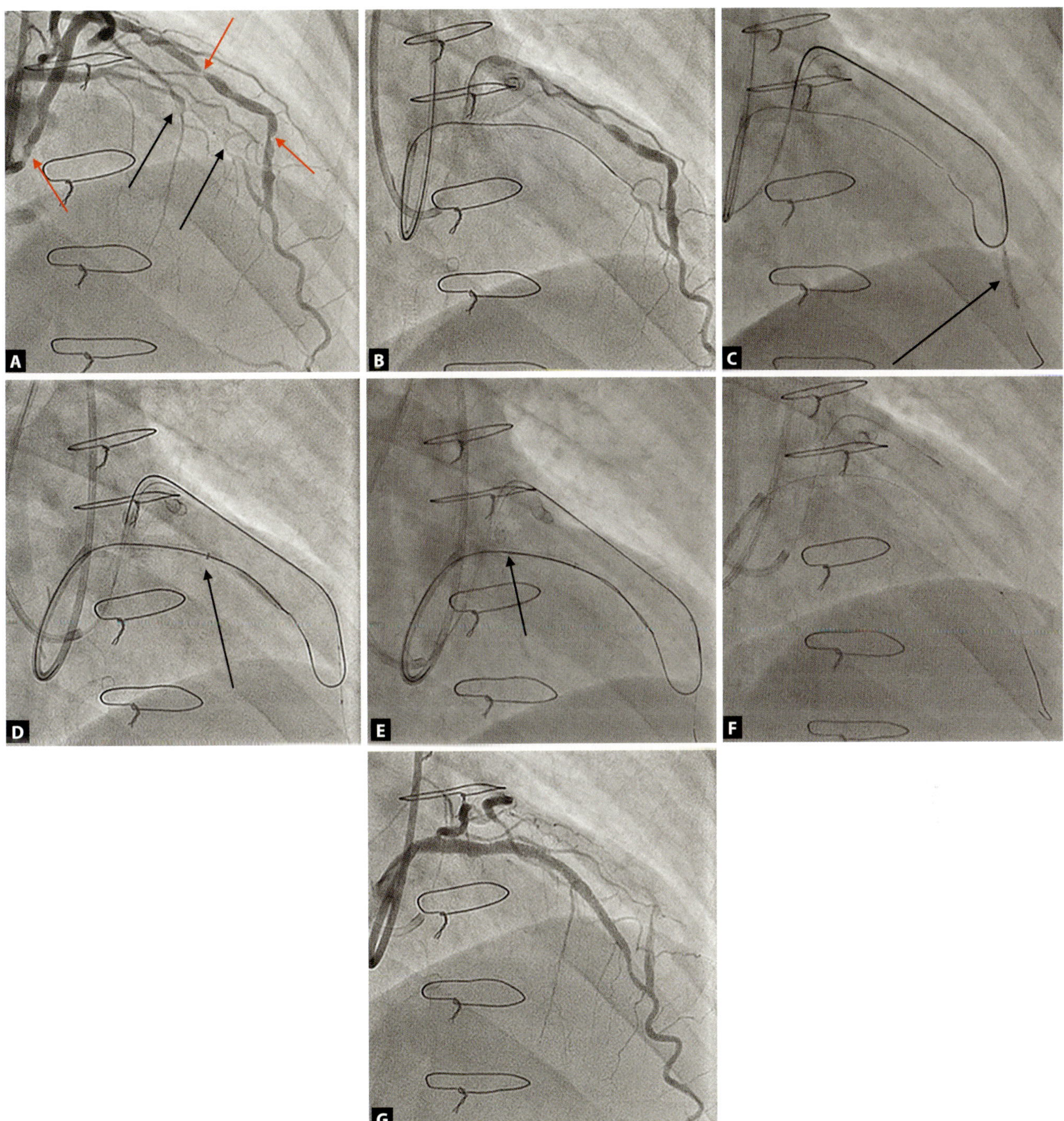

Figs 13.26A to G A case of reverse CART technique using the guide extension catheter. (A) The LAD had a CTO at the midportion (black arrows) having degenerated the saphenous vein graft (SVG). (red arrows); (B) The antegrade wiring using the XT-A (Asahi Intecc.) was performed, but migrated into the subintimal space at the CTO exit; (C) Consequently, retrograde approach via the SVG using the Gaia 2nd with the Caravel microcatheter support was performed. The anchoring balloon technique at the distal LAD was concomitant used for the aiming at stabilization of the retrograde guide catheter and screening protrusion the retrograde microcatheter to the distal LAD (black arrow); (D) Performance of the reverse CART technique concomitant use of the guide extension catheter: The 2.25 mm sized balloon was advanced into the CTO segment, after the 6Fr Guidezilla (Boston scientific) was navigated into the mid LAD in front of the CTO entry (black arrow); (E) The retrograde wire was successfully passed through the CTO segment and put into the Guidezilla catheter (black arrow); (F) After wire externalization using the RG3 in the retrograde manner, the antegrade wire navigated to the distal LAD via the OTW port of the Crusade microcatheter; (G) Complete the CTO-PCI procedure after two drug-eluting stents deployment

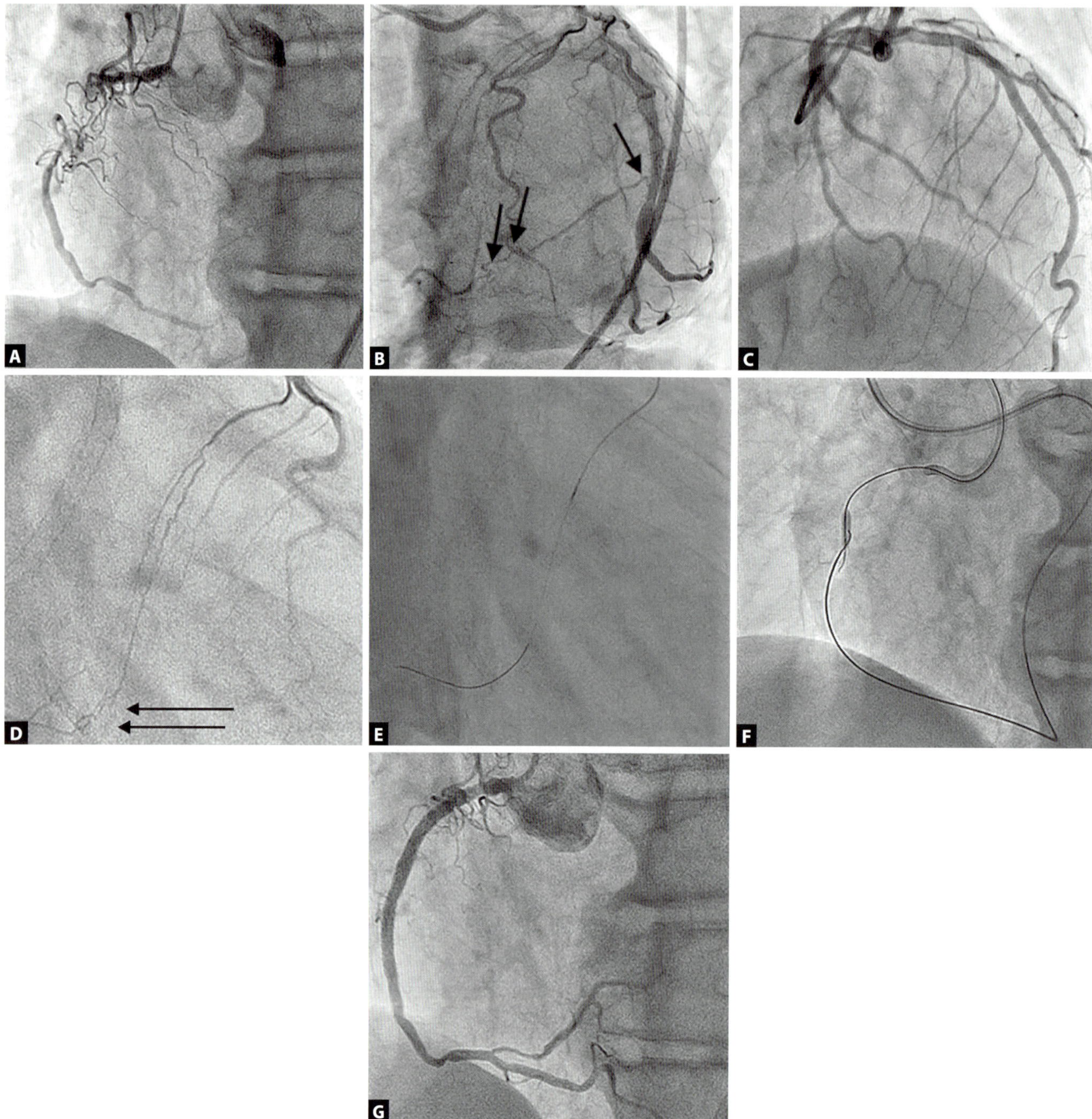

Figs 13.27A to G A case of proximal RCA-CTO having rich bridge collaterals. (A) Both of the entry and the exit of the CTO were unclear due to these rich collaterals; (B) The main collateral (black arrows) was found from the AC branch of the left circumflex (LCX) via an AV groove to the RCA PL branch, but it had tortuous morphology; (C) Trans-septal collaterals to the PD branch of the RCA were invisible and unclear whether there were connecting to the PD branch of the RCA or not; (D) From the tip injection via the 3rd septal branch using the Caravel microcatheter was visualized the connection to the distal RCA, although it was tiny and bend (black arrows); (E) Careful wire manipulation using the Sion black with the Caravel microcatheter support was successfully negotiated and passed through this trans-septal collateral; (F) Performance of reverse CART technique using 2.5 mm balloon. After performance of the IVUS-guided reverse CART, the retrograde wire was successfully passed through the CTO segment; (G) Successful interventional revascularization was achieved by two drug-eluting stents deployment

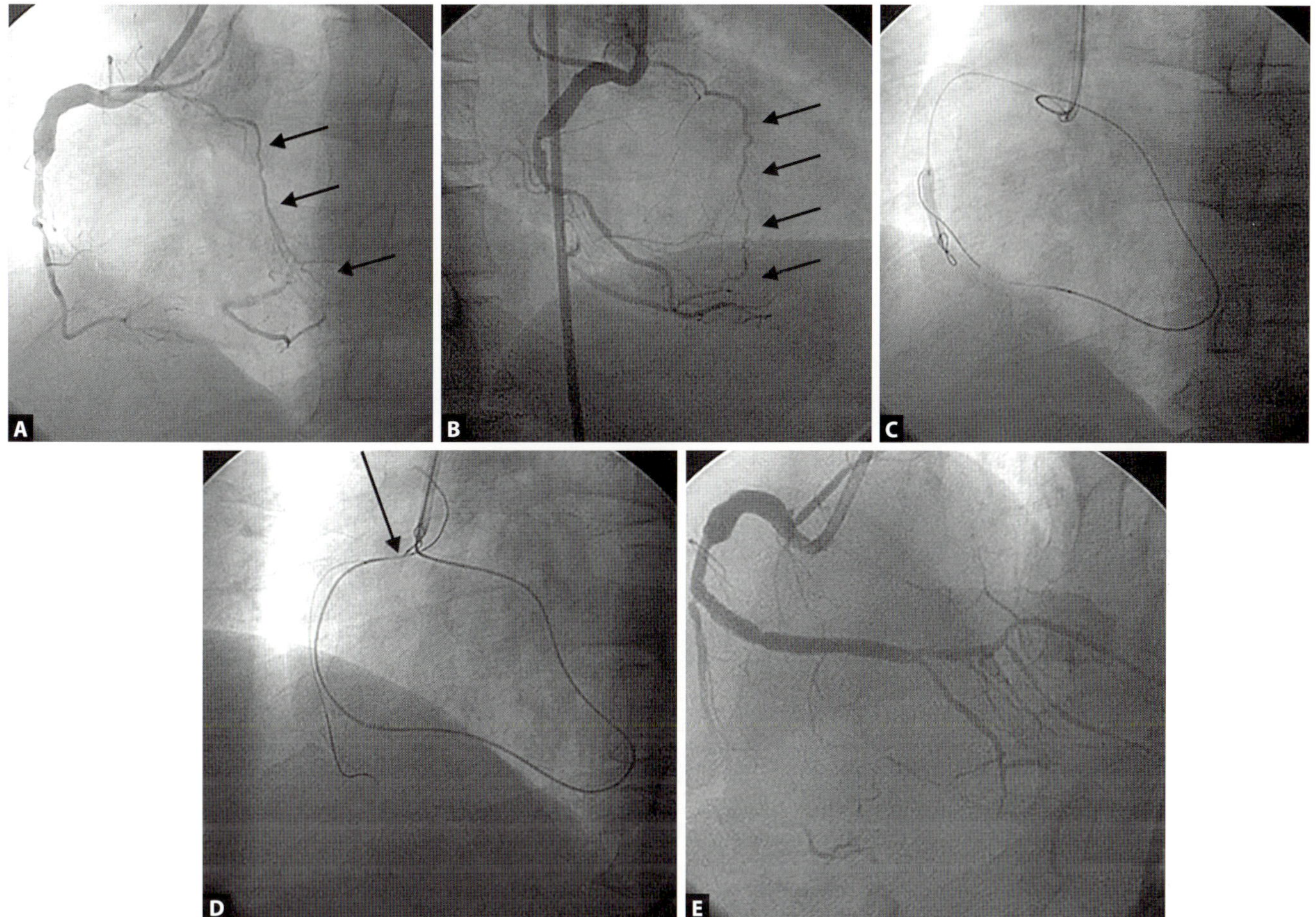

Figs 13.28A to E A case of reverse CART technique via a Kugel's artery. (A and B) The RCA had a CTO from the mid to the distal bifurcation. There was a fair ipsilateral collateral via the Kugel's network (black arrows). Contralateral collaterals were not found at all; (C) The antegrade wire was migrated into the subintimal space within the CTO segment due to hard plaque. The retrograde wire was also migrated into the subintimal space and had poor wire controllability in this ipsilateral collateral's negotiation. A reverse CART technique was performed using the 3.5 mm balloon dilatation; (D) The retrograde wire was caught by the antegrade Soutenir (Asahi Intecc) snare device (black arrow), since it was difficult to put the retrograde wire into the guide catheter in itself due to poor stability of the guide catheter; (E) After successful snaring and wire externalization in the retrograde manner, interventional revascularization was achieved with two drug-eluting stents implantation as a final result

as it enters the enlarged subintimal space that communicates with the true lumen (Figs 13.27 and 13.30).

Occasionally, a guide catheter extension (Figs 13.26A to G) such as the Guideliner or the Guidezilla, can be advanced over the antegrade guide catheter or the guidewire to form a proximal target for the retrograde guidewire and facilitate entry into the guide catheter. In the 'stent reverse CART' technique (Figs 13.30A to I), a stent is placed in the proximal true lumen into the subintimal space to facilitate retrograde wiring into the stent.

Collateral Crossing with a Guidewire

Three elements should be kept in mind for successful collateral crossing: (a) channel selection; (b) wire tip curve, and (c) wire handling. The best collateral channel for retrograde wire crossing is clearly visualized, less tortuous collaterals by super-selective injection, exemplified by Werner's collateral connection (CC) grade 1 or 2 (CCs are graded as follows: CC0, no continuous connection; CC1, continuous thread-like connection; and CC2, continuous, small side branch-like connection). On the other hand, major obstacles of wire crossing are acute angulations, sharp bends, branching, corkscrew morphology, calcification, and nonvisibility of the CC connection with the recipient vessel.

As mentioned previously, retrograde wiring of septal collaterals is preferred for epicardial collaterals because septal collaterals are usually multiple and are relatively straight. Injury or perforation of septal collaterals is less likely to cause acute myocardial infarction, myocardial hematoma, or

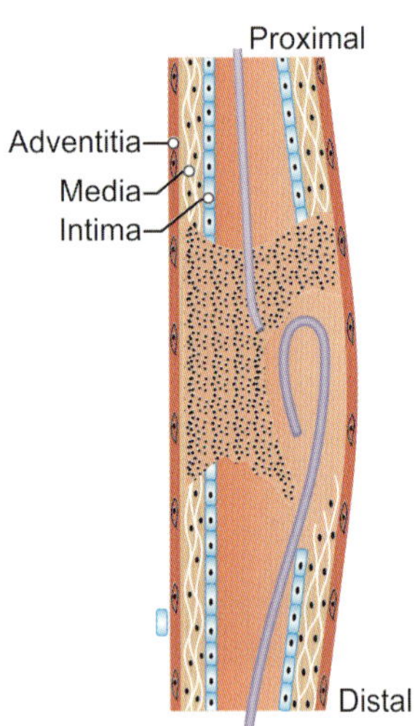

Fig. 13.29 Knuckle wire technique image
Reproduced with permission from Joyal et al.

tamponade compared to perforation of epicardial collaterals. On the other hand, epicardial collaterals are less preferred for retrograde CTO-PCI, because they are usually more tortuous than septal collaterals and their perforation could lead to rapid tamponade or their hematomas may cause cardiac chamber compression and subsequent tamponade. Moreover, if epicardial collaterals are the only source of collateral blood supply and they are occluded during the CTO procedure, acute ischemia and myocardial infarction may occur. In the case of patients with prior coronary bypass graft surgery, use of epicardial collaterals may be safer, as the adhesions may prevent tamponade in the case of perforation.

Despite these limitations, with increasing experience and rapid progress in retrograde equipment, including dedicated guidewires and microcatheters, the use of epicardial collaterals has been increasing (Figs 13.16 and 13.31).

In such cases that may only appear to have epicardial collaterals, septal collaterals may appear in the setting that epicardial collaterals have become occluded. Selective tip injection of the septal branches may also allow visualization of previously invisible collaterals (Figs 13.27A to G). Another option for crossing invisible septal collaterals is the 'surfing' technique, in which septal collaterals are probed and crossed without contrast injection.

If the interventional collateral for the retrograde approach enters the vessel close to the distal cap, there may not be enough space to allow manipulation of the guidewire and delivery of a microcatheter distal to the CTO. Accordingly, the retrograde interventional collateral that enters the vessel is preferred more distally in such cases.

With regard to the wire tip curve, an extremely small tip curve (<1.0 mm) is recommended after the microcatheter is navigated to the proximal segment of the collateral channel by a normal floppy wire. As the tips of these wires are soft, gentle tapping of the wire tip on the insertion needle would be the best method to create a curve in the same way as shaping a guidewire tip curve for CTO-PCI (Fig. 13.6).

Wire handling should be gentle with slow rotation, and should advance and halt once a series of ventricular premature contractions has developed or migration to the side branch is noticed. Forceful advancement and rotation could result in channel rupture, vessel perforation, and eventual septal hematoma. Therefore, utmost care should be paid to manipulate the wire in the collateral channels. Exceptionally, in the setting of the septal surfing technique, the guidewire is advanced rapidly until it either buckles or advances into the distal target vessel. However, if the wire buckles, it is withdrawn instantaneously and redirected.

Whenever the wire position is in doubt, the microcatheter should be advanced and the wire pulled back to perform 'repeated' tip injection with contrast medium (as little as 2 mL) to determine the correct direction to follow. In so doing, it is crucially important to confirm some retrograde drops of blood from the tail of the microcatheter to avoid channel injuries due to excessive pressurized injection by wedge conditions. When an injection reveals washout of the contrast agent, the channel is connected to either the right ventricular or the left ventricular cavity. When the contrast agent remains in the channel, it infers local disruption (focal perforation). These are examples in which no further treatment is required and other channels should be explored.

In CTO lesions with fair ipsilateral collaterals, such as septal collaterals from the proximal to the distal LAD, or diagonal or obtuse marginal left-to-left collaterals, it is feasible to perform the retrograde approach via these collateral channels (Figs 13.28, 13.24, 13.31, 13.34).[18] However, in the setting of retrograde CTO-PCI using ipsilateral collaterals, the retrograde wire may take a sharp turn to return into the proximal vessel, which can lead to difficulty advancing equipment, or more importantly, to collateral rupture, which occurs more frequently with ipsilateral than contralateral collaterals. If the CTO lesion is successfully passed through the ipsilateral collateral, then the second ipsilateral guide catheter may be beneficial for trapping or externalizing the wire (Figs 13.31A to G), because if the retrograde wire is inserted into the antegrade guiding catheter, delivery of the following microcatheter is more difficult through the same guide catheter.

Knuckled Wire Technique

If the antegrade or retrograde wire escalation strategy technique fails, or if the CTO lesion is long or its trajectory is poorly understood due to vessel ambiguity, or devices cannot

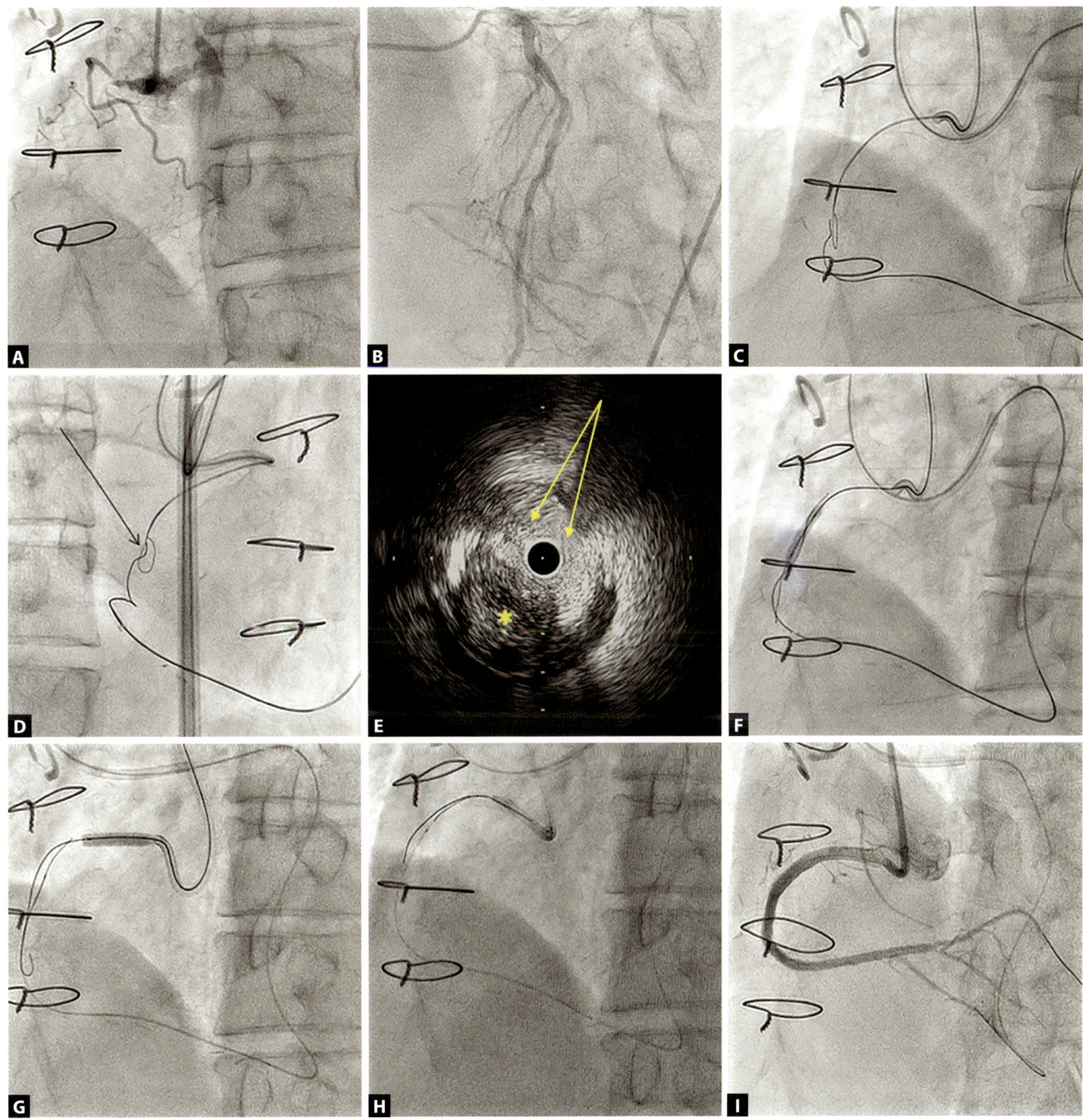

Figs 13.30A to I A case of knuckle wire technique. (A and B) The RCA had a very long CTO. The CTO entry was the proximal portion after branching the Conus artery. And the CTO exit, which was dyed by trans-septal collateral from the LAD, was found was just before the distal bifurcation; (C) The antegrade wire was advanced with a looped wire tip using the Pilot 200 with the Corsair support pushed deeper into the CTO segment, because of poor antegrade wire handling due to long CTO length and bending; (D) Subsequently, the retrograde wire using the Gaia 2nd progressed toward the looped wire tip. (Looped wire tips were shown by black arrow); (E) It showed that large subintimal space made by knuckle wire technique (yellow arrows) was compressing the intima of the CTO segment (asterisk) in the ultrasound image; (F) The conventional reverse CART technique was performed using a 3.5 mm balloon for aiming to make subintimal connection, however it did not work; (G) Thereby, the stent CART technique was performed for connect subintimal space and true lumen at the CTO entry point; (H) The retrograde wire was succeeded in passing through all the CTO segment and advanced into the proximal stent strut; (I) Final result; complete revascularization to the very long RCA-CTO was achieved with four drug-eluting stents implantation

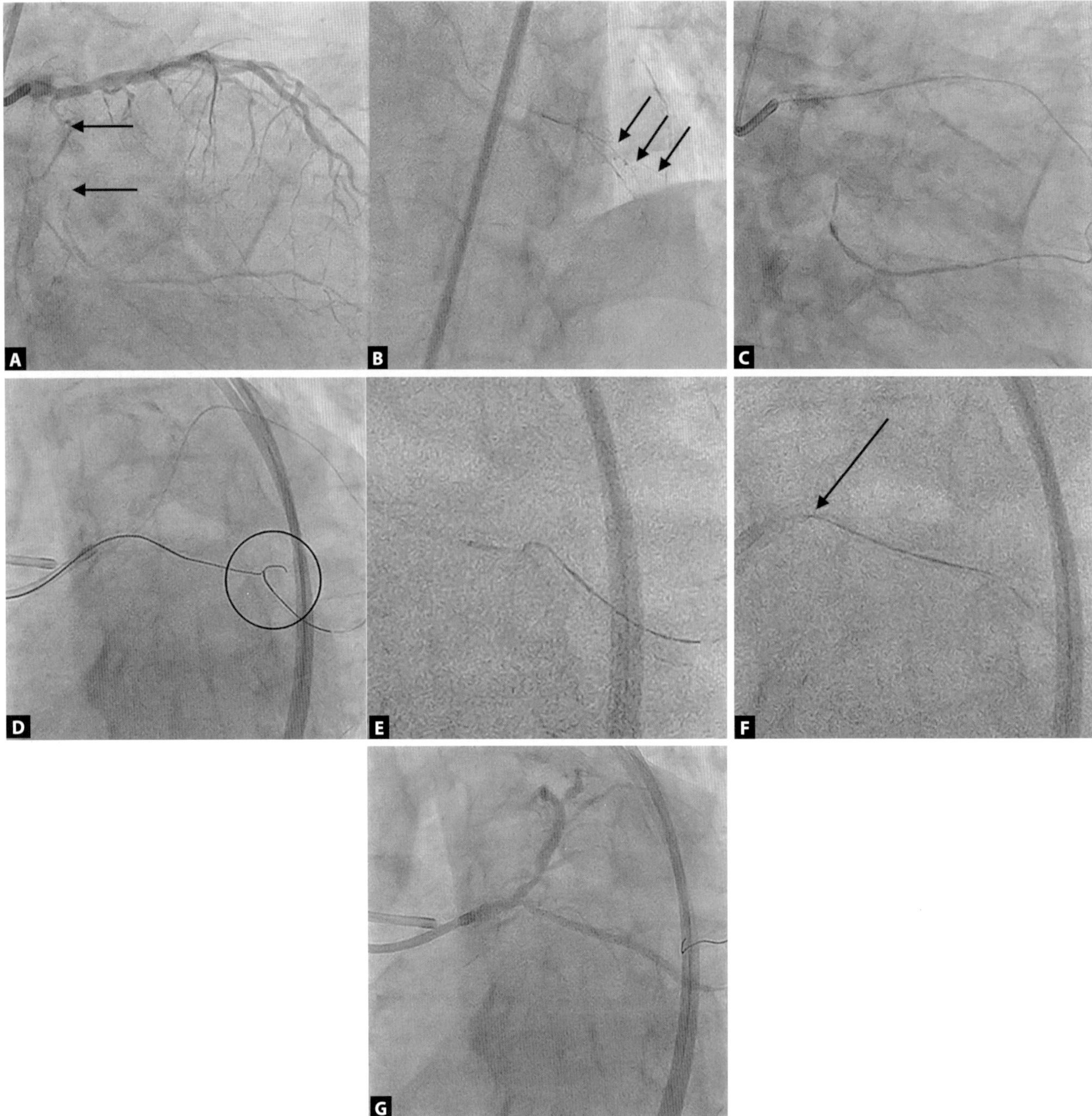

Figs 13.31A to G A case of wire rendezvous technique: (A) The LCX had a CTO at the proximal portion (black arrows showed the CTO entry and the exit); (B and C) The selective injection via the Caravel microcatheter. The ipsilateral epicardial collaterals were found via the 2nd diagonal branch. Careful wire manipulation against the proximal channel of this epicardial collateral using the Sion black (black arrows) was successful in negotiation; (C) The tip injection via the retrograde Caravel microcatheter, which was also successfully passed through this epicardial collateral; (D) Performance of bilateral wiring. The antegrade wiring using the UB3 with the Corsair microcatheter support advanced the CTO segment of the intimal plaque and reached the CTO exit. However, it was unable to pass through the bending of the CTO exit (black circle); (E) Performance of the wire rendezvous technique: The retrograde wire (Gaia 2nd) was attempting to put into the antegrade Corsair at the intima of the CTO distal segment; (F) Successful wire rendezvous: The retrograde wire tip was successfully inserted into the wire lumen of the antegrade Corsair which was inserted from the another antegrade guide catheter (Black arrow pointed the tip of the retrograde wire). After successful wire rendezvous, which means bilateral microcatheters on the same retrograde wire and kisses each other (Kissing micro technique). The subsequent CTO-PCI was continued in an antegrade manner after the antegrade microcatheter advanced over the CTO segment; (G) Complete the CTO-PCI procedure after two drug-eluting stents deployment

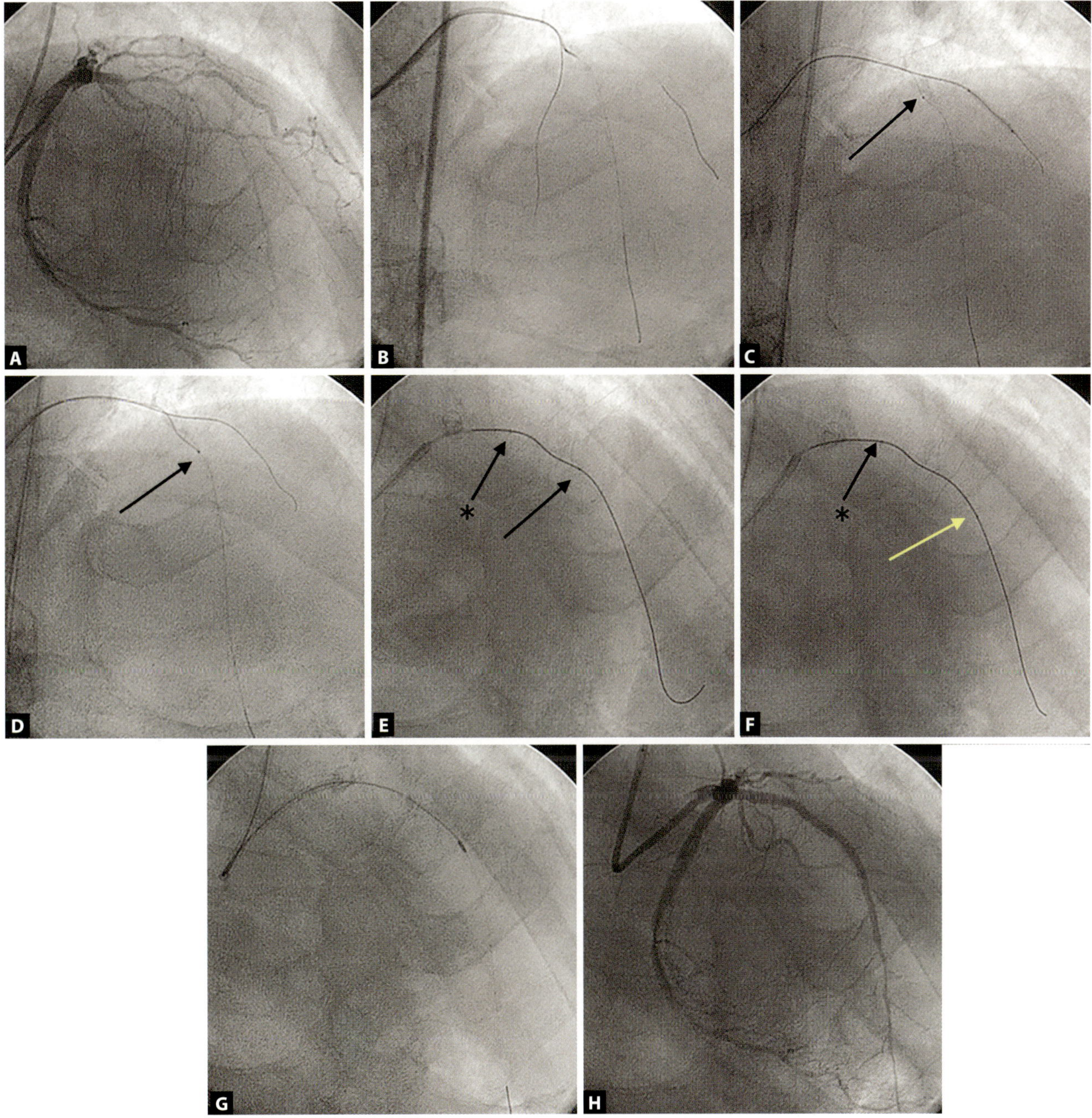

Figs 13.32A to H A case of PCI to LAD-CTO having 'devices uncrossable'. (A) Baseline coronary angiogram. The LAD had a CTO with heavy calcification at the midportion just after branching the 1st major septal and the 1st diagonal. There were not fair interventional collaterals; (B) Antegrade wiring using the Pilot 200 (Abbott vascular) with the Corsair support was able to pass through the LAD CTO segment successfully; (C) 'Balloon uncrossable' within the CTO segment (black arrow) due to heavy calcification under the side branch anchor balloon technique in the first diagonal branch; (D) 'Device uncrossable' at the bending portion within the CTO segment (black arrow) of the LAD-CTO under the drilling procedure using the Tornus pro; (E) Performance of the drilling procedure using the Tornus pro. (black arrow) under the child-in-mother technique using the 5Fr ST-01 catheter (Terumo) simultaneously (black arrow with asterisk); (F) Accordingly, the Tornus pro was successfully passed through the heavy calcified CTO segment (yellow arrow); (G) Performance of rotational atherectomy with a 1.25 mm burr against heavily calcified plaque within the CTO segment; (H) Complete revascularization to the heavy calcified LAD-CTO was achieved with three drug-eluting stents implantation to overcome 'devices uncrossable'

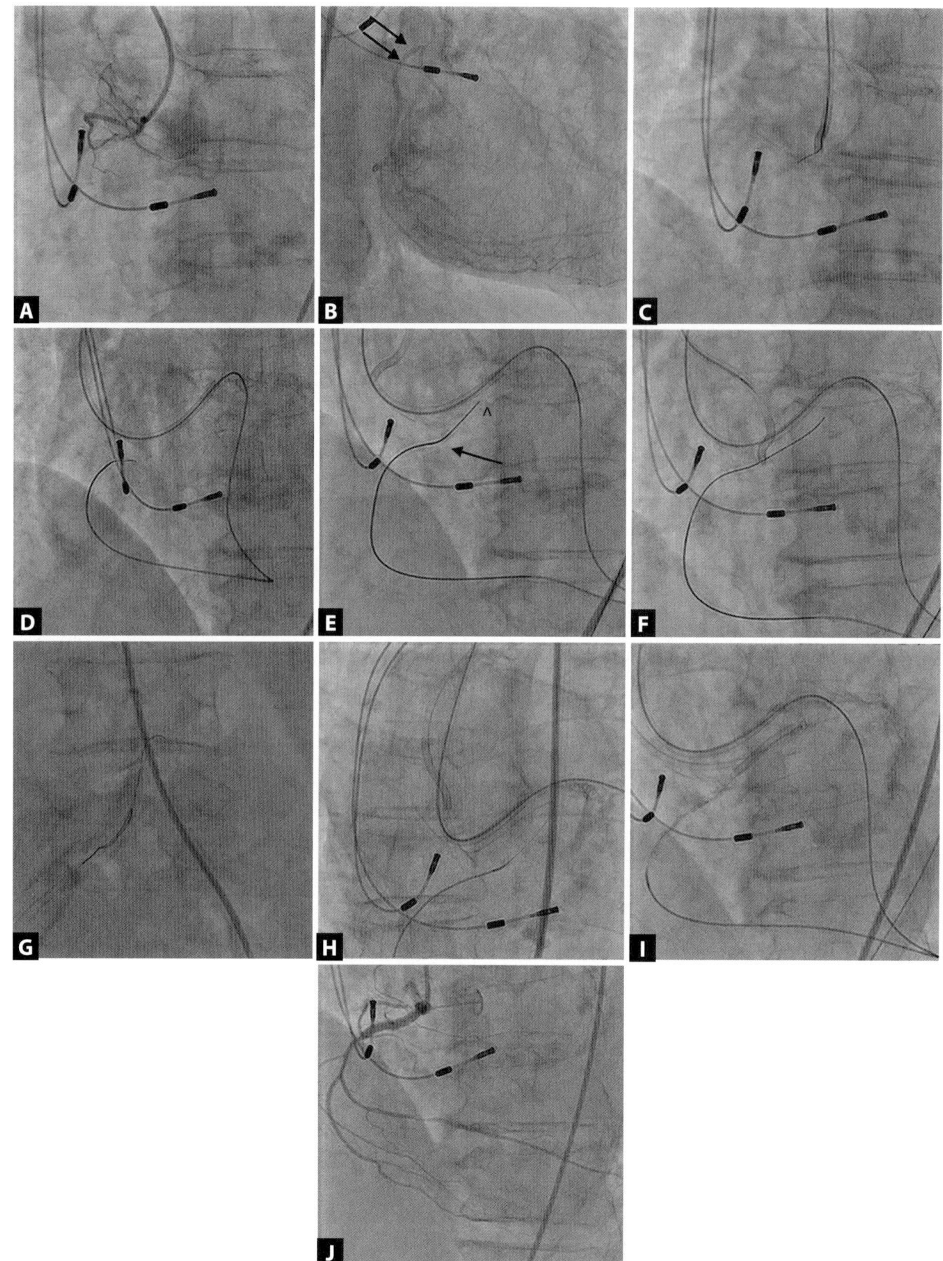

Figs 13.33A to J A case of retrograde approach and snaring technique against "devices uncrossable": (A) The RCA had CTO at the proximal portion and diffuse stenosis from the aortic ostium with heavy calcification; (B) The RCA was dyed with contrast media up to the midportion retrogradely (black arrows) via trans-septal collaterals; (C) Firstly, PCI to RCA-CTO was started by the antegrade approach, but it did not work, since an antegrade guide catheter was unable to stably engage due to severe stenosis with heavy calcification from the aortic ostium as well as anterior take-off; (D) The retrograde Corsair microcatheter managed to progress to the CTO exit via the septal collateral channel; (E) The retrograde Ultimate Bros. 3 was able to pass through all CTO segments and reached the ascending aorta directly (Arrowhead). However, the Corsair microcatheter could not cross due to the heavily calcified plaque within the CTO segment (black arrow); (F) To overcome this situation, the retrograde wire was changed to the RG3 wire. Consequently, the RG3 was retrogradely successful in passing through the CTO segment again, and approached the ascending aorta directly. However, the wire tip was unable to be inserted into the antegrade guide catheter; (G) Retrograde guidewire trapping technique at the terminal aorta: The tip of the RG3 wire was pushed forward to the terminal aorta in its present condition, and was caught by the 10 mm Amplatz GooseNeck snare system (Covidien Corp) and brought into the antegrade guide catheter at this point; (H) The antegrade guide catheter was reinserted to the RCA ostium with navigation by the RG3 shaft; (I) The dedicated low-profile 1.5 mm balloon (Ikazuchi zero, Kaneka medix) was successful in crossing through the whole CTO segment beyond the heavily calcified segment thanks to construction bilateral approach after wire externalization; (J) The final angiogram showed optimal results after a DES stent implantation with restoration of flow in the RCA

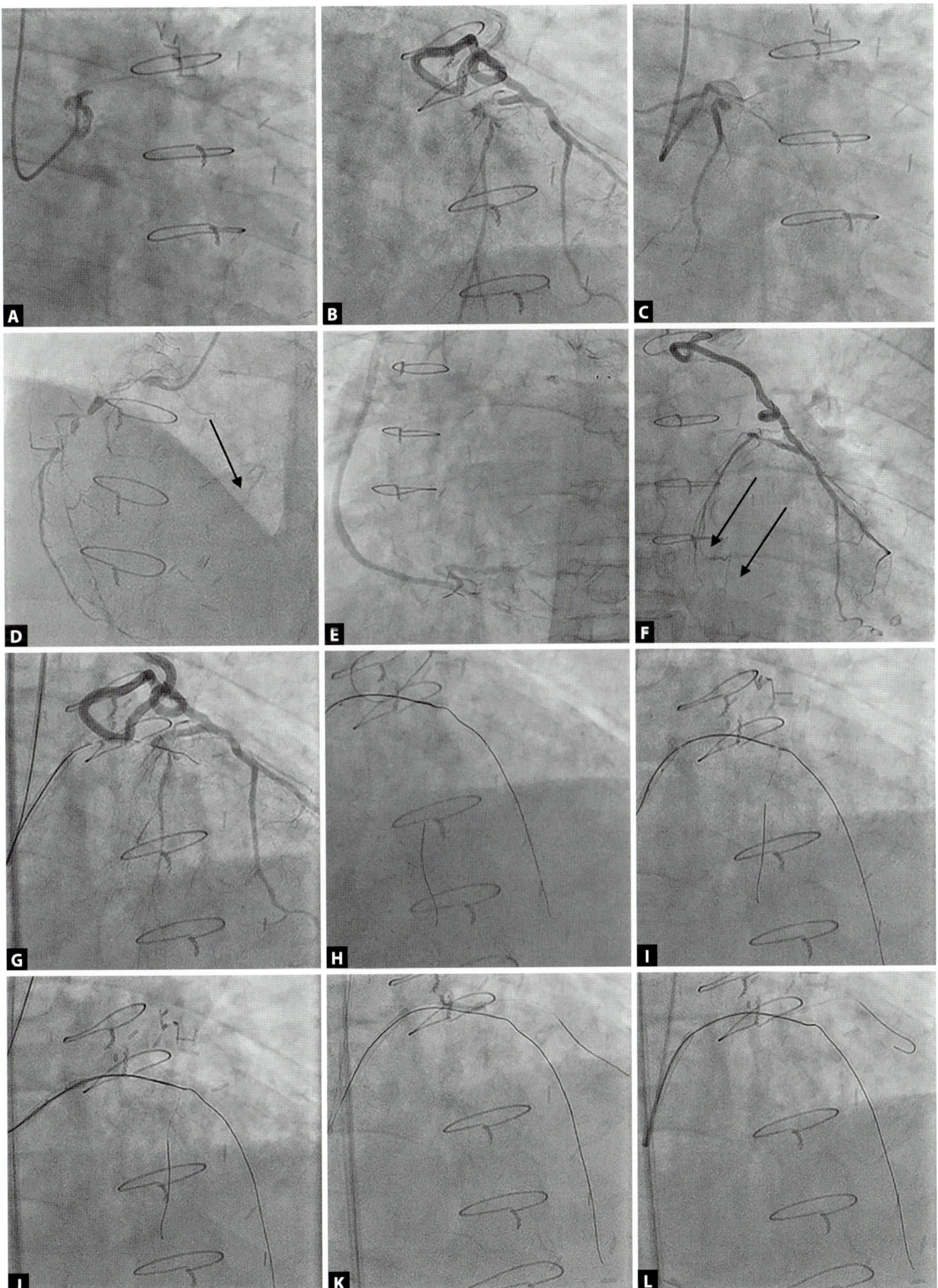

Figs 13.34A to L

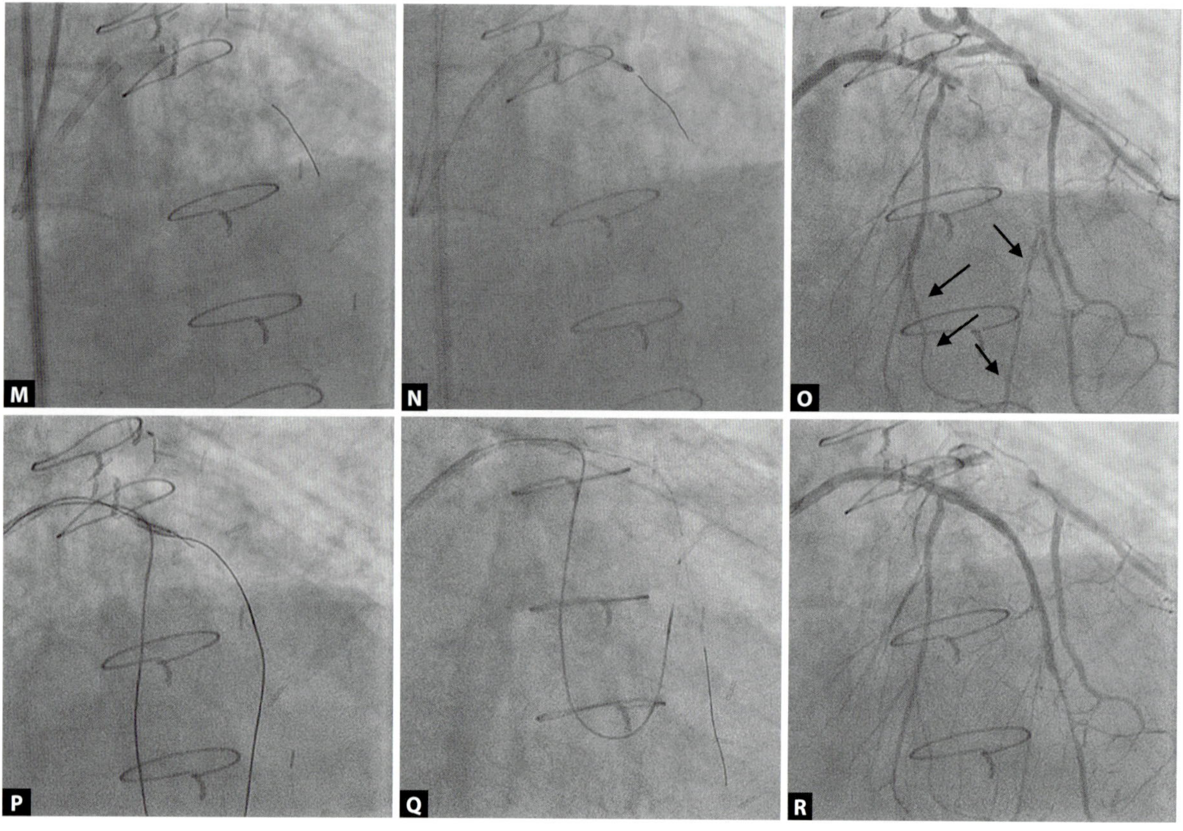

Figs 13.34M to R

Figs 13.34A to R A case of PCI to LAD double CTOs that was required hybrid procedural management against "devices uncrossable": staged Baseline coronary angiogram; (A and B) Two CTO lesions of native LAD; the proximal CTO was near the ostium and the distal CTO was just after the bifurcation to the first septal branch. LITA graft that was anastomosed to the first diagonal branch was patent; (C) Small circumflex artery that had significant stenosis with severe tortuosity at the proximal portion; (D) Totally occluded RCA at the middle portion. A main collateral to the distal LAD via the conus branch (black arrow); (E) SVG-right posterior descending artery that had no trans-septal collateral to the distal LAD; (F) From 'the island' sandwiched between two CTOs, a tiny ipsilateral intraseptal collateral via the first septal branch was found (black arrows). Staged 1st attempt PCI to LAD-CTOs; Successful antegrade guidewire crossing to the proximal LAD-CTO (G) and the distal LAD-CTO (H) using the Gaia 2nd with the Corsair microcatheter; (I) "balloon uncrossable" at the entry of the distal LAD-CTO; (J) The cracking technique using stiff wires, without passing through; (K) The side branch anchor balloon technique in the first diagonal branch; (L) The anchor Tornus technique without successful passing through; (M) As a final resort, the wire exchange to the Rotawire floppy was not able to pass through the distal CTO lesion completely, but was advanced over the entry of the distal CTO; (N) Performance of rotational atherectomy with a 1.5 mm burr from the protruding heavily calcified plaque at the bifurcation of the first septal branch to the entry of the distal LAD-CTO limit as plaque modification. Accordingly, the first attempt CTO-PCI was concluded as successful revascularization of the proximal LAD-CTO lesion only. Staged 2nd attempt PCI to distal LAD-CTO; (O) Growth of the ipsilateral intraseptal collateral due to recanalization of the proximal LAD-CTO was found (black arrows); (P) Reverse CART technique using a 2.0 mm balloon via this ipsilateral intraseptal collateral with manipulating Gaia 2nd guidewires bilaterally; (Q) Successful antegrade wiring with the Crusade microcatheter after wire externalization; (R) Final result.

Abbreviations: LITA, left internal mammary artery; SVG, saphenous vein graft

pass into the CTO lesion but the guidewire tip can, the 'knuckle-wire' technique may be considered (Figs 13.29 and 13.30).[19] This entails creating a small loop with polymer-jacketed wire, such as Sion black (Asahi Intecc) or Pilot 200 (Abbott Vascular, Santa Clara, CA) for dissection within the subintimal space (occasional occurring within the intimal space) either retrogradely or antegradely, and hence prepare an opportunity to connect the proximal lumen with the distal lumen within the CTO segment using the reverse CART technique. With regard to the handling of the knuckle-wire, rotation may cause wire knotting, making it impossible to retrieve, and therefore it should be only pushed and never rotated.

Wire Rendezvous Technique

Although the retrograde wire has been passed through the CTO segment, occasionally the retrograde microcatheter may be unable to advance within the CTO segment due to hard plaque and advancement of the retrograde microcatheter carries a risk of channel injury due to tiny size, bending, and fragility of its collateral channel. In such situations, the wire rendezvous technique (also referred to as the kissing microcatheter technique)[20,21] is useful (Fig. 13.31).

The key feature of this technique is placing the retrograde wire tip into the antegrade microcatheter either within the CTO segment or outside of it, such as the proximal lumen of the CTO and inside of the antegrade guiding catheter. The retrograde microcatheter and antegrade microcatheter are on the same retrograde wire. After advancing the antegrade microcatheter until both tips 'kiss' each other, the antegrade microcatheter is advanced to the distal portion of the CTO lesion, pulling back the retrograde microcatheter. The retrograde guidewire is pulled out and an antegrade guidewire is advanced to the distal true lumen through the antegrade microcatheter and subsequent CTO-PCI is continued in an antegrade manner.

Management of 'Device-Uncrossable' CTO Lesions

The inability of guidewire passage through CTO lesions is the most common reason for failure of CTO-PCI. On the other hand, 'balloon and device-uncrossable' CTO lesions, even after successful guidewire passage, account for 10–15% of all CTO-PCI procedural failures[22] and are most often due to heavy calcification at the occlusion site.

To overcome these conditions, several bailout strategies have been proposed, and can be roughly divided into two categories: (1) strategies that increase guide catheter support and (2) strategies that provide plaque modification.

The former include changing the guide catheter to provide better support or deep engagement of the guide catheter, utilization of various child-in-mother techniques, such as the Guideliner catheter,[23] 4Fr KIWAMI ST-01 (Terumo) (Figs 13.32A to H), and 4.5 Fr CoKatte (Asahi Intecc), etc. with utilization of various anchor techniques.[24,25]

The latter include advancing low-profile balloons as far as possible into the lesion in an attempt to modify the proximal cap, utilization of various microcatheters (e.g. Corsair, Caravel, Finecross, etc.), drilling techniques utilizing Tornus catheters,[26,27] (Fig. 13.32) the anchor-Tornus technique[25] (Figs 13.32 and 13.34) (which simultaneously drills into the lesion utilizing the Tornus catheter under anchor ballooning), buddy (occasionally triple) wire technique, cracking technique utilizing stiff wires,[28] (Fig. 13.32) the anterograde dissection and reentry device (although these are not commercially available in Japan at present), utilization of excimer laser coronary atherectomy, and rotational atherectomy (Figs 13.32 and 13.34).[27,29] However, rotational atherectomy should be considered as a final resort because rotational atherectomy requires wire exchange for a 0.009 inch stemless steel guidewire, which may not always be feasible through CTO lesions.

The retrograde approach is also considered to be an effective alternative method for cases with 'balloon-uncrossable' CTO lesions,[29,30] as it has become a safe and reliable approach for CTO intervention. In cases of complete wire externalization by a retrograde guidewire crossing through the CTO segment despite inability to pass 'devices', strong backup support is provided by bilateral guide catheter anchor (Figs 13.33 and 13.34). Performance of the reverse CART technique may also provide ideal plaque modification by avoidance of the hard plaque of the CTO segment through subintimal tracking (Figs 13.34A to R).

Management of Complications

The risk of coronary perforation from the antegrade and retrograde approach was 0.4% in the J-CTO registry.[31] With regard to the retrograde approach, the rate of complications requiring treatment was 2.1% in the Japanese Retrograde Summit registry.[32]

Specific complications associated with the retrograde approach are collateral channel rupture, thrombus formation, and global ischemia.

Pericardiocentesis is occasionally required and should be considered when rapid hemodynamic compromise occurs. Collateral channel rupture is potentially fatal. Septal collateral rupture usually results in self-limiting septal hematoma and may be managed conservatively except in cases of serious growing septal hematoma. Epicardial collateral rupture is more serious, in which definitive hemostasis via a microcatheter and often requires pericardial drainage followed by antegrade and retrograde coiling to complete hemostasis. Coils should be available and operators should be familiar with their use.

Thrombus formation is also prevented by flushing of the guiding catheter with saline and by maintenance of activated clotting time >300 s, checked every 30–60 minutes. Global ischemia can be minimized by careful manipulation of the retrograde system in relation to the retrograde guide catheter engagement. Therefore, when there is substantial coronary stenosis on route to the collaterals of the donor side, advance treatment with a stent allows for safer and stable retrograde instrumentation. Further, catheter-induced dissection, which can occasionally occur due to deep insertion or excessive backup force of guide catheters, may be prevented by constant pulling of the guide catheter to disengage from the ostium.

In addition, contrast volume is monitored closely and should be minimized at all times. Routine radiation minimization techniques are particularly important with prolonged procedures. This involves monitoring the patient's skin dose, reducing fluoroscopy frame rates, and angulation changes of the image intensifier at regular intervals to prevent intensified skin doses. Intraprocedural bleeding should be minimized by careful attention to Y-adapter hemostasis. Overtreatment of distal disease should be avoided. Chronic underfilling makes it difficult to assess true vessel size. With time, vasodilation and remodeling may result in significant improvements.

CONCLUSION

In summary, CTO-PCI has undergone marked evolution in recent years. Excellent results can be achieved with high success rates and low complication rates in experienced centers and operators using all available techniques.

Future prospective randomized controlled trials comparing conservative strategies with percutaneous revascularization are required to provide reliable real-world clinical evidence.

REFERENCES

1. Bagnall A, Spyridopoulos I. The Evidence Base for Revascularisation of Chronic Total Occlusions. Current Cardiology Reviews. 2014;10:88-98.
2. Valenti R, Vergara R, Migliorini A, Parodi G, Carrabba N, Cerisano G, et al. Predictors of reocclusion after successful drug-eluting stent-supported percutaneous coronary intervention of chronic total occlusion. J Am Cooll Cardiol. 2013;61:545-50.
3. Habara M, Tsuchikane E, Muramatsu T, Kashima Y, Okamura A, Mutoh M, Yamane M, et al. Comparison of percutaneous coronary intervention for chronic total occlusion outcome according to operator experience from the Japanese retrograde summit registry. Catheter Cardiovasc Interv. 2016;87(6): 1027-35.
4. Touma G, Ramsey D, Weaver J. Chronic total occlusions—Current techniques and future directions. IJC Heart and Vasculature. 2015;7:28-39.
5. Yamane M. Current percutaneous recanalization of coronary chronic total occlusion. Rev Esp Cardiol. 2012;65:265-77.
6. Sumitsuji S, Inoue K, Ochiai M, Tsuchikane E, Ikeno F. Fundamental wire technique and current standard strategy of percutaneous intervention for chronic total occlusion with histopathological insights. JACC Cardiov Interv. 2011;4(9): 941-51.
7. Sakakura K, Nakano M, Otsuka F, Yahagi K, Kutys R, Ladich E, et al. Comparison of pathology of chronic total occlusion with and without coronary artery bypass graft. European Heart J. 2014;35:1683-93.
8. Morino Y, Abe M, Morimoto T, Kimura T, Hayashi Y, Muramatsu T, et al. Predicting successful guidewire crossing through chronic total occlusion of native coronary lesions within 30 minutes: the J-CTO (Multicenter CTO Registry in Japan) score as a difficulty grading and time assessment tool. JACC Cardiovasc Interv. 2011;4(2):213-21.
9. Newell MC, Schwartz RS. Utility of CT coronary angiography for planning CTO Intervention. Cardiac Intervention Today. 2009;3:25-8.
10. Alaswad K, Menon RV, Christopoulos G, Lombardi WL, Karmpaliotis D, Grantham JA, et al. Transradial approach for coronary chronic total occlusion interventions: Insights from a contemporary multicenter registry. Catheter Cardiovasc Interv. 2015;85(7):1123-9.
11. Mitsudo K, Yamashita T, Asakura Y, Muramatsu T, Doi O, Shibata Y, et al. Recanalization strategy for chronic total occlusions with tapered and stiff-tip guidewire. The results of CTO new techniQUE for STandard procedure (CONQUEST) trial. J Invasive Cardiol. 2008;20:571-7.
12. Fujita S, Tamai H, Kyo E, Kosuga K, Hata T, Okada M, et al. New technique for superior guiding catheter support during advancement of a balloon in coronary angioplasty: The anchor technique. Catheter Cardiovasc Interv. 2003;59:482-8.
13. Colombo A, Mikhail GW, Michev I, Iakovou I, Airoldi F, Chieffo A, et al. Treating chronic total occlusions using subintimal tracking and reentry: the STAR technique. Catheter Cardiovasc Interv. 2005;64:407-11.
14. Sekiguchi M, Yamazaki M, Kurabayashi M. Retrograde percutaneous coronary intervention via critically degenerated saphenous vein grafts for chronic total occlusion in native coronary arteries. World J Cardiovasc Dis. 2013;03:261-5.
15. Surmely JF, Tsuchikane E, Katoh O, et al. New concept for CTO recanalization using controlled antegrade and retrograde subintimal tracking; the CART technique. J of Invasive Cardiology. 2006(18):334-8.
16. Tsuchikane E, Katoh O, Kimura M, Nasu K, Kinoshita Y, Suzuki T, et al. The first clinical experience with a novel catheter for collateral channel tracking in retrograde approach for chronic coronary total occlusions. JACC Cardiovasc Interv. 2010;3: 165-71.
17. Rathore S, Katoh O, Tsuchikane E, Oida A, Suzuki T, Takase S, et al. A novel modification of the retrograde approach for the recanalization of chronic total occlusion of the coronary arteries intravascular ultrasound-guided reverse controlled antegrade and retrograde tracking. JACC Cardiovasc Interv. 2010;3: 155-64.
18. Otsuji S, Terasoma K, Takiuchi S. Retrograde recanalization of a left anterior descending chronic total occlusion via an ipsilateral intraseptal collateral. J Invasive Cardiol. 2008;20(6):312-6.
19. Joyal D, Thompson CA, Grantham JA, Buller CEH, Rinflet S. The retrograde technique for recanalization of chronic total occlusions A step-by-step approach. JACC Cardiovasc Interv. 2012;5:1-11.
20. Muramatsu T, Tsukahara R, Ito Y. "Rendezous in coronary" technique with the retrograde approach for chronic total osslusion. J Invasive Cardiol. 2010;22(9):E179-182.
21. Funatsu A, Kobayashi T, Nakamura S. Use of the kissing microcatheter technique to exchange a retrograde wire for an antegrade wire in the retrograde approach to intervention in chronic total occlusion. J Invasive Cardiol. 2010;22(5):E74-7.

22. Pagnotta P, Brigouri C, Mango R, Visconti G, Focaccio A, Belli G, et al. Rotational atherectomy in resistant chronic total occlusions. Catheter Cardiovasc Interv. 2010;76(3):366-71.
23. Kovacic JC, Sharma AB, Roy S, Li JR, Narayan R, Kim DB, et al. GuideLiner mother-and child guide catheter extension: a simple adjunctive tool in PCI for balloon uncrossable chronic total occlusions. J Interv Cardiol. 2013;26(4):343-50.
24. Michael TT, Banerjee S, Brilakis ES. Subintimal distal anchor technique for "Balloon-uncrossable" chronic total occlusions. J Invasive Cardiol. 2013;25(10):552-4.
25. Kitane AJ, Stone GW. The Anchor-Tornus technique: a novel approach to "uncrossable" chronic total occlusions. Catheter Cardiovasc Interv. 2007;70(4):554-7.
26. Brilakis ES, Banerjee S. Crossing the "balloon uncrossable" chronic total occlusion: tornus to the rescue. Catheter Cardiovasc Interv. 2011;78(3):363-5.
27. Pagnotta P, Briguori C, Ferrante G, et al. Tornus catheter and rotational atherectomy in resistant chronic total occlusions. Int J Cardiol. 2013;167(6):2653-6.
28. Ohya H, Katoh O. A Case of Successful Cracking of Calcified Fibrous Cap of Totally Occluded Left Anterior Descending Artery by Using Cutting Balloon. J Am Coll Cardiol. 2014;63(12): S135-6.
29. Tanabe M, Wada A, Doi O. Successful interventional revascularization utilizing hybrid procedural steps of rotational atherectomy and retrograde approach via an ipsilateral collateral. Cardiovasc Interv and Ther. 2016;31(4):309-15.
30. Tanabe M, Kunitomo T, Doi O. Successful interventional recanalization against heavily calcified chronic total occlusion of proximal right coronary artery utilizing retrograde guidewire trapping technique at the terminal aorta. J Cardiovasc Dis Diagn. 2016;4:231-4.
31. Morino Y, Kimura T, Hayashi Y, Muramatsu T, Ochiai M, Noguchi Y, et al. In-hospital outcomes of contemporary percutaneous coronary intervention in patients with chronic total occlusion insights from the J-CTO Registry (Multicenter CTO Registry in Japan). JACC Cardiovasc Interv. 2010(2)3:143-51.
32. Okamura A, Yamane M, Muto M, Matsubara T, Igarashi Y, Nakamura S, et al. Complications during retrograde approach for chronic coronary total occlusion: Sub-Analysis of Japanese Multicenter Registry. Catheter Cardiovasc Interv. 2016;88(1): 7-14.

CHAPTER

14

Primary Angioplasty in Myocardial Infarction

Ajit S Mullasari

INTRODUCTION

Sudden thrombotic occlusion of major epicardial coronary artery in the absence of adequate collaterals is the culprit for acute ST elevation myocardial infarction (STEMI). The sudden thrombotic occlusion of a coronary artery is triggered by fibrous cap disruption of an atherosclerotic plaque or surface erosion in the absence of fibrous cap disruption.[1] The aim of treatment for acute ST elevation myocardial infarction (STEMI) is to restore complete antegrade blood flow in the infarct related artery (IRA) and minimize ischemic damage to the myocardium. Options of treatment include thrombolysis and primary percutaneous coronary intervention (PPCI). Primary percutaneous emergency coronary intervention or primary angioplasty in myocardial infarction (PAMI) is the treatment of choice in view of good success rates in restoring antegrade blood flow, limiting infarct size and lower rates of recurrent ischemia or infarction.[2,3] Though there has been a decline in STEMI mortality in the last two decades 30% of patients still do not get acute reperfusion therapy.[4] PAMI is the preferred reperfusion strategy for patients with STEMI if it can be performed in a timely manner and by experienced operators.[5]

Fibrinolytic therapy is an alternative to primary percutaneous coronary intervention (PCI), but as many as 40% of patients are ultimately resistant to infarct artery reperfusion.[6]

STRATEGIES IN ACUTE STEMI

Various strategies[7] that have been used to achieve reperfusion in acute STEMI include:

- *Pharmacological reperfusion:* Thrombolysis
- *Mechanical reperfusion:* Primary Angioplasty thrombosuction and stenting-PAMI
- Rescue PCI for failed thrombolysis
- *Facilitated PCI:* Administration of pharmacological measures and immediate transfer for angiography and PCI
- *Pharmacoinvasive strategy:* Immediate transfer and or routine angiography with adjunctive PCI within 3–24 hours of successful pharmacological reperfusion.
- Ischemia/Symptom guided PCI. The definitive goal in STEMI management is early, complete, and sustained reperfusion, which in turn results in better short-term and long-term outcomes.[8]

ADVANTAGE OF PRIMARY PCI OVER THROMBOLYTIC THERAPY

Primary PCI was compared with thrombolysis as reperfusion strategy for patients of acute STEMI in 23 randomized trials involving more than 7,500 patients. A meta-analysis[3] of these trials showed that primary PCI resulted in a 25% reduction in death, a 64% reduction in reinfarction, a 95% reduction in intracranial hemorrhage, and a 53% reduction in stroke in compared with fibrinolysis. Primary PCI was found to be superior in reducing short-term mortality (21 lives saved per 1,000 patient treated), nonfatal reinfarction, and stroke across all subgroups (elderly, women, diabetics, anterior or inferior MI, or prior MI), which was maintained on long-term follow-up. The benefit was maximum in patients with highest risk like patients in cardiogenic shock. Frequency of achieving TIMI 3 flow in infarct related artery was also significantly higher in primary PCI with significantly lower bleeding risk.[9] Moreover, reperfusion injury and hemorrhagic transformation of a bland infarction, which occurs after fibrinolytic therapy, occur rarely after primary PCI; hemorrhagic stroke occurred in 0.05% of patients after primary PCI which is also significantly lower than fibrinolysis (1.1%).[10]

Primary PCI should be the universal "dominant default strategy" for prompt early reperfusion if there are no resource or logistical constraints.

The American College of Cardiology/American Heart Association (ACC/AHA) and European Society of Cardiology (ESC) STEMI guidelines Recommend PCI as the initial approach to management of STEMI, at centers with a skilled PCI laboratory with rapid initiation.[11,12]

The Danish Acute Myocardial Infarction-2 (DANAMI-2) trial showed that primary PCI when compared with thrombolysis reduced the risk of reinfarction (13% versus 18.5%; hazard ratio [HR], 0.66; 95% confidence interval [CI], 0.49–0.89) and mortality (26.7% versus 33.3%; HR, 0.78; 95% CI, 0.63–0.97) among patients randomized at invasive centers within 120 minutes.[13] Comparison of angioplasty and prehospital thrombolysis in acute myocardial infarction (CAPTIM)[14] and PRAGUE-2 (Primary Angioplasty in Patients Transported from General Community Hospitals to Specialized PTCA Units with or without Emergency Thrombolysis 2)[15] trials have shown that there is no strong. Preference between PCI and thrombolysis in STEMI patients who present within 3 hours after symptom onset, as the mortality is similar or lower in both groups.[14,15] An analysis of 21 trials showed that as PCI-related time delay increased, absolute mortality reduction at 4–6 weeks favoring primary PCI versus thrombolysis decreased (0.94% decrease per additional10-minute delay; $p < 0.006$).[16]

STEMI guidelines indicate that thrombolysis is generally preferred over primary PCI when the door-to-balloon time minus door-to-needle time exceeds 1 hour.[11] According to the ACC/AHA 2013 guidelines in non PCI capable hospitals it is indicated to thrombolyse when a >120 minutes time delay is expected from point of first medical contact (FMC) to primary PCI. The current ACC/AHA guidelines strongly recommend that all PCI hospital systems achieve a median door-to-balloon time for primary PCI of 90 minutes. The proposed timings for PPCI as per the national STEMI program is shown in Figure 14.1.

INTERVENTIONS DURING PAMI

In the majority of patients undergoing primary PCI for STEMI routine stent implantation with or without thrombosuction with or without prior balloon dilatation is performed according to current guidelines.[11,12]

However, a substantial number of patients may not achieve tissue level perfusion even after successful recanalization of the epicardial coronary artery. Inadequate myocardial perfusion of a given coronary segment without angiographic evidence of epicardial vessel obstruction, flow limiting dissection, conduit vessel spasm, or apparent in-situ thrombosis is described as no-reflow. This condition is also known as micro vascular obstruction (MVO).[17] This ominous phenomenon is caused by various mechanisms (Fig. 14.2 and Table 14.1) and has been shown to be associated with increased morbidity and mortality following acute myocardial infarction (AMI) perfusion.[18] No-reflow phenomenon is the Achilles heel in PAMI interventions and hence recognition and prevention of distal embolization and no-reflow is of utmost importance.

PREVENTION OF DISTAL EMBOLIZATION IN PAMI

As shown by Yip et al. patients who present with angiographic high Thrombus load have a higher risk of no-reflow and epicardial artery distal embolization which clearly translates into a higher cardiac mortality rate at 30 days.[19] The thrombus load and occurrence of no-reflow in an era of drug eluting stent implantation for acute myocardial infarction is of major interest since safety concerns are still unresolved following registry reports of a higher rate of stent thrombosis in these high risk acute myocardial infarction patients.[20]

Currently, there are several strategies available for 'fighting' distal embolization of coronary thrombus:[21]

- Use of adjunctive mechanical devices (thrombus aspiration and embolic protection devices)
- Pharmacologic approaches to dissolve the thrombus [with a special role for glycoprotein IIb/IIIa inhibitors (GPIs)]
- Dedicated stent for thrombus entrapment (e.g. MGuard stent).

Thrombus Aspiration

There are two approaches available for thrombus aspiration (Figs 14.3A to F):

1. Mechanical thrombus aspiration (MT) with AngioJet, X-Sizer, Rinspirator catheters, etc.
2. Manual thrombus aspiration (MTA) with Export, Thrombuster II, Diver, Eliminate catheters.

The randomized evaluation of the effect of mechanical reduction of distal embolization by thrombus-aspiration in primary and rescue angioplasty (REMEDIA) was the first trial that assessed the role of thrombectomy with a simple manual aspiration catheter.[22] The use of thrombus aspiration catheters has been widely adopted in almost all PPCI procedures due to the results of the thrombus aspiration during percutaneous coronary intervention in acute myocardial infarction study (TAPAS) trial.[23]

TAPAS was a single center study of thrombus aspiration in 1071 STEMI patients with export catheter which showed that thrombosuction is applicable in a large majority of STEMI patients and results in a better reperfusion parameter shown by a lower proportion of patients achieving MBG 0 or 1 compared to conventional PCI group (17.1% versus 26.3%, $p < 0.001$). Moreover, one year mortality was significantly lower in the thrombus aspiration group compared to conventional PCI without aspiration (3.6% versus 6.7%, $p = 0.02$).[24] This study provided the necessary evidence to

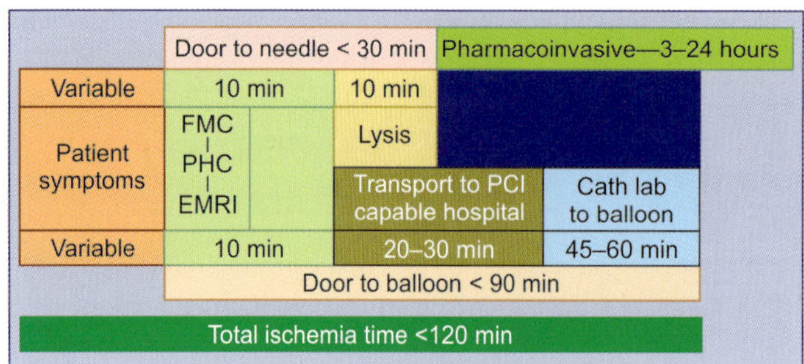

Fig. 14.1 Proposed timings in PPCI
(*Courtesy:* National STEMI programme)
Abbreviations: FMC, first medical contact; PHC, primary health center; EMRI, ambulance service

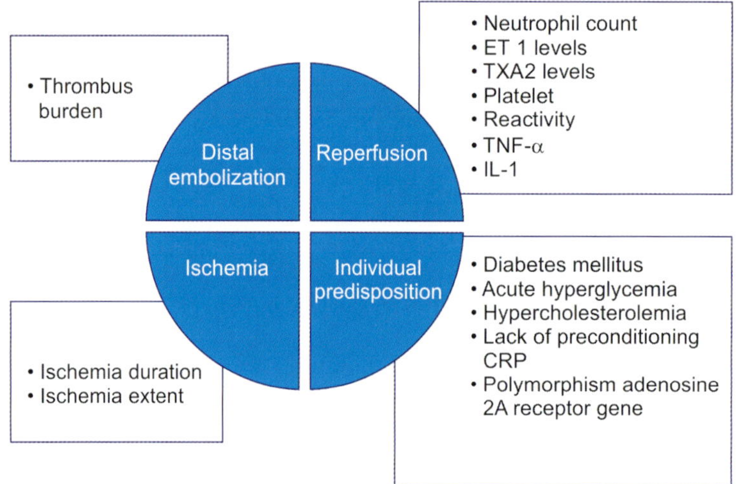

Fig. 14.2 Cascade of mechanisms of no-reflow as targets for prevention in PAMI

include thrombosuction as a class IIa indication with level of evidence B in the ACC/AHA 2013 STEMI guidelines as well as the ESC 2012 STEMI guidelines.[25] The TAPAS study compared a strategy of aspiration plus direct stenting versus balloon predilatation followed by stenting. The use of predilatation only in the control arm has been claimed to be a flaw in the TAPAS study by its detractors.

After the publication of TAPAS, many investigators have reported varying results with manual aspiration. There is considerable disagreement between various meta-analysis performed by different authors. The most recently published meta-analysis of the trials evaluating manual thrombus aspiration (MTA) and manual thrombectomy (MT) by De-Luca suggests that both of these methods appear to exert mild beneficial effect on embolization, ST resolution, TIMI flow and myocardial perfusion when compared to standard therapy.[26] However, a similar meta-analysis by Mongeon demonstrates no beneficial effects on TIMI flow, re-infarction or mortality and a concerning trend towards increased stroke.[27] A meta-analysis by Bavry suggests a benefit of thrombosuction in PPCI but suggests a 3-fold increase in stroke rates when MTA or MT are used (RR = 3.01, p = 0.024).[28] On the other hand, the use of mechanical thrombus aspiration has failed to show a clinical benefit compared to the manual aspiration catheter as shown by a pooled analysis of individual patient data from 11 STEMI trials involving 2686 patients by Burzotta.[29]

The effect of manual thrombus aspiration on the no-reflow phenomenon as measured with contrast-enhanced MRI has also been demonstrated in the EXPIRA (Thrombectomy with Export Catheter in Infarct-Related Artery During Primary Percutaneous Coronary Intervention) trial.[30] At 3 months the infarct size was considerably reduced in the manual thrombectomy group (Fig. 14.4).

In 2010 the INFUSE AMI multicenter randomized trial (which enrolled exclusively proximal or mid-LAD primary PCI) MTA did not improve infarct size at 30 days (by MRI),

Table 14.1 Predictors of no-reflow in primary PCI

- *Baseline demographics/medical history:*
  - Male sex
  - Older age
  - Diabetes mellitus
  - Low GFR
- *Indicators of disease severity:*
  - Infarct size
  - Higher cardiac biomarkers
  - Lower baseline ejection fraction
  - Killips classification ≥ 2
- *Investigations:*
  - Higher initial WBC count/neutrophil count
  - Endothelin-I level
  - C-reactive protein level
  - Thromboxane A2 level
  - Platelet count/reactivity
- *Therapeutic implications:*
  - Absence of preinfarction angina
  - Longer time-to-reperfusion
  - Elevated blood glucose level
  - Elevated total cholesterol level
- *Angiographic indicators:*
  - Anterior MI/LAD lesion
  - Thrombus burden
  - Thrombus cut off pattern
  - Thrombus >5 mm proximal to occlusion
  - Floating thrombus
  - Persistent dye stasis distal to obstruction
  - Infarct related artery diameter >4 mm
  - Reduced pre-PCI TIMI flow grade

Abbreviations: GFR, glomerular filtration rate; WBC, white blood cell; LAD, left anterior descending, MI, myocardial infarction, TIMI, thrombolysis in myocardial infarction; PCI, percutaneous coronary intervention

ST resolution, myocardial perfusion, TIMI flow, death or any other clinical endpoint. If anything there was a trend toward worse ST resolution with MTA.[31]

Compared to single center studies, multicenter aspiration trials have largely been negative.[32] Based on the data from the TAPAS and EXPIRA RCTs and the meta-analysis by Bavry the 2013 ACC/AHA and the 2012 ESC STEMI guideline gives a class IIa indication for manual thrombus aspiration with level of evidence B.[11,12]

The thrombus aspiration during ST-segment elevation (TASTE) myocardial infarction, which included more than 7000 participants was unable to document a mortality benefit from aspiration thrombectomy.[33] However, aspiration thrombectomy was associated with a marginal reduction in recurrent myocardial infarction ($p = 0.09$) and stent thrombosis at 30 days ($p = 0.06$). One year follow-up also did not show any reduction in rate of death, re-hospitalization for myocardial infarction or stent thrombosis by routine thrombus aspiration pre PCI in STEMI.[34] Also the results from the randomized trial of routine aspiration thrombectomy with PCI versus PCI Alone (TOTAL)[35] in patients with STEMI undergoing primary PCI did not show any reduction in primary outcomes of cardiovascular death or recurrent myocardial infarction. The 2014 ESC ESC/EATS guidelines on myocardial revascularization gives a class IIb indication for thrombosuction in selected cases after considering the TASTE trial results.[25] However, critics of the above two trials point to the low thrombus burden and operator dependency of the procedure as important factors in determining the efficacy of thrombosuction and should not mitigate the use of thrombosuction in high-risk STEMI with huge thrombus burden.[36] Dr Kumbhani and co investigators carried out meta-analysis[37] of 18 randomized trials with 3,836 patients who were randomized to aspiration device and conventional primary PCI and other 7 trials that randomized 1,598 patients to mechanical thrombectomy devices. The weighted mean follow-up period was 6 months. The authors have taken all the trials into account except the recently published TASTE trial. The meta-analysis conclusively showed that:

- Mechanical devices do not offer any benefit
- Thrombus aspiration catheter not only provided 30 days benefit but also reduced all cause mortality at 6 months (Figs 14.5A to D).

COVERED STENTS

The MGuard™ stent consists of bare metal stent (BMS) platform covered with a polyethylene terephthalate mesh that aims to trap thrombus and hence prevent distal embolization showed a trend towards reduced one year mortality in patients of STEMI undergoing primary PCI in the MASTER trial.[38]

EMBOLIC PROTECTION DEVICES

Embolic distal protection devices in the EMERALD and PROMISE trials did not show benefit in terms of ST resolution, final infarct size or the incidence of MACE at 6 months.[39]

GLYCOPROTEIN IIB/IIIA INHIBITORS

Glycoprotein IIB/IIIA inhibitors (GPIs) are effective and potent intravenous platelet aggregation inhibitors that have been studied in the wide spectrum of acute coronary syndrome, especially in the setting of PCI with highly thrombotic lesions; abciximab (large molecule), eptifibatide and tirofiban (small

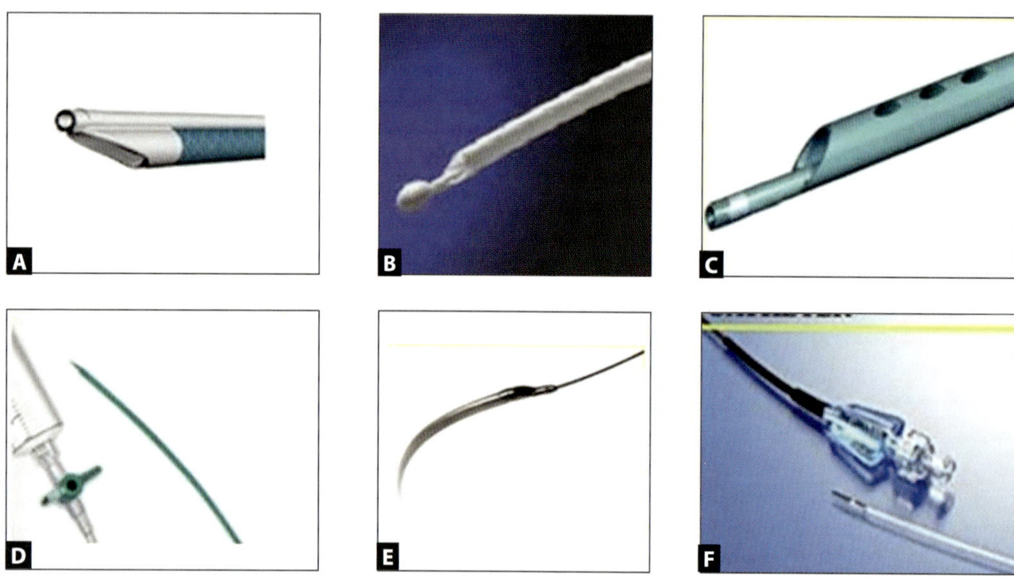

Figs 14.3A to E Commonly used thrombosuction catheters: (A) Export® catheter; (B) Pronto® catheter; (C) Diver-CE™ catheter; (D) FETCHM® catheter; (E) Eliminate™ catheter; (F) Thrombuster® catheter

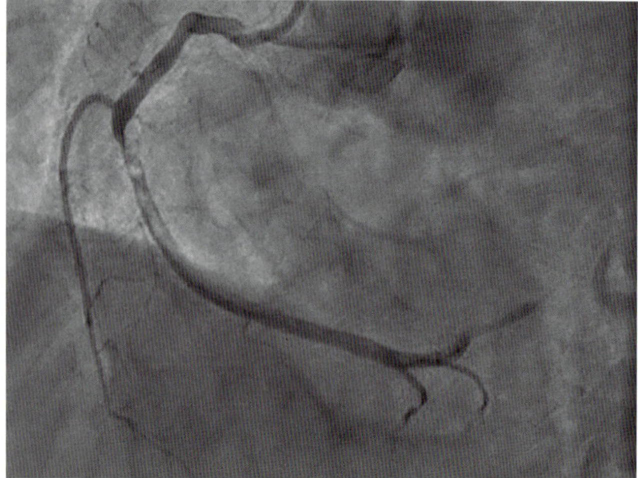

Fig. 14.4 Angiogram showing large thrombus burden in RCA with distal cutoff

molecule) are the available GPI agents.[40] The statement from the 2011 American College of Cardiology/American Heart Association/Society for Cardiovascular Angiography and Interventions (ACCF/AHA/SCAI) PCI guideline executive summary mentions that "In patients undergoing PPCI treated with UFH [unfractionated heparin], it is reasonable to administer a GP IIb/IIIa inhibitor (abciximab, double bolus eptifibatide or high bolus dose tirofiban), whether or not patients were pretreated with clopidogrel" as class IIa indication.[41] This statement has clearly put the same position for all three GPIs.

In various randomized trials in patients with acute MI, the IIb/IIIa inhibitors abciximab, eptifibatide and tirofiban improved infarct size, ST resolution, TIMI flow grade, MBG, no-reflow by cardiac magnetic resonance imaging (MRI), myocardial contrast echocardiography (MCE) perfusion score at 1 month, ejection fraction at 1 month, and left ventricular remodeling at 6 months.[42-47] GPI were particularly effective when administered in patients with initial TIMI flow grades 0/1, in the emergency room versus after PCI, and intracoronary versus intravenous.[46,47]

TIMING OF GPI ADMINISTRATION

Various trials have showed conflicting reports about the timing of administration of GPI (early or delayed). The ON-TIME 2 study (n = 984) by van't Hof et al. has further emphasized the routine (early) pre-hospital initiation of high bolus dose tirofiban to improved ST segment resolution and clinical outcome after PPCI, without increasing the bleeding risk.[45] The Leiden MISSION study (n = 179) was in favor of early in-ambulance abciximab administration and this was associated with a smaller infarct size, improved left ventricular function and a lower risk of heart failure during clinical follow-up compared to in-hospital abciximab administration. However, another study, the recently published MISTRAL trial (n = 256), failed to demonstrate a clinical benefit of

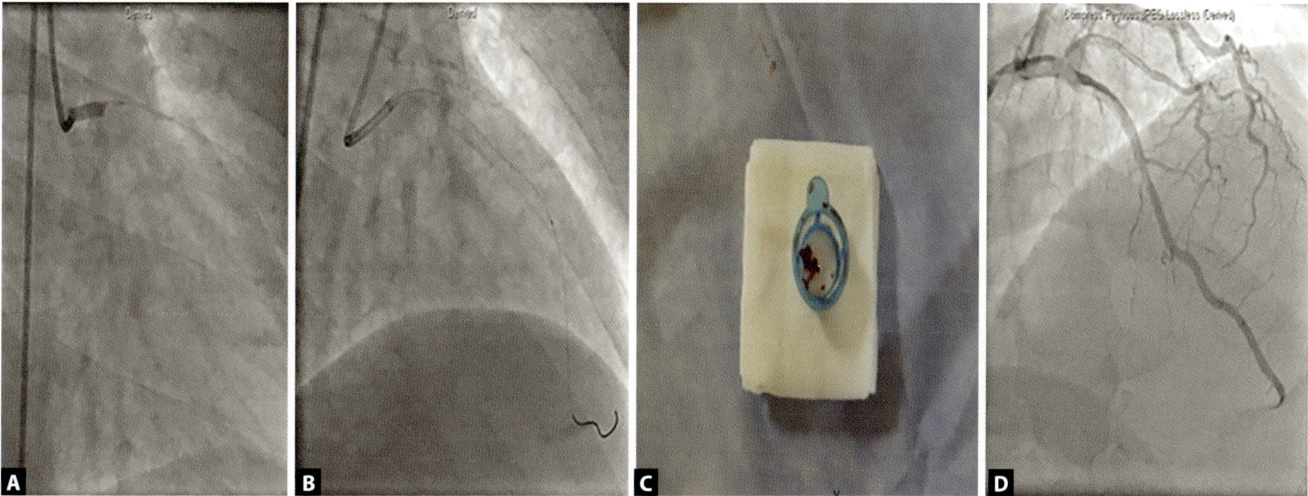

Figs 14.5A to D Thrombosuction in occluded LAD1. (A) Occluded LAD; (B) Thromosuction; (C) Clot in bowl; (D) Flowing LAD

early in-ambulance administration of abciximab in STEMI patients. Because of the conflicting results, the 2011 ACCF/AHA/SCAI PCI guideline executive summary[42] has indicated GPI administration as class III indication for routine pre-catheterization laboratory (e.g. ambulance or emergency room) as part of an upstream strategy for patients with STEMI undergoing PCI, while the recent 2012 European Society of Cardiology (ESC) guideline on STEMI has indicated it as class IIb.[12] Larger randomized trials are needed to analyze further the proper timing of GPIs.

INTRACORONARY VERSUS INTRAVENOUS GPI ADMINISTRATION

A higher local GPI concentration by intracoronary administration might disrupt platelet cross-linking, thus augmenting thrombus disaggregation forms the basis for intracoronary GPI administration. The recently published INFUSE-AMI Trial showed that infarct size at 30 days was significantly reduced by bolus intracoronary abciximab delivered to the infarct lesion site compared to the no abciximab group (p=0.03).[32] A meta-analysis of 6 randomized trials with 1246 patients reported enhanced survival with intracoronary abciximab.[48] However, the CICERO trial[49] showed no improvement in myocardial reperfusion as assessed by ST segment resolution in the intracoronary group compared to intravenous GPI administration during PPCI and the same incidence of 30 days MACE.[49] The AIDA STEMI trial found nearly identical rates of MACE with bolus and intracoronary and intravenous abciximab.[50] The recent guideline on PCI has given class IIb indication for intracoronary abciximab administration in PPCI.[41]

In conclusion GPI reduced no-reflow and improved left ventricular ejection fraction (LVEF) if administered early and via an intracoronary route.

INTRACORONARY PHARMACOTHERAPY IN PAMI

Patients with high-risk of no-reflow on the basis of the presence of predictors of reperfusion-related injury can be treated with drugs like Nicorandil, Nitroprusside, Adenosine and Verapamil.

The Clear Way Rx ™ infusion catheter (Atrium Medical, Hudson, NH-Fig. 14.6) can be used as rapid exchange on 0.014 inch coronary wire to occlude flow with balloon and contain thrombus as also to infuse drugs into the coronary artery.

Nicorandil

Nicorandil is a hybrid ATP-sensitive potassium channel opener which decreases infarct size possibly by suppressing free radical generation and by modulating neutrophil activation.[51] In an RCT by Ito et al. the frequency of sizable MCE defined no-reflow phenomenon was significantly lower in a group treated by nicorandil than in the control group (15% versus 33%, p <0.05).[52] In a larger RCT with 368 patients, intravenous nicorandil 12 mg given over 20–30 minutes prior to PPCI showed better ST-segment resolution (79.5% and 61.2%) as well as fewer events at 2.4 years of follow-up.[53] Studies have shown that intracoronary administration of nicorandil can decrease baseline index of microcirculatory resistance (IMR) and improve coronary flows in primary PCI.[54]

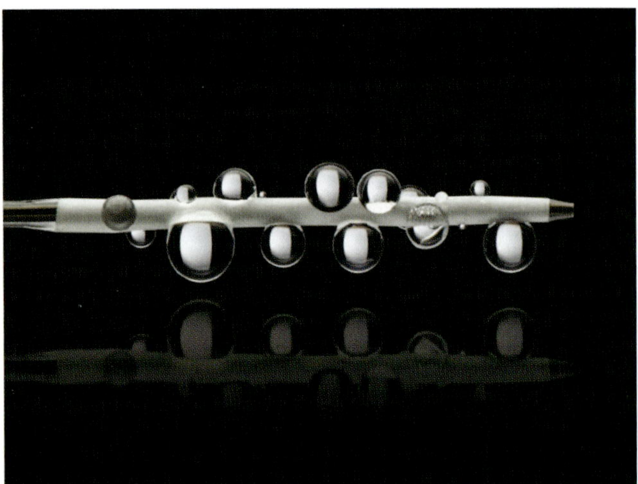

Fig. 14.6 Clearway infusion catheter™

Nitroprusside

Sodium nitroprusside is a direct nitric oxide donor and very effective microvascular vasodilator. Initial observational studies of the use of this agent for treatment of no-reflow were encouraging.[55] However, the selective injection of the drug (60 μg diluted in 5 mL as intracoronary bolus) in the IRA as primary prevention of no-reflow remains debatable since an RCT showed no improvement in ST segment resolution, myocardial blush score despite improvement in clinical outcomes at 6 months.[56] On the other hand in an observational study with 120 patients, Shinozaki et al. reported a 60% reduction in the incidence of no-reflow as well as improvement in other parameters of epicardial coronary flow.[57] A dose of 120 μg was used in this study suggesting a better effect of nitroprusside at such a higher dose, however these findings this will need to be confirmed in an adequately powered RCT.

Adenosine

Adenosine is an endogenous nucleoside mainly produced by the degradation of adenosine triphosphate, which antagonizes platelets and neutrophils, reduces calcium overload and oxygen free radicals, and induces vasodilation.[58] In a randomized trial, intracoronary administration of 4 mg of adenosine before complete vessel reopening resulted in a lower rate of no-reflow as compared with the control arm.[59] Intravenous adenosine has been tested in 2 large randomized trials (AMISTAD [Acute Myocardial Infarction Study of Adenosine] I and II).[58,59] Both studies showed a reduction of incomplete STR with a 3 hour infusion of adenosine, but in-hospital and 6-month clinical outcome were similar to those observed in the placebo group.

IC Fibrinolytics

Theoretically the postulated role of intracoronary fibrinolytics in STEMI interventions is to improve tissue level perfusion by dissolving thrombi at the micro vascular level.[60] In the pilot study Sezer et al.[60] randomized 41 STEMI patients undergoing PCI to receive either 250 kU of IC streptokinase or no additional therapy and found that the measured various indices of micro vascular function were better in the streptokinase arm at end of two days after PCI. However, the initial enthusiasm with intracoronary thrombolysis with or without PCI was met with minimal success and high complication rates.

The Delivery of thrombolytics before thrombectomy in patients with ST-segment elevation myocardial infarction undergoing primary percutaneous coronary intervention (DISSOLUTION) trial (n = 102) compared IC thrombolytic delivery (urokinase at 200,000 U) via a micro catheter prior to aspiration thrombectomy compared with IC normal saline control via micro catheter prior to aspiration thrombectomy in patients with large thrombus.[61] It showed that patients treated with IC thrombolytic up front prior to aspiration thrombectomy compared to control showed a higher rate of TIMI 3 flow (90 versus 66%; $p = 0.008$), higher rate of MBG 2 or 3 (68 versus 45%; $p = 0.028$) and higher rate of STR >70% (82 versus 55%, $p = 0.006$). It also showed a significantly lower rate of MACE at six months in the upfront IC thrombolytic group compared to control (6 versus 21%; $p = 0.044$) but this was entirely driven by a reduction in re-hospitalization for heart failure. Thrombolysis prior to thrombectomy allowed greater volume of aspirate from manual thrombectomy. Further larger randomized trials are needed to validate these findings and test safety and efficacy of IC lytics as an adjunct to PCI.

Stenting in PAMI-BMS VS DES, Newer Generation DES, Role of BVS

Stenting is recommended over plain old balloon angioplasty as class IA indication in the latest 2014 ESC/EATS guidelines on myocardial revascularization. Direct stenting and low pressure dilatation by avoiding balloon-induced thrombus fragmentation and by entrapping the atherothrombus under the stent struts has been suggested as a possible technique to reduce distal embolization. It has been shown to be superior to balloon predilatation followed by stenting irrespective of aspiration in previous studies.[62] Loubeyre and colleagues have shown that direct stenting decreases the rate of no-reflow and improves micro vascular perfusion compared to balloon predilatation followed by stenting.[62] However, only a specific subset of patients in whom good visualization of IRA occurs after guidewire passage through the culprit lesion are suitable for direct stenting.

BARE-METAL STENTS VERSUS DRUG-ELUTING STENTS

Thrombus is a major component of coronary artery occlusion in STEMI. PCI in this setting with DES could therefore theoretically increase the rate of stent thrombosis but the data on this issue are conflicting. A number of randomized clinical trials comparing first-generation DES with BMS in STEMI were conducted—most did not confirm increased mortality after DES implantation and reported reduction in repeat revascularizations.

In one of the first, MULTISTRATEGY, patients were randomized to receive Tirofiban or abciximab and subsequently sirolimus-eluting stents (SES) or BMS.[63] The number of major adverse cardiac events after 8 months was significantly lower in the SES group (7.8%) than in the BMS group (14.5%), mainly due to reduction of repeat revascularizations with comparable frequency of in-stent thrombosis. Similar results were reported in the TYPHOON study, in which 712 patients were randomized to SES or BMS.

Combined end-point consisting of death, myocardial infarction and repeat target vessel revascularization (TVR) was 7.3% in the SES group and 14.3% in the BMS group ($p = 0.004$) after 12 months of observation, similarly due to TVR reduction. The SESAMI study showed reduction of restenosis in the SES group in comparison to the BMS group (11.1 versus 15.4%; $p = 0.12$) after 12 months with no difference in the frequency of other cardiovascular incidents in 320 patients. The PASSION study compared paclitaxel-eluting stents (PES) with BMS in 619 patients with STEMI. One-year observation did not demonstrate significant differences in terms of cardiac death, myocardial infarction, repeated target lesion revascularization (TLR) or in-stent thrombosis with a preserved trend towards benefit of PES use (RR = 0.63, $p = 0.09$). The MISSION study analyzed the frequency of stent malapposition and late lumen loss after SES and BMS implantation in 310 patients with STEMI. Late lumen loss after 9 months was higher in the BMS group and stent malapposition after 12 months was more frequent in the SES group (37.5 versus 12.5%; $p < 0.001$), which however did not translate into higher frequency of cardiac incidents and led to less need for repeat revascularization (SES 2.5% versus BMS 7.9%; $p = 0.03$). Another large randomized study, DEDICATION, compared the use of DES (PES, SES, ZES) and BMS with or without distal protection in 626 patients.[64] Late lumen loss was significantly lower after DES use and the combined end-point consisting of cardiac death, myocardial infarction and TLR occurred significantly less often in the DES group (8.9 versus 14.4%; $p = 0.03$). Despite some differences in the construction of the described studies, regarding also the concomitant therapy, there was no significant difference in the number of deaths, myocardial infarctions or incidents of in-stent thrombosis between studied groups with reduction of the need for repeated revascularization (TVR or TLR) after DES use in most of these studies.

NEWER GENERATION DES

Newer generation DES include more compatible biological polymers (less pro-inflammatory or endothelium damaging) or biodegradable polymers, or do not have a polymer. They elute new substances such as everolimus, zotarolimus or biolimus.

Safety of new-generation DES (everolimus coated) in STEMI was confirmed in the EXAMINATION study (Evaluation of Xience V Stent in acute myocardial infarction). An advantage of this study was less restrictive inclusion criteria (the so-called "all comers"), so the studied group was similar to the population of patients treated on a daily basis.[65] In comparison to cobalt-chromium stents there were no differences in combined end-point (death, myocardial infarction, any repeated revascularization) with less frequent occurrence of in-stent thrombosis and repeated TLR in patients treated with everolimus-eluting stents at 1-year observation. Even more encouraging results were observed in the COMFORTABLE-AMI study (Comparison of Biomatrix Versus Gazelle in ST-Elevation Myocardial Infarction).

The 2013 meta-analysis[66] by Bangalore et al. Analyzed data from twenty-eight randomized, controlled clinical trials including 14,740 STEMI patients and 34,068 patient-years of follow-up. SES, PES and EES, compared with BMS, were associated with a reduction in rates of TVR (53%, 31% and 57%, respectively). Compared with BMS, no DES (data were unavailable for the ZES-R) were associated with an increased risk of death. There was a 64% probability that Everolimus eluting stents (EES) produced the lowest death rate compared with all other stent types.

Furthermore, compared with BMS, no DES were associated with an increased rate of MI. There was a 48% and a 44% probability that ZES-R and ZES yielded the lowest MI rate compared with all other stent types. Compared with BMS, EES were associated with a 58% reduction in the rate of any ST and 62% and 61% reductions compared with SES and PES, respectively. EES were comparable to other DES.

The ESC guidelines 2012 and ACC 2013 guidelines on the management of patients with STEMI from recommend the use of DES as class IIa indication in all patients without contraindications to prolonged use of dual antiplatelet therapy. The 2014 ESC/EATS myocardial revascularization give a class I A indication for newer generation DES over BMS in primary PCI.

The newer bioresorbable scaffold (BVS) have been evaluated in primary PCI in small non-randomized trials and the registry data from PRAGUE-19 Registry shows encouraging results. Results of ongoing randomized trial are required before they are to be used routinely in primary PCI.

PRIMARY PCI IN SPECIAL SITUATIONS: NONCULPRIT ARTERY PCI IN STEMI

The timing of revascularization of severe non-culprit vessel lesions in multivessel disease undergoing PPCI has long been debated. The ACC/AHA guidelines state definitely that PCI should not be performed in a noninfarcted artery at the time of PPCI in patients without hemodynamic compromise based on the data from the large scale contemporary and prospective international HORIZONS-AMI trial. The 2013 ACC guideline also notes a clear trend toward lower rates of adverse outcomes when PPCI is limited to infarct related artery. The ESC guidelines also state that PPCI for STEMI should be limited to the culprit lesion except in patients with cardiogenic shock. The recently published PRAMI trial[67] recruiting 485 patients concluded that a strategy of preventive PCI in non-infarcted coronary arteries with major stenosis significantly reduced risk of adverse CV events as compared with PCI limited to the infarct artery. The CvLPRIT trial of 276 patients published in 2015 showed that in patients presenting with acute STEMI index admission complete revascularization significantly lowered primary end points. However, this finding needs to be confirmed in larger adequately powered randomized clinical trials.

LEFT MAIN CORONARY ANGIOPLASTY IN PPCI

Acute left main coronary artery (LMCA) occlusion in patients with acute STEMI is a rare angiographic finding seen in 0.37 to 2.96% of patients and is associated with extensive multivessel CAD in more than 75% patients. These patients either succumbed to illness before reaching hospital or present in critical condition with cardiogenic shock or pulmonary edema, malignant arrhythmias or acute cardio respiratory arrest. ACC/AHA has no given specific guidelines in view of lack of randomized data. These patients are to be treated as STEMI with cardiogenic shock with emergency revascularization by PCI, surgery or thrombolysis with IABP support and have high mortality rates. Kalaichelvan et al.[68] have reported successful primary percutaneous thrombus aspiration alone as definitive intervention for LMCA occlusion presenting with STEMI in a case series of 3 patients.

PPCI IN THE ELDERLY PATIENT

Age is an independent predictor of mortality in STEMI. The elderly with STEMI often have significant co morbidities, absence of clear symptoms, delayed presentation, multi-vessel or calcified disease, impaired left ventricular function, and there is often a reluctance on part of the treating team to be aggressive. Benefits from PPCI are due to reduced risk of intracranial bleeding, re-ischemia and re-infarction. It is difficult to define the elderly age group with various classifications according to age, e.g. 65–70 years, young elderly 70–80 years, retired elderly 80–90 years, very elderly and >90 years, extreme elderly. Thrombolysis is associated with a very high-risk of intracranial hemorrhage making PPCI an even more beneficial alternative in octogenarian as shown in the PAMI seniors registry. There are hardly any trials involving octogenarians in STEMI and the perceived benefits are extrapolated from younger patients. It is difficult to determine how old is too old for PPCI and the interventional cardiologist should take into consideration various factors like co morbidities, family preference, mental emotional issues of the patient and quality of life issues before deciding which patient to be taken for PPCI.[69]

PPCI IN CARDIOGENIC SHOCK

STEMI with cardiogenic shock has 25–50% mortality despite the best efforts to revascularise the patient. PPCI with mechanical support, e.g.: IABP/Impella/ECMO offers the best chance of survival for these patients and hence patients with cardiogenic shock should be offered early revascularization. Current ACC/AHA guidelines carry a class I indication for primary PCI in cardiogenic shock for patients <75 years old and class IIa for patients >75 years old. Immediate transfer for cardiogenic shock or severe acute HF is a class I indication for transfer for CAG irrespective of time delay from MI onset as per the 2013 ACC/AHA STEMI guidelines.

PPCI IN CARDIAC ARREST SURVIVORS/ UNCONSCIOUS PATIENT

Likely scenarios would include 3 of the following:

1. Out of hospital cardiac arrest with successful resuscitation
2. In hospital cardiac arrest with successful resuscitation
3. STEMI with stroke.

The extent of neurological damage and the chances of cerebral recovery would ultimately determine the prognosis in such cases. It would be extremely difficult to take up for PPCI without adequate assessment of cerebral damage. Length of CPR, electrical and hemodynamic stability and neurological status would determine suitability to undergo PPCI. In patients with clear cut features of stroke it would be reasonable to defer PPCI as heparin/GPI/dual antiplatelets are likely to worsen the neurological scenario.

Patients with in hospital cardiac arrest with brief CPR having a good chance of neurological recovery can be offered PPCI if within the window of STEMI.

PPCI AT HOSPITALS WITHOUT ONSITE CARDIAC SURGERY

Performing PPCI in hospitals without onsite cardiac surgery is an alternative approach to expand the use of PPCI. Onsite cardiac surgery is required in only 2–5% of STEMI patients undergoing PPCI. PCI with stenting is the management strategy for 95–98% patients who can be benefitted by early revascularization in centers without onsite cardiac surgery but with a provision for emergency transfer facility for patients requiring surgery to a tertiary care hospital.[70] The Cardiovascular Patient Outcomes Research Team (C-PORT) trial showed a significant reduction in reinfarction with lower mortality and stroke in the primary PCI group than fibrinolysis at nonsurgical hospitals. The current ACC guidelines provides a class IIa recommendation for PPCI without onsite surgical capabilities.

CURRENT STATUS OF PRIMARY PCI IN INDIA AND CHALLENGES FOR STEMI SYSTEM OF CARE IN INDIA[71,72]

Primary PCI is the gold standard for treatment for STEMI the world over but is available to less than 10% STEMI patients in India. Data from the NIC database shows that PPCI comprises of just 17% of all interventional cardiac procedures in India in 800 interventional centers across India. Only about of half of these centers provide round the clock services and more than half of them had no surgical capability.

The most complete data about contemporary trends in STEMI patients come from CREATE, a large clinical registry of acute coronary syndrome patients from 89 large hospitals in 10 regions and cities across India.[72]

Among the more than 20,000 patients enrolled in CREATE, over 60% had STEMI a proportion that is substantially higher than in North American and European registries. STEMI patients also were younger and had a lower socioeconomic status when compared with non-STEMI patients. The median time from the onset of symptoms to hospital arrival was 300 min in STEMI patients, again more than double the delay reported in developed countries.

Finally, approximately 60% received fibrinolytic therapy and only 8% underwent percutaneous coronary intervention (PCI) during their hospitalization, suggesting substantial room for improvement in the use of acute reperfusion therapy.

There are several challenges unique to the Indian context. These include long time delay in reaching the hospital due to initial patient lack of awareness, traffic congestion/lack of transfer facilities. The third delay is possible within the tertiary care hospital due to various factors viz. finances, obtaining consent, round the clock man power and available of PCI lab in busy hours. Inadequate private and public insurance results in patients having to self finance PPCI and hence resulting in underutilization of therapy.

Despite these challenges recent clinical advances and policy changes like the development of 108/GVK EMS, state sponsored PPCI programs, development of novel integrated regional pilot projects like the Kovai-Erode/TN STEMI project which triage patients into pharmacoinvasive arms versus PPCI arms based on first medical contact to balloon times target of 90–120 minutes based from the spoke to hub hospitals have striven to improve reperfusion in STEMI. As a proof-of-concept study it was demonstrated that by linking several smaller, peripheral 'spoke' hospitals with a centrally located, PCI-capable 'hub' hospital, the use and timelines of reperfusion therapy could be improved. Encouraged by these results, now a broader 'hub-and-spoke' model in other areas of Tamil Nadu: the TN-STEMI program is being proposed (Fig. 14.7).

OCT-BASED CHARACTERIZATION OF PLAQUE MORPHOLOGY IN MANAGEMENT OF STEMI

Occlusive luminal thrombosis is the mechanism underlying most acute coronary syndromes (ACS). As many as 75% of autopsy studies after fatal ACS relate thrombotic occlusion to atherosclerotic plaque rupture; most of the remainder involve plaque erosion. Less common mechanisms involve thrombosis of a calcified nodule.[73] Atherosclerotic lesions associated with plaque rupture may produce hemodynamically significant obstruction and typically contain a large necrotic core beneath a ruptured fibrous cap (RFC) that is attenuated and inflamed (Figs 14.8 and 14.9).

Discontinuity of the fibrous cap brings circulating platelets into contact with the highly thrombogenic plaque core, leading to acute thrombus formation that occludes the arterial lumen. In contrast, erosion of plaque rich in proteoglycans and smooth muscle cells predisposes to thrombus formation over an intact fibrous cap (IFC). Because the pathogenesis of ACS in patients with an RFC differs from that in patients with an IFC, it is possible that clinical management of these 2 groups of patients may differ.

Intracoronary optical coherence tomography (OCT) provides superior resolution (10–15 m), allowing more detailed analysis of plaque morphology,[74] including discriminating IFC from RFC in patients with ACS.

Plaque rupture and plaque erosion in the culprit lesions of patients with ACS can be distinguished as discrete syndromes on the basis of an RFC (ACS-RFC) and IFC (ACS-IFC).[74]

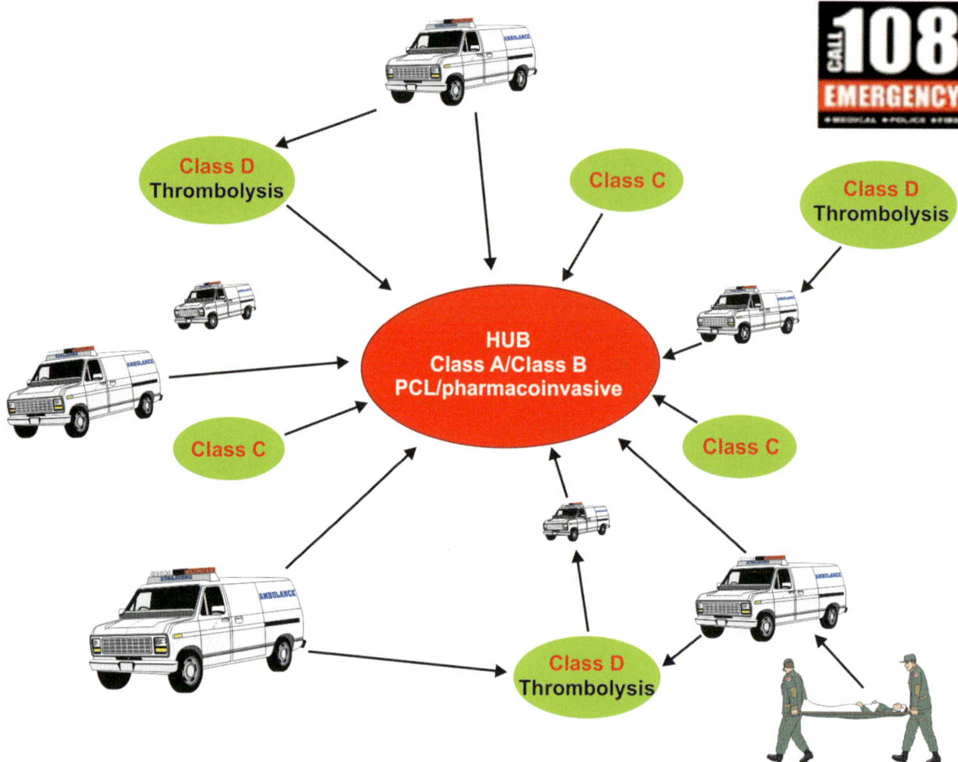

Fig. 14.7 Spoke and hub model of TN STEMI program

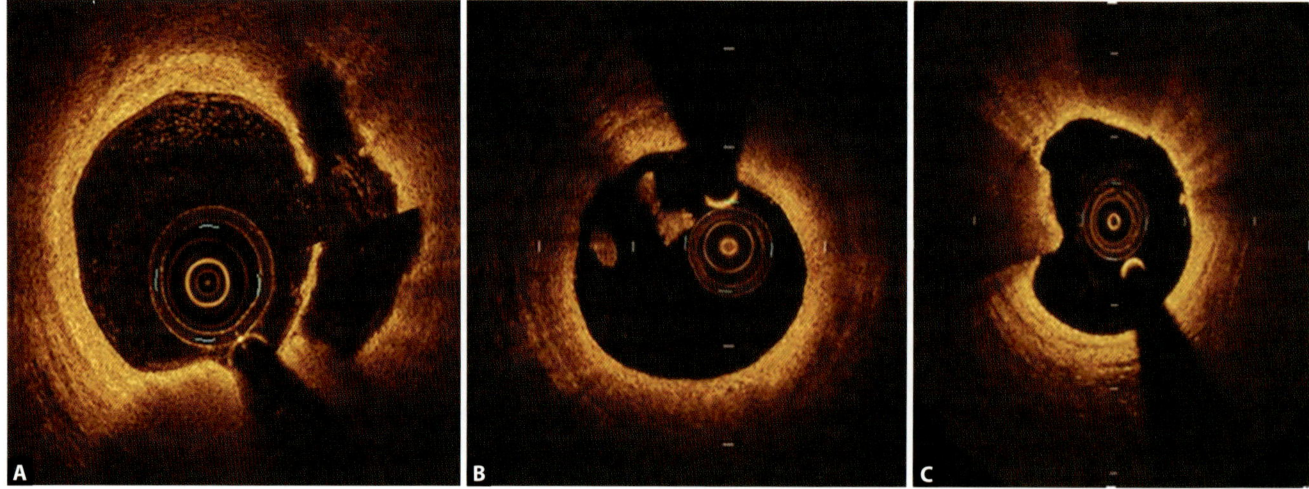

Figs 14.8A to C OCT-based characterization of plaque morphology in STEMI. (A) Ruture plaque; (B) Plaque erosion; (C) Calcific nodule

Plaque erosion is an entity distinct from plaque rupture.[73,74] Most erosive lesions are devoid of necrotic core, and, when present, the core does not communicate with the lumen because of a thick fibrous cap. Such lesions have been reported in younger individuals, including premenopausal women, with smoking as the most prevalent risk factor. Many of these lesions display relatively minor luminal narrowing, and thrombus removal without balloon dilation or stent implantation may be sufficient to restore vessel patency. The luminal thrombosis in plaque erosion has been attributed

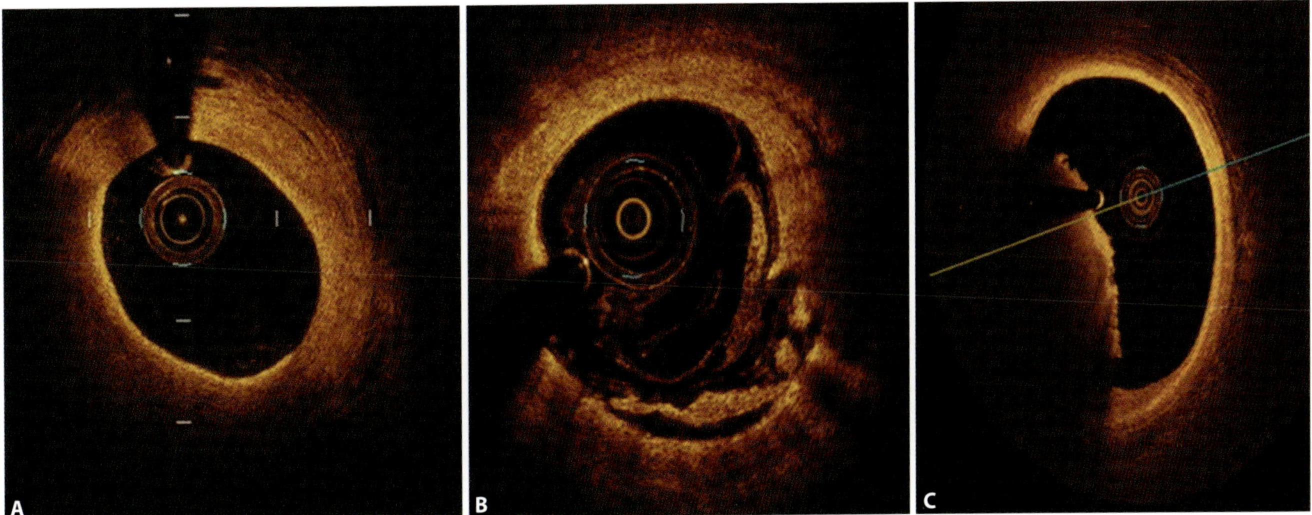

Figs 14.9A to C OCT characterization of plaque and thrombus, (A) TCFA; (B) White thrombus; (C) Red thrombus

to apoptosis or degradation of endothelial cells lining the plaque surface.

Therefore, after thrombus removal, treatment with antiplatelet drugs may allow healing of the endothelial layer. The mechanisms involved may be similar to re-endothelial ization after stent implantation. Avoiding stent deployment could potentially reduce the risks of both early (dissection, embolism, occlusive thrombosis) and late (restenosis, neoatherosclerosis, thrombosis) complications. Prati et al.[75] in their provocative series of 31 patients who underwent thrombus aspiration for STEMI and then had an OCT to document IFC showed that TLR, re MI and HF in the group that was not stented and managed medically was same as the group that was stented.

They demonstrated in a limited number of patients with ACS that characterization of plaque morphology by OCT could identify non obstructive lesions amenable to treatment with an antiplatelet strategy alone, without angioplasty or coronary stent deployment, and result in satisfactory clinical outcomes. The clinical benefits of routine OCT during STEMI have not been properly established. OCT might provide valuable data before and after the procedure, mostly related to vessel size, plaque morphology, plaque protrusion, residual dissections, and adequate stent-vessel wall apposition. Adding routine OCT to every single STEMI to look for erosion will increase procedural time, with the risk of increasing complications in this group of potentially unstable patients. The risk/benefit ratio of doing routine OCT to identify plaque erosion (<15% of STEMI lesions) and treating them with thrombosuction alone is controversial.[76]

Randomized trials will be needed, however, to clarify the role of aspiration thrombectomy and catheter-directed lytic therapy without stent implantation in cases of OCT-verified ACS-IFC and further evaluate the long-term outcomes of an alternative management strategy for such unique cause of ACS.

CONCLUSION

The prognosis and outcomes of patients developing STEMI can be markedly improved with timely reperfusion therapy. Primary PCI with appropriate use of thrombosuction, stents with adequate platelet inhibition is the best strategy in the management of Acute STEMI. Outcomes can be improved by creating patient awareness along with rapid triage/transport to appropriately equipped and staffed PCI capable hospitals. Access to primary angioplasty can also be expanded by allowing appropriately trained centers to perform PPCI without onsite surgical backup and instituting systematic transfer of patients to tertiary centers. The major challenge is to make primary angioplasty available to the general population in a cost effective and timely manner with development of infrastructure, increasing awareness and strategies to reduce door to balloon time. The need for development of regional integrated care for STEMI is therefore of paramount importance.

REFERENCES

1. Falk E, Shah AC, Fuster V. Coronary plaque disruption. Circulation. 1995;92:657-71.
2. Weawer WD, Simes RJ, Betriu A, Grines CL, Zijlstra F, Garcia E, et al. Comparison of primary coronary angioplasty and intravenous thrombolytic therapy for acute myocardial infarction: A quantitative review. JAMA. 1997;278:2093-8.

3. Keeley EC, Boura JA, Grines CL. Primary angioplasty versus Thrombolytic therapy for acute myocardial infarction: A quantitative review of 23 randomized trials. Lancet. 2003;361:13-20.
4. Eagle KA, Goodman SG, Avezum A, et al. Practice variation and missed opportunities for reperfusion in ST-segment-elevation myocardial infarction: findings from the Global Registry of Acute Coronary Events (GRACE). Lancet. 2002;359:373-7.
5. Van de Werf F, Bax J, Betriu A, et al. Management of acute myocardial infarction in patients presenting with persistent ST segment elevation: the Task Force on the Management of ST Segment Elevation Acute Myocardial Infarction of the European Society of Cardiology. Eur Heart J. 2008;29:2909-45.
6. The GUSTO Investigators. The effects of tissue plasminogen activator, streptokinase, or both on coronary-artery patency, ventricular function, and survival after acute myocardial function. N Engl J Med. 1993;329:1615-22.
7. Pakshirajan B, Vijaykumar S, Ajit S Mullasari. Pharmaco Invasive Management in STEMI Intervent Cardiol Clin. 2012.pp.409-19.
8. Ndrepepa G, Mehilli J, Schulz S, et al. Prognostic significance of Epicardial blood flow before and after percutaneous coronary intervention in patients with acute coronary syndromes. J Am Coll Cardiol. 2008;52:512-7.
9. Anderson JL, Karagounis LA, Califf RM. Meta-analysis of five reported studies on the relation of early coronary patency grades with mortality and outcomes after acute myocardial infarction. Am J Cardiol. 1996;78:1-8.
10. Grines CM, Ellis S, Jones M, et al. Primary coronary angioplasty versus thrombolytic therapy for acute myocardial infarction. Long term follow-up of ten randomized controlled trials. Circulation. 1999;100:1-499.
11. O'Gara PT, Kushner FG, Ascheim DD, Casey DE Jr, Chung MK, de Lemos JA, et al. 2013 ACCF/AHA guideline for the management of ST-elevation myocardial infarction: a report of the American College of Cardiology Foundation/American Heart Association Task Force on Practice Guidelines. Circulation. 2013;127:1-88.
12. Steg PG, James SK, Atar D, Blömstrom-Lundqvist C, Borger MA, Di Mario C, et al. 2012 ESC guidelines for the management of acute myocardial infarction in patients presenting with ST segment elevation. Eur Heart J. 2012;33:2569-619.
13. Nielsen PH, Maeng M, Busk M, et al. Primary angioplasty versus fibrinolysis in acute myocardial infarction, long-term follow-up in the Danish Acute Myocardial Infarction 2 trial. Circulation. 2010;121:1484-91.
14. Steg PG, Bonnefoy E, Chabaud S, et al. Impact of time to treatment on mortality after prehospital fibrinolysis or primary angioplasty: data from the CAPTIM randomized clinical trial. Circulation. 2003;108:2851-6.
15. Widimsky´ P, Budesı´nsky´ T, Vora´c D, et al, 'PRAGUE' Study Group Investigators. Long distance transport for primary angioplasty vs. immediate thrombolysis in acute myocardial infarction: final results of the randomized national multicenter trial 'PRAGUE-2'.Eur Heart J. 2003;23:94-104.
16. Nallamothu BK, Bates ER. Percutaneous coronary intervention versus fibrinolytic therapy in acute myocardial infarction: is timing (almost) everything? Am J Cardiol. 2003;92:824-6.
17. Jaffe R, Charron T, Puley G, Dick A, Strauss BH. Micro vascular obstruction and the no reflow phenomenon after percutaneous coronary intervention. Circulation. 2008;117:3152-6.
18. Reffelmann T, Kloner RA. The "no-reflow" phenomenon: basic science and clinical correlates. Heart. 2002;87:162-8.
19. Yip HK, Chen MC, Chang HW, Hang CL, Hsieh YK, Fang CY, et al. Angiographic morphologic features of infarct-related arteries and timely reperfusion in acute myocardial infarction: predictors of slow-flow and no-reflow phenomenon. Chest. 2002;122: 1322-32.
20. Sianos G, Papafaklis MI, Daemen J, Vaina S, van Mieghem CA, van Domburg RT, et al. Angiographic stent thrombosis after routine use of drug-eluting stents in ST-segment elevation myocardial infarction: the importance of thrombus burden. J Am Coll Cardiol. 2007;50:573-83.
21. Dharma S, Kedev S, Jukema JW. Thrombus management in the catheterization laboratory in the setting of primary percutaneous coronary intervention: what is the current evidence. Heart. 2013;99:279-84.
22. Burzotta F, Trani C, Romagnoli E, Mazzari MA, RebuzziAG,De Vita M et al. Manual thrombus aspiration improves myocardial reperfusion: the randomized evaluation of the effect of mechanical reduction of distal embolization by thrombus-aspiration in primary and rescue angioplasty (REMEDIA) trial. J Am Coll Cardiol. 2005;46:371-6.
23. Svilaas T, Vlaar PJ, van der Horst IC, Diercks GF, de Smet BJ, van den Heuvel AF, et al. Thrombus aspiration during primary percutaneous coronary intervention. N Engl J Med. 2008;358: 557-67.
24. Vlaar PJ, Svilaas T, van der Horst IC, Diercks GF, Fokkema ML, de Smet BJ, et al. Cardiac death and reinfarction after 1 year in the Thrombus aspiration during Percutaneous Coronary Intervention in Acute Myocardial Infarction Study (TAPAS): a 1-year follow-up study. Lancet. 2008;371:1915-20.
25. Stephan W, Philippe K, Fernando A, et al. 2014 ESC/EATS guidelines of myocardial revascularization. Eur Heart J. 2014 1;35(37):2541-619.
26. De Luca G, Dudek D, Sardella G, Marino P, Chevalier B, Zijlstra F. Adjunctive manual thrombectomy improves myocardial perfusion and mortality in patients undergoing primary percutaneous coronary intervention for ST-elevation myocardial infarction: a meta-analysis of randomized trials. Eur Heart J. 2008;29:3002-10.
27. Mongeon FP, Belisle P, Joseph L, Eisenberg MJ, Rinfret S. Adjunctive thrombectomy for acute myocardial infarction: A Bayesian meta-analysis. Circ Cardiovasc Interv. 2010;3:6-16.
28. Bavry AA, Kumbhani DJ, Bhatt DL. Role of adjunctive thrombectomy and embolic protection devices in acute myocardial infarction: a comprehensive meta-analysis of randomized trials. Eur Heart J. 2008;29:2989-3001.
29. Burzotta F, De Vita M, Gu YL, Isshiki T, Lefèvre T, Kaltoft A, et al. Clinical impact of thrombectomy in acute ST-elevation myocardial infarction: an individual patient-data pooled analysis of 11 trials. Eur Heart J. 2009;30:2193-203.
30. Sardella G, Mancone M, Bucciarelli-Ducci C, Agati L, Scardala R, Carbone I, et al. Thrombus aspiration during primary percutaneous coronary intervention improves myocardial reperfusion and reduces infarct size: the EXPIRA (thrombectomy with export catheter in infarct-related artery during primary percutaneous coronary intervention) prospective, randomized trial. J Am Coll Cardiol. 2009;53(4): 309-15.

31. Stone GW, Maehara A, Witzenbichler B, GodlewskiJ, Parise H, Dambrink JH, et al. INFUSE-AMI Investigators. Intracoronary Abciximab and aspiration thrombectomy in patients with large anterior Myocardial infarction: the INFUSE-AMI randomized trial. JAMA. 2012;307:1817-26.
32. Inaba Y, Chen JA, Mehta N, Bergmann SR. Impact of single or multicenter study design on the results of trials examining the efficacy of adjunctive devices to prevent distal embolization during acute myocardial infarction. Euro Intervention. 2009;5:375-383.
33. Frobert O, Lagerqvist B, Olivecrona GK, et al. Thrombus aspiration during ST segment elevation myocardial infarction. N Engl J Med. 2013;369:1587-97.
34. Lagerqvist B, Frobert O, Olivecrona GK, et al. Outcomes 1 year after Thrombus aspiration for Myocardial infarction. N Engl J Med. 2013;371:1111-20.
35. Jolly SS, Cairns JA, Yusuf S, et al. Randomized trial of Primary PCI with or without routine manual thrombectomy. N Engl J Med. 2015;372:1389-98.
36. Colin Berry, Matthew Lee, Nadeem Ahmed. Thrombus aspiration during myocardial infarction. N Engl J Med. 2013;370:674.
37. Kumbhani DJ, Bavry AA, Desai MY, et al. Role of aspiration and mechanical thrombectomy in patients with acute myocardial infarction undergoing primary angioplasty: an updated meta-analysis of randomized trials. J Am Coll Cardiol. 2013;62: 1409-18.
38. Dariusz Dudek, Artur Dziewierz, Sorin J. Brener, et al. Mesh-covered embolic protection stent implantation in ST-segment-elevation myocardial infarction. Circulation: Cardiovascular Interventions. 2015;8:e001484.
39. Stone GW, Webb J, Cox DA, Brodie BR, Qureshi M, Kalynych A, et al. Distal microcirculatory protection during percutaneous coronary intervention in acute ST segment elevation myocardial infarction: a randomized controlled trial. JAMA. 2005;293: 1063-72.
40. Boersma E, Harrington RA, Moliterno DJ, White H, Théroux P, Van de Werf F, et al. Platelet glycoprotein IIb/IIIa inhibitors in acute coronary syndromes: a meta-analysis of all major randomized clinical trials. Lancet. 2002;359:189-98.
41. Levine GN, Bates ER, Blankenship JC, Bailey SR, Bittl JA, Cercek B, et al. 2011 ACCF/AHA/SCAI guideline for percutaneous coronary intervention: executive summary. A report of the American College of Cardiology Foundation/American Heart Association Heart Association Task Force on Practice Guidelines and the Society for Cardiovascular Angiography and Interventions. J Am Coll Cardiol. 2011;58:e44-122.
42. de Lemos JA, Antman EM, Gibson CM, McCabe CH, Giugliano RP, Murphy SA, et al. Abciximab improves both epicardial flow and Myocardial reperfusion in ST elevation myocardial infarction. Observations from the TIMI 14 trial. Circulation. 2000;101:239-43.
43. Petronio AS, De CM, Ciabatti N, Amoroso G, Limbruno U, Palagi C, et al. Left ventricular remodeling after primary coronary angioplasty in patients treated with abciximab or intracoronary adenosine. Am Heart J. 2005;150:1015.
44. Gibson CM, Morrow DA, Murphy SA, Palabrica TM, Jennings LK, Stone PH, et al. A randomized trial to evaluate the relative protection Against post-percutaneous coronary intervention micro vascular dysfunction, ischemia, and inflammation among antiplatelet and antithrombotic agents: the PROTECT-TIMI-30 trial. J Am Coll Cardiol. 2006;47:2364-73.
45. Van't Hof AW, ten Berg J, Heestermans T, Dill T, Funck RC, van Werkum W, et al. Prehospital initiation of tirofiban in patients with ST-elevation myocardial infarction undergoing primary angioplasty (On-TIME2): a multicentre, double blind, randomized controlled trial. Lancet. 2008;372:537-46.
46. Thiele H, Schindler K, Friedenberger J, Eitel I, Furnau G, Grebe E, et al. Intracoronary compared with intravenous bolus abciximab application in patients with ST-elevation myocardial infarction undergoing primary percutaneous coronary intervention: the randomized Leipzig immediate percutaneous coronary intervention abciximab IV versus IC in ST-elevation myocardial infarction trial. Circulation. 2008;118:49-57.
47. Maioli M, Bellandi F, Leoncini M, Toso A, Dabizzi RP. Randomized Early versus late abciximab in acute myocardial infarction treated with primary coronary intervention (RELAX-AMI Trial). J Am Coll Cardiol. 2007;49:1517-24.
48. Navarese EP, Kozinski M, Obonska K, Margheri M, Gurbel PA, Kubica J, et al. Clinical efficacy and safety of intracoronary vs. intravenous abciximab administration in STEMI patients undergoing primary percutaneous coronary intervention: a meta-analysis of randomized trials. Platelets. 2012;23:274-81
49. Gu YL, Kampinga MA, Wieringa WG, Fokkema ML, Nijsten MW, Hillege HL, et al. Intracoronary versus intravenous administration of abciximab in patients with ST-segment elevation myocardial infarction undergoing primary percutaneous coronary intervention with thrombus aspiration: the comparison of intracoronary versus intravenous abciximab administration during emergency reperfusion of ST-segment elevation myocardial infarction (CICERO) trial. Circulation. 2010;122:2709-17.
50. Thiele H, Wöhrle J, Hambrecht R, Rittger H, Birkemeyer R, Lauer B, et al. Intracoronary versus intravenous bolus abciximab during primary percutaneous coronary intervention in patients with acute ST-elevation myocardial infarction: a randomized trial. Lancet. 2012;379:923-31.
51. Ohno Y, Minatoguchi S, Uno Y, Kariya T, Arai M, Yamashita K, et al. Nicorandil reduces myocardial infarct size by opening the K (ATP) channel in rabbits. Int J Cardiol. 1997;62:181-90.
52. Ito H, Taniyama Y, Iwakura K,Nishikawa N, Masuyama T, Kuzuya T et al. Intravenous nicorandil can preserve micro vascular integrity and myocardial viability in patients with reperfused anterior wall myocardial infarction. J Am Coll Cardiol. 1999;33:654-60.
53. Ishii H, Ichimiya S, Kanashiro M. Impact of a single intravenous administration of nicorandil before reperfusion in patients with ST-segment-elevation myocardial infarction. Circulation. 2005;112:1284-8.
54. Ito N, Nanto S, Doi Y, Sawano H. High index of Microcirculatory resistance level After Successful Primary Percutaneous Coronary Intervention Can Be Improved by Intracoronary administration of Nicorandil. Circulation J. 2010;74:909-15.
55. Pasceri V, Pristipino C, Pelliccia F,Granatelli A, Speciale G, Roncella A, et al. Effects of the nitric oxide donor nitroprusside on no-reflow phenomenon during coronary interventions for acute myocardial. Am J Cardiol. 2005;95:1358-61.
56. Amit G, Cafri C, Yaroslavtsev S. Intracoronary nitroprusside for the prevention of the no-reflow phenomenon after primary

percutaneous coronary intervention in acute myocardial infarction. A randomized, double-blind, placebo-controlled clinical trial. Am Heart J. 2006;152:887 e9-14.

57. Shinozaki N, Ichinose H, Yahikozawa K, Shimada H, Hoshino K. elective intracoronary administration of nitroprusside before balloon dilatation prevents slow reflow during. 2007;48:423-33.
58. Marzilli M, Orsini E, Marraccini P, Testa R. Beneficial effects of intracoronary adenosine as an adjunct to primary angioplasty in acute myocardial infarction. Circulation. 2000;101:2154-9.
59. Mahaffey KW, Puma JA, Barbagelata NA, DiCarli MF, Leesar MA, Browne KF, et al. Adenosine as an adjunct to thrombolytic therapy for acute myocardial infarction: results of a multicenter, randomized, placebo-controlled trial: the Acute Myocardial Infarction Study of Adenosine (AMISTAD) trial. J Am Coll Cardiol. 1999;34:1711-20
60. Sezer M, Olfaz H, Goren T, et al. Intracoronary streptokinase after primary PCI. N Engl Med. 2007;356:1823-34.
61. Greco C, et al. Usefulness of local delivery of thrombolytics before thrombectomy in patients with ST-segment elevation myocardial infarction undergoing primary percutaneous coronary intervention (the delivery of thrombolytics before thrombectomy in patients with ST-segment elevation myocardial infarction undergoing primary percutaneous coronary intervention [DISSOLUTION] randomized trial). AM J Cardiol. 2013;112:630-5.
62. Loubeyre C, Morice MC, Lefevre T, Piéchaud JF, Louvard Y, Dumas P. A randomized comparison of direct stenting with conventional stent implantation in selected patients with acute myocardial infarction. J Am Coll Cardiol. 2002;39:15-21.
63. Valgimigli M, Campo G, Percoco G, et al. Comparison of angioplasty with infusion of tirofiban or abciximab and with implantation of sirolimus-eluting or uncoated stents for acute myocardial infarction: the MULTISTRATEGY randomized trial. JAMA. 2008;299:1788-99.
64. Kelbaek H, Thuesen L, Helquist S, et al. Drug-eluting versus bare metal stents in patients with ST-segment-elevation myocardial infarction: eight-month follow-up in the Drug Elution and Distal Protection in Acute Myocardial Infarction (DEDICATION) trial. Circulation. 2008;118:1155-62.
65. Sabate M, Cequier A, Iniguez A, et al. Rationale and design of the EXAMINATION trial: a randomized comparison between everolimus eluting stents and cobalt-chromium bare-metal stents in ST-elevation myocardial infarction. Euro intervention. 2011;7:977-84.
66. Sripal Bangalore, Nicholas S, Mario F et al. Outcomes with various Drug eluting or bare metal stents in patients with STEMI. Circ Cardiovas Interv. 2013;6:1-14.
67. David S Wald, Alexander J C, Richard J E et al. Randomized trial of preventive angioplasty in myocardial infarction. N Eng J Med. 2013;369(12):1115-23.
68. Kalaichelvan U, Vijaykumar S, Balaji P, et al. Primary percutaneous thrombus aspiration alone as definitive intervention for left main coronary artery occlusion presenting as acute anterior wall STEMI. Heart Lung Circulation. 2014;23:166-170.
69. Patel M, Jeremias A. Primary Angioplasty in the very elderly-how old is too old? J Invasive Cardiol. 2010.pp.479-480.
70. Stone W, Brodie BR, Griffin JJ, et al. The role of cardiac surgery in the hospital phase management of patients treated with primary angioplasty for acute myocardial infarction. Am J Cardiol. 2000;85:1292-6.
71. Alexander T, Mehta S, Mullasari A, Nallamothu BK. Systems of care for ST-elevation myocardial infarction in India. Heart. 2012;98:15e17.
72. Xavier D, Pais P, Devereaux PJ, et al, CREATE Registry Investigators. Treatment and outcomes of acute coronary syndromes in India (CREATE): a prospective analysis of registry data. Lancet. 2008;371:1435-42.
73. Burke AP, Farb A, Malcom GT, LiangYH, Smialek J, Virmani R. Coronary risk factors and plaque morphology in men with coronary disease who died suddenly. N Engl J Med. 1997;336:1276-82.
74. Ozaki Y, Okumura M, Ismail TF, et al. Coronary CT angiographic characteristics of culprit lesions in acute coronary syndromes not related to plaque rupture as defined by optical coherence tomography and angioscopy. Eur Heart J. 2011;32:2814-23.
75. Prati F, Uemura S, Souteyrand G, et al. OCT-based diagnosis and management of STEMI associated with intact fibrous cap. J Am Coll Cardiol Img. 2013;6:283-7.
76. David R. Holmes J, Amir Lerman, Pedro R. Moreno,Spencer B. King III, MD, Samin K. Sharma, MD Diagnosis and Management of STEMI Arising From Plaque Erosion. JACC CV imaging. 2013;3:283-7.

CHAPTER

15

Complications in Coronary Angioplasty

Vilas P Magarkar

INTRODUCTION

Percutaneous transluminal coronary angioplasty (PTCA) is becoming increasingly safer due to ongoing improvements in the hardware and improving skills in the operating staff. PTCA is now well-accepted interventional procedure, among the general population, thanks to continuous medical education, increased awareness about the safety and efficacy of the procedure and wide spread availability of skilled interventional cardiologists. It is nowadays relatively safer procedure, except few complex substrates. In spite of all this success stories of PTCA, the complications are inevitable to some extent. It is necessary to know the likely complications, anticipate them, to prevent them and to manage them. Treatment of the complications should be in the cath lab as far as possible, as most of the issues can be solved in the cath lab itself. If required, the help of cardiovascular surgeon or other specialties can be taken in the best interest of the patient. PTCA has the ability to relieve symptoms in chronic ischemic heart disease and alter the natural history in acute coronary syndromes. Adverse procedural outcomes, known as complications, can occur as a direct result of intervention itself. Complication can happen despite the application of best practices and result in unsatisfactory clinical outcomes. Operator can predict the patients at risk for complications but still those can happen due to human error and system failure.[1]

PROCEDURAL COMPLICATION CATEGORIES[2,3]

- Nonfatal myocardial infarction (related to the procedure regardless of mechanism)
- Ischemia, requiring emergency bypass surgery
- Coronary perforation and tamponade
- No flow, dissection
- Air embolism
- Side branch closure
- Arrhythmias
- Stroke
- Vascular access site complications
- Contrast-induced nephropathy
- Excessive blood loss requiring blood transfusion
- Death
- Acute and subacute stent thrombosis
- Retained equipment
- Sepsis.

Contemporary Complications Rates for Percutaneous Coronary Intervention (PCI)[4]

Taken from NY state PCI registry mention in detail in Table 15.1 and Fig. 15.1.

IMPORTANT TIPS BEFORE GOING FOR PERCUTANEOUS TRANSLUMINAL CORONARY ANGIOPLASTY

- Any intervention, however easy, it appears to be, should have a clear indication that justifies the risk, no matter how small it is. Avoiding an unnecessary procedure may, in turn, avoid the complication.[7]
- Assessment should be done to judge the feasibility of PTCA, based on combination of individualized risk benefit analysis, lesion technical and patient comorbid characteristics.
- The key point is to plan strategy as much as possible before starting.
- Patients' clinical characteristics should be assessed. Advanced age, urgent intervention, diabetes mellitus, electrolyte imbalance, severe LV dysfunction, peripheral vascular disease and arrhythmias are patients' characteristic with more likelihood of complications.

Table 15.1 Complications of percutaneous coronary intervention

Complication	*Rate (n = 23,339 procedures)*
Death one month	0.6
Death in catheter laboratory	0.047
Stroke	0.29
Cardiac perforation	0.29
Acute myocardial infarction	0.74
Emergent surgery	0.15
Stent thrombosis <1 month	0.53
Renal failure	0.28
Hemodialysis	0.17
Retroperitoneal bleed	0.18
Vascular complication or bleeding	0.79
Any complication	3.36

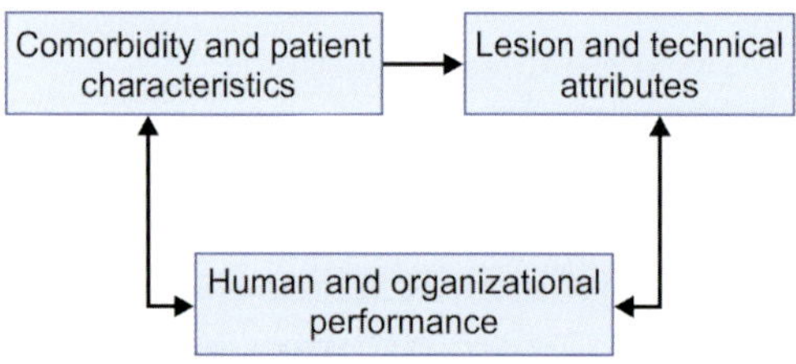

Fig. 15.1 Simplified conceptual framework for the genesis of PCI complications[5,6]

VASCULAR COMPLICATIONS

Prediction of vascular access-related complications is important. Following are the substrates who are prone for vascular complications.

Female gender, advanced age, small body surface area, prior instrumentation, anticoagulation, peripheral vascular disease, diabetes mellitus, suboptimal technique of puncture and closure are the risk predictors.

Vascular access is either femoral or radial. Nowadays there is increased trend toward radial access, in view of early mobilization and less hemorrhagic complications, atleast in severe obesity, chronic obstructive pulmonary disease, primary PTCA. Results from the radius versus femoral percutaneous coronary intervention access in unstable angina or MI (RIVAL) randomized control trial comparing femoral and radial access have shown clear mortality benefit in primary PCI subgroup with radial approach (Fig. 15.1).[8]

How to Reduce Transfemoral Access Complications?

- Access using fluoroscopy (or ultrasound)
- Puncture site or below centerline of the femoral head
- Femoral angiogram [right anterior oblique (RAO) 30° and left anterior oblique (LAO) 60°] prior to closure
- PCI and anticoagulate only if the 'safe zone' (elective patients).

Complications from Femoral Access for PCI

- Retroperitoneal hemorrhage
- Pseudoaneurysm
- AV fistula
- Infection
- Hematoma
- Neuropraxia
- Lower limb ischemia (thrombosis or embolism)
- Dissection.

Reported Complications from Transradial Access for PCI

- Vasospasm
- Pseudoaneurysm
- Puncture site granuloma
- Dissection
- Perforation/forearm or chest wall hematoma
- Compartment syndrome.

How to Reduce Transradial Access Complications?

- Hydration and anxiolysis
- Vessel 'cocktail' (usually calcium channel antagonist and/or nitrate)
- Heparin (at least 3-5,000 units)
- Avoid puncture through the flexor retinaculum
- Perfusion hemostasis.

Management of Femoral Vascular Complications

Acute Ischemia

Arterial thrombosis or embolism of the femoral artery is a limb threatening complication. Any sign of acute limb ischemia (pulseless, pale, painful, paresthetic foot) should prompt emergency referral to a vascular surgeon for assessment.

Hematoma

The most common complication encountered is that of a hematoma. This is a palpable mass over the puncture site and must be distinguished from ecchymosis. Management consists of manual or mechanical compression. Ultrasound examination is mandatory if there is persistent discomfort or audible bruit.

Retroperitoneal Hemorrhage (RPH)

A large (>110,000 patients) cotemporary retrospective analysis, informs us that this complication is uncommon after PTCA and its incidence is <0.1%. Although associated with high femoral puncture, sometimes, it can occur with ideally situated punctures owing to movement of blood along the fascial planes.[9] They typically present within 3 hours of the index procedure and should be suspected if there is recurrent hypotension (in association with bradycardia or tachycardia), flank or abdominal pain ipsilateral to the puncture site following PCI. Initially management is with fluid resuscitation and only once the patient is stable, should definitely in the form of a CT pelvis/abdomen be undertaken. The vast majority (>90%) of RPH is managed conservatively, however, there is a significant mortality (6%) compared with those without this complication.[10] Although medical management is common, recurrent clinical signs of hypovolemia and/or radiographic signs of active extravasation merit surgical consultation with a view to open exploration or interventional therapy, including the deployment of a covered stent via contralateral femoral artery.

Pseudoaneurysm

Pseudoaneurysms are the result of punctures that fail to heal completely leaving a cap of hematoma over the puncture site. These frequently involve punctures below the femoral bifurcation as they can be difficult to compress effectively post procedure. They are typically tender, pulsatile and expansile and have an audible bruit. However, the latter depends on the position of the defect, with posterior or lateral pseudoaneurysms frequently being silent. Management consists of manual compression with an ultrasound and administration of opiate analgesia. If unsuccessful and an accessible track can be located to the neck of the aneurysm, then ultrasound fibrin injection to thrombose the neck is commonly undertaken.

Arteriovenous Fistulae

Arteriovenous fistulae are uncommon iatrogenic complication comprising <1% of transfemoral cardiac catheterizations. Prospective large-scale cohort analysis (n = 10,272) identifies left femoral puncture (with right-handed operators), female gender, intensity of anticoagulation (warfarin and heparin) and hypertension as predictive factors.[11] Puncture below the common femoral bifurcation may provide an anatomical substrate as at this level the femoral vein lies posterior to the superficial femoral artery rather than medial. These complications are not associated with limb injury, symptoms or right heart failure (owing to universally low associated shunt volumes <500 mL/min). More than one third close spontaneously within a year, and so despite a number of invasive solutions (e.g. covered stent deployment and open surgery), an initial conservative approach with ultrasound-guided compression is supported by the observational data.

Neuropraxia

Neuralgic complications involving the femoral nerve can be very symptomatic but non life threatening but have a good prognosis. They are always neuropraxias rather than transections and so will heal, late most by six months.

Infection

This complication is very rarely seen. It occurs at the site of vascular access, particularly in presence of failure of aseptic precautions and baseline local skin problems. Needs to be taken care with appropriate antibiotics and local care.

Management of Radial Vascular Complications

Compartment Syndrome

This syndrome is caused by raised pressures within a closed ossieo-facial anatomical space. It triggers ischemia of forearm muscles. Cardinal sign is pain on passive stretch (hand dorsiflection). Prompt application of proximal compression for any hematoma will help mitigate against this complications. If there is any sign of neurovascular deficit, then emergency referral to a vascular surgeon is needed.

Vessel Perforation or Injury

Dissection and perforation of forearm vessels will produce sudden intense pain. It heals spontaneously more than often but a close observation is required for compartment syndrome.

Severe Vasospasm

Radial, ulnar or axillary arteries with equipment passing from those arteries, can produce severe vasospasm, at any site of the arterial course. Sedation, analgesia, additional nitrates

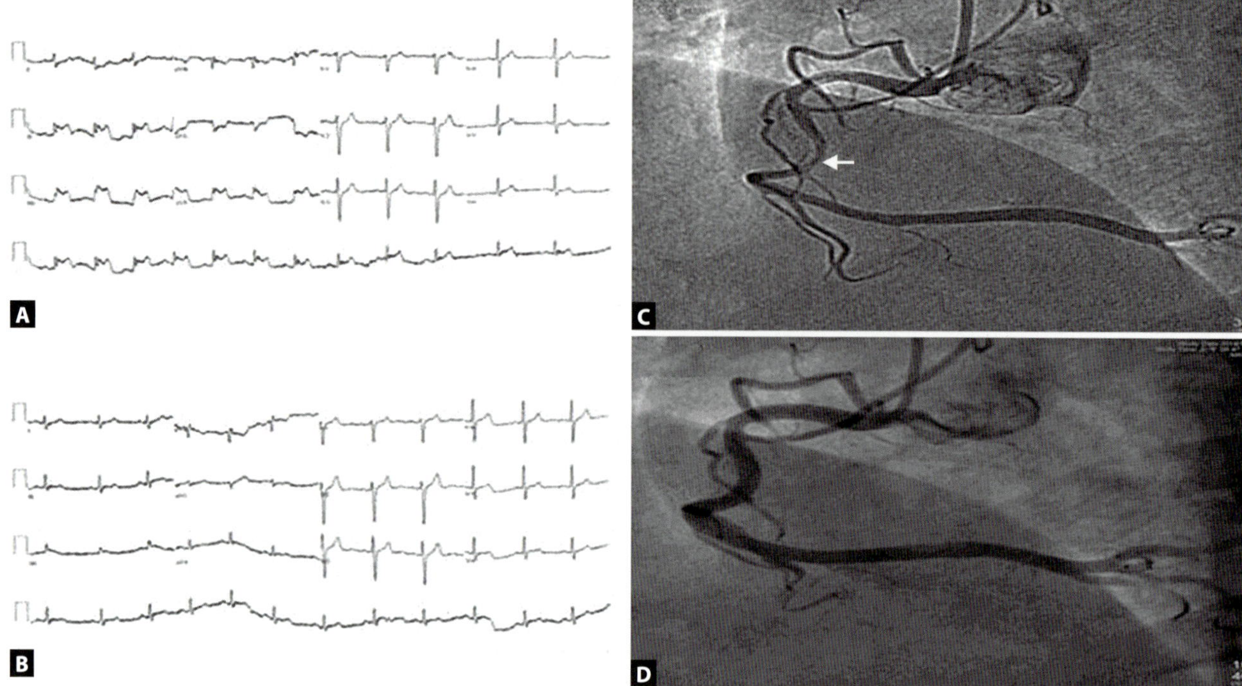

Figs 15.2A to D Vasospasm of mid-right coronary artery

and calcium channel antagonist help to relieve the spasm. Occasionally, regional anesthetic block or deep sedation is required to remove the entrapped equipment, in presence of severe spasms.

COMPLICATIONS RELATED TO CORONARY BLOOD FLOW

Acute Myocardial Ischemia during Coronary Angioplasty

Vasospasm, dissection of the coronary artery, abrupt closure of the vessel, perforation of the coronary artery, acute thrombus formation, air embolism, side branch occlusion, no flow phenomenon and retained equipment into the coronary tree and sometimes prolonged ischemia leading to myocardial infarction, urgent coronary artery bypass graft surgery (CABG) are the important complications responsible for acute myocardial ischemia during the coronary angioplasty.

Vasospasm

Patients with Prinzmetal's angina can have vasospasm with normal coronaries.[12] Female gender, ostial lesions, tortuous vessels and chronic smokers are more prone for vasospasm. Intracoronary nitroglycerin or calcium channel antagonist with watch on hypotension is the treatment of choice (Figs 15.2A to D).

Dissection of the Coronary Artery

Types A and B dissection are benign and managed conservatively. Type C to F are considered major dissections and need treatment (Fig. 15.3).

Several key elements are:

- Selection of the optimal guiding catheter with proper alignment.
- Good tactile and visual feedback during guidewire manipulation.
- Proper-sized balloon and stent.
- Special care during calcified and tortuous lesions.
- If dissection is suspected but cannot be confirmed by multiple projections, then intravascular ultrasound (IVUS) can be used.

If the dissection is flow-limiting, it needs to be mostly sealed with overlapping stents or sometimes, managed with prolonged balloon dilatations and GP blockers with watchful observation.

Ostial dissection is an emergency, as the entire territory is potentially threatened. Iatrogenic dissection of the left main ostium is rare but critical condition and warrants emergency measures, which involves stenting and hemodynamic management. Incidence in various studies is less than 0.01%.

The National Heart, Lung and Blood Institute (NHLBI) classification system for intimal tears

Type A dissections represent minor radiolucent area within the coronary lumen during contrast injection with little or no persistence of contrast after the day had cleared

Type B dissections are parallel tracts or a double lumen separated by a radiolucent area during contrast injection, with minimal or no persistence after dye clearance

Type C dissections appear as contrast outside the coronary lumen (extraluminal cap) with persistence of contrast after dye had cleared form the lumen

Type D dissections represent spinal (barber shop pole) luminal filling defects, frequently with excessive contrast staining of the dissected false lumen

Type E dissections appear as new, persistent filling defects within the coronary lumen

Type F dissections represent those that lead to total occlusion of the coronary lumen with distal antegrade flow

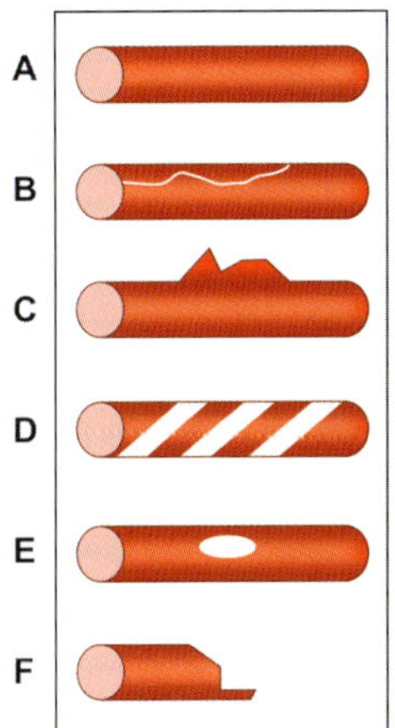

Fig. 15.3 Dissection of the coronary artery[13]

Ostial right coronary dissection can be sometimes disastrous and needs to be managed with emergency temporary pacemaker and multiple overlapping stents.

Abrupt Closure of the Vessel

During coronary angioplasty while manipulation of the hardwares, there can occur abrupt closure of the vessel. This can produce sudden hemodynamic compromise and arrhythmias along with severe symptoms. Acute thrombus formation, which could due to inadequate heparin or antiplatelets, dissection of the vessel, embolization of the clot, no flow phenomenon, air embolism, etc. are responsible for abrupt closure of the vessel.

Adequate use of heparin, antiplatelets, GP blockers is necessary during angioplasty. Intermittent watch on ACT, every 30–60 minutes in cases of prolonged duration of angioplasty is necessary. Adequate flushing of the hardware before introducing is also important. When using thrombus aspiration catheter, it is necessary to back bleed the catheter adequately.

Perforation of the Coronary Artery

Perforation is an anatomical breach in the integrity of the tunica adventitia of epicardial artery leading to extravasation of blood, either into myocardium, pericardium or cardiac chamber. It can be caused by oversized balloons or stents, balloon rupture leading to jet effect, aggressive post dilation of stent, laser therapy, excessive rotablation or due to guide-wire exit. High-risk clinical and morphological predictors are females, elderly population, previous CABG, PCI for unstable syndromes, tortuous, calcified and small vessels and seen in CTO interventions (Figs 15.4A to C).[14]

Numerous studies have reported a overall low incidence of coronary perforation ranging from 0.1% to 1% of all angioplasties.[15,16]

Prevention

- Avoiding oversizing of balloons.
- Careful manipulation of guidewires.
- Do not perform angioplasty if distal vessel is not visualized.
- Careful handling temporary pacemaker, as it can lead to perforation of right ventricle.

Diagnosis and Management

Adapted angiographic classification of coronary perforation:

- *Type I:* Extraluminal crater without jet extravasation
- *Type II:* Pericardial or myocardial blushing without jet extravasation
- *Type III:* Active jet extravasation
- *Type IV:* Cavity spilling
- *Type V:* Distal perforation.[17]

Type I and type II are generally benign and seal after balloon after inflation can be left untreated. Type III perforation needs emergency pericardiocentesis and hemodynamic stabilization with covered stent to the perforated segment. Type IV often needs conservative management and it seals spontaneously. Type V perforation may require distal embolization using coils, gel, foams, thrombin.

Careful watch on the hemodynamics and, if required, reversal of heparin should be thought of. GP blocker needs to be stopped. Autologous tamponade blood transfusion and correction of hypovolemia is needed.

If all attempts are unsuccessful in locating the pericardium or in restoring hemodynamic stability, then a surgeon is required to salvage the situation.

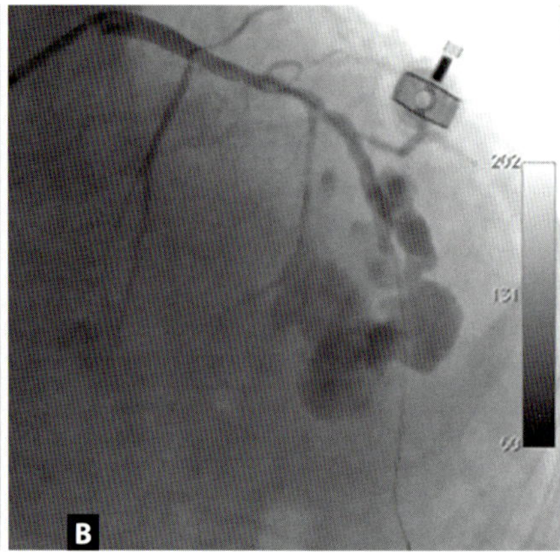

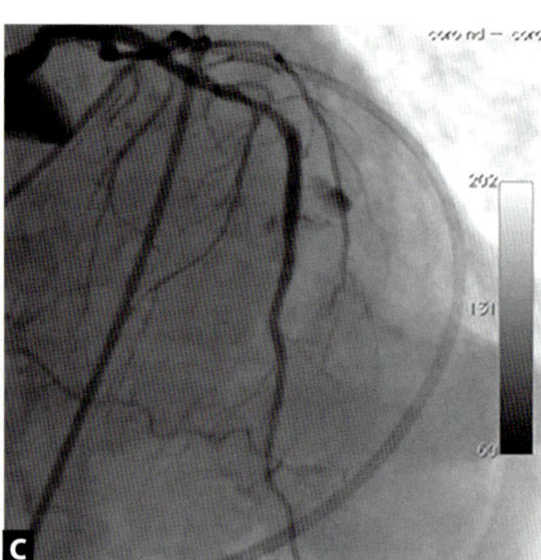

Figs 15.4A to C Perforation of coronary artery

THROMBUS FORMATION

Preventive Pharmacotherapy

Adequate anticoagulation and antiplatelet therapy are key determinants of complication rates and a variety of acceptable options exist. These therapies alone will not, however, always compensate for suboptimal technique. Any foreign material into the vascular system is thrombogenic. Clot forming in introducer sheaths and equipment when outside the patient are potential source of embolism and also a potent catalyst for thrombosis when reintroduce. All material exchanges must, therefore, be frequently and methodically wiped down with saline, introducer sheaths regularly flushed and equipment dwell times kept to a minimum. A damped pressure trace with poor back-bleed is an early sign of partially occluded catheter and warrants removal without injections.

Avoiding Iatrogenic Coronary Thrombus

- Keep equipment dwell times to a minimum
- Wipe down all exteriorized equipment before reintroduction
- Flush introducer and catheters frequently and thoroughly
- Load unfractionated heparin before PCI equipment is used
- Keep ACT >250–400 seconds with regular checks
- Use weight-adjusted heparin dosing.

Management of Thrombus Formation

- If there is a dampening of the pressure tracing and no back-bleed, take out the catheter and flush it outside the patient's body. Another catheter should be used after checking ACT levels (Figs 15.5A and B).
- Check ACT and correct with heparin.
- Sometimes urgent thrombus aspiration or GP blockers may be needed.

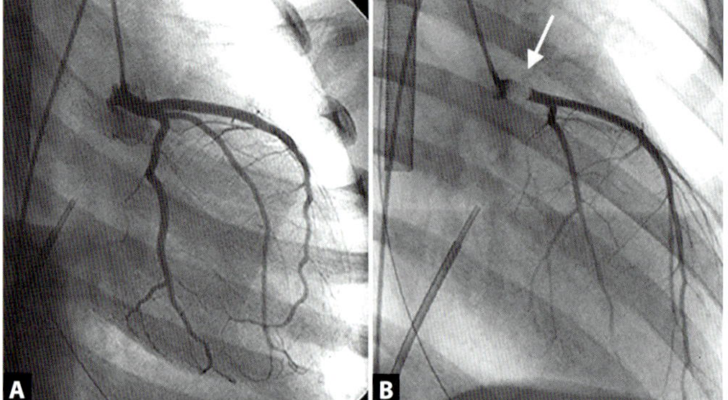

Figs 15.5A and B Thrombus formation

- Refractory thrombus with hemodynamic compromise warrants IABP or CABG.

AIR EMBOLISM

Retrospective data suggest that inadequate technique is the predominant cause with junior operators, particularly in the first months of training, more prone than senior; and events more common during PCI than diagnostic catheterization.[18] The incidence of air embolism in various studies is approximately 0.1–0.3%. Conventional manual injection using a stopcock-manifold, equipment exchanges that can entrain air (venturi effect) via the Tuohy-Borst connector (Y connector), inadequate aspiration of the catheters and balloon rapture are all potential risks for the inadvertent introduction of air into the coronary circulation (Fig. 15.6).

Coronary air embolism underlies the importance of ensuring that all catheters and devices inserted into the vascular system are saline or contrast filled and competent at all times. Furthermore, any exchange of equipment should be followed by a visual check that the back bleeding through the Y connector has occurred. The latter is especially relevant during aspiration catheter exchanges in primary PCI.

Treatment of Air Embolism

More than half of this embolic events are asymptomatic. Severe form of air embolism can even lead to cardiac arrest and may need prolonged resuscitation until the air is reabsorbed into the venous system. Symptoms of chest pain and transient ST elevation may be accompanied by severe bradycardia leading to asystole or ventricular fibrillation. This may need fluids, atropine, vasopressors, temporary pacemaker or DC version, as per the hemodynamics. Sometimes patient may need to be ventilated with 100% oxygen. If refractory to high doses of vasopressors then intra-aortic balloon pump (IABP) may be used.

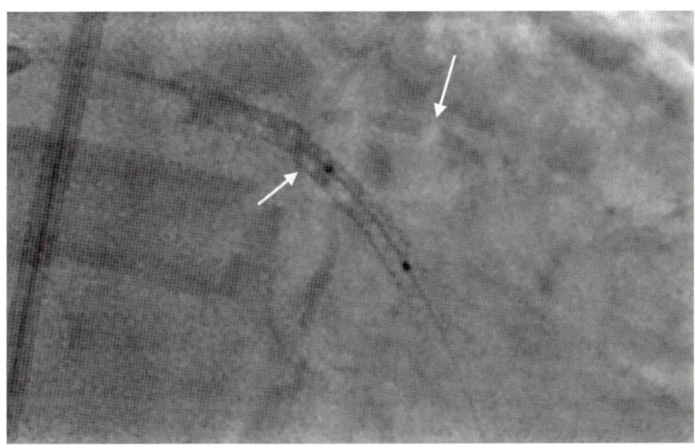

Fig. 15.6 Air embolism

No-reflow Phenomenon

The no-reflow phenomenon is defined as inadequate myocardial perfusion in a territory subtended by the given epicardial coronary artery without angiographic evidence of mechanical vessel obstruction.[19] It typically accompanies primary percutaneous coronary intervention (PCI) and complex lesion intervention, particularly vein graft intervention or when rotational artherectomy devices are used. This manifestation of microvascular injury must be distinguished from several mimics (thrombus, air embolism, dissection and severe spasm) (Figs 15.7A and B).

The incidence of no-reflow phenomenon ranges from 0.6% to 2% and is more frequently observed when using stents or artherectomy and when performing PCI in saphenous vein grafts (SVGs).[20] Risk factors for no-reflow phenomenon include the angiographic presence of thrombus, cardiogenic shock, increased reperfusion time, hyperglycemia, and leukocytosis.[21] Diagnosis of no reflow is made angiographically.

Treatment

Intracoronary adenosine (10–20 ug bolus), verapamil (100–200 ug bolus or 100 ug/min up to 1000 ug total with temporary pacemaker on standby), papaverine (10–20 ug), sodium nitroprusside (50–200 ug bolus, up to 1000 ug total dose), abciximab, cyclosporine, epinephrine (50–200 ug) and nicorandil (2 mg) have all been used as treatment after the development of no-reflow with success.

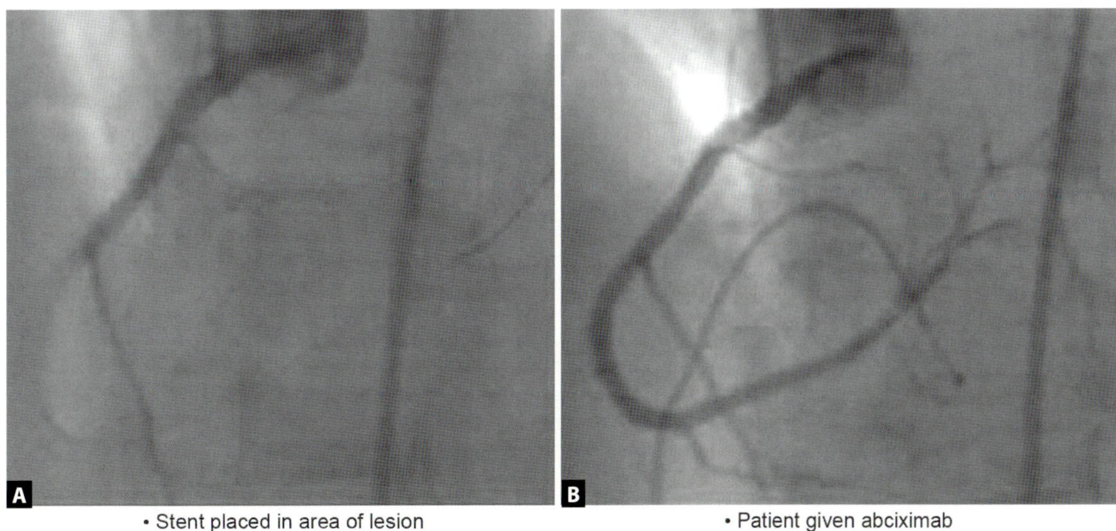

Figs 15.7A and B Case presentation—No reflow B

The first-line treatment for no-reflow phenomenon primarily consists of delivery of vasodilators especially adenosine, calcium channel blockers, and/or nitroprusside into the coronary microcirculation. Should the dye column stop at midvessel, distal contrast injections through balloon or microcatheters should be performed to exclude dissection. Injection of vasodilators through an infusion catheter close to the distal bed may improve microcirculation drug delivery. No role has been found for referral for emergent CABG or thrombolytic therapy (Box 15.1).

Retained Equipment into the Coronary Tree

PCI equipment retained within the circulation is rare and includes stents, guidewire fragments, catheter fragments, misplaced intravascular coils and any diagnostic equipment used for PCI. Stent loss and embolization, although infrequent (<1% of PCI) since factory crimping was introduced, has not been eliminated entirely. The most vulnerable stage for this event occurs when the stent-balloon assembly is pulled back into the guiding catheter following failure to reach or pass the target lesion. There is, therefore, an association with poor guiding support, lack of coaxial guide catheter position, vessel tortuosity, calcification and absence to predilatation. A stent can be stripped off its delivery balloon at the lesion or, more commonly, a deformed stent strut can prevent reentry into the guide catheter. If not anticipated inadvertent pulling on the stent, the catheter will cause the mouth of the guide to displace the stent off the delivery balloon. Retrospectively analysis[21] of over 4,000 stent implantations has revealed higher embolization rate for manually crimped stents (1% vs 0.3% {$p < 0.01$}) than factory crimped devices (Figs 15.8A to C).

Box 15.1 Prevention of no-reflow phenomenon

- Use distal protection devices when treating saphenous vein graft lesions.
- When performing rotational artherectomy, routinely use nitroglycerin, verapamil, and heparin in combination with the flush solution.
- Consider pretreatment with a glycoprotein IIb/IIIa inhibitor during percutaneous coronary intervention in patient with acute coronary syndromes.
- Minimize balloon inflation and consider direct stenting in patients with bulky atheroma or saphenous vein grafts.
- Pretreat with verapamil or adenosine.
- Aspiration thrombectomy for thrombus-laden lesions.

Nonsurgical Stent Retrieval

The key principle for retrieval is to bring the foreign body down to iliac artery as this removes the risk of embolization to the cerebrovascular system and, or thrombosis in a coronary artery (Figs 15.9A and B).

Stent Retrieval with Guidewire within the Stent

It is done as a first attempt. Low profile 1.5 or 2 mm diameter balloon is advanced on the guidewire and passed through the unexpanded stent and inflated at 2 atm pressure and then the balloon is pulled gently. Once the stent is secured between

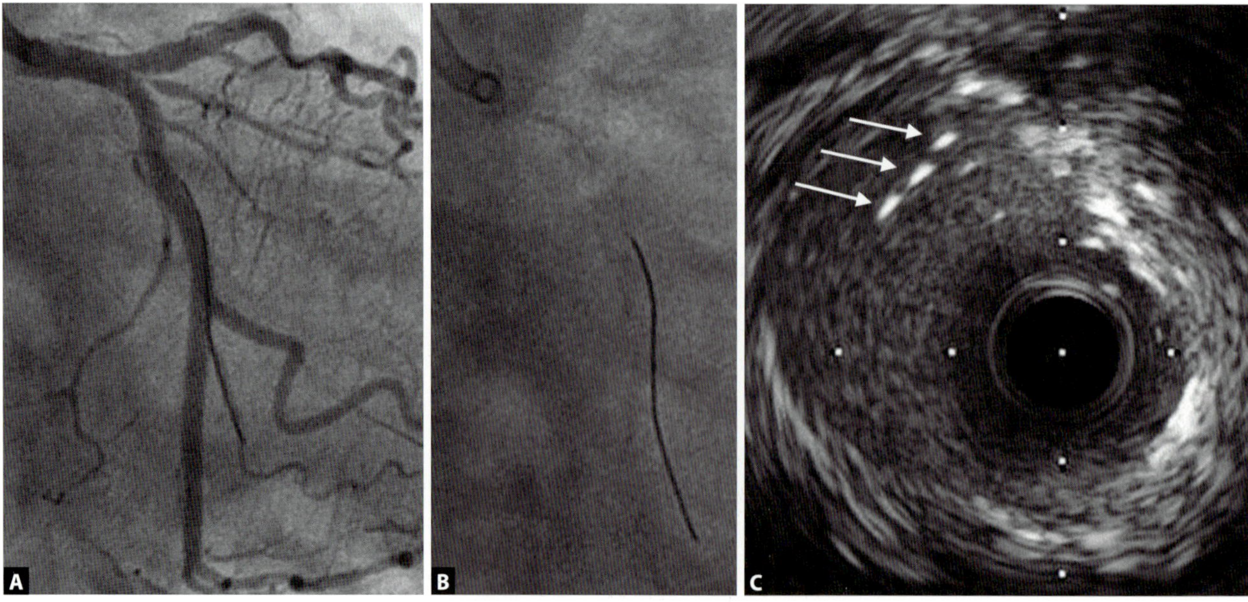

Figs 15.8A to C Dislodgement of guidewire in circumflex artery

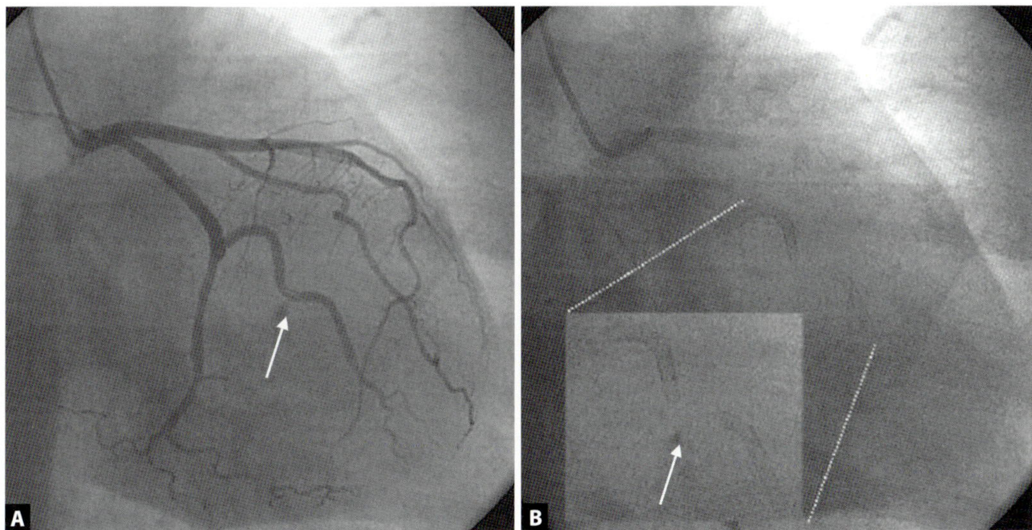

Figs 15.9A and B Dislodged stent into coronary tree

the balloon and guide catheter, then entire assembly is pulled back to iliac artery and removed en bloc through the sheath. If the stent does not come back, then the technique should be abandoned.[22]

Second alternative of retrieval is to inflate the balloon inside the stent. That will allow the operator to advance the stent directly and deploy it at the target lesion or in nonconsequential location.

Third alternative is use of stiff wire with snare, which is passed parallel to the stent and distal tip is passed through the dislodged stent and micro-snare is advanced into the exchange catheter. Then remove the exchange catheter and loop of the snare is retracted to hold the stent and pull back the assembly.[23,24]

Stent Retrieval without Guidewire within the Stent

Commercially available snares like 'gooseneck' snares can be used to capture the free end of the stent.[25]

Double or multiwire technique can be used for retrieval of stent. Two or multiple wires outside the guiding catheter are rotated with torquer for 15-20 times until the wires are observed twisting together near the proximal end of the stent. Then the twisted wires are pulled back together and guide catheter is advanced. The whole assembly consisting of trapped stent is pulled out gently.

Stent-crush Technique

If all the attempts of the retrieval of the stent are unsuccessful, the stent can be crushed at the site of dislodgement against the coronary wall. Very often this is the easiest solution but has a potential thrombosis risk.

Forceps Removal

Retrieval using this feasible if the stent is present within the most proximal part of the left main or right coronary arteries but cannot be recommended as a first-line option as it is aggressive. If employed, then use of small French (pediatric sized) myocardial biotomes is best (3 Fr–1.3 mm).

Prolonged Ischemia Leading to Myocardial Infarction, Urgent CABG and Death

Various reasons are responsible for prolonged ischemia. Prolonged vasospasm, coronary dissection, coronary perforation, dislodgement of the stent into left main or proximal part of the major coronary artery, major side branch occlusion, severe air embolism, severe refractory no flow phenomenon, etc. are the common reason for prolonged ischemia or myocardial infarction. Rarely, patient needs to be referred for CABG. Occasionally, in spite of all the efforts, patient can die (Figs 15.10 and 15.11).

Emergency CABG

The incidence of emergency CABG has decreased from 3.7% during the balloon angioplasty era to near 0% in the most recent National Heart, Lung, and Blood Institute (NHLBI) registry. Individual single center registries showed an incidence of 0.4–0.5%.

Emergent CABG following PCI is associated with significant morbidity and mortality with a death rate ranging from 7.8% to 14% among three single center studies.

Preprocedural myonecrosis during PCI is common and occurs with a 0–47% incidence based on reported series.[26] The definition of MI varies among studies with respect to

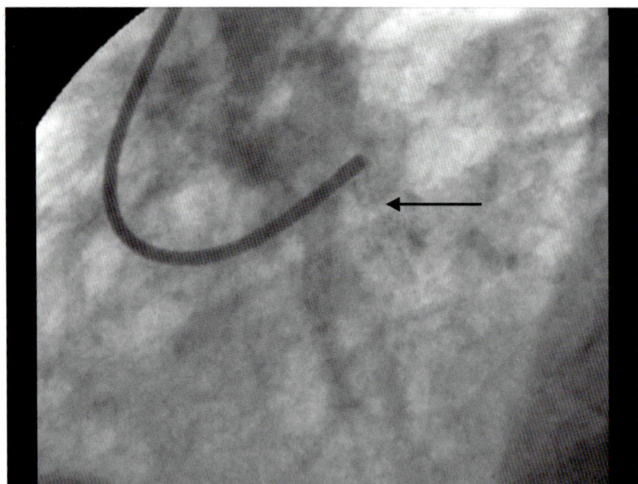

Fig. 15.10 Dislodged stent in coronary tree. Arrow demonstrated at high magnification on fluoroscopy

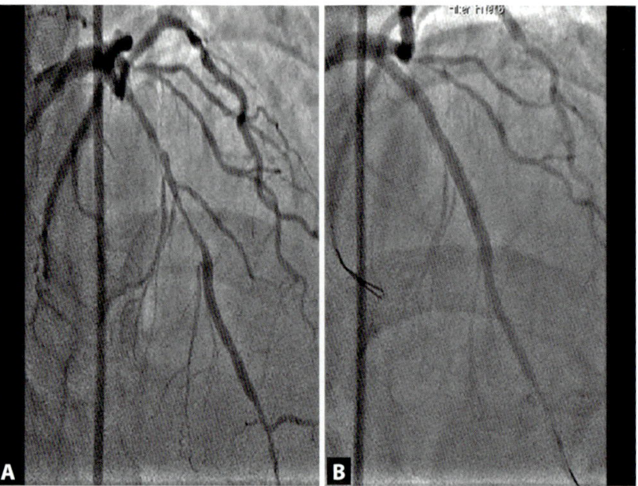

Figs 15.11A and B Side-branch occlusion

biomarkers assay, threshold value, frequency of blood, specimen, sampling and use of ECG data among studies, which results in wide ranges of reported incidence.[27]

Radiocontrast Hypersensitivity

Since the advent of low osmolar nonionic agents, the incidence of contrast hypersensitivity is reduced. The risk of allergy to ionic contrast agents was 4–12% and with nonionic contrast, it is around 1%.[28] Treatment of anaphylactoid reactions to contrast media is as follows:

Mild

Nausea, vomiting, rash—observation.

Moderate

Laryngeal edema and bronchospasm. Epinephrine 1:10,000 dilution at 1–3 mL IV.

Severe

Respiratory or cardiac arrest—ACLS resuscitation (airway, breathing, circulation) and epinephrine.

Bleeding

Proper use of heparin, bivaluridin, GP blockers, antiplatelets and low molecular weight heparin is important. If required, frequent checks in activated clotting time (ACT), are required. In case of bleeding complications necessary management to stop bleeding and revert anticoagulation in consideration with no increase in coronary thrombosis is very important. One has to consider issue of stent thrombosis while reverting the heparin.

Stroke

Cerebrovascular complications are amongst the most devastating that can occur during PCI and has a frequency of 0.1–0.4%.[29]

Transcranial Doppler cerebral MRI and CT scan of the brain evaluates the complication. Neurologist should be actively involved in the management of stroke.

Contrast-induced Nephropathy (CIN)

Refer Box 15.2 for details.

MINIMIZING THE RISK OF ACUTE KIDNEY INJURY

Patients with CKD often have existing comorbidities that may complicate their procedure and postprocedure management. As always developing a systemic approach that reviews the patient's history, physical examination, and laboratory studies, is critical.

Periprocedural Hydration

The most important preventive strategy to lower the risk of contrast-induced acute kidney injury (CI-AKI) is to ensure adequate hydration at the time of contrast administration.

Box 15.2 Risk factor for the development of contrast-induced nephropathy
Clinical factors
Chronic kidney disease
Diabetes mellitus
Advanced age
Female gender
Peripheral vascular disease
Hypertension
Ejection fraction less than 40%
Presenting factors
Acute coronary syndrome
Hypotension
Heart failure
Volume depletion
Concomitant nephrotoxic medications
Anemia
Procedural factors
Intra-aortic balloon pump placement
Multivessel disease
Contrast amount
Contrast type

Medications

Several medications have been investigated as potential preventive therapies for CI-AKI. The most extensively studied agent is N-acetylcysteine, which has been evaluated in more than 20 randomized clinical trials.[30] The premise behind the use of N-acetylcysteine is that it acts as a scavenger of reactive oxygen species and promotes vasodilatory effects in the renal medulla. The first major trial reported by Tepal and colleagues,[31] evaluated its use in 83 patients who received IV contrast agents for computed tomography (CT). This study found an approximately 90% relative risk reduction in CI-AKI with the use of N-acetylcysteine. However, a recent large, multicenter, randomized trial by the acetylcysteine for contrast-induced nephropathy trial (ACT) investigators studied 2308 patients with at least one risk factor for CI-AKI undergoing elective coronary or peripheral vascular angiography and found no difference in the incidence of CI-AKI or the need for dialysis at 30 days in patients treated with N-acetylcysteine versus placebo.[32]

Another important medication that has been studied extensively in randomized clinical trials is fenoldopam, which works as dopamine receptor antagonist and is believed to preserve renal blood flow despite insults from contrast agent exposure. A series of small clinical studies had suggested significant benefits in terms of reduction of CI-AKI, particularly in high-risk patients.[33] However, enthusiasm for the use of fenoldopam has fallen since publication of a large, multicenter trial by Stone and colleagues in 2003.[34] In this study, no benefit was seen with fenoldopam in 315 patients who had glomerular filtration rate (GFRs) below 60 mL/min and underwent cardiac catheterization.

Ascorbic acid has antioxidant properties that have led to investigation into its use for preventing CI-AKI. A recent meta-analysis of nine small, randomized controlled trial of 1536 patients treated with ascorbic acid (usually 1–3 g the night before, the day of, and daily, 1 for 2 days after cardiac catheterization) showed a 33% relative risk reduction of CI-AKI compared with that patients given placebo or an alternative therapy.[35] The finding should be confirmed with larger clinical trials, but ascorbic acid is a well tolerated, low-risk, inexpensive therapy that may be worth considering for selected patients.

Intraprocedural Strategies

Intraprocedural strategies for approaching patients with CKD largely depend on three things:

- The choice of contrast agent.
- Minimizing the volume that is used as much as possible.
- Avoiding use of potentially nephrotoxic medications.

Although useful, these strategies must always be used without sacrificing the operator's ability to adequately and safely perform the procedure. This requires a careful balance to weigh the clinical risks and benefits of different approaches. For example, appropriate visualization of the lesion and adjacent coronary anatomy is essential for success during PCI and should not be scarified.

The Choice and Use of Contrast Agents

The choice of contrast agent is an important Intraprocedural consideration that has evolved considerably over the last several years with the development of low-osmolor and isosmolar contrast agents. The introduction of iodixanol, an isosmolar contrast agent has raised the question of whether the incidence of CI-AKI can be further reduced. In a widely cited study of patients with CKD and diabetes mellitus, the use of isosmolar contrast reduces the incidence CI-AKI by over 90% when compared with low-osmolar contrast agent.[36]

Regardless of the selection of a contrast agent, it is imperative to use least amount of volume required for adequate visualization of the coronary artery and technical success of the procedure.

Ten Golden Rules to Prevent Complications

Rule #1: Select the patient and lesion carefully, plan well and anticipate problems.
Rule #2: Do not fall victim to the 'oculostenotic reflex'.
Rule #3: Select a good guide catheter.
Rule #4: Acquire adequate angiographic views prior to and post-intervention.
Rule #5: The procedure should be kept as simple as possible.
Rule #6: One must have excellent knowledge of the equipment.
Rule #7: Know your own limitations.
Rule #8: Know when to stop.
Rule #9: Always maintain the highest level of concentration.
Rule #10: Learn from one's own and other's mistakes and misfortunes.

Stent thrombosis (acute, subacute, late), stent restenosis and sten-related future adverse events are not included in this chapter.

CONCLUSION

Risk stratification and technical expertise are vital to prevent or mitigate against complications but the human and organizational components of a procedure or institutional program seldom taken into consideration or evaluated. Professionals working in a hazardous environment are prone to errors and these are the cause of adverse events. One must try and prevent the complications. If it happens, then it needs to be treated on priority in a very methodical approach. Most of the complications in the cath lab can be solved in the cath lab only. But if required one should not hesitate to take the help of cardiac surgeon or other specialties.

REFERENCES

1. Rodney De Palma, Christian Roguelov, Adel Aminian, Olivier Muller, Tito Kabir, Eeric Eeckhout. Chapter on prevention and management of complications during percutaneous coronary intervention. The PCR EAPCI textbook.
2. Levine GN, Bates ER, Blankenship JC, Bailey SR, Bittl JA, Cercek B, Chambers CE, Ellis SG, Guyton RA, Hollenberg SM, Khot UN, Lange RA, Mauri L, Mehran R, Moussa ID, Mukherjee D, Nallamothu BK, Ting HH. ACCF/AHA/SCAI guidelines for PCI. 2011.
3. Bredlau CE, Roubin GS, Leimgruber PP, Douglas JS, King SB III, Gruentzig AR. In-hospital morbidity and mortality in patients undergoing elective coronary angioplasty. Circulation. 1985;72:1044-52.
4. Stathopoulos I, Jimenez M, Panagopoulos G, Kwak EJ, Losquadro M, Cohen H, Iyer S, Ruiz C, Roubin G, Garratt K. The decline in PCI complication rate - 2003-2006 versus 1999- 2002. Hellenic J Cardiol. 2009;50:379-85.
5. Allnutt MF. Human factors in accidents. Br J Anaesth. 1987;59:856-64.
6. Gaba DM. Anesthesiology as a model for patients safety in healthcare. BMJ. 2000;320:785-8.
7. Patel MR, Dehmer GJ, Hershfeld JW, Smith PK, Spertus JA. ACCF/SCAI/STB/AATS/AHA/ASNC—2009. Appropriate criteria for coronary revascularization. NEJM. 2009;360:213-4.
8. Jolly SS, Yusuf S, Cairns J, Niemela K, Xavier D, Widimsky P, Budaj A, Niemela M, Valentin V, Lewis BS, Avezum A, Steg PG, Rao SV, Gao P, Afzal R, Joyner CD, Chrolavicius S, Mehta SR, RIVAL trial group. Radial versus femoral access for coronary angiography and intervention in patients with acute coronary syndromes (RIVAL): a randomized, parallel group, multicentre trial. Lancet. 2011;377:1409-20.
9. Trimarchi, Santi, Smith, Dean E, Share, David, Jani, Sandeep M, O'Donnell, Michael, McNamara, Richard, Riba, Arthur, Kline Rogers, Eva, Gurm, Hitinder S, Moscucci, Mauro. On behalf of the BMC2 registry, Retroperitoneal Hematoma after Percutaneous Coronary Intervention: Prevalence, risk factors, management, outcomes, and predictors of mortality: A report from the BMC2 (Blue cross blue shield of Michigan Cardiovascular Consortium) registry. J Am Coll Cardiol Intv. 2010;3:845-50.
10. Farouque HM, Omar Tremmel, Jennifer A, Shabari, Farshad Raissi, Aggrawal Meenakshi, Fearon, William F, Ng, Martin KC, Rezaee, Mehrdad, Yeung, Alan C, Lee, David P. Risk factors for the development of retroperitoneal hematoma after percutaneous coronary intervention in the era of glycoprotein IIb/IIIa inhibitors and vascular closure devices. J Am Coll Cardiol. 2005;45:363-36.
11. Kelm M, Perings SM, Jax T, Lauer T, Schoebel FC, Heintzen MP, Perings C, Strauer BE. Incidence and clinical outcomes of iatrogenic femoral arteriovenous fistulas: implication for risk stratification and treatment. J Am Coll Cardiol. 2002;40:291-7.
12. Uren NG, Crake T, Lefroy DC, de Silva R, Davies GJ, Maseri A. Reduced coronary vasodilator function in infarcted and normal myocardium after myocardial infarction. NEJM. 1994;331:222-7.
13. Klein LW. Coronary complication of percutaneous coronary intervention; a practical approach to the management of abrupt closure. Catheter. Cardiovasc. Interven. 2005;64:395-401.
14. Cohen BM, Weber VJ, Reisman M, Casale A, Dorros G. Coronary perforation complicating rotational ablation: the US multicenter experience. Cathet Cardiovasc Diagn. 1996;3:55-9.
15. Ajluni SC, Glazier S, Blankenship L, O'Neil WW, Safian RD. Perforations after percutaneous coronary interventions: clinical, angiographic, and therapeutic observations. Cathet Cardiovasc Diagn. 1994;32:206-12.
16. Gruberg L, Pinnow E, Flood R, Bonnet Y, Tebeica M, Waksman R, Satler LF, Pichard AD, Kent KM, Leon MB, Lindsay Jr. Incidence, management, and outcome of coronary artery perforation during percutaneous coronary intervention. Am J Cardiol. 2000;86:680-2.
17. Ellis SG, Ajluni S, Arnold AZ, Popma JJ, Bittl JA, Eigler NL, Cowley MJ, Raymond RE, Safian RD, Whitlow PL. Increased coronary perforation in the new device era. Incidence, classification, management, and outcome. Circulation. 1994;90:2725-30.
18. Dib J, Boyle AJ, Chan M, Rear JR, Coronary air embolism: A case reported and review of the literature. Cathet Cardiovasc Diagn. 2006;68:897-900.
19. Eeckhout E, Kern M, The coronary no-reflow phenomenon: a review of mechanisms and therapies. Eur Heart J. 2001;22:729-39.

20. Abbo KM, Dooris M, Glazier S, et al. Features and outcome of no-reflow after percutaneous coronary intervention. Am J Cardiol. 1995;75:778-82.
21. Iwakura K, Ito H, Kawano S, et al. Predictive factors for development of the no-reflow phenomenon in patients with repurfused anterior wall myocardial infarction. J Am Cardiol. 2001;38:472-7.
22. Eggbrecht H, Haude M, Von Birgelen C, von Birgelen C, Oldenburg O, Baumgart D, Herrmann J, Welge D, Bartel T, Dagres N, Erbal R. Nonsurgical retrieval of embolized coronary stents. Cath Cardiovasc Intervent. 2000;51:432-40.
23. Cishek MB, Laslett L, Gershony G. Balloon catheter retrieval of dislodged coronary stents; a novel technique. Cath Cardiovasc Diagn. 1995;34:350-2.
24. Borgart DB, Jung SJ, Dislodged stent: A simple Retrieval Technique. Cath Cardiovasc Interv. 1999;47:323-4.
25. Watson LE. Snare loop technique for removal of broken steerable PTCA wire. Cath Cardiovasc Diagn. 1987;13:44-9.
26. Hermann J. Peri-procedural myocardial injury: 2005 update. Eur Heart J. 2005;26:2493-519.
27. Thygesen K, Alpert JS, White HD, et al. Universal definition of myocardial infarction. Circulation. 2007;116:2634-53.
28. Fayed AM, White CJ, Ramee SR, Jenkins JS, Collins TJ, Carotid and cerebral angiography performed by cardiologists: Cerebrovascular complications. Catheter Cardiovasc Interv. 2002;5:277-80.
29. Kawamura A, Lombardi DA, Tilem ME, Gossman DE, Piemonte TC, Nesto RW, Stroke complicating percutaneous coronary intervention in patients with acute myocardial infarction. Circ J. 2007;71:1370-5.
30. Nallmothu BK, Shojania KG, Saint S, et al. Is acetylcysteine effective in preventing contrast-related nephropathy? A met analysis. Am J Med. 2004;117 (12):938-47.
31. Tepel M, van der Giet M, Schwarzfeld C, et al. Prevention of radiographic contrast agent-induced reduction in renal function by acetylcysteine. N Engl J Med. 2000;343(3):180-4.
32. ACT Investigators: Acetylcysteine for prevention of renal outcomes in patients undergoing coronary and peripheral vascular angiography: main results from the randomized Acetylcysteine for contrast-induced nephropathy trial (ACT). Circulation. 2011;124(11):1250-9.
33. Kini AS, Mitre CA, Kamran M, et al. Changing trends in incidence and predictors of radiographic contrast nephropathy after percutaneous coronary intervention with use of fenoldopam. Am J Cardiol. 2002;89(8):999-1002.
34. Stone GW, McCullough PA, Tumlin JA, et al. Fenoldopam mesylate for the prevention of contrast induced nephropathy: a randomized controlled trial. JAMA. 2003;290(17):2284-91.
35. Sadat U, Usman A, Gillard JH, Boyle JR, Does ascorbic acid protect against contrast-induced acute kidney injury patients undergoing coronary angiography? A systemic review with meta-analysis of randomized, controlled trials. J Am Coll Cardiol. 2013;62(23):2167-75.
36. Aspelin P, Aubry P, Fransson SG, et al. Nephrotoxic effects in high risk patients undergoing angiography. N Engl J Med. 2003;348(6):491-9. doi: 10.1056/NEJMoa021833.

CHAPTER

16

Non-left-main Bifurcation Angioplasty

Rajiv G Bhagwat, Ronak V Ruparelia, Jaideep Rajebahadur

INTRODUCTION

Approximately 15–20% of all coronary interventions are performed to treat bifurcations.[1,2] Bifurcation lesion is a stenosis involving the origin (or close proximity to origin—i.e. 2-3 mm) of a 'significant' side branch.[3] The stenosis can involve a larger main branch, the smaller side branch or both.

True bifurcation lesions are those with significant involvement (>50%) of both main branch and side branch. While partial/false bifurcation are all other lesions involving bifurcation.

Factors to consider before planning a bifurcation strategy include extent of disease in side branch (whether it is limited to ostium or extending beyond), size of side branch (>2.5 mm reference diameter) and distribution of side branch. Implantation of one single stent on main branch is most widely used approach at present and should be considered the default approach. 2-stent strategy as "intention to treat" should be considered when disease extends beyond the ostium in side branch and larger sized side branch with larger territory.

HISTORY

Long before the nomenclature of lesion complexity matured, side branch involvement was recognized as an unfavorable determinant of angioplasty success. Miere and associates[4] were amongthefirsttodefinetheriskofsidebranchocclusionassociated with parent vessel angioplasty, emphasizing the importance of plaque extension into the side branch as predictor of percutaneous coronary intervention (PCI).

PATHOPHYSIOLOGY

Several important factors such as anatomic variation, angulation between branches, downstream territory and extent of plaque burden should be taken into consideration when addressing the bifurcation lesion to choose the most appropriate approach and achieve an optimal result.

Atherosclerosis within coronary bifurcation most frequently occurs in the lateral walls of both the main vessel and side branch. Atherosclerotic involvement of Carina is substantially low.[5-11] Histopathology has shown that the degree of intimal thickening and necrotic core formation in the carina is considerable less than that of the lateral walls (Fig. 16.1).[12]

Endothelial Shear Stress

It is the tangential force exerted on the endothelial surface that results from the friction of the flowing blood. It is calculated as the product of the blood viscosity (μ) and the radial gradient of axial blood velocity (dv/dy) at the endothelial surface (i.e. μ × dv/dy) and is expressed in units of force per area, N/m^2 or Pascal or dyne/cm^2. (1 N/m^2 = 1 Pascal = 10 dyne/cm^2).

Endothelial shear stress is determined by complex geometric configuration of the coronary arteries and the pulsatile nature of the arterial blood flow in coronary tree.[13-15] Shear stress is characterized by direction and magnitude. In relatively straight arterial segment, endothelial shear stress is unidirectional with magnitude that varies within a range of 15–70 dyne/cm^2 over the cardiac cycle and yields a positive time average. In contrast, in geometrically irregular regions in which laminar flow is disturbed, pulsatile flow generates low and/or oscillatory endothelial shear stress.[16-18] 'Low endothelial shear stress' typically occurs at the inner areas of curvatures as well as upstream of stenosis.[19] 'Oscillatory endothelial shear stress' is characterized by significant changes in direction (is bidirectional) and in magnitude between systole and diastole, resulting in a very low time average that is usually close to zero. Oscillatory endothelial shear stress occurs primarily downstream of stenosis, at the lateral walls of bifurcations and in the vicinity of branch points.[13,18-20] In addition to these temporal oscillations,

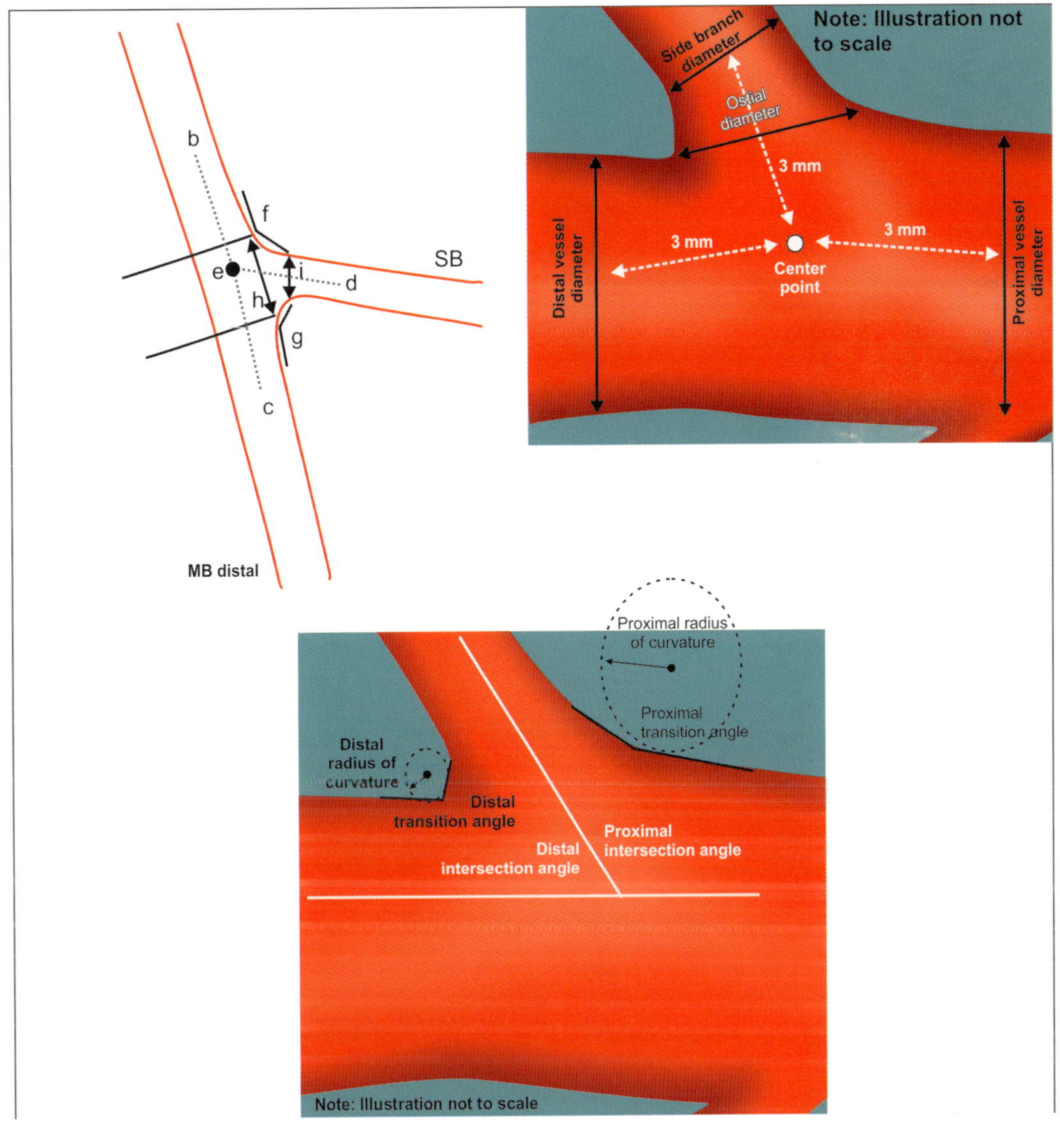

Fig. 16.1 Location of vessel measurements. (A) Vessel diameters. (B) "Intersection" angles, "transition zone" angles, and radii of curvatures

significant spatial oscillation in endothelial shear stress can occur over short distance, especially in geometrically irregular regions, resulting in high spatial gradients, which are also involved in the development and progression atherosclerosis (Fig. 16.2).[20-23]

Low endothelial shear stress reduces the bioavailability of nitric oxide by decreasing eNOS messenger ribonucleic acid and protein expression, thereby exposing the endothelium to the atherogenic effect of local and systemic risk factors.[24-27] Low shear stress downregulates prostacyclin, and endothelial vasodilator[5-16] while upregulates endothelin-1,[16,26,27] thus precipitating atherosclerosis. Low endothelial shear stress furthermore promotes permeability and the uptake of low-density lipoprotein (LDL) cholesterol and enhancing oxidative stress, which further promotes inflammation. Low endothelial shear stress also promotes vascular smooth muscle cell migration, differentiation and proliferation and extracellular matrix degradation in the vascular wall and plaque fibrous cap.[28]

CLASSIFICATION OF BIFURCATION LESIONS

Various classifications had been proposed for bifurcation lesions (Fig. 16.3). Few of them are:

- Medina
- Duke
- Sanborn

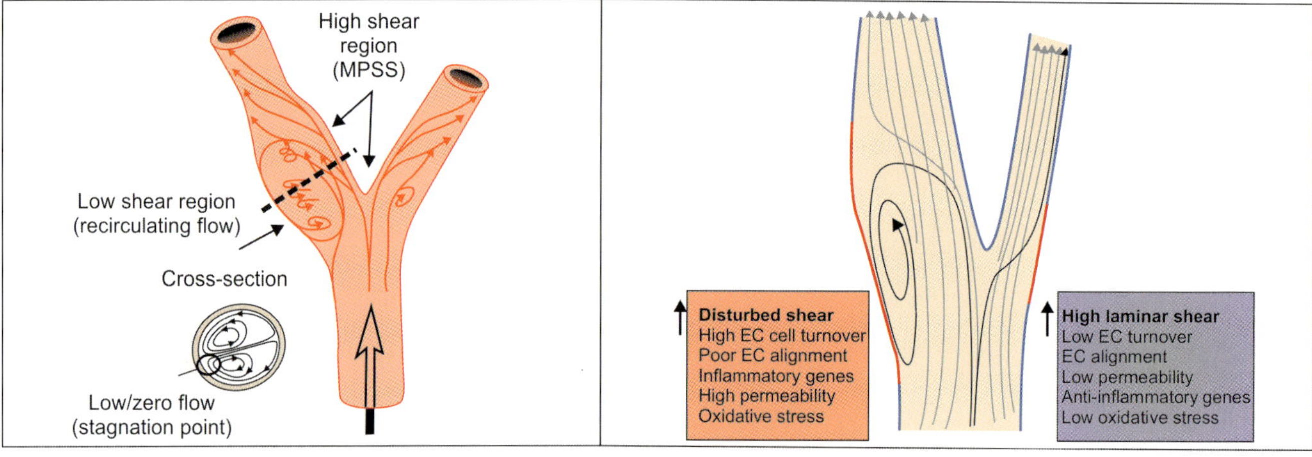

Fig. 16.2 Endothelial shear stress

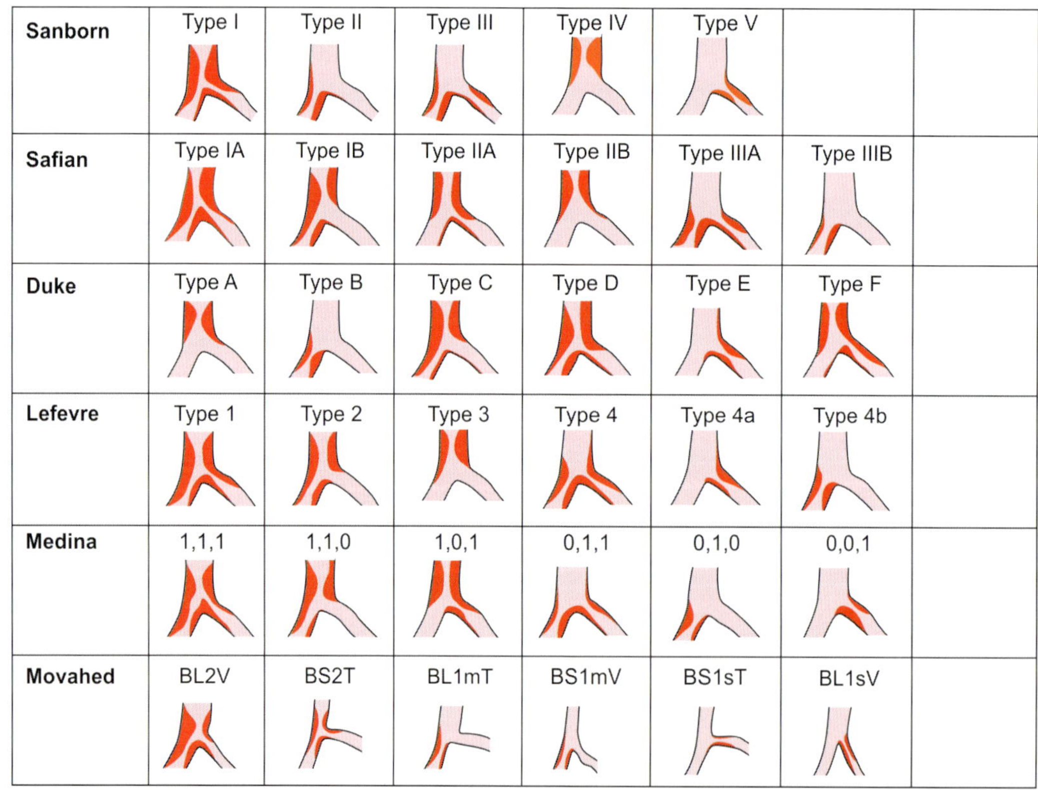

Fig. 16.3 Classification of bifurcation lesion

- Lefevre
- Safian
- Movahed.

VARIOUS TECHNIQUES OF BIFURCATION STENTING

Many techniques have been described and used successfully in the treatment of bifurcation lesion. Classification of treatments has been complicated and has caused confusion in the past. The European Bifurcation Club has suggested a MADS (Main, Across, Distal, Side) classification, taking into account initial stent deployment, which often corresponds to a technical strategy related to the importance of the vessel that is treated first.[29] MADS is a family classification system that facilitates the description of techniques by listing only the variants of each individual technique, allowing comparisons between techniques in various anatomic and clinical setting (Fig. 16.4).

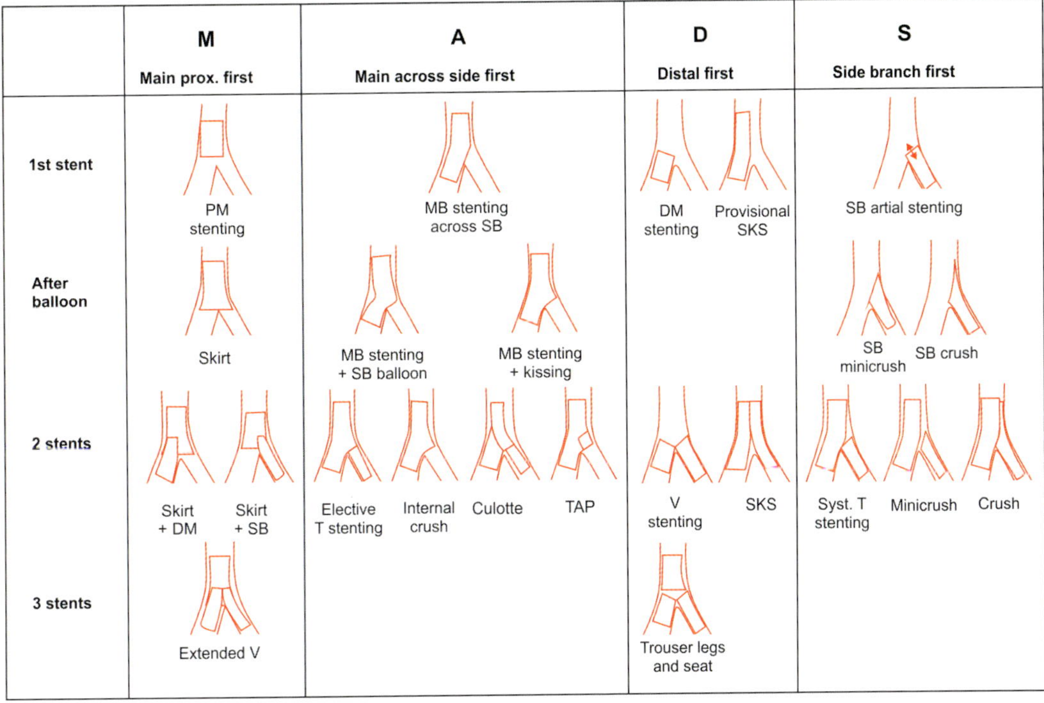

Fig. 16.4 MADS classification of bifurcation techniques

The first family of technique (M) starts by stent implantation in the proximal **M**ain vessel relatively close to the carina. The opening of the stent toward both branches may follow this initial step, with subsequent successive or simultaneous stent placement in one or both distal branch. The second family (A) starts with the stenting of the proximal main vessel to the distal main branch **A**cross the side branch. This may be the first and the last step of the procedure but may also be followed by the opening of the stent struts, delivery of a second stent in the side branch and with or without kissing balloon inflation. The third family (D) involves the **D**istal branches and historically starts with simultaneous stent placement at the ostium of both distal branches (V stenting). A recent variant consist of creating a new carina by stent implantation in the proximal segment (i.e. SKS). The fourth family (S) involves **S**trategies in which the side branch is stented first, either at the ostium level or with relatively pronounced protrusion into the proximal main vessel. The side branch stent may be crushed with a balloon inflated in the main vessel, or a second stent may be deployed in the main vessel across the side branch.[29]

The MADS classification does not exhaustively describe all technical aspect of interventional techniques, including the use of wires, lesion preparation, single balloon inflation, kissing balloon inflation, or using one or two stents. Therefore, Movahed and Stinis[30] have suggested classifying the most common bifurcation techniques with regard to stenting into six categories: one stent technique, stent with balloon technique, kissing stent technique, T stent technique, crush stent technique and culotte stent technique.

The most important issue in bifurcation intervention is selecting the most appropriate strategy for an individual bifurcation and optimizing the performance of this technique.

MAIN BRANCH STENTING ONLY

This strategy is used when the side branch has ostial or diffuse disease and is not suitable (too small) for stenting or is clinically irrelevant.[31] Two wires should be place in most bifurcations, and the side branch guidewire should be jailed in most of them after deployment of the stent in the MB. It is important in protecting the side branch from closure because of plaque shift and/or obstructing stent struts after MB stenting. Careful handling of the guiding catheter to prevent deep migration into the ostium of the coronary vessel is important to allow for the safe removal of the jailed guidewire.

PROVISIONAL SIDE BRANCH TECHNIQUE

This is the most frequently utilized technique for bifurcation lesions.

Approach

- Both MB and SB are wired after pre-dilatation (if required).
- Stenting of MB with proximal optimization technique

- Re-crossing into SB with wire (note: Jailed SB wire should not be removed until recrossing is done with another wire, alternatively the MB wire can be used for this purpose. The stenting procedure on the MB is completed, including postdilatation, after recrossing wire in SB). Caution has to be taken to retrieve this jailed wire because guiding catheter tends to be pulled in while retrieving this wire, which can damage coronary ostia and the stent.

Proximal optimization technique (POT)

Inflating a short bigger balloon just proximal to the carina.
It is useful in following ways:

- Solves the problem of underdeployment of proximal part of MB stent.
- The original anatomical configuration of the bifurcation is restored in compliance with Muray and Finet law.[32]
- Changes the ostium of SB favorable for rewiring/ballooning/stenting.

POT is of utmost importance when the SB is large and there is a great difference between the dimension of distal MB and proximal MB.

- Crossing with a balloon in SB
- Kissing balloon inflation with moderate pressure in SB until the balloon is fully expanded
- Final kissing balloon inflation (FKBI).

FKBI

It allows SB ostium treatment and apposition of the MB stent struts on the SB ostium. It also facilitates correction of stent distortion and correction of inadequate apposition in the MB.

How to do FKBI?:

- Balloon must be sufficiently short to avoid inflation outside the stent in MB and disease free area in SB
- Diameter of balloon must match with that of 2 distal branch
- Balloon inflated in MB first and then in SB in order to achieve strut projection in the ostium
- Use of noncompliant balloon allow improved stent expansion in MB while reducing risk of dissection in SB

Problem with FKBI: It increases procedural complexity, ovalization of stent, proximal dissection and suboptimal deployment of proximal stent segment.

Nordic-Baltic Bifurcation Study III[33] and CORPAL KISS[34] did not reveal any significant difference in FKBI vs No-FKBI group in terms of death, nonprocedural related MI, target lesion revascularization and stent thrombosis. However, angiographic restenosis was significantly reduced with FKBI.

- Second stent in SB to be done only if the result is inadequate.

Indications for second stent are:

- SB >2.5 mm (with TIMI flow < Grade III or FFR < 0.75)
- Threatening flow limiting dissection
- Hemodynamically significant SB
- 75% residual stenosis

Note: FFR may be helpful in decision-making when there is significant residual lesion in SB after provisional stenting[32]

TWO-STENT STRATEGY AS INTENTION TO TREAT

It requires correct patient selection, accurate assessment of the lesion severity, distribution of SB territory, extension of SB lesion and presence of concomitant disease.

It should be reserved for true bifurcation with SB that:

- Relatively large in diameter (>2.5 mm)
- Larger territory of distribution
- Severe disease that extends well beyond ostium (>10–20 mm)
- Unfavorable angle for re-crossing after MB stent implantation

Various 2-stent strategies are as follows:

T-stenting

- Most frequently used to shift from provisional stenting to stenting of SB
- It is best when angle between MB and SB is close to 90° (Fig. 16.5).

Classical T-stenting

- Both branches are wired and dilated
- Stent is deployed at the ostium of SB carefully to avoid stent protrusion into the MB while at the same time trying to minimize any possible gap
- Balloon from the SB is removed with wire in place
- Advance and deploy the stent in the MB
- Rewiring of the SB
- SB balloon dilatation
- Final kissing inflation

Modified T-stenting

- Performed by simultaneously positioning stent at the SB and MB, with the SB stent minimally protruding into the MB[35,36]
- The SB stent is deployed first and then after wire and balloon removal from the SB, the MB stent is deployed. The procedure is completed with a final kissing balloon inflation

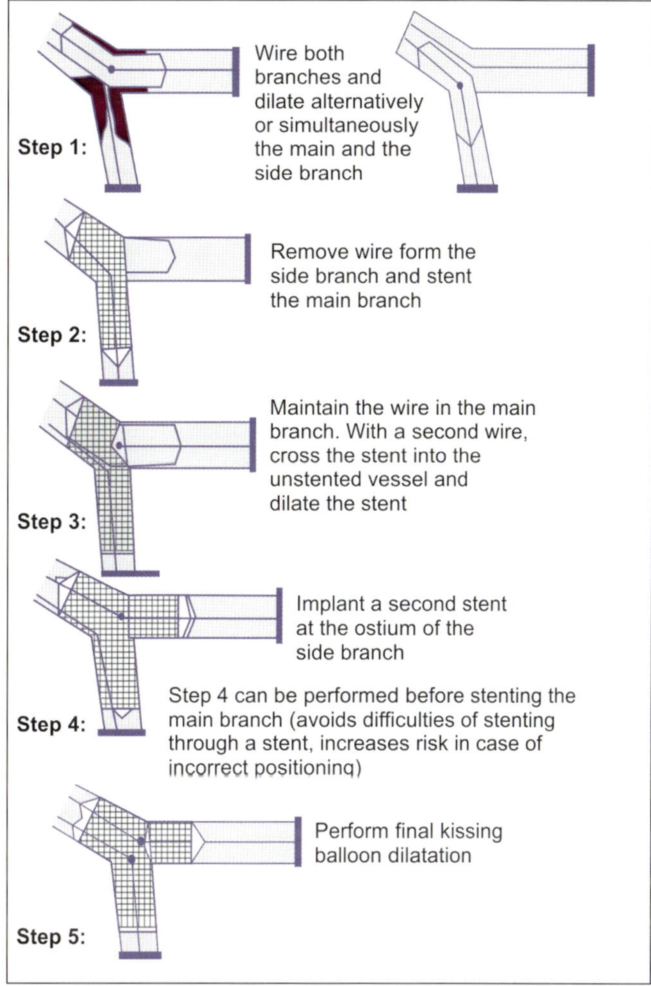

Fig. 16.5 T-stenting technique

Reverse T-stenting

- Best suitable bailout technique after initial MB stenting
- Rewiring the SB through the MB stent struts
- Ballooning and stenting of the SB
- Final kissing balloon is recommended for optimal result

Limitation (Above 3 techniques) Possibility of stent gap between MB and SB stent.

T-stenting and protrusion

- Used to enhance SB ostial coverage
- Initial steps are similar to T-stenting except the position of the SB stent, which is intentionally kept protruding in MB.
- Rest of the steps remains same as of classical T stenting
- The kissing balloon inflation reorients the protruding SB stent struts, resulting in a small neocarina.[37]

Advantage of T stenting: Easy and not technically demanding

Limitations of T-stenting: 90° angle between MB and SB is infrequent in non-left main coronary bifurcation. Not easy to recross wire following TAP in narrow angle.

V- and SKS Technique

- This technique includes inflating 2 stents simultaneously.[38,39]
- In V-stenting both the stents are pulled back as close as possible to create new carina as close as possible to original one.

While in SKS technique, 2 stents protrude into the MB with the creation of double barrel and a very proximal carina (Fig. 16.6).

Advantages

- Operator will never loose access to any of 2 branches.
- When final kiss is done, no need to recross any stent.

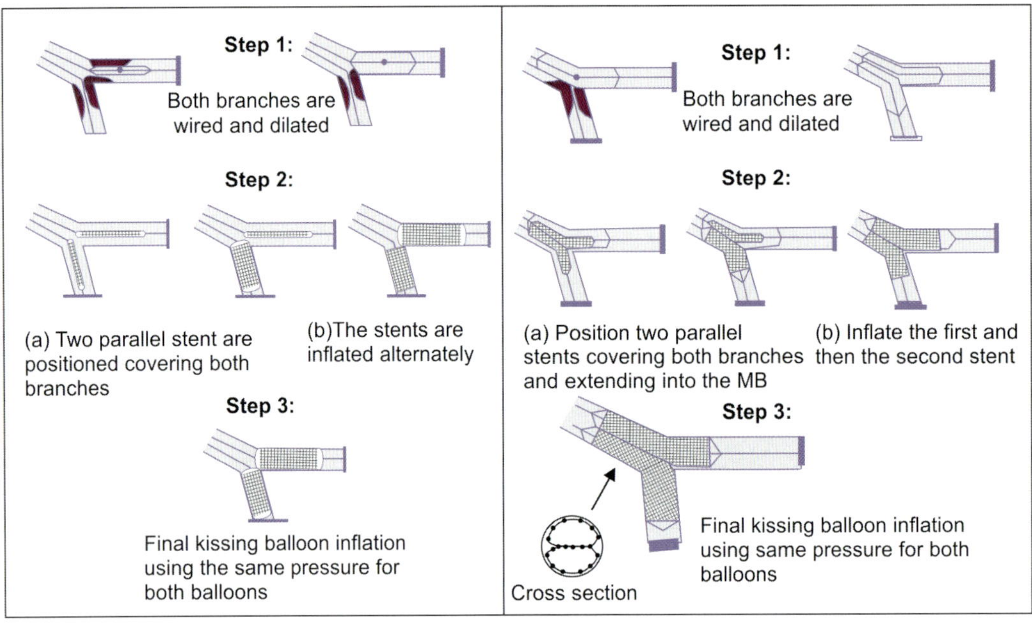

Fig. 16.6 V and SKS stenting technique

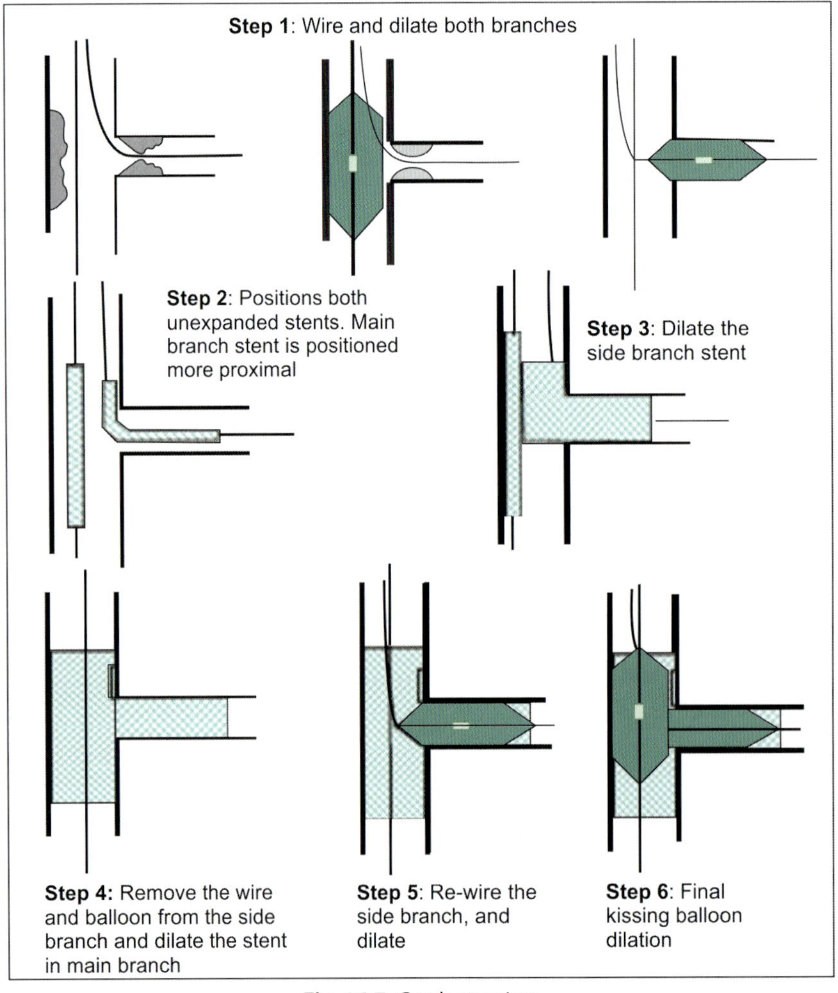

Fig. 16.7 Crush stenting

Limitations

- Incomplete proximal alignment of 2 stents
- Limited ability to effectively treat proximal dissections
- Difficult to recross stent with guidewire (if required).

Crush Technique (Fig. 16.7)

Standard crush

- 7Fr or 8Fr guiding catheter
- Both branches are wired and fully dilated
- Both SB and MB stents are advanced
- SB stent is positioned so that significant amount of stent protrudes within the MB
- SB stent is deployed at least at 12 atm and balloon is removed
- Angiogram is done to verify that the SB has an appropriate lumen and normal flow and there is no distal dissection or residual lesion. If additional stent is needed in the SB, this is the time to perform that
- Wire is removed from the SB and the stent in the MB is fully deployed at high pressure, usually above 12 atm
- Balloon removed from the MB and angiogram is taken
- Wire is reintroduced in SB and balloon dilatation of the SB done at high pressure (>12 atm)[40]
- Kissing dilatation with second balloon in the MB with an inflation pressure of 8–10 atm[41,42]

Step crush

- Used when there is need for 2-stent and 6Fr guiding is the only available option (e.g. radial approach)
- Both branches are wired and fully dilated
- Each stent is advanced and deployed separately
- First a stent is advanced into the SB protruding a few millimeters into the MB
- A balloon, rather than a second stent, is advanced into the MB
- Stent in the SB is deployed and the stent balloon is removed
- Angiography is performed and if the SB result is adequate, the wire is also removed
- MB balloon is then inflated to crush the protruding SB stent
- MB stent is advanced and deployed
- Remaining steps are similar as classical crush
- The result is identical to that obtained with the standard crush technique, except tat each stent is advanced and deployed separately

Mini crush

- 7Fr or 8Fr guiding catheter
- Both branches are wired and fully dilated
- Both SB and MB stents are advanced
- SB stent is positioned so that about 1–2 mm of the proximal end (minicrush) is within the MB
- Rest of the steps are similar to standard crush

Minicrush is associated with more complete endothelialization and in turn, less stent thrombosis, as well as easier recrossing of the crushed stent[51]

Double kissing (DK) crush technique

Modification of the step crush procedure, in which a balloon kissing inflation is performed twice: First after a MB balloon crushes the SB stent and then the standard final kissing inflation. 5 basic steps of DK crush are:

- SB stenting
- Balloon crush
- First kissing
- MB stenting and crushing
- Final kissing

DK crush may be superior to the classic crush technique with respect to acute procedural results and clinical outcomes by facilitating successful final kissing inflation in all patients.[43]

Reverse (Internal) crush

An option in the setting of provisional SB stenting using a 6Fr-guiding catheter:

- After stenting of MB, if the SB result is suboptimal internal crush could be an option to deploy a second stent in SB
- Guidewire is inserted into SB through stent and struts are dilated
- Second stent us advanced into the SB and left in position without deployed
- A balloon is advanced in MB at the level of the bifurcation making sure to stay inside the stent previously deployed in the MB
- Stent in SB is retracted about 2–3 mm into MB and deployed
- Stent balloon is removed and an angiogram is obtained to verify that a good result is present at the SB
- Wire from SB is removed and balloon in MB is inflated to high pressure
- Remaining steps are similar to those of crush technique

Advantages

- Immediate patency of both branches is assured
- Important when SB is functionally relevant or difficult to be wired
- Confirms to vessel geometry and there is complete coverage of carina especially with DK crush technique.

Limitations

- Need to recross multiple struts with wire and balloon
- An angle of 50° or more between the two branches have been suggested to be an independent predictor of major adverse cardiac events after crush stenting.[44]
- Ormiston et al.[45-47] stated that appropriate SB and MB dilatation is needed to fully expand the stent at SB ostium to widen gaps between stent strut overlying the SB and minimize stent distortion.

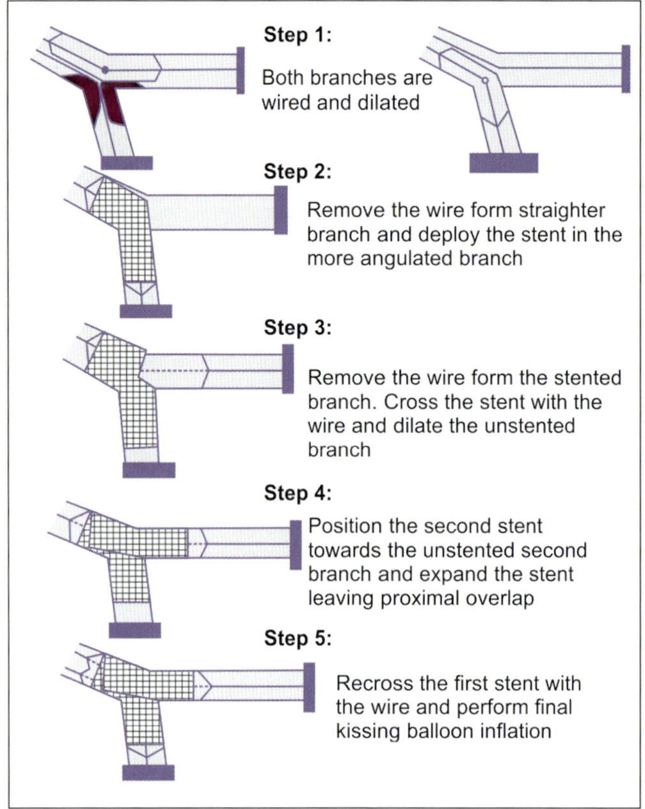

Fig. 16.8 Culotte technique

Table 16.1 Comparison between various bifurcation techniques[52]

Study	*Year*	*Technique*	*N*	*Follow-up (months)*	*MACE (%)*	*TVR (%)*	*Definite ST (%)*
Ferenc et al.[24]	2008	T stent vs provisional	202	9	11.9 vs 12.9	8.9 vs 10.9	2 vs 1
CACTUS[8]	2009	Crush vs provisional	350	6	15.8 vs 15	7.9 vs 7.5	1.7 vs 1.1
BBC ONE[2]	2010	Crush/culotte vs provisional	500	9	15.2 vs 8	5.6 vs 7.2	2.0 vs 0.4
DKCRUSH-11[4]	2011	DK crush vs provisional	370	12	10.3 vs 17.3	6.5 vs 14.6	2.2 vs 0,5
NOROIC-III[3]	2011	FKBI vs no FKBI	477	6	2,5 vs 3	1.3 vs 1.7	0.4 vs 0.4
NORDIC[6]	2013	Simple vs complex	413	60	15.8 vs 21.8	13.4 vs 18.3	3 vs 1.5
NORDIC-11[40]	2013	Crush vs culotte	424	36	22 vs 19.1	11.5 vs 6.5	1.4 vs 4.7
DK-III[25]	2013	DK crush vs culotte	419	12	6.2 vs 16.3	4.3 vs 11	0 vs 1

Culotte Technique (Fig. 16.8)

- It is referred as Y-stenting or trouser legs
- Was associated with high restenosis rate in past, but has regained popularity in the DES era[48,49]
- It gives maximum coverage at bifurcation at the expense of an excess of metal covering the proximal MB[50]
- Can be used in all true bifurcation lesions irrespective of the bifurcation angle and provide more homogeneous drug distribution at the side of the bifurcation.
- The only anatomic limitation is when there is a large mismatch between the proximal MB and SB diameter, which may lead to malapposition of the SB stent within the proximal part of the MB.[51]

Culotte technique
Can be performed using a 6Fr-guiding catheter
• Both branches are wired and predilated
• First a stent is deployed across the smaller, more angulated branch, usually the SB

- The nonstented branch is the rewired through the stent struts and dilatation is performed to facilitate passage of the second stent
- Stent is advanced and expanded into the nonstented branch, usually the MB
- Finally kissing balloon inflation is performed with preferably noncompliant balloons and each limb of the culotte should be dilated at high pressure individually before simultaneously inflating both balloons to nominal pressure.

When rewiring the other branch after stent placement, it is reasonable always to first place the guidewire distal into the stented branch to ensure that the wire has not passed under the stent struts before recrossing into the non stented branch.

Limitation of culotte with use of some closed cell stents (e.g. Cypher), the opening of the struts toward the branches may only reach a maximum diameter of 3 mm because of this, culotte technique should only be used with stents that have design allowing full opening of the struts toward both branches or when the expected size of the SB <3 mm.

Advantage

It guarantees the complete coverage of the SB ostium.

Limitations

- Double stent layer at the proximal MB and at the level of the carina.
- This technique is not advisable when there is large discrepancy between the size of the proximal MB and the SB due to the risk of incomplete wall apposition of the SB stent in the proximal MB segment
- Require rewiring of both branches through the stent strut, which can be technically demanding and time consuming.

GUIDELINES

Consensus from a meeting of the European bifurcation technique with regard to 2-stent strategies was.[53]

- Provisional T-stenting remains the gold standard technique for most bifurcations
- Large SB with ostial disease extending >5 mm from the carina are likely to require a 2-stent strategy.
- SB whose access is particularly challenging should be secured by stenting once accessed
- Kissing balloon inflation for carina reconstruction is mandatory in 2-stent techniques
- Noncompliant balloon are recommended for kissing inflation
- Individual noncompliant high-pressure "ostial" postinflations are mandatory in complex stenting techniques to achieve full stent expansion
- High-pressure proximal stent inflation using a short noncompliant balloon should be considered for correction of possible proximal stent distortion after kissing balloon inflation.

2011 ACC/AHA/SCAI[54] guidelines for percutaneous coronary interventions, recommendations for bifurcation lesion treatment:

- *Class I:* Provisional SB stenting should be the initial approach in patients with bifurcation lesions when the SB is not large and has only mild or moderate focal disease at the ostium (Level of evidence A)
- *Class IIa:* It is reasonable to use elective double stenting in patients with complex bifurcation morphology involving a large SB where the risk of side-branch occlusion is high and the likelihood of successful side-branch re-access is low (Level of evidence B).

BIORESORBABLE SCAFFOLDS IN BIFURCATION LESIONS

Bifurcation management with bioresorbable scaffolds (BRS) remains challenging.

Potential advantage of BRS is that it restores vessel patency without implanting a permanent prosthesis, which may be especially important for bifurcation treatment. On the other hand, limitations with BRS are its bulky profile, limited expansion capacity, length of time for complete resorption of the absorb (approx. 4 years) an creation of neointimal bridge on jailed struts.[55] Another potential drawback of BRS is increased early scaffold thrombosis as demonstrated by two large all-comers registries the GHOST-EU and AMC.[56,57]

Generally provisional stenting is the preferred technique when BRS is used for treatment of bifurcation.[58]

Determining Size of BRS

The main problem is the restriction of dilatation of the BRS above 0.5 mm of the reference diameter. One approach is to select the stent according to the distal reference of the MB. This strategy suffers restriction of postdilating proximal MB due to mechanical limitation of expanding the stent. Another strategy could be to select the stent according to the proximal MB and to deploy at low pressure in order to avoid damaging the distal vessel, followed by adequate postdilatation of the proximal segment.[58,59] However, the decision on sizing the stent according to the proximal or distal reference diameter depends on the individual coronary anatomy of the patient and is, in the end, the decision of the operator. Importantly an absorb BRS should not be used in bifurcations in which the proximal MV diameter is greater than the maximal recommended diameter of the BRS.[58]

Optimization Strategies

Proximal optimization technique (POT) is recommended with BRS but the restricted to NC balloons 0.5 mm larger than the reference for BRS. NC balloon is positioned with the distal balloon marker just proximal to the carina, and then inflated to expand to the diameter of the proximal segment.[58]

SB Ostial Dilatation

This results in distortion of BRS inside the MB and also some protrusion of struts into the SB.[59,60] To avoid strut fracture, a side branch dilatation with a 3.0 mm NC balloon at a maximum of 10 atm could be used for a 3.0 mm absorb BRS.[59] Final POT with an adequately sized NC balloon should be performed in the proximal MB to correct any scaffold malapposition created by SB opening (the sequential strategy is PSP: POT + side branch opening + final POT.

Routine FKBI is not recommended

Two Stent Technique

Bench studies and several case report have demonstrated the feasibility of a number of planned 2 stent techniques utilizing either 2 BRS or a combination of BRS and DES.[61-67]

When SB stenting is required as a crossover from provisional, metallic DES or BRS implantation can be used. T-stenting is the preferred technique.[58,68] Preliminary experience with TAP has also demonstrated sufficient SB lumen area without compromising the MB.[61-66] BRS may be considered for SB >2.5 mm and if the angle with the MB is favorable for T technique. Mini crush and culotte technique results in MB and SB lumen obstruction and these techniques should be avoided in order to prevent scaffold strut fractures and excessive overlap related to the thickness of the struts.[58,59] In the case of culotte stenting, 300 μm scaffold remains in the overlapped region of the proximal MB and in the case of mini crush the triple layer create approximately 450 μm of scaffold on one side, though for a short distance.

SUMMARY

Though the ideal approach to bifurcation lesions is provisional stenting, which coincides with the minimalist approach to angioplasty. When provisional approach is not feasible leads to 2-stent techniques as an intention to treat. Often a lesion can be treated with more than one approach. Each technique has its advantages and disadvantages. The DK Crush techniques by enlarge appears superior in restoring vessel geometry with complete coverage of the lesion and carina though Culotte procedure is very close. For 2-stent techniques, the operator should be well versed with the guiding catheter ID/OD, wires, use of noncompliant balloons and the stent platform, which is very vital in the final result. The introduction of BRS adds a new dimension. At the moment technical limitations of the BRS restricts its use. Provisional probably is the best approach with BRS. Future generations of the BRS should offer more flexibility.

REFERENCES

1. Myler RK, Shaw RE, Stertzer SH, et al. Lesion morphology and coronary angioplasty: current experience and analysis. J Am Coll Cardiol. 1992;19:1641-52.
2. Steigen TK, Maeng M, Wiseth R, et al. Randomized study on simple versus complex stenting of coronary artery bifurcation lesions: the Nordic bifurcation study. Circulation. 2006;114: 1955-61.
3. Louvare Y, Thomas M, Dazavik V, et al. Classification of coronary artery bifurcation lesions and treatments: time for a consensus! Catheter Cardiovasc Interv. 2008;71:175
4. Meier B, Gruentzig AR, King SB, et al. Risk of side branch occlusion during coronary angioplasty. Am J Cardiol 1984;53: 10-4.
5. Toggweiler S, Urbanek N, Schoenenberger AW, et al. Analysis of coronary bifurcations by intravascular ultrasound and virtual histology. Atherosclerosis. 2010;212:524-7.
6. Svindland A. The localization of sudanophilic and brous plaques in the main left coronary bifurcation. Atherosclerosis. 1983;48:139-45.
7. Grottum P, Svindland A, Walloe L. Localization of atherosclerotic lesions in the bifurcation of the main left coronary artery. Atherosclerosis. 1983;47:55-62.
8. Fox B, James K, Morgan B, et al. Distribution of fatty and brous plaques in young human coronary arteries. Atherosclerosis. 1982;41:337-47.
9. Oviedo C, Maehara A, Mintz GS, et al. Intravascular ultrasound classification of plaque distribution in left main coronary artery bifurcations: where is the plaque really located? Circ Cardiovasc Interv. 2010;3:105-12.
10. Colombo A, Al-Lamee R. Bifurcation lesions: an inside view. Circ Cardiovasc Interv. 2010;3:94-6.
11. Medina A, Martin P, Suarez de Lezo J, et al. Vulnerable carina anatomy and ostial lesions in the left anterior descending coronary artery after floating-stent treatment. Rev Esp Cardiol. 2009;62:1240-9.
12. Nakazawa G, Yazdani SK, Finn AV, et al. Pathological findings at bifurcation lesions: the impact of flow distribution on atherosclerosis and arterial healing after stent implantation. J Am Coll Cardiol. 2010;55:1679-87.
13. Ku DN, Giddens DP, Zarins CK, et al. Pulsatile flow and atherosclerosis in the human carotid bifurcation: positive correlation between plaque location and low oscillating shear stress. Arteriosclerosis. 1985;5:293-302.
14. Feldman CL, Stone PH. Intravascular hemodynamic factors responsible for progression of coronary atherosclerosis and development of vulnerable plaque. Curr Opin Cardiol. 2000; 15:430-40.
15. Papaioannou TG, Karatzis EN, Vavuranakis M, et al. Assessment of vascular wall shear stress and implications for atherosclerotic disease. Int J Cardiol. 2006;113:12-8.

16. Malek AM, Alper SL, Izumo S. Hemodynamic shear stress and its role in atherosclerosis. Jama. 1999;282:2035-42.
17. Stone PH, Coskun AU, Yeghiazarians Y, et al. Prediction of sites of coronary atherosclerosis progression: in vivo profiling of endothelial shear stress, lumen, and outer vessel wall characteristics to predict vascular behavior. Curr Opin Cardiol. 2003;18:458-70.
18. Gimbrone Jr MA, Topper JN, Nagel T, et al. Endothelial dysfunction, hemodynamic forces, and atherogenesis. Ann N Y Acad Sci. 2000;902:230-9.
19. Ku DN. Blood flow in arteries. Annu Rev Fluid Mech. 1997;29:399-434.
20. Soulis JV, Giannoglou GD, Chatzizisis YS, et al. Spatial and phasic oscillation of non-Newtonian wall shear stress in human left coronary artery bifurcation: an insight to atherogenesis. Coron Artery Dis. 2006;17:351-8.
21. Nagel T, Resnick N, Dewey Jr CF, et al. Vascular endothelial cells respond to spatial gradients in fluid shear stress by enhanced activation of transcription factors. Arterioscler Thromb Vasc Biol. 1999;19:1825-34.
22. Giannoglou GD, Soulis JV, Farmakis TM, et al. Haemodynamic factors and the important role of local low static pressure in coronary wall thickening. Int J Cardiol. 2002;86:27-40.
23. Buchanan JR Jr, Kleinstreuer C, Truskey GA, et al. Relation between nonuniform hemodynamics and sites of altered permeability and lesion growth at the rabbit aorto-celiac junction. Atherosclerosis. 1999;143:27-40.
24. Gambillara V, Chambaz C, Montorzi G, et al. Plaque-prone hemodynamics impair endothelial function in pig carotid arteries. Am J Physiol Heart Circ Physiol. 2006;290:H2320-H2328.
25. Cheng C, van Haperen R, de Waard M, et al. Shear stress affects the intracellular distribution of eNOS: direct demonstration by a novel in vivo technique. Blood. 2005;106:3691-8.
26. Ziegler T, Bouzourene K, Harrison VJ, et al. Influence of oscillatory and unidirectional flow environments on the expression of endothelin and nitric oxide synthase in cultured endothelial cells. Arterioscler Thromb Vasc Biol. 1998;18:686-92.
27. Qiu Y, Tarbell JM. Interaction between wall shear stress and circumferential strain affects endothelial cell biochemical production. J Vasc Res. 2000;37:147-57.
28. Chatzizisis YS, Coskun AU, Jonas M, et al. Role of endothelial shear stress in the natural history of coronary atherosclerosis and vascular remodeling: molecular, cellular, and vascular behavior. J Am Coll Cardiol. 2007;49:2379-93.
29. Louvard Y, Thomas M, Dzavik V, et al. Classification of coronary artery bifurcation lesions and treatments: time for a consensus! Catheter Cardiovasc Interv. 2008;71:175-83.
30. Movahed MR, Stinis CT. A new proposed simplified classification of coronary artery bifurcation lesions and bifurcation interventional techniques. J Invasive Cardiol. 2006;18:199-204.
31. Movahed MR. Coronary artery bifurcation lesion classifications, interventional techniques and clinical outcome. Expert Rev Cardiovasc Ther. 2008;6:261-74.
32. Lefevre T, Darremont O, Albiero R. provisional side branch stenting for the treatment of bifurcation lesions. Eurointervention 2010;6 (Suppl J):J65-71.
33. Niemela M, Kervinen K, Erglis A, et al. Randomized comparison of final kissing balloon dilatation versus no final kissing balloon dilatation in patients with coronary bifurcation lesions treated with main vessel stenting: the Nordic-Baltic Bifurcation Study III. Circulation. 2011;123:79-86.
34. Pan M, Medina A, Suarez de Lezo J, et al. Coronary bifurcation lesions treated with simple approach (from the Cordoba & Las Palmas [CORPAL] Kiss Trial) Am J Cardiol. 2011;107:1460-5.
35. Colombo A, Stankovic G, Orlic D, et al. Modified T-stenting technique with crushing for bifurcation lesions: immediate results and 30-day outcome. Catheter Cardiovasc Interv. 2003; 60:145-51.
36. Kobayashi Y, Colombo A, Akiyama T, et al. Modified "T" stenting: a technique for kissing stents in bifurcational coronary lesion. Catheterization and Cardiovascular Diagnosis. 1998;43:323-6.
37. Burzotta F, Gwon HC, Hahn JY, et al. Modified T-stenting with intentional protrusion of the side-branch stent within the main vessel stent to ensure ostial coverage and facilitate final kissing balloon: the T-stenting and small protrusion technique (TAP-stenting). Report of bench testing and first clinical Italian-Korean two-centre experience. Catheter Cardiovasc Interv. 2007;70: 75-82.
38. Schampaert E, Fort S, Adelman AG, Schwartz L. The V stent: a novel technique for coronary bifurcation stenting. Cathet Cardio vasc Diagn. 1996;39:320-6.
39. Sharma SK, Simultaneous kissing drug-eluting stent technique for percutaneous treatment of bifurcation lesions in large-size vessels. Catheter Cardiovasc Interv. 2005;65:10-16.
40. Ormiston JA, Currie E, Webster MW, et al. Drug-eluting stents for coronary bifurcations: insights into the crush technique. Catheter Cardiovasc Interv. 2004;63:332-336.
41. Ge L, Airoldi F, Iakovou I, et al. Clinical and angiographic outcome after implantation of drug-eluting stents in bifurcation lesions with the crush stent technique: importance of final kissing balloon post-dilation. J Am Coll Cardiol. 2005;46:613-20.
42. Ge L, Tsagalou E, Iakovou I, et al. In-hospital and nine-month outcome of treatment of coronary bifurcational lesions with sirolimus-eluting stent. Am J Cardiol. 2005;95:757-60.
43. Chen SL, Zhang JJ, Ye F, et al. Study comparing the double kissing (DK) crush with classical crush for the treatment of coronary bifurcation lesions: the DKCRUSH-1 Bifurcation Study with drug-eluting stents. Eur J Clin Invest. 2008;38:361-71.
44. Dzavik V, Kharbanda R, Ivanov J, et al. Predictors of long-term outcome after crush stenting of coronary bifurcation lesions: importance of the bifurcation angle. Am Heart J. 2006;152:762-9.
45. Ormiston JA, Webster MW, El Jack S, et al. Drug eluting stents for coronary bifurcations: bench testing of provisional side-branch strategies. Catheter Cardiovasc Interv. 2006;67:49-55.
46. Ormiston JA, Currie E, Webster MW, et al. Drug-eluting stents for coronary bifurcations: insight into the crush technique. Catheter Cardiovasc Interv. 2004; 63:332-6.
47. Ormiston JA, Webster MW, Webber B, Stewart JT, Ruygrok PN, Hatrick RI. The "crush" technique for coronary artery bifurcation stenting: insight from microcomputed tomographic imaging of bench deployments. JACC Cardiovasc Interv. 2008;1:351-7.
48. Chevalier B, Glatt B, Royer T, et al. Placement of coronary stents in bifurcation lesions by the "culotte" technique. Am J Cardiol. 1998;82:943-9.
49. Erglis A, Kumsars I, Niemela M, et al. Randomized comparison of coronary bifurcation stenting with the crush versus the culotte technique using sirolimus eluting stents: the Nordic Stent Technique Study. Circ Cardiovasc Interv. 2009;2:27-34.

50. Chevalier B, Glatt B, Royer T, Guyon P. Placement of coronary stents in bifurcation lesions by the "culotte" technique. Am J Cardiol. 1998;82:943-9.
51. Latib A, Colombo A, Moussa I, et al. When are two stents needed? Which technique is the best? How to perform? Euro-Intervention. 2010;6(Suppl. J):J81-7.
52. Felipe Fuchs, Vladimír Džavík. Coronary artery bifurcation lesions: a review of contemporary techniques in percutaneous coronary intervention. EMJ Int Cardiol. 2014;1:73-80.
53. Hildick-Smith D, Lassen JF, Albiero R, et al. Consensus from the 5th European Bifurcation club meeting. Eurointervention. 2010; 6:34-8.
54. Glenn NL, Eric RB, James C, et al. 2011 ACCF/AHA/SCAI Guideline for Percutaneous Coronary Intervention. J Am Coll Cardiol. 2011;58(24):e44-e122.
55. Okamura T, Onuma Y, Garcia-Garcia HM, et al. 3-Dimensional optical coherence tomography assessment of jailed side branches by bioresorbable vascular scaffolds: a proposal for classification. JACC Cardiovasc Interv. 2010;3:836-44.
56. Kraak RP, Hassell ME, Grundeken MJ, et al. Initial experience and clinical evaluation of the Absorb bioresorbable vascular scaffold (BVS) in real-world practice: the AMC Single Centre Real World PCI Registry. Euro Intervention. 2015;10:1160-8.
57. Capodanno D, Gori T, Nef H, et al. Percutaneous coronary intervention with everolimus-eluting bioresorbable vascular scaffolds in routine clinical practice: early and midterm outcomes from the European multicentre GHOST-EU registry. Euro Intervention. 2015;10:1144-53.
58. Lassen JF, Holm NR, Stankovic G, et al. Percutaneous coronary intervention for coronary bifurcation disease: consensus from the first 10 years of the European Bifurcation Club meetings. Euro Intervention. 2014;10:545-60.
59. Ormiston JA, Webber B, Ubod B, et al. Absorb everolimus-eluting bioresorbable scaffolds in coronary bifurcations: a bench study of deployment, side-branch dilatation and post-dilatation strategies. EuroI ntervention. 2015;10:1169-77.
60. Ormiston JA, Webster MW, Ruygrok PN, et al. Stent deformation following simulated side- branch dilatation: a comparison of five stent designs. Catheter Cardiovasc Interv. 1999;47:258-64.
61. Attizzani GF, Ohno Y, Capranzano P, et al. Initial experience of percutaneous coronary intervention in bifurcations with bioresorbable vascular scaffolds using different techniques-insights from optical coherence tomography. Int J Cardiol. 2013;170:e33-5.
62. Grundeken MJ, Hassell ME, Kraak RP, et al. Treatment of coronary bifurcation lesions with the absorb bioresorbable vascular scaffold in combination with the Tryton dedicated coronary bifurcation stent: evaluation using two- and three-dimensional optical coherence tomography. Euro Intervention. 2014.
63. Fernandez D, Brugaletta S, Martin-Yuste V, et al. First experience of a bioresorbable vascular scaffold implantation in left main stenosis. Int J Cardiol. 2013;168:1566-8.
64. Dzavik V, Muramatsu T, Crooks N, et al. Complex bifurcation percutaneous coronary intervention with the absorb bioresorbable vascular scaffold. Euro Intervention. 2013;9:888
65. Jim MH. No-kiss sleeve: a technical modification of the sleeve technique to treat true bifurcation lesions in the bioresorbable vascular scaffold era. Int J Cardiol. 2014;176:532-4.
66. Miyazaki T, Costopoulos C, Sato K, et al. Strategy for optimal side-branch positioning of bioresorbable vascular scaffolds in dedicated 2-stent techniques: insights from optical coherence tomography. Cardiovasc Revasc Med. 2014;15:298-300.
67. Miyazaki T, Latib A, Colombo A. Provisional hybrid 2-stent strategy utilizing bioresorbable vascular scaffold and drug-eluting metal stent; 'T-stenting and small protrusion' technique. Catheter Cardiovasc Interv. 2014.
68. Motreff P, Darremont O, Leymarie JL, et al. BVS Bench Testing. 10th European Bifurcation Club Meeting, Bordeaux, October 17-18, 2014. http://*www.bifurc.net/files/medtool/webmedtool/icpstool01/stud0638/pdf00001.pdf*

CHAPTER

17

Saphenous Vein Graft Intervention

Anil Dhall, Salil Garg, Ajay Joshi, Anup Banerji

INTRODUCTION

In 1969, Favalaro described the first use of coronary artery bypass surgery (CABG) for the treatment of myocardial ischemia due to coronary artery disease. Subsequent advances led to improvements in outcomes and the widespread use of CABG. It has been proven that CABG improves long-term prognosis in high-risk subsets, those with significant left main, triple vessel disease and with decreased left ventricular function. The internal mammary artery (IMA) and other arterial conduits revolutionized CABG because of the relative resistance of arterial conduits to accelerated atherosclerosis compared with saphenous vein bypass grafts. In post-CABG patients recurrent ischemia can be due to progression of disease in native vessel. But, the most common cause of adverse cardiac events in the post-CABG patient is atherosclerosis and attrition of saphenous vein graft (SVG). One year after surgery, up to 15% of SVG are occluded and only 61% of SVG are patent at 10 years. And those with patent SVG, many are diffusely diseased. It has been seen that repeat CABG is associated with increased morbidity and mortality. Therefore, PCI is the preferred revascularization strategy for SVG disease. But their a substantial risk of major adverse cardiac event (MACE) which is caused mainly by periprocedural myocardial infarction (MI) as a result of distal embolization and no-reflow. The postprocedure ischemia is graded as:

Very Early Postoperative Ischemia (<1 Month)

The most common cause of ischemia within hours or days of surgery is acute vein graft thrombosis (60%). Other causes are incomplete surgical revascularization (10%) are due to, kinked grafts, focal stenosis at the proximal or distal anastomotic sites, spasm or injury, insertion of graft to a vein causing AV fistula, or bypass of the wrong vessel.

Early Postoperative Ischemia (1 Month–1 Year)

Recurrent angina between 1 month and 1 year after the surgery is most often due to peri-anastomotic stenosis, graft occlusion, or mid-SVG stenosis from fibrous intimal hyperplasia. Recurrence of angina at about 3 months postoperatively is also highly suggestive of a distal graft anastomotic lesion and should, in most cases, lead to evaluation for PCI.

Late Postoperative Ischemia (>3 Years after Surgery)

At this stage, the most common cause of ischemia is due to formation of new atherosclerotic plaques in the SVG. However, these plaques have less fibrocollagenous tissue and calcification, so they are softer, more friable, of larger size, and frequently associated with thrombus.

Very Late Postoperative Ischemia

This generally is due to fibrotic or calcific disease.

The percutaneous treatment of patients with obstructive atherosclerotic disease in SVG remains a challenge in interventional cardiology. Patients undergoing SVG intervention are often older, and have multiple comorbidities. Moreover, SVG usually present a degenerated pattern of atherosclerosis, with complex, friable, thrombotic-prone lesions. SVG interventions carry a higher risk of acute complications, mainly distal embolization, and poorer long-term out comes, mainly restenosis, than do native coronary vessel interventions.

The predictors of one-month major adverse cardiac events after SVG intervention have been explored. The degree of SVG degeneration assessed by the SVG degeneration score, the estimated plaque volume, angiographic evidence of thrombus, and increasing patient age are the correlates associated with the 30-days composite outcome of death, myocardial infarction (MI) and target lesion revascularization (TLR). The important reason for poorer outcomes PCI of SVG is the embolization of atherothrombotic debris into the native coronary circulation, often resulting in reduced antegrade flow (no-reflow). Strategies for addressing this distal embolization problem include both proximal and distal protection devices, as well as adjunctive pharmacology and stenting approaches.

The embolic protection devices have demonstrated value in decreasing the risk of embolization and postprocedural myocardial enzyme elevation after SVG intervention. While stenting has definitely been proved to be superior to balloon-only angioplasty or the treatment of SVG lesions, the choice of the type of stent bare metal stent versus drug-eluting stent is still a matter of debate. Drug-eluting stents appear promising for the management of SVG disease; however, available long-term safety and effectiveness data are conflicting and give reason for caution.[1-3] Mesh covered stents at one time appeared to be the ideal way forward, but data has not shown remarkable advantage. Long-term studies in the use of current generation Bioabsorbable Vascular Scaffold is not available and the Octopus study has just observed six patients for a period of 12 months.

NATURAL HISTORY OF SVG DISEASE

The SVG disease process involves three interlinked pathophysiological phenomena that lead to progressive degeneration: Thrombosis, intimal hyperplasia, and atherosclerosis.

THROMBOSIS

About 10% of SVG occlude, with or without symptoms, within the first month after coronary artery bypass graft (CABG) surgery. This early phenomenon seems to be related to severe endothelial cell loss and medial damage during harvesting. In addition, this prothrombotic stage of SVG may be amplified by technical factors that reduce graft flow, such as intact venous valves, anastomotic stricture, and graft anastomosis proximal to diseased segments.

INTIMAL HYPERPLASIA

Accumulation of smooth muscle cells and extracellular matrix in the intimal space (intimal hyperplasia) is the main disease process that occurs during the first months after venous bypass grafting. The increase in wall stress by exposure to arterial pressures seems to be an important factor inducing this phenomenon. This process represents the foundation for later development of SVG atherosclerosis.

ATHEROSCLEROSIS

In the first years after CABG, atherosclerosis is the dominant process involved in SVG disease, but recurrent symptoms due to SVG disease rarely occur before three years after grafting. Morphologically, vein graft atherosclerosis tends to be diffuse, concentric, and friable with a poorly developed or absent fibrous cap and little evidence of calcification.

INDICATIONS FOR INTERVENTION

Due to the increased risk of periprocedural MI related to SVG interventions, PCI of the native grafted vessel if technically feasible is usually preferred over PCI of the degenerated SVG. However, when PCI of the native vessel is not possible, the clinical benefit of a high-risk SVG intervention should be balanced against the risk of morbidity and mortality of repeat CABG. In addition, repeat CABG is less effective in terms of complete revascularization and symptom control when compared to the first procedure.

The latest updated guidelines on this topic recommend PCI in the following circumstances.[4]

- Early ischemia (usually within 30 days) after CABG, when technically feasible.
- Ischemia that occurs one to three years after CABG in patients with discrete lesions and preserved LV function.
- Also in patients with diseased SVGs older than three years with patent left internal mammary artery (IMA) and significant obstruction in other vessels.

Percutaneous coronary intervention (PCI) is not recommended in patients with total SVG occlusions, or multiple target lesions (native/SVG disease) and impaired LV function, unless repeat CABG poses excessive risk. CABG is usually reserved for patients who cannot have adequate percutaneous revascularization or for those who may gain an additional benefit from CABG, such as those with previously unused left IMA to left anterior descending artery.

Thus to summarize, PCI is usually preferred over repeat CABG for early recurrent symptoms after CABG (<3 years). For late graft failure, because of the initial higher mortality of redo CABG and the comparable long-term mortality, PCI is the preferred revascularization strategy in patients with patent left IMA and amenable anatomy. However, most symptomatic post-CABG patients present with extensive native and graft disease where the revascularization strategy must be based on careful risk/benefit assessment of the procedure and the local experience. The most important factors involved in the choice of repeat CABG are more extensive SVG/native disease, lower left ventricular ejection fraction, longer interval from first CABG, more total occlusion of native arteries, and the absence of patent IMA graft. It is prudent for redo CABG the IMA be the graft of choice.

DIFFICULTIES AND METHODS

When dealing with a percutaneous intervention for an SVG lesion. Dual antiplatelet therapy and statins are mandatory, unless clearly contraindicated. Periprocedural glycoprotein IIb/IIIa inhibitors do not seem to be effective in SVG interventions.[5] However, in cases of acute myocardial infarction due to acute graft closure and the possibly high burden of acute, non-organized thrombus, they can be used.

ACCESS SITE AND GUIDING CATHETER CHOICE

For SVG there is no specific recommendation to choose either the radial or the femoral approach besides the known risks/benefits of each access site, the choice of the patient and the experience of the operator (Fig. 17.1). In our experience, when using radial access, a left radial approach is more suitable for SVG, originating from the left anterior wall of the aorta and directed to the left coronary artery. For these SVG, mainly if their aortic anastomosis is high in the ascending aorta, the right radial approach offers poor support and the choice of the guiding catheter remains complicated and poorly predictable. On the other hand, for SVG from the right or posterior wall of the aorta (usually directed to the right coronary artery or sometimes to the circumflex territory) right and left radial approaches are equivalent. Choosing the correct guiding catheter is a very important step. In our experience, for SVG to the right coronary artery, originating most of the time from the right anterior surface of the aorta, the multipurpose catheter has the best alignment and support when performing the procedure via either the femoral or the radial artery. Engagement of the catheter can be performed in the left anterior oblique view. For vein grafts originating from the left anterior surface (usually to the left anterior descending/diagonal or marginal/circumflex arteries), we prefer Judkins right or left coronary bypass catheters (the best fitting catheter can be tested during the diagnostic angiography) in case of femoral access. If additional support is needed, Amplatz left catheters can be used. Engagement is feasible in the right anterior oblique view. When approaching these bypasses via the radial approach, as previously mentioned, we recommend choosing the left radial artery. Guiding catheters of choice can be extra back-up shaped or Amplatz left catheters. Sometimes vein grafts to the circumflex originate from the posterior surface of the aorta. In this case, Amplatz left or multipurpose guiding catheters are preferred, and engagement is performed in the right anterior oblique view.

The use of the RAO view to engage the grafts has a possible advantage in that the grafts to the left coronary are usually anterior whereas those to the right coronary are usually posterior in origin.

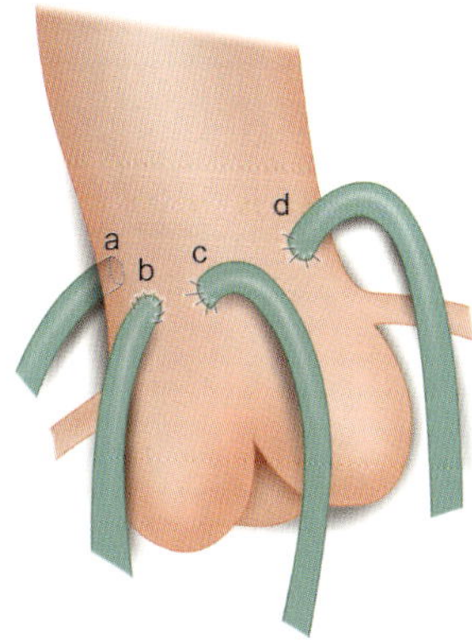

Fig. 17.1 Radial and femoral access no specific benefit, but for anterior left sided grafts left radial approach better than right radial approach. Guide catheter choice for different graft location. (a) MP, AL, JR, AR; (b) MP, AL, JR; (c) HS, AL, JR; (d) AL, JR

Abbreviations: AL, amplatz left; AR, amplatz right; HS, hockey stick; JR, judkins right; MP, multipurpose

EMBOLIC PROTECTION

The "mechanical" protection of the vasculature distal to the treated SVG lesion is the only strategy, up to now, soundly proven to reduce distal embolization and periprocedural MI. Indeed PCI of SVG should always be performed under embolic protection device. So far, three types of device have been developed.

The first to be tested in SVG was a distal occlusion device (Figs 17.2 to 17.4). Its mechanism is as follows. A compliant balloon, directly present in the distal tip of a guidewire specifically made with this feature, is positioned distal to the lesion before the PCI and is inflated at low pressure during the procedure.

Distal filters have the same rationale but a different mechanism of action from the distal occlusion device (Figs 17.5A and B). A distal filter is a porous filter, which is placed distally to the lesion before the PCI in order to collect embolic material and retrieve it after the procedure.[6,7] The value of the first commercialized filter has been proven in the Filter wire Randomized Evaluation (FIRE) trial, a large randomized study, in which the filter was shown to be noninferior to the previously described "occlusion and aspiration" system.[8] Several filters have recently been released onto the market, some with proven non-inferiority as compared with the approved protection devices (Table 17.1),[9] some without clear evidence of benefit (Fig. 17.6).[10,11] The last embolic protection device is the proximal protection device (Figs 17.7A to E). This is a catheter with a specific protection balloon on its distal tip, guided inside a standard guiding catheter up to the ostium of the vein graft proximal to the lesion site similar to a mother-and-child technique. At this level the balloon is inflated temporarily, occluding blood flow and creating a column of stagnant blood, so that the debris dislodged during the PCI which is performed through the device itself can then be aspirated from the vessel through the same catheter. The Proximal Protection During saphenous vein graft intervention using the Proxis Embolic Protection System (PROXIMAL) trial compared this proximal protection device with currently available distal protection devices (either occlusion-based or filters) showing non-inferiority of the study device.[12] Despite this large body of evidence and the guidelines, embolic protection devices remain underutilized in daily practice. The elevated cost of these devices seems to be a major explanation for their low utilization. Moreover, the fact that there is a learning curve can also play a role in the speed of their adoption in clinical practice. We recommend that operators select a couple of embolic protection devices that they can utilize regularly to build up experience with and confidence in their use. Protection devices can eventually be avoided in cases of very focal lesions in small (<3.5 mm) grafts. In this case, a soft-tip coronary guidewire and direct stenting without predilatation and post-dilatation should be the recommended strategy.

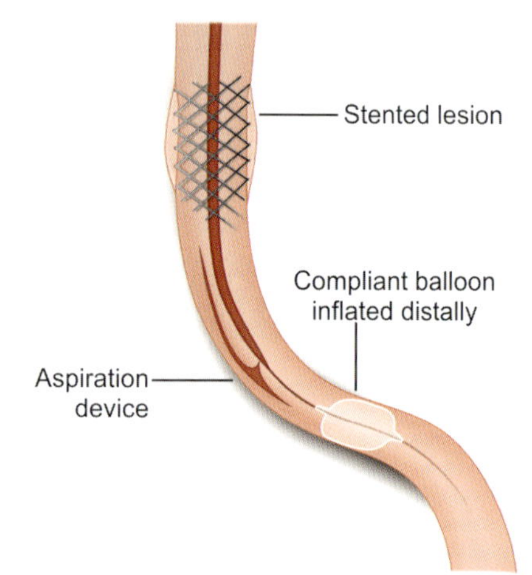

Fig. 17.2 Depicting a distal balloon occlusion device

Choosing the type of protection device depends mainly on the location of the lesion, on the tolerance of the patient to prolonged ischemia and on the operator's personal experience with the device (Fig. 17.8). In cases of proximal or ostial lesions, distal protection devices should be recommended. In cases of distal lesions, a proximal protection device fits better. The theoretical background for these choices relies on the fact that every protection device needs a vein graft disease-free landing zone of around 3–5 cm. In case of lesions in the mid body of the graft, any type of protection device is usable. In this instance, an important consideration for the choice of the device is the tolerance of the patient to ischemia. Indeed, proximal protection devices and distal occlusion devices require a prolonged time of ischemia (in our experience, usually two to four minutes) due to the temporary occlusion of the SVG by means of the inflated low-compliance balloon. On the contrary, filters allow performance of the procedure without interruption of blood flow and should be preferred in

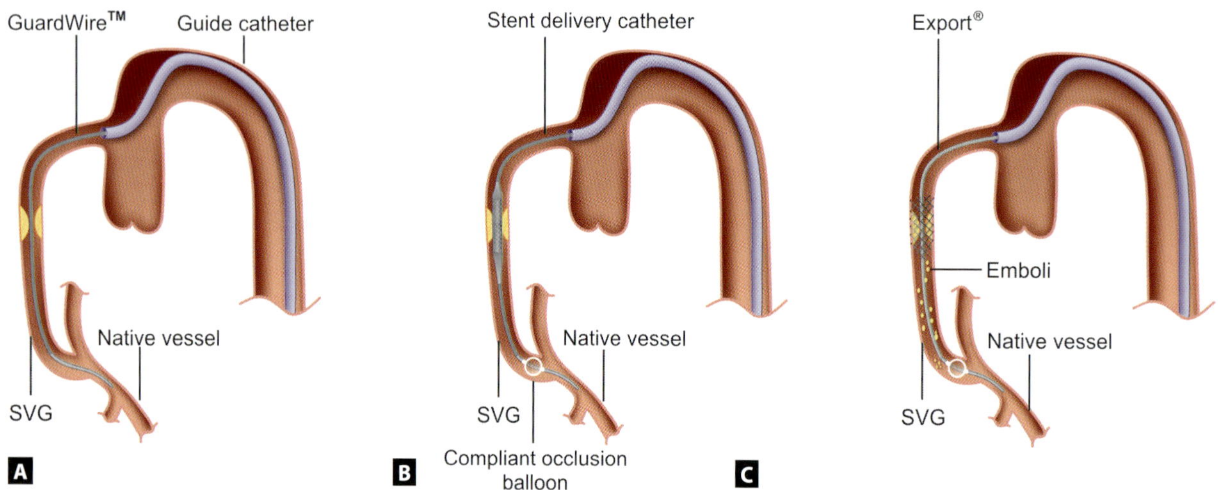

Figs 17.3A to C Distal balloon occlusion device. (A) Lesion crossed with wire; (B) Balloon protection device inflated distally and PCI performed; (C) Balloon inflated till use of export catheter

Abbreviation: SVG, saphenous vein graft

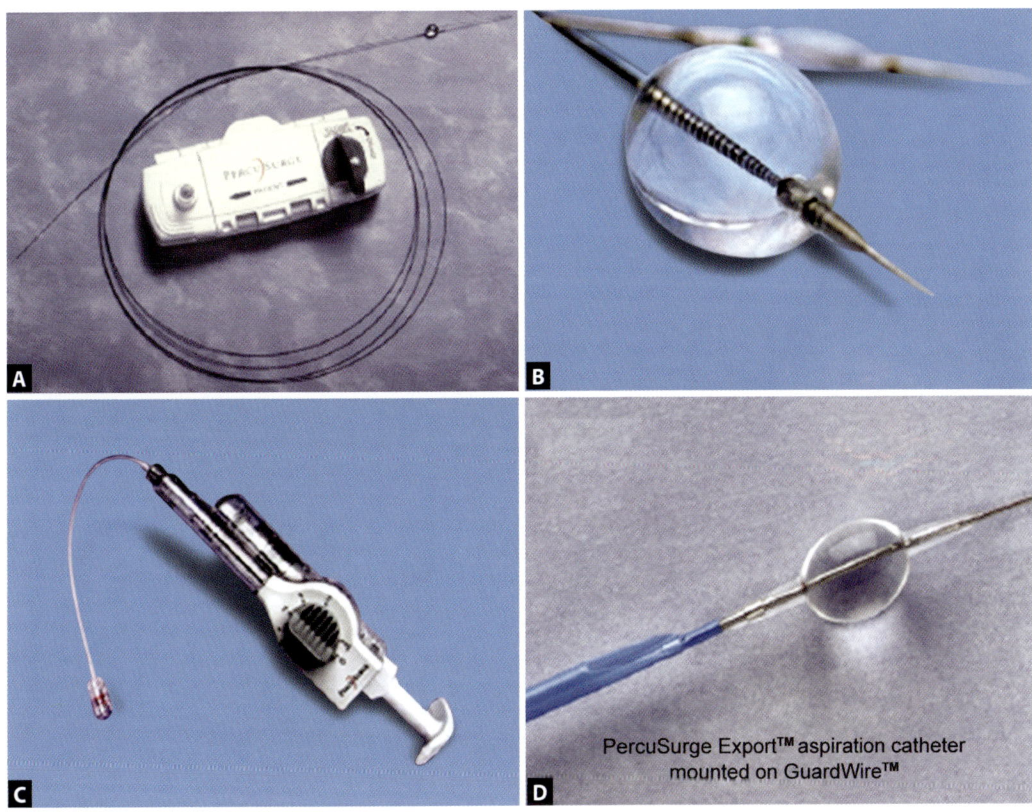

Figs 17.4A to D PercuSurge GuardWire distal protection system (Medtronic). (A) Miniature valve within the hypo tube controlled with microseal adaptor which keeps the distal balloon inflated during the procedure; (B) Distal occlusion balloon inflated over a 0.014 inch nitinol based hypotube guidewire; (C) EZ-flator inflates the balloon to stop distal flow; (D) Export aspiration catheter removes debris while the occlusion is inflated

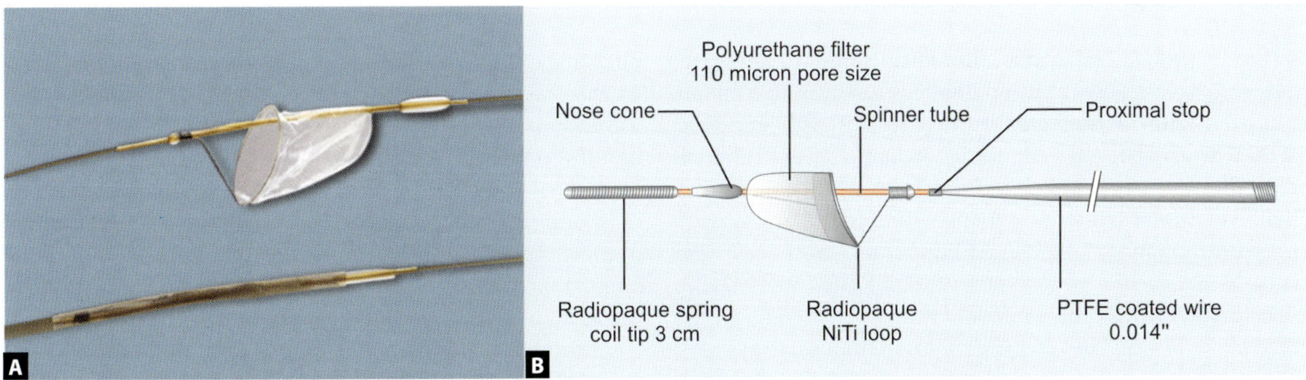

Figs 17.5A and B Filter wire EZ (Boston scientific). (A) Filter wire is composed of polyurethane filter basket preloaded on a delivery sheath; (B) Filter wire is compatible with a 6 F guide catheter available in wire length of 190 and 300 cm. A landing zone of >30 mm is required and a retrieval sheath is required for capture and removal of the filter
Abbreviation: PTFE, polytetrafluoroethylene.

more unstable patients with poorer left ventricular function, or in SVG with a very large area of myocardium downstream When using a protection device, the careful positioning of the device itself (the low-compliance balloon or the filter) in an angiographically disease-free zone is the first step. If possible, the proximal protection device can be tracked in the SVG to approximate the lesion, thus improving the support of the catheter itself or the procedure. In case of proximal or distal

Table 17.1 Comparison of different distal embolic protection devices

	EZ	*Accunet*	*Nav 6*	*Spider*	*Fibernet*
ø ≥6 mm	No	Yes	Yes	Yes	Yes
Tight stenosis	++	++	+++	++±	+
Small landing zone	+	+	++	+	+++
Angulations	++	++	++±	+++	+
Curved landing	+	++	++	+	+++
Complex crossing	+	+	++	+++	+

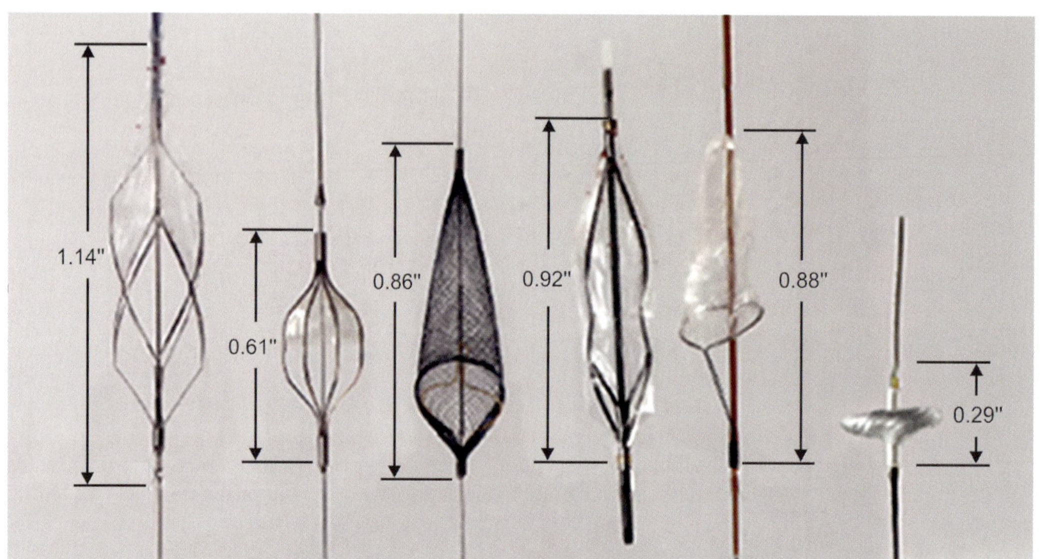

Fig. 17.6 Different shape and sizes of distal filter protection devices with different pore size from 80 uM to 200 uM

occlusion protection devices, the effectiveness of adequate and complete vessel occlusion should be assured. This means that a column of stagnant blood (checked with contrast) should be evident once the device is in place and inflated. If a filter is used, we recommend securing appropriate deployment of the filter (good apposition to the vessel wall) in two orthogonal views. An additional tip, in case of filter use and in case of a poorly supportive guiding catheter, is to place an additional conventional coronary guidewire in the SVG before placing the filter. This helps to stabilize the system and improves track ability of subsequent devices. Once the protection device is in place, we always recommend direct stenting and, in case the stent remains significantly under deployed, high-pressure postdilatation must be done with a protection device in place.

Once the stenting procedure is finished, care should be given to the collection of debris from the protection device and to retrieval of the device itself. With proximal device placement, direct aspiration of at least 5 cc of blood from the device should be performed before releasing the occlusion. In case of distal occlusion device use, the specific manual aspiration device should be used, and two syringes of 20 cc of blood should be aspirated. If a filter is used, careful, complete closure of the filter with a dedicated retrieval catheter is necessary before retrieval of the filter. We recommend performing the complete procedure under fluoroscopy. Final angiographic control of the stenting procedure without a device in place is mandatory in at least two orthogonal views.

Although definitive data coming from randomized trials are lacking, "pharmacologic" protection targeted at improving microvascular flow dynamics with intra-graft administration of vasodilators (such as adenosine, nitroprusside, verapamil or nicardipine) is considered another possible prophylactic treatment for the prevention of no-reflow. Currently, due to the lack of clear evidence about these agents, we do not perform routine prophylactic administration of these agents before SVG PCI, but only as "bail-out" in case of proven no-reflow just after PCI.

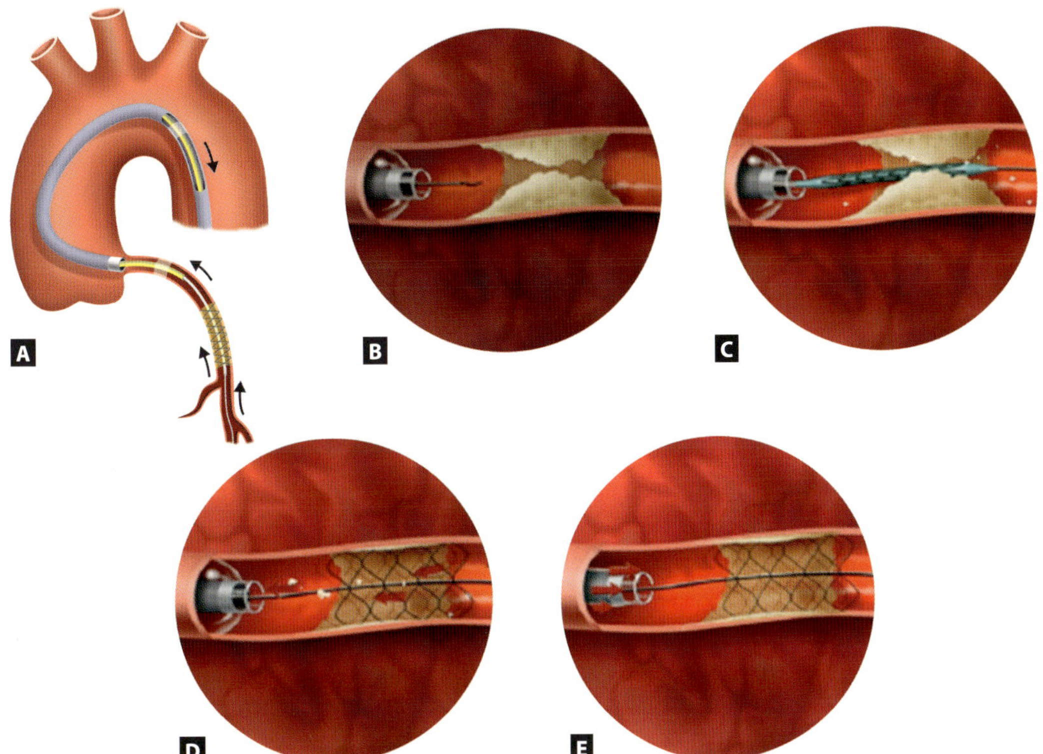

Figs 17.7A to E Proxis proximal embolic protection device (St jude). (A) Proximal embolic protection device before crossing the lesion with guidewire; (B) Balloon inflated in SVG to suspend the blood flow; (C) SVG intervention performed after guidewire is advanced across the lesion; (D) Embolic debris is aspirated from the SVG after stenting; (E) Balloon is deflated, restoring flow in the SVG

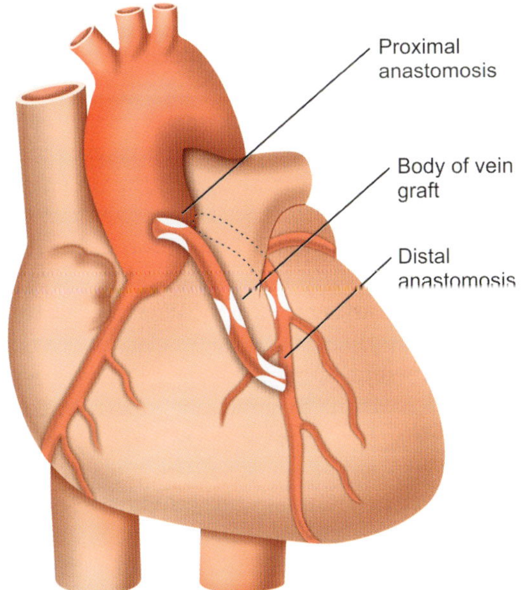

Fig. 17.8 For ostio or proximal lesions distal protection devices and for distal lesion proximal device fits better and for mid body or shaft any device is better. Distal embolic filters need a distal landing zone of more than 30 mm

CHOICE OF STENT

While stenting has been definitely proven superior to balloon-only angioplasty in SVG intervention,[13] the specific type of stent (bare metal or drug-eluting) is still a matter of debate. In almost all pivotal randomized trials, SVG lesions were excluded. The mechanisms of the in-stent restenotic process in SVG are different when compared to native arteries. Furthermore, the problem of higher local prothrombotic conditions in SVG and the expected delay in endothelial healing after drug-eluting stent (DES) placement are claimed to be possible drawbacks of DES implantation in SVG, as they can potentially lead to a higher risk of stent thrombosis. Thus, clear and available data concerning the safety and the efficacy of these devices in SVG are needed before a routine application of DES in this lesion subset can be approved.

There are currently three randomized studies specifically performed in SVG: the single-center double-blind "Reduction of Restenosis. In Saphenous vein grafts with Cypher stent" (RRISC) trial, comparing in 75 patients sirolimus-eluting stents and the respective uncoated bare metal stents (BMS),[14] the multicentre single-blind "Stenting of Saphenous Vein Grafts"(SOS) trial, comparing in 80 patients paclitaxel-eluting stents and the respective BMS,[15] and the multicenter "Is Drug-Eluting-Stenting Associated with Improved Results in Coronary Artery Bypass Grafts" (ISAR CABG) trial comparing in 610 patients three different DES (sub-randomized to paclitaxel-eluting stents, permanent polymer sirolimus-eluting stents, or biodegradable-polymer sirolimus-eluting stents) versus BMS.[16]

All these trials showed significant reduction of angiographic and clinical restenosis with DES compared with BMS at one-year follow-up. However, longer-term follow-up and analyses of the RRISC and of the SOS trials showed conflicting clinical results. The SOS trial reported sustained benefit; with DES significantly reducing repeated revascularization procedures without any significant difference in mortality.[17] The RRISC trial showed a notable increase in mortality with DES, also with attrition in revascularisation difference that disappeared at three-year follow-up.[18] The long-term results of the much larger ISAR CABG trial are eagerly awaited and will shed additional light on the topic.

At a lower level of evidence with respect to randomized trials, several registries have assessed the mid-term and long-term safety and effectiveness of DES in SVG. Overall, while in all studies with follow-up <1 year the benefits of DES in terms of reduction of repeated revascularization procedures seem evident, at longer term several studies have not shown significantly different revascularization outcomes between DES and BMS, while a few studies have demonstrated only moderate advantages, clearly not comparable to the benefits shown in native coronary arteries. On the other hand, safety issues, such as those seen in the long-term follow-up of the RRISC trial, have never been confirmed.

All these data underline the fact that DES can be considered effective and safe at short-term (one year) follow-up as consistently shown in several studies; however, long term follow-up of adequately performed studies is required to confirm that DES remain safe and effective also after one year. While awaiting these studies, our policy is to implant BMS as first choice for *de novo* SVG lesions and in case of restenosis, which in any case has a different, less thrombus-prone physiopathological substrate than native in graft disease.

Concerning the implantation strategy, independently from the type of stent chosen, we almost always definitely recommend attempting direct stenting. In case of failure, we also suggest a low threshold for switching to balloon predilatation. Significantly undersized balloons should be favored in case of predilatation in order to minimize plaque embolization. In case of temporary occlusion of the SVG during direct stent placement and the impossibility of visualizing with contrast the distal landing zone of the SVG, the clips present around the SVG can often be used as landmarks to improve accuracy in stent positioning and deployment, even without the help of contrast injections. Other types of stent, so-called "covered" stents, have also been tested in SVG lesions (Fig. 17.9). The rationale behind this type of stent was to prevent distal embolization, as the stent itself, covered by a layer of polytetrafluoroethylene (PTFE), was supposed to trap friable plaque between the stent and the SVG wall. However, this theory proved false: PTFE-covered stents, in comparison to BMS, did not reduce the amount of distal embolization and the rate of periprocedural MI, and showed no different, or even worse, clinical and angiographic restenosis. Thus, the use of PTFE-covered stents in the treatment of SVG cannot be recommended. None the less, new developments in the same concept have recently been undertaken. Preliminary experience using a newly developed system comprising a BMS platform with a polymeric net attached to its surface (supposed liable to entrap fibro-thrombotic material), appears to be a potentially interesting innovation to prevent distal embolization and no-reflow in SVG PCI. However, these data are preliminary and based on a small number of patients: once again, therefore, larger trials are definitely needed. In the meanwhile, this device should be used only in the setting of clinical studies. A 22% rate of progression from moderate non-ischemic lesions to clinically severe stenosis was shown in only one year in the group treated conventionally, with medical therapy only. This indeed proves the rapidly evolving nature of SVG disease.

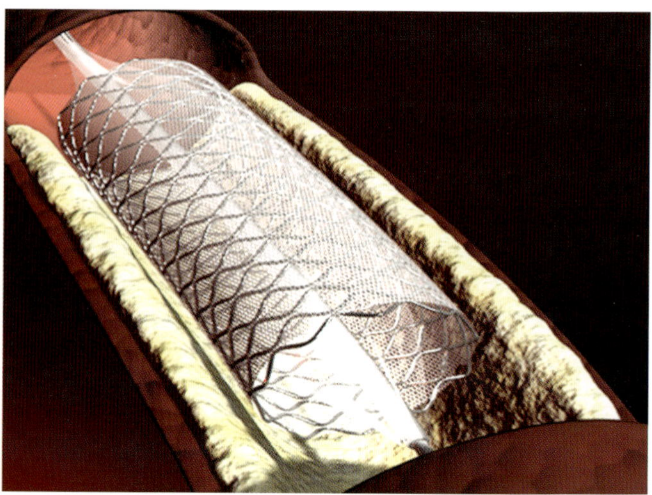

Fig. 17.9 Covered stent polytetrafluoroethylene (PTFE) should be the answer to friable bulky atheroma by trapping it in the graft wall and preventing distal embolization. It has failed to show benefit as compared to BMS in SVG except in perforation. There is also increased risk of in-stent restenosis associated with it

PLAQUE SEALING IN SVG

Atherosclerosis in SVG is known to be markedly accelerated. The progression, in the short term, of SVG segments from previously non-significant lesions to new severe stenosis accounts for a considerable rate of SVG failure post PCI. Thus, the idea of treating SVG lesions before they become ischemic ("plaque sealing") definitely remains appealing in SVG. This interesting concept has been tested in the small randomized "Moderate Vein Graft Lesion Stenting with the Taxus stent and intravascular ultrasound" (VELETI) pilot trial with promising results. In our routine, we tend to treat lesions in SVG in case they are angiographically >50% (and in case the PCI is technically feasible with an *a priori* low chance of having major complications), in the presence of proven ischemia to the specific myocardial territory vascularized by the diseased SVG.

Some issues with SVG interventions remain unresolved:

- Post CABG MI; addressing native CTO or recently occluded graft ?
- Adequate vasodilator pretreatment to prevent slow flow
- Optimal treatment of slow flow
- Antiplatelet strategy
- Role of bivaluridin
- GPI in SVG interventions; identifying subset who would benefit
- FFR in borderline lesions; conduit distensibility may differ from native vessel
- Embolic protection when landing zone is inadequate especially as Proxis has been withdrawn
- Role of thromboaspiration
- Role of intracoronary imaging, safety considerations and disease profile
- Focal or diffuse treatment of degenerated grafts
- Role of covered stents such as M Guard or Papyrus PK
- Additional benefit with drug-eluting stents
- Plaque or disease sealing
- Ideal stent especially for ectatic SVG
- Handling SVG rupture may require understanding of pericardial adhesions and regional tamponade
- Post-SVG PCI follow-up
- Stent sizing and criteria for optimal stent expansion with reference to undersized stents.

REFERENCES

1. Frimerman A, Rechavia E, Eigler N, Payton MR, Makkar R, Litvack F. Long-term follow-up of a high risk cohort after stent implantation in saphenous vein grafts. J Am Coll Cardiol. 1997;30:1277-83.
2. Pucelikova T, Mehran R, Kirtane AJ, Kim YH, Fahy M, Weisz G, et al. Short- and long-term outcomes after stent-assisted percutaneous treatment of saphenous vein grafts in the drug-eluting stent era. Am J Cardiol. 2008;101:63-8.
3. Coolong A, Baim DS, Kuntz RE, O'Malley AJ, Marulkar S, Cutlip DE, et al. Saphenous vein graft stenting and major adverse cardiac events: a predictive model derived from a pooled analysis of 3958 patients. Circulation. 2008;117:790-7.
4. Task Force on Myocardial Revascularization of the European Society of Cardiology (ESC) and the European Association for Cardio-Thoracic Surgery (EACTS); European Association for Percutaneous Cardiovascular Interventions (EAPCI), Wijns W, Kolh P, Danchin N, Di Mario C, Falk V, Folliguet T, Garg S, Huber K, James S, Knuuti J, Lopez-Sendon J, Marco J, Menicanti L, Ostojic M, Piepoli MF, Pirlet C, Pomar JL, Reifart N, Ribichini FL, Schalij MJ, Sergeant P, Serruys PW, Silber S, Sousa Uva M, Taggart D. Guidelines on myocardial revascularization. Eur Heart J. 2010;31:2501-55.
5. Roffi M, Mukherjee D, Chew DP, Bhatt DL, Cho L, Robbins MA, et al. Lack of benefit from intravenous platelet glycoprotein IIb/IIIa receptor inhibition as adjunctive treatment for percutaneous interventions of aortocoronary bypass grafts: a pooled analysis of five randomized clinical trials. Circulation. 2002;106:3063-7.
6. Baim DS, Wahr D, George B, Leon MB, Greenberg J, Cutlip DE, et al. Randomized trial of a distal embolic protection device during percutaneous intervention of saphenous vein aorto-coronary bypass grafts. Circulation. 2002;105:1285-90.
7. Carrozza JP, Mumma M, Breall J, Fernandez A, Heyman E, Metzger C. Randomized evaluation of the TriActiv balloon-protection flush and extraction system for the treatment of saphenous vein graft disease. J Am Coll Cardiol. 2005;46:1677-83.
8. Stone GW, Rogers C, Hermiller J, Feldman R, Hall P, Haber R, et al. Randomized comparison of distal protection with a filter-based catheter and a balloon occlusion and aspiration system during percutaneous intervention of diseased saphenous vein aorto-coronary bypass grafts. Circulation. 2003;108:548-53.
9. Kereiakes DJ, Turco MA, Breall J, Farhat NZ, Feldman RL, McLaurin B, et al. A novel filter-based distal embolic protection device for percutaneous intervention of saphenous vein graft lesions: results of the AMEthyst randomized controlled trial. JACC Cardiovasc Interv. 2008;1:248-57.
10. Dixon SR, Mann JT, Lauer MA, Casale PN, Dippel EJ, Strumpf RK, et al. A randomized, controlled trial of saphenous vein graft intervention with a filter-based distal embolic protection device: TRAP trial. J Interv Cardiol. 2005;18:233-41.
11. Holmes DR, Coolong A, O'Shaughnessy C, Chauhan M, Van Langenhove G, Hall P, et al. Comparison of the CardioShield filter with the guardwire balloon in the prevention of embolisation during vein graft intervention: results from the CAPTIVE randomised trial. Euro Intervention. 2006;2:161-8.
12. Mauri L, Cox D, Hermiller J, Massaro J, Wahr J, Tay SW, et al. The PROXIMAL trial: proximal protection during saphenous vein graft intervention using the Proxis Embolic Protection System: a randomized, prospective, multicenter clinical trial. J Am Coll Cardiol. 2007;50:1442-9.
13. Mehilli J, Pache J, Abdel-Wahab M, Schulz S, Byrne RA, Tiroch K, et al. Drug-eluting versus bare-metal stents in saphenous vein graft lesions (ISAR-CABG): a randomised controlled superiority trial. Lancet. 2011;378:1071-8.
14. Brilakis ES, Lichtenwalter C, Abdel-karim AR, de Lemos JA, Obel O, Addo T, et al. Continued benefit from paclitaxel-eluting compared with bare-metal stent implantation in saphenous vein graft lesions during long-term follow-up of the SOS (Stenting of Saphenous Vein Grafts) trial. JACC Cardiovasc Interv. 2011;4:176-82.
15. Vermeersch P, Agostoni P, Verheye S, Van den Heuvel P, Convens C, et al. Increased late mortality after sirolimus-eluting stents

versus bare-metal stents in diseased saphenous vein grafts: results from the randomized DELAYED RRISC Trial. J Am Coll Cardiol. 2007;50:261-7

16. Testa L, Agostoni P, Vermeersch P, Biondi-Zoccai G, Van Gaal W, Bhindi R, et al. Drug eluting stents versus bare metal stents in the treatment of saphenous vein graft disease: a systematic review and meta-analysis. Euro Intervention. 2010;6:527-36.
17. Costa JR Jr, Abizaid A, Feres F, Costa R, Staico R, Siqueira D, et al. One-year results of the INSPIRE trial with the novel MGuard stent: serial analysis with QCA and IVUS. Catheter Cardiovasc Interv. 2011;78:1095-100.
18. Rodés-Cabau J, Bertrand OF, Larose E, Déry JP, Rinfret S, Bagur R, et al. Comparison of plaque sealing with paclitaxel-eluting stents versus medical therapy for the treatment of moderate nonsignificant saphenous vein graft lesions: the moderate vein graft lesion stenting with the taxus stent and intravascular ultrasound (VELETI) pilot trial. Circulation. 2009;120: 1978-86.

CHAPTER

18 Interventions from the Upper Limb: Transradial Approach

Cherukupalli Raghu

Bleeding is one of the major complications of percutaneous coronary interventions (PCI). Majority of these bleeds happen at the vascular access site and cause substantial morbidity, mortality and costs. The most effective strategy to reduce bleeding risk from PCI is to use the radial artery instead of the femoral artery. Multiple observational and randomized trials performed to date have shown an association between radial access and reduced risk for bleeding and vascular complication.[1] Other studies have shown an association between radial approach and reduced costs,[2] increased patient satisfaction,[3,4] and reduced mortality in high-risk patient subgroups like those with ST-segment elevation myocardial infarction (STEMI).[5] Disadvantages include increased radiation exposure to the operator during the learning curve, limitation of guide catheter size in some patients, and radial artery occlusion.

Transradial interventions (TRI) has become popular in India over the past decade and become the default access in majority of the centers. TRI has contributed to the exponential increase in the procedures in India as the procedures have become simple, safe and most importantly cost-effective. Countries like India have an impetus on cost containment and TRI is an important step in that direction. In this chapter we present the various practical issues and complications along with solutions that we can encounter during TRI.

CHALLENGES IN TRANSRADIAL INTERVENTIONS

Despite being a simple and safe technique there are certain important barriers for the acceptance of this technique on a large scale in various countries importantly USA. The major limitations are the lack of a structured transradial training during residency, mindset to change from femoral to radial access, getting radial access, avoiding spasm, traversing the upper limb vasculature, choosing an appropriate guide catheter, manipulating a 'slender' guide catheter etc. A single-center study examined the mechanism of TRI procedural failure in 2100 procedures (≤6F catheter) performed by low- to intermediate-volume operators. Procedural failure occurred in 98 (4.7%) patients. The mechanism of TRI failure included inability to advance guide catheter to ascending aorta in 50 (51%), inadequate guide catheter support in 35 (36%), and unsuccessful radial artery puncture in 13 (13%) patients.[6]

RADIAL ARTERY ACCESS

Patient Selection

Most patients referred for cardiac catheterization or peripheral endovascular procedures are candidates for TRI. Tests such as Allen's test for assessing the intactness of collateral circulation are rapidly losing their relevance.[7] Specific patients that seem less suitable for TRI are limited to patients with scleroderma, due to the risk of diffuse spasm leading to ischemia, and patients with ipsilateral dialysis access.

Patient Set-up

In a typical catheterization laboratory, the patient is prepped in a supine position, with the right hand gently extended. The right hand is usually placed in a supinated position next to the patient's trunk. For left radial access, a similar preparation is sufficient, and arterial puncture is accomplished with the operator standing either on the patient's right side or on the patient's left side. Once the guidewire is placed above the elbow joint, the left upper extremity could be adducted over to the patient's midline and the procedure performed with the operator standing on the patient's right side.

Radial Artery Puncture

After local infiltration with 1–2 mL of lidocaine, the radial artery is punctured, ideally 2–3 finger breadths above the

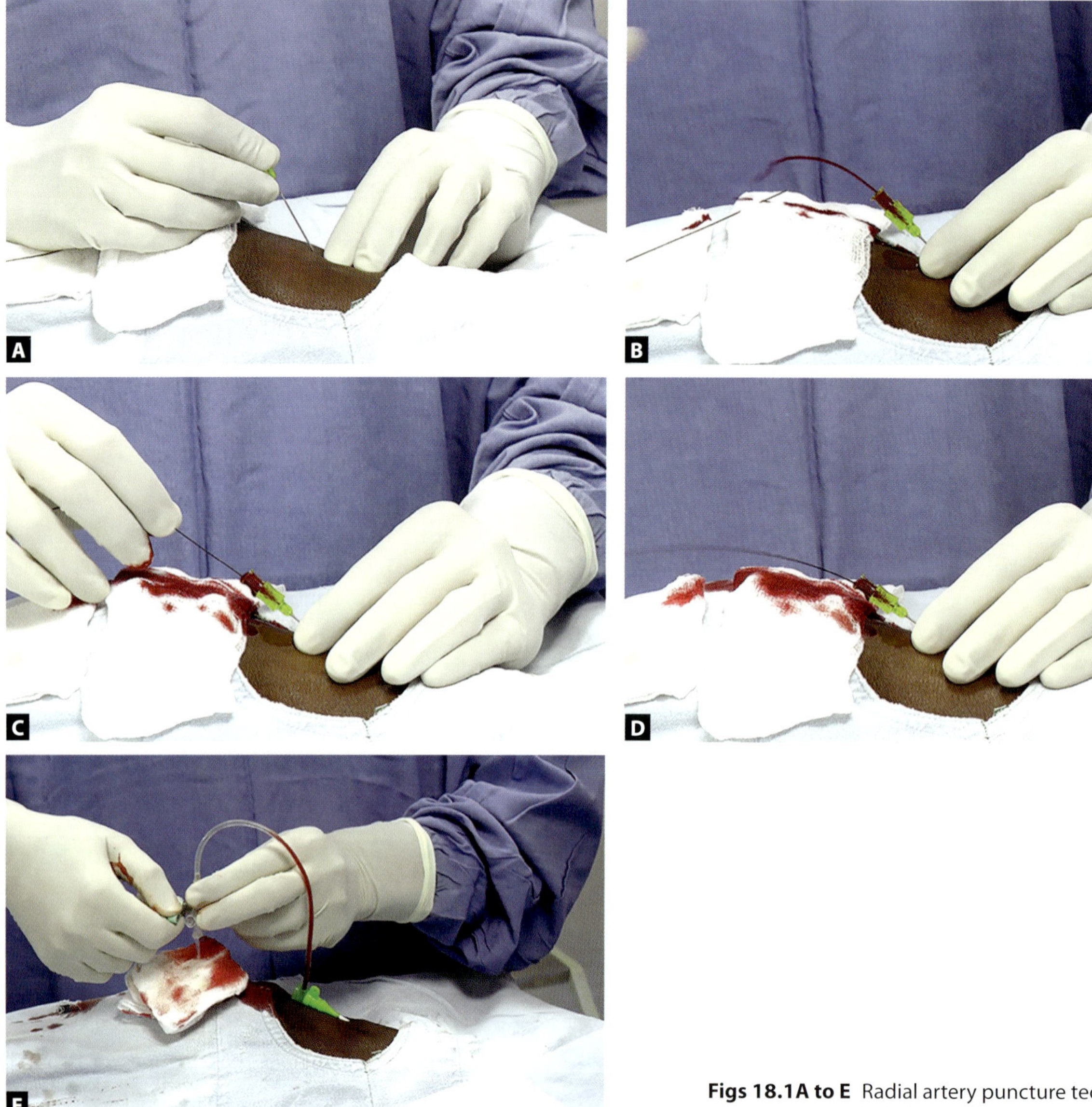

Figs 18.1A to E Radial artery puncture technique: Anterior puncture

radial styloid process. A micro-puncture needle is used in most instances. Either a bare needle or a Teflon-sheathed needle may be used. The traditional anterior puncture technique may be used (Figs 18.1A to E), where the operator, after puncturing the anterior wall of the radial artery and visualizing bleeding from the needle hub, immobilizes the needle and advances the guidewire.

The other commonly used technique is the counter-puncture technique (Figs 18.2A to F) where, after appearance of blood in the needle hub, indicating anterior wall puncture, the needle is advanced through the lumen and the posterior wall is punctured. The needle is then gently withdrawn into the arterial lumen, and the guidewire is advanced once continuous or pulsatile flow of blood is seen. When a Teflon-sheathed needle is used, the inner stylet is removed after needle stabilization and a similar procedure is used. Counter-puncture technique has been shown faster and more likely to succeed at first attempt and has not been associated with an increase in bleeding or radial artery occlusion (RAO).

Arterial Access

After placement of a micro-puncture guidewire (0.018-in or 0.021-in) in the radial artery lumen, an introducer sheath is inserted. Hydrophilic-coated introducer sheaths have been associated with less spasm and found easier to remove. After placement of an introducer sheath, a vasodilator cocktail is administered intra-arterially. Nitrates and/or calcium channel blockers are common ingredients of the vasodilator cocktail; 5000 units of UFH are usually administered to

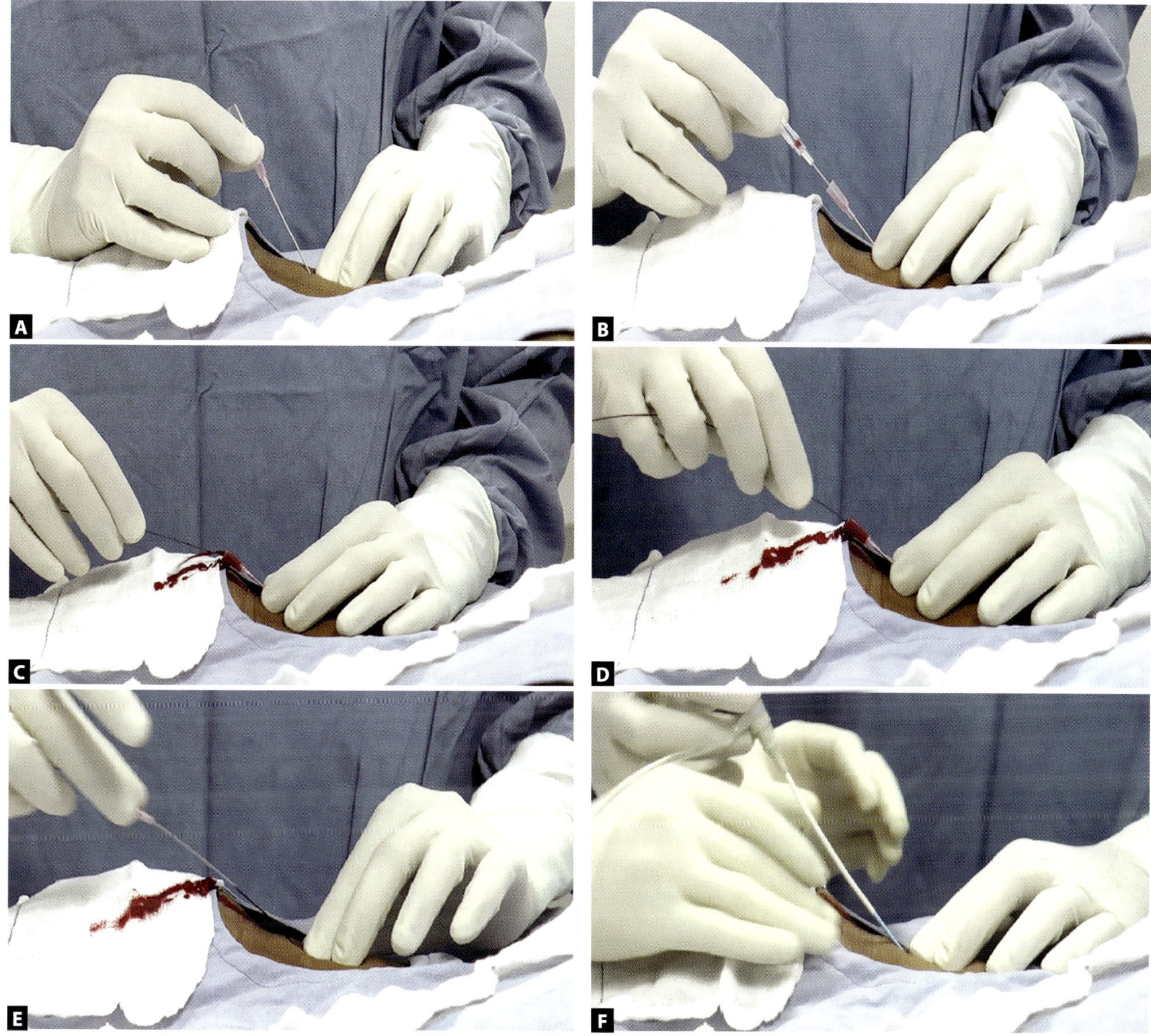

Figs 18.2A to F Radial artery puncture technique: Counter puncture

lower the incidence of RAO. UFH can be administered intra-arterially or intravenously with equivalent prophylactic efficacy.

Technique of Hemostasis

Radial artery hemostasis can be achieved fairly easily by local manual compression. The firm and flat base of the radius bone is ideally suitable for compression and in conjunction with a thick-walled structure of the radial artery; bleeding at the puncture site can be stopped by application of modest pressure.

Several hemostatic compression practices are prevalent, ranging from manual compression-to-compression dressings and, recently, the increasing use of circumferential bands capable of applying titratable pressure. All of these modalities are highly effective in achieving hemostasis. The bands allow for patients to be free and ambulate immediately post procedure. Caution should be exercised to apply the center point of the bands at the site of arterial puncture (usually proximal to the skin entry site) to prevent bleeding complications when practicing low-pressure hemostasis.

Cannulating the Coronaries: Techniques and Tips

Advancing the catheter into the ascending aorta:

Inability to reach the ascending aorta is the major cause for TRI failure. Understanding the obstacle and adopting a tailor made solution for the same can overcome this problem.

Redundancy and loop of the subclavian artery can be overcome by asking the patient to take a deep breath and hold the breath. This maneuver will straighten the loop and makes the brachiocephalic artery and ascending aorta aligned.

Owing to the angle at which brachiocephalic artery is originating from the arch of aorta the catheter can have difficulties in reaching the ascending aorta and might be repeatedly reaching the descending aorta.

Gaining Access to the Ascending Aorta (Figs 18.3A to E)

- *Step 1*: The 0.035" Teflon coated guidewire needs to be allowed to pass into the descending aorta and the catheter advanced over the same (Fig. 18.3A).
- *Step 2*: The guidewire is pulled back into the catheter (Fig. 18.3B).
- *Step 3*: The patient is asked to take a deep breath and hold it (Fig. 18.3C).
- *Step 4*: Catheter is now pulled back from the descending aorta to the arch of aorta gradually. At the junction of brachiocephalic artery to arch of aorta there is a sudden jump of catheter into the ascending aorta (Fig. 18.3D).
- *Step 5*: At this step, the catheter alone (not the guidewire) will be pushed gently forward to reach the ascending aorta (Fig. 18.3E).

Catheter Choice in Case of Difficulty to Reach the Ascending Aorta

In case the dedicated radial or Judkin's left catheter are unable to reach the aorta we need to exchange the catheter to a short tip catheter such a Judkin's right catheter.

Guidewire of Choice

To traverse a redundant subclavian loop the wire of choice is a 150 cm hydrophilic wire of 0.035" diameter. This will allow the catheter to reach the ascending aorta. To exchange the catheter subsequently, the wire of choice would be a 260 cm guidewire that needs to be parked in the ascending aorta over which the exchange can take place. A super stiff wire is also an important part of the tool kit for exchanging the catheters in case of severe tortuosity.

Angiogram in the left anterior oblique projection is another simple solution to overcome the challenges in reaching the ascending aorta.

Catheter Selection for TRI

For coronary engagement, finesse is required rather than force. Active catheter holding is recommended because there may be multiple friction points in the subclavian and the aorta. Small (finger-based) clockwise and counterclockwise torqueing movements are suggested. Extensive torqueing and manipulation can cause catheter kinking and knotting.

Diagnostic Catheter Selection

The diagnostic catheter of choice in majority of cath labs is the Tiger catheter (Optitorque Terumo, Somerset, NJ). This is a single catheter for cannulating both coronaries.

But operators shifting from femoral to radial can use the Judkin's left and right catheters. But the choice of the secondary curve size for TRI on the left side has to be at least 0.5 less.

Cannulating with a Judkin's left catheter (Fig. 18.4)

- *Step 1*: Leaving the 0.035-in guidewire inside the catheter (but not protruding) prevents the catheter from curling up during manipulation.
- *Step 2*: The JL catheter is gently torqued clockwise as it navigates through the ascending aorta pointing toward the left coronary cusp. The patient is encouraged to take a deep breath and hold it during this step. A sudden jump of the catheter from the noncoronary to the left sinus is noticed.
- *Step 3*: When close to the left coronary ostium, final torqueing movements usually allow for selective cannulation.

Alternate Strategy (Fig. 18.5)

- *Step 1*: If the tip of catheter points below the ostium, advancing the catheter gently prolapses the secondary curve of the catheter into the sinus of Valsalva and points the tip up toward the ostium. This advancement has to be with a gentle push and counter clock rotation of the catheter. Always remember that there is a lag for the transmission of torque to the tip of catheter. So the torqueing of catheter has to be gradual.
- *Step 2*: Once engaged, a slight catheter pull back with gentle clockwise torque allows for more coaxial engagement. This is an important step without which at the time of contrast injection the catheter flips off.

Right Coronary Cannulation (Fig. 18.6)

To engage the right coronary artery (RCA), JR4 still remains the most common catheter. Catheter manipulation for RCA engagement is similar to the femoral approach. The JR catheter is advanced into the right coronary cusp and then pulled back while torqueing clockwise until the catheter finds the ostium of the RCA.

Single Catheter Strategy

A 'single-catheter' approach where one catheter is used to engage both coronary ostia and is possible with various catheter shapes and has various benefits:

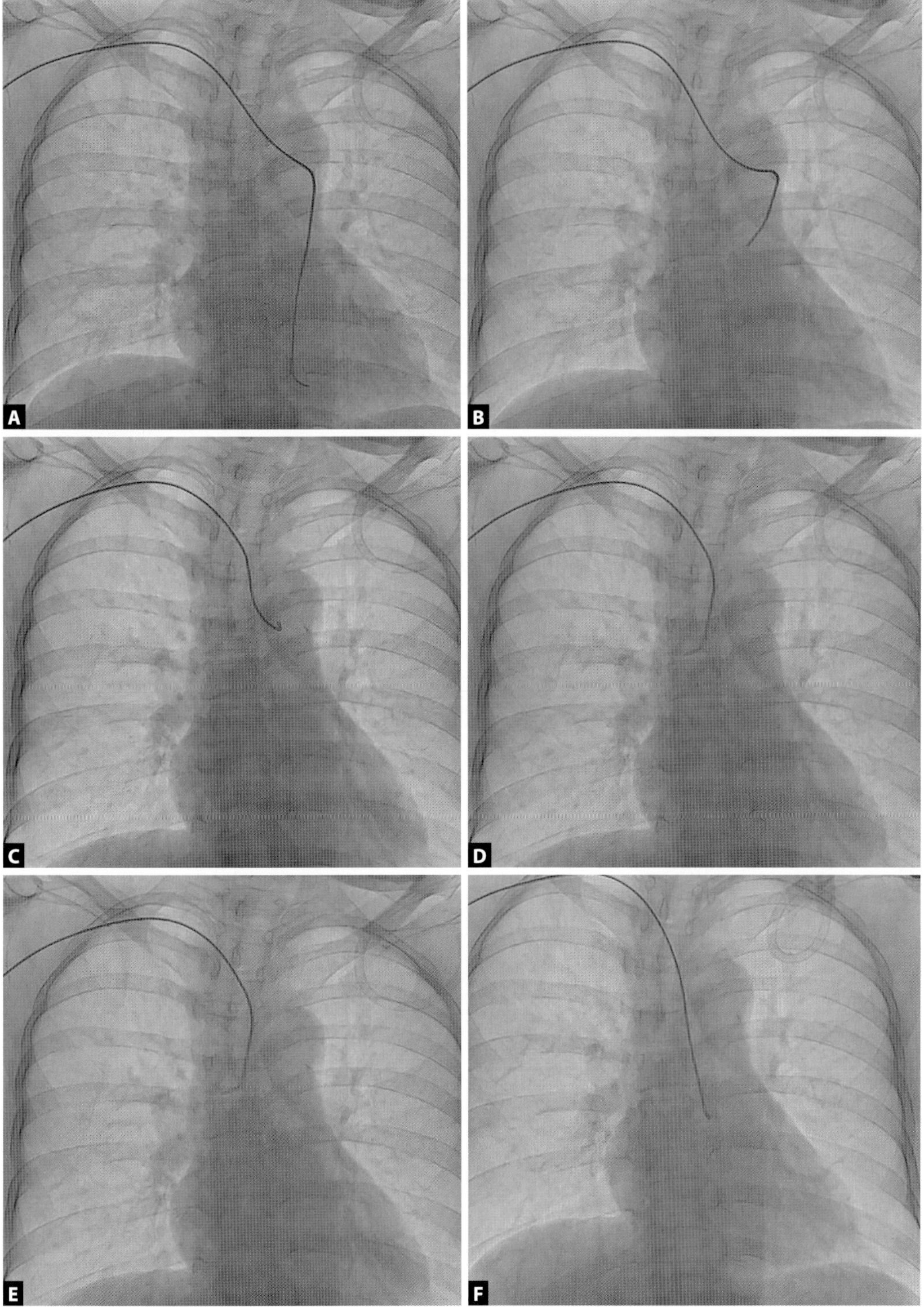

Figs 18.3A to E Gaining access to the ascending from descending aorta; (A) Guidewire and catheter in descending aorta; (B) Guidewire pull back to the catheter; (C) Deep breath by patient; (D) Sudden jump into ascending aorta; (E) Advancing catheter alone into the ascending aorta

- Decrease in catheter exchanges and manipulation reduces the occurrence of vasospasm
- Increases patient comfort
- Reduction in procedure and fluoroscopy time
- Reduction in radiation exposure,
- Use of fewer catheters.

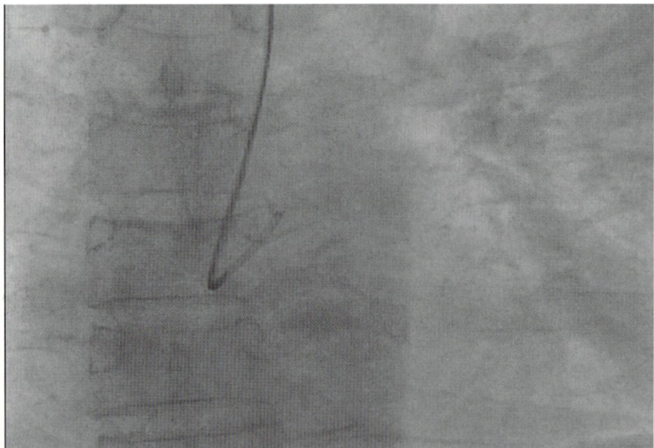

Fig. 18.4 Cannulating left coronary with a Judkin's left catheter

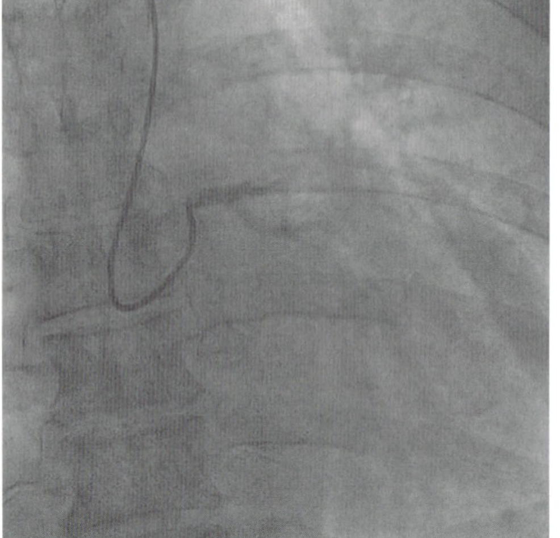

Fig. 18.5 Alternate strategy for cannulating left coronary

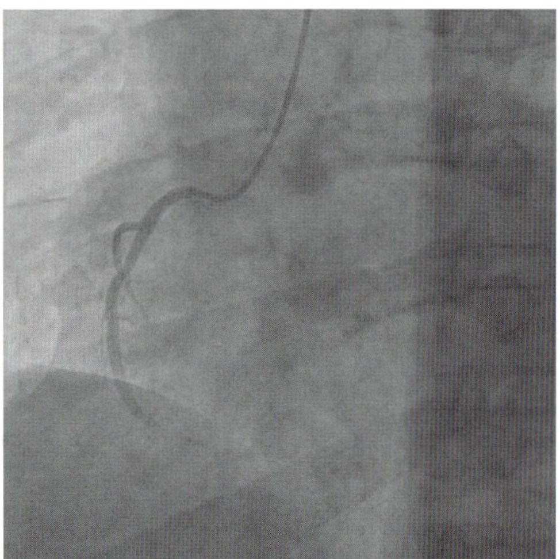

Fig. 18.6 RCA cannulation with Judkin's catheter

One drawback to a single-catheter strategy remains the ability to engage both coronary ostia completely coaxially every time.

Various catheter shapes have now been designed that allow for the single-catheter strategy and include the Kimny, Tiger, Jacky, and Ikari catheters. The Tiger (Optitorque Terumo, Somerset, NJ) is a double-braided catheter with a flat segment in the third portion of the loop, which provides contralateral backup support, and a side hole just proximal to the tip.

Left Coronary Cannulation with Tiger Catheter (Fig. 18.7)

Engagement of the LCA with the Tiger or Jacky (Optitorque Terumo) catheter is somewhat similar to the engagement with the JL and is performed as follows:

- *Step 1*: Keep the 0.035-in wire within the catheter.
- *Step 2*: Place the tip of the catheter just below the LCA and facing left.
- *Step 3*: Pull back the wire slowly, making the tip of the catheter point upward to engage the left main coronary ostium.
- *Step 4*: Slight clockwise or counterclockwise torque can be applied for more selective and coaxial cannulation.

Right Coronary Cannulation with Tiger Catheter (Fig. 18.8)

Engaging the RCA is performed by applying clockwise motion until the tip enters the right sinus of Valsalva and eventually engages the RCA.

Guide Catheter Selection for TRI

Most TRI can be successfully accomplished with 5F or 6F guiding catheters. All current stent technologies (including

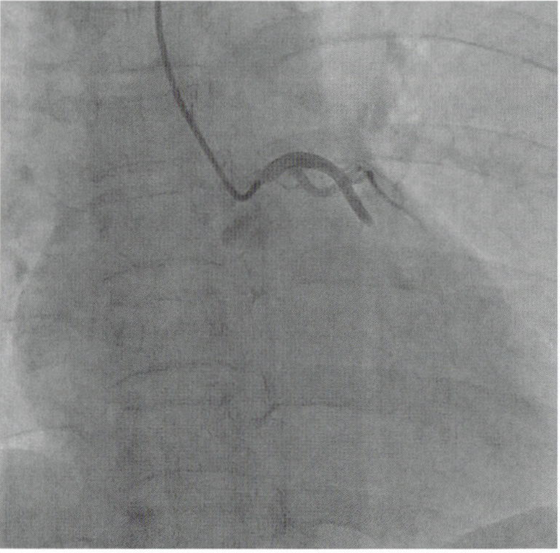

Fig. 18.7 LCA cannulation with tiger catheter

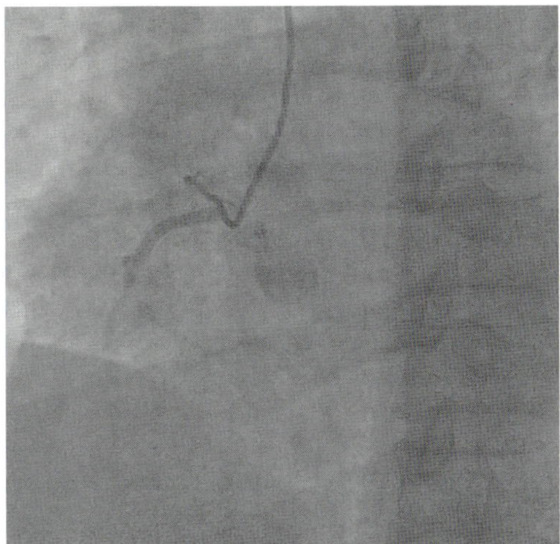

Fig. 18.8 RCA cannulation with tiger catheter

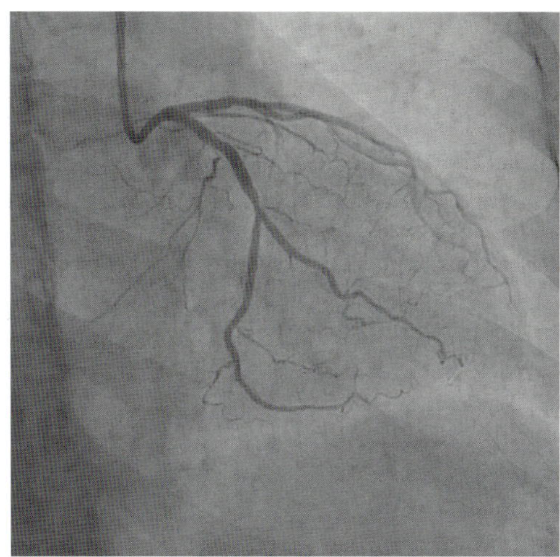

Fig. 18.9 AL catheter for left circumflex lesion—short left main coronary artery

covered stents), rotational atherectomy, and/or intravascular ultrasound catheters can be delivered safely and efficiently through 5F to 6F guiding catheters. These guides and equipment still allow for the treatment of simple or even the most complex lesions (i.e. bifurcation or chronic total occlusion). Soft-tip guides can provide greater safety during deep-seating maneuvers.

Left Coronary Guide Catheter Selection for TRI

Most curves designed for the femoral approach (Judkins, Amplatz, and extra backup catheters) remain well suited for TR PCI. The JL catheters, however, provide less backup support for TR PCI than when used via femoral approach. The angle between the opposite wall of the aorta and the catheter is an important determinant of backup support. The wider the angle between the aortic wall and the catheter, the greater the backup support. As such, JL catheters are only suited for straightforward interventions for proximal disease where minimal backup support is expected to be required. For ostial left main coronary lesions the Judkins catheters remain a good option. For interventions requiring more support, the extra backup catheters (EBU, Voda, or XB) are adequate and remain the most popular. However, a catheter curve that is usually 0.5 cm smaller than what would be used in femoral procedures (3F or 3.5F vs 3.5F or 4F, respectively) may be needed.

Engagement into the left main artery is also different from the femoral approach and is cannulated from below the ostium with counterclockwise movement. These catheters provide passive backup support from the contralateral sinus of Valsalva and offer appropriate deep-seating capability. Fine manipulation is usually required to obtain a stable coaxial position in the LCA.

The Amplatz left catheters (1 or 2) provide great passive backup support and may be the catheters of choice for complex coronary interventions (i.e. calcified lesions, chronic total occlusion). In the authors' experience Amplatz catheters are ideal for performing a complex left circumflex angioplasty in a situation of short left main (Fig. 18.9).

Right Coronary Guide Catheter Selection for TRI

The JR guide catheter remains the workhorse catheter used for most TR PCI. It is manipulated in a way similar to that for the femoral approach, with gentle clockwise rotation applied to engage the RCA. It may be preferred for ostial lesions. However, although the JR catheter shape provides some passive backup, it provides little active backup force because it does not contact the contralateral aortic wall. So although for PCI of 'simple' RCA lesions the JR may be adequate, for complex lesions that require additional backup, such as lesions with significant calcification, tortuosity, or chronic occlusions, the JR may be insufficient. A deep coronary intubation can sometimes be helpful for further support and is obtained by careful clockwise rotation and advancement of the guide over an interventional device (wire or balloon) sometimes as deep as the mid segment. But care should be exercised with this aggressive maneuver (Fig. 18.10).

Dilated aortic roots and/or RCAs that arise anteriorly also pose a particular problem because the JR catheters often do not have sufficient reach to engage the coronary ostium adequately, coaxial engagement may be limited and PCI may be cumbersome. In this situation, an Amplatz right (1 or 2) or Amplatz left (0.75 or 1) may be a better selection and provide better support. The Amplatz left guide catheter provides

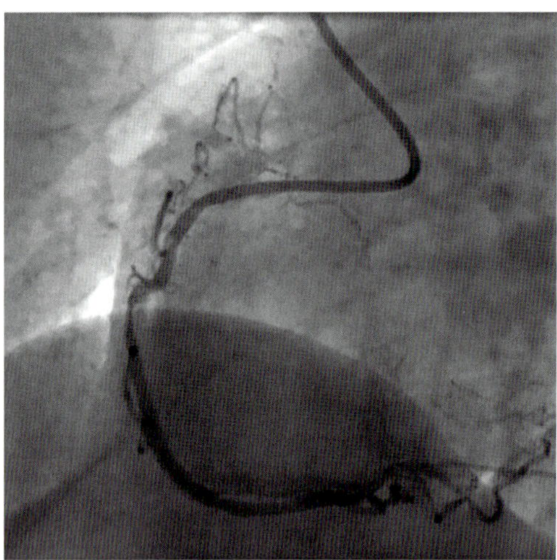

Fig. 18.10 Deep cannulation of RCA with Judkin's right catheter

further passive support, with more aggressive engagement, which is particularly useful for RCAs with shepherd's crook configuration. Amplatz left catheters may not be the first choice for very proximal or ostial lesions, and carries the risk of catheter-induced traumatic injury to the vessel or aortic wall.

Enhancing the Guide Catheter Back-up Support

Deep intubation of the coronary artery can reliably be obtained with soft-tip and smaller-diameter guide catheters. However, this carries a risk of traumatic injury to the proximal vessel, particularly if there is significant disease. In some situations, a larger guide catheter may provide more stability and 'passive backup'.

A buddy wire, a stiffer extra support wire, or placing a second stiff wire in the left anterior descending while intervening in the left circumflex (or vice versa) may also be useful for further support. An anchoring balloon can be placed in a proximal small side branch and inflated at low pressure during advancement of interventional devices.

A 'mother-child' hybrid system has also been proposed as a way to enhance the backup support of 6F catheters and also allow for the use of smaller guide catheters to perform deep intubation maneuvers to treat lesions with extreme proximal tortuosity or heavy calcification.

An analogous option is the use of extension catheters, such as the Guide Liner (Vascular Solutions, Inc, Minneapolis, MN) or Guidezilla (Boston Scientific, Marlborough). These devices are a 'rapid-exchange' version of the mother-child system and consist of a 20 cm soft-tipped catheter connected with a metal collar to a 115 cm stainless steel shaft for advancement and positioning. These extensions allow for safer, deep intubation of the target vessel, which provides additional support during complex PCI when there is difficulty in advancing equipment, such as balloon and/or stents across the target lesion. Additionally, for PCI of chronic total occlusion it can help reestablish a reentry plane in the case of retrograde crossing or reverse controlled anterograde and retrograde.

TRANSRADIAL PROCEDURES: TRAVERSING LOOPS AND TORTUOSITIES

Anatomic complexities of arm and chest vasculature play an important role in cases of TRA failure. Using a simple framework to classify the anatomic or functional problem and approaching these challenges in a logical sequence should facilitate management and increase the success rate for TRA/I.

Tortuosity of the Radial or Brachial Artery (Fig. 18.11)

Identification of the anatomy of the tortuosity is the first step. This can be by performing a local angiogram, which delineates the loop and aids in choosing the appropriate hardware. If the RA diameter is small and the tortuous segment is long, it should be crossed using a 0.025-in or 0.032-in J-shaped hydrophilic guidewire or a 0.014-in soft-tip PTCA guidewire. Carefully negotiate a catheter over the wire using a slow corkscrew movement under fluoroscopic guidance. Once the segment is crossed with the assembly, the procedure can be finished in the usual fashion.

Antebrachial Loop in TRI (Fig. 18.12)

Loops and curvatures are to be expected, and a radial operator needs to have a plan to work through this challenge. A consistent plan will reduce the apprehension of a new radialist and give additional confidence to an experienced operator.

The loop can be either a simple loop or a complex one. Performing a local angiogram with diluted contrast does differentiation of these. Complex loops may need additional oblique views. If there is resistance to the passage of a regular 0.035-inch Teflon guidewire, the wire can be changed to a 0.025-inch hydrophilic-coated wire or even a 0.014-inch PTCA guidewire in case of a complex loop.

Once the loop has been crossed with the guidewire the catheter needs to be downsized to a 4 or 5 F catheter. This will facilitate the catheter advancement to the aortic root. Subsequent catheter exchanges can be done over an exchange length angiographic guidewire or a super-stiff guidewire.

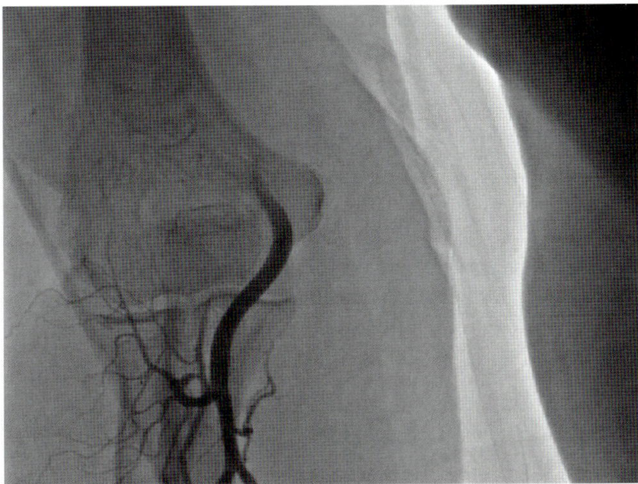

Fig. 18.11 Tortuosity of the radial artery

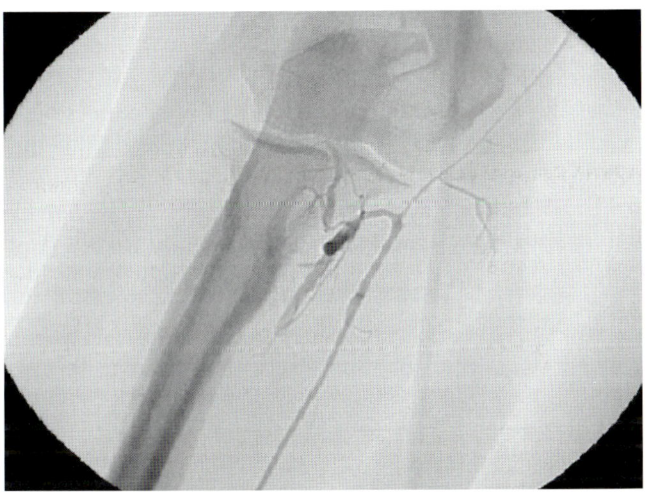

Fig. 18.12 Antebrachial loop

Subclavian Loops and Tortuosities

At this location, a simple maneuver of taking a deep breath pulls the diaphragm down along with the thoracic contents, resulting in favorable change in the course of the vessel. This will allow the catheter to enter the ascending aorta.

In case the loop is complex to be crossed by this maneuver, using 0.025-in or 0.032-in hydrophilic guidewire should be successful. At times, deep inspiration facilitates the entry of the guidewire and catheter in the ascending aorta.

COMPLICATIONS AND MANAGEMENT

Radial Artery Occlusion

Radial artery occlusion (RAO) is a well-recognized complication of transradial catheterization with variable reported incidence rates of anywhere from 1% to 38%.[8] Endothelial injury from sheath insertion and cessation of radial artery flow create an environment conducive to thrombosis, which is thought to be the underlying process responsible for RAO.[9] RAO typically occurs early in the post-procedure setting, with many patients having spontaneous re-canalization within 1–3 months. RAO is silent clinically, given the dual blood supply to the hand from the radial and ulnar arteries. The incidence of symptomatic RAO requiring medical attention has been reported as 2% in the RIVAL study.[10] Several studies have identified independent predictors of RAO, which include sheath size and sheath to artery ratio, post-procedure compression time, presence of anterograde flow during hemostasis, and use of systemic anticoagulation.[11]

Strategies to treat RAO include, compression of ipsilateral ulnar artery for one hour,[12] utilization of intra-arterial heparin 5000 U and post-procedure low-molecular weight heparin for few days.[13]

Radial Artery Spasm

Radial artery spasm (RAS) is another well-recognized complication of transradial catheterization procedures especially during the learning curve. Although RAS rarely results in serious complications, RAS decreases procedural success owing to difficulty obtaining radial access and increases difficulty of sheath removal upon case completion. Several studies have identified independent predictors of RAS including younger age, female gender, small radial artery size, anomalous radial artery anatomy, more than 3 catheter changes, and moderate to severe pain during cannulation.[14] Strategies to prevent occurrence of RAS include administration of intra-arterial vasodilators, utilization of hydrophilic-coated sheaths, and adequate operator training and experience with the transradial approach.

Treatment strategies for sheath removal and resolution of RAS include repeat administration of intra-arterial vasodilator, additional sedation/analgesia, reinsertion of the introducer and guidewire, and often times merely operator patience.

Forearm Hematoma and Compartment Syndrome

The radial artery is a fairly superficial structure and thus has limited surrounding space to contain bleeding. If not controlled, bleeding can progress rapidly to hematoma formation. Female sex, sheath size, and procedure duration are factors associated with hematoma formation. The progression from hematoma to forearm compartment syndrome is very rare.[15]

Prevention of compartment syndrome includes adequate vasodilator therapy before sheath removal, application of a sphygmomanometer cuff over the arm inflated to 10–20 mm Hg more than the systolic blood pressure, prompt recognition and treatment of hematomas, and continued monitoring of the patient for any worsening swelling or pain.

Radial Artery Perforation

Radial artery perforation is another rare complication seen with the transradial approach. Perforation occurs more often in elderly, short-statured women as well as in patients with tortuous and atherosclerotic arteries. Anatomic variations such as radial loops, a high radial–ulnar bifurcation, and a short ascending aorta also increase the risk of perforation. Various approaches can be used in the management of radial artery perforation include utilization of a long sheath,[16] sealing the perforation with guide catheter[17] and prolonged balloon inflation.[18]

Pseudoaneurysm

The incidence of radial artery pseudoaneurysm has been shown to be < 0.1% in a large case series.[19] Pseudoaneurysms usually present as a pulsatile mass with or without localized swelling and pain in the wrist, ante-cubital fossa, or forearm. Diagnosis is made using Doppler ultrasonography or angiography. Although there have been no systematic studies analyzing the risk factors for radial artery pseudoaneurysms, systemic anticoagulation and inadequate compression have been suggested as risk factors.

Management of radial pseudoaneurysms includes firm prolonged mechanical pressure (4–6 hours) with a radial hemostasis device, ultrasound-guided compression, thrombin injection, or surgical repair.

Arteriovenous Fistula Formation

Arteriovenous fistula formation in transradial procedures is an extremely rare complication given the superficial course of the vessel and the surrounding small caliber veins.[20] While obtaining radial access, the initial puncture may deviate through a venous tributary and can lead to arteriovenous communication. These communications typically seal spontaneously; however, if they remain patent an arterio-venous fistula can form. Pain and swelling at the site can be seen with a palpable thrill. Surgical options vary depending on the size and location of the arteriovenous fistula. These options include partial resection, ligation, excision, and repair. Given the relatively benign course of most arteriovenous fistulas, conservative management in the absence of increasing size or neurovascular insufficiency is the mode of treatment.[21]

Catheter Entrapment

Excessive catheter manipulation and tortuous vascular anatomy can lead to catheter kinking and subsequent catheter entrapment. Operator experience and early identification of catheter kinking are crucial in the avoidance of catheter entrapment.[22] In such cases, gentle traction allows typically for straightening of the catheter. Additional support from a guidewire can also be useful.

LEARNING CURVE IN TRANSRADIAL PROCEDURES

Interventional cardiologist, both novice and experienced, will need to learn this technique to remain competitive, and PCI training programs need to offer this skill to attract the top candidates. Expert interventional cardiologists wishing to adopt this approach should plan accordingly keeping in mind the learning period. Latest data suggest a minimum of 50 procedures to deliver transradial PCI in a safe effective manner.[23] However, the authors feel that these numbers are too small for a proficiency in transradial procedures. Louvard and colleagues (unpublished data)[24] suggested a minimum number of 1000 cases to have a less than 2% failure rate to reach ascending aorta from the radial access. In addition, the initial failure is due to puncture issues and subsequent failures seem to be their inability to traverse the arm vasculature and aortic loops. When starting initially, it is advisable to use a stepwise approach, starting with diagnostic angiography and simple PCI in patients with favorable anatomy, before proceeding to more complex procedures and patients with less favorable anatomy. For training programs, the trainees should be exposed to radial and femoral access in a parallel manner.

CONCLUSION

Transradial procedures are being increasingly accepted by various operators, invasive and interventional, because of the huge potential to reduce vascular complications, minimize the hospital stay and patient preference. Despite the steep learning curve, it has replaced transfemoral procedures to a large extent in many cath labs of India, Japan and Europe. Operators embarking upon a transradial program must understand the science behind transradial procedures and tailored solutions for the various obstacles. This will help them to complete the procedure successfully. Finally with the recent burgeoning interest of the US interventional community in transradial procedures we are bound to see many original research article that will provide strong data on why everyone should be a 'radialist'.

REFERENCES

1. Jolly SS, Amlani S, Hamon M, Yusuf S, Mehta SR. Radial versus femoral access for coronary angiography or intervention and the impact on major bleeding and ischemic events: A systematic review and meta-analysis of randomized trials. Am Heart J. 2009;157:132-40.
2. Caputo RP, Tremmel JA, Rao S, et al. Transradial arterial access for coronary and peripheral procedures: Executive summary by the Transradial Committee of the SCAI. Catheter Cardiovasc Interv. 2011;78:823-39.
3. Cooper CJ, El-Shiekh RA, Cohen DJ, et al. Effect of transradial access on quality of life and cost of cardiac catheterization: A randomized comparison. Am Heart J. 1999;138:430-6.
4. Jolly SS, Yusuf S, Cairns J, et al. Radial versus femoral access for coronary angiography and intervention in patients with acute coronary syndromes (RIVAL): A randomised, parallel group, multicentre trial. Lancet. 2011;377:1409-20.
5. Joyal D, Bertrand OF, Rinfret S, Shimony A, Eisenberg MJ. Meta-analysis of ten trials on the effectiveness of the radial versus the femoral approach in primary percutaneous coronary intervention. Am J Cardiol. 2012;109:813-8.
6. Dehghani P, Mohammad A, Bajaj R, et al. Mechanism and predictors of failed transradial approach for percutaneous coronary interventions. JACC Cardiovasc Interv. 2009;2:1057-64.
7. Hermann H, Valgimigli M, et al. Is the allen test necessary before transradial artery catheterization. J Am Coll Cardiol. 2014.
8. Uhlemann M, Möbius-Winkler S, Mende M, et al. The Leipzig prospective vascular ultrasound registry in radial artery catheterization: impact of sheath size on vascular complications. JACC Cardiovasc Interv. 2012;5(1):36-43.
9. Kotowycz MA, Dzavik V. Radial artery patency after transradial catheterization. Circ Cardiovasc Interv. 2012;5(1):127-33.
10. Jolly SS, Yusuf S, Cairns J, et al. Radial versus femoral access for coronary angiography and intervention in patients with acute coronary syndromes (RIVAL): a randomised, parallel group, multicentre trial. Lancet. 2011;377(9775):1409-20.
11. Stella PR, Kiemeneij F, Laarman GJ, et al. Incidence and outcome of radial artery occlusion following transradial artery coronary angioplasty. Cathet Cardiovasc Diagn. 1997;40(2):156-8.
12. Bernat I, Bertrand OF, Rokyta R, et al. Efficacy and safety of transient ulnar artery compression to recanalize acute radial artery occlusion after transradial catheterization. Am J Cardiol. 2011;107(11):1698-701.
13. Zankl AR, Andrassy M, Volz C, et al. Radial artery thrombosis following transradial coronary angiography: incidence and rationale for treatment of symptomatic patients with low molecular-weight heparins. Clin Res Cardiol. 2010; 99(12): 841-7.
14. Jia DA, Zhou YJ, Shi DM, et al. Incidence and predictors of radial artery spasm during transradial coronary angiography and intervention. Chin Med J (Engl). 2010;123(7):843-7.
15. Tizon-Marcos H, Barbeau GR. Incidence of compartment syndrome of the arm in a large series of transradial approach for coronary procedures. J Interv Cardiol. 2008;21(5):380-4.
16. Calvino-Santos RA, Vazquez-Rodrıguez JM, Salgado-Fernandez J, et al. Management of iatrogenic radial artery perforation. Catheter Cardiovasc Interv. 2004;61(1):74-8.
17. Gunasekaran S, Cherukupalli R. Radial artery perforation and its management during PCI. J Invasive Cardiol. 2009;21(2):E24-6.
18. Rigatelli G, Dell'Avvocata F, Ronco F, et al. Successful coronary angioplasty via the radial approach after sealing a radial perforation. JACC Cardiovasc Interv. 2009;2(11):1158-9.
19. Sanmartin M, Cuevas D, Goicolea J, et al. Vascular complications associated with radial artery access for cardiac catheterization. Rev Esp Cardiol (Engl Ed). 2004;57(6):581-4.
20. Spence MS, Byrne J, Haegeli L, et al. Rare access site complications following transradial coronary intervention. Can J Cardiol. 2009; 25(6):e206.
21. Dehghani P, Culig J, Patel D, et al. Arteriovenous fistula as a complication of transradial coronary angiography: a case report. J Med Case Rep. 2013;7:21.
22. Kim JY, Moon KW, Yoo KD. Entrapment of a kinked catheter in the radial artery during transradial coronary angiography. J Invasive Cardiol. 2012;24(1):E3-4.
23. Hess CN, Peterson ED, Neely ML, et al. The learning curve for transradial percutaneous coronary intervention among operators in the United States: a study from the National Cardiovascular Data Registry. Circulation. 2014;129(22):2277-86.
24. Guedes A, Dangoisse V, Gabriel L, Jamart J, Ghenu P, Marchandise B, Schroeder E. Low rate of conversion to transfemoral approach when attempting both radial arterial for coronary angiography and percutaneous coronary intervention. J Invasive Cardiol. 2010;22(9):391-7.

CHAPTER

19

Radial and Groin Care after Percutaneous Coronary Intervention

Kaushik Sheth

INTRODUCTION

While most of the attention during percutaneous coronary intervention (PCI) is directed to executing the complex intervention in most appropriate way and giving perfect angiographic outcome, from a patient's perspective, he wants a painless and uncomplicated outcome. Vascular access site is easily visualized and any untoward outcome at the site diminishes patient's confidence in the procedure.

Vascular access site complications may be seen in up to 6% of cases. These can range from retroperitoneal hemorrhage, pseudoaneurysm, AV fistula, infection, hematoma, neuropraxia, lower limb ischemia to dissection of the artery at femoral site. At the radial access site, complications are vasospasm, pseudoaneurysm, puncture site granuloma, dissection, forearm hematoma and compartment syndrome.

Predictors of vascular access site complications are female gender, advanced age, small body surface area, prior intervention, peripheral vascular disease, diabetes mellitus, anticoagulation and inappropriate technique of puncture.

Common femoral artery should be punctured 5–14 mm inferior to the center of femoral head to avoid puncture site complications.[1,2] This avoids femoral bifurcation and inferior passage of inferior epigastric artery. Effective manual compression is also possible at this site. Femoral angiography may be performed in cases deemed at high vascular risk. Use of groin skin crease as the landmark for femoral puncture should be strongly discouraged (Fig. 19.1).

SITE-RELATED COMPLICATIONS

We will go through few of the access site-related complications:

Femoral Access Site-related Complications (Tables 19.1, 19.2 and Figs 19.2A and B)[3]

- *Acute limb ischemia:* This is limb threatening complication. Pale, pulseless, painful, paresthetic limb should prompt urgent referral to vascular surgeon.
- *Hematoma:* A palpable mass at puncture site is most common complication. This should be distinguished from ecchymosis, which has discoloration due to extravasated blood. Doppler of the limb is necessary if prolonged pain or bruit at the site. Prolonged manual or mechanical compression is the treatment of choice.
- *Retroperitoneal hemorrhage:*[4] This complication is seen in <1% of all PCI. This is caused by high puncture site (above the center of femoral head). Patients complain of ipsilateral groin or flank pain, develop refractory hypotension and occur within 3 hours of the procedure. After initial fluid resuscitation, CT abdomen and pelvis is investigation of choice to confirm this complication. Most of these hemorrhages are managed medically, though around 10% will need surgery or covered stent deployment via contralateral femoral approach.
- *Pseudoaneurysm:* Complications of "low stick" (below femoral bifurcation) puncture, this presents as tender, pulsatile, expansile swelling with a bruit. These puncture sites do not heal completely and continue to expand with

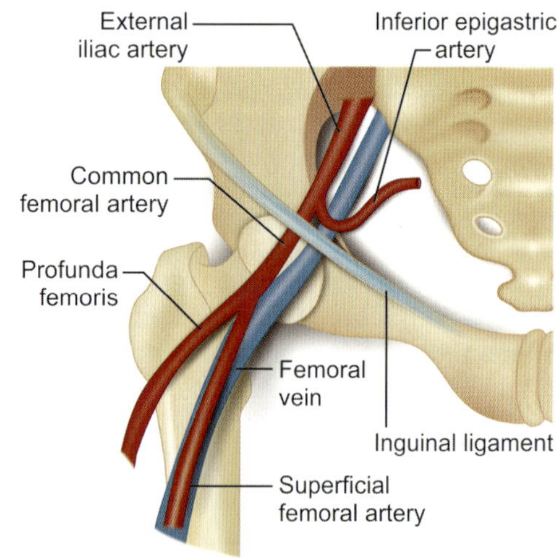

Fig. 19.1 Anatomy of femoral vessels

Table 19.1 Femoral puncture location aid associated complications

Femoral puncture location: Definition	*Complications*
Low stick: Puncture below the femoral bifurcation	Pseudoaneurysm
	Hematoma
	Arteriovenous fistula
High stick: Puncturing the inferior epigastric artery	Retroperitoneal hemorrhage
Posterior wall puncture: Puncture through the back wall of the artery	Retroperitoneal hemorrhage

each systole. Doppler ultrasound is used to detect this complication as well as to apply pressure at puncture site. Thrombin may be injected in the pseudoaneurysm to close it. Patients usually require opiate analgesics for pain control.

- *AV fistulae:* Rare (<1%). Usually seen with puncture below common femoral bifurcation as femoral vein lies posterior to superficial femoral artery at this location. Predictor of this complication includes left groin puncture, female gender, prior anticoagulation and hypertension. One-third of these close spontaneously over first year, allowing observation or ultrasound compression as approach of choice compared to surgery.
- *Neurapraxia to femoral nerve:* Patients complain of shooting pain or anesthetic patch on lateral aspect of thigh which usually recovers over a period of 6 months.

Radial Access Site-related Complications

- *Compartment syndrome:*[5] Rare but dreaded complication. This is caused by raised pressure within a closed osseo-facial anatomic space. Pressure >30 mm Hg or within 30 mm Hg of diastolic pressure is sufficient to trigger ischemia of forearm muscles. Hand dorsiflexion causes stretch on forearm muscles and causes severe pain. Proximal compression for any suspected hematoma will prevent this complication. If any neurodeficit develops, urgent vascular surgery reference is necessary.
- *Granuloma at puncture site:* Extremely rare.
- *Pseudoaneurysm:* Inadequate compression following sheath removal leads to this complication. Management is already discussed.
- *Perforation of vessel:* Presents as sudden discomfort during procedure. Occurs in small branches of forearm or axillary vessels. Close follow-up is required to look for possible compartment syndrome.
- *Vasospasm:* Radial artery is rich in vasoconstrictor alpha receptors (alpha 1 and 2). Multiple punctures, prolonged procedural duration, multiple catheter exchanges and anxious female patients are common subset of patients who develop vasospasm. Analgesia, local nitrates and calcium channel blockers and/or sedation may be required for removal of catheter and to overcome vasospasm.
- *Asymptomatic radial artery occlusion:* Occurs in 3–5% of cases. This can be avoided by use of procedural heparin (3000–5000 units), use of small sized sheaths and using "Patent Hemostasis" technique at the end of procedure.

We will discuss various methods for femoral vascular site compression: Manual versus Mechanical.

Using manual compression to achieve hemostasis requires using 2 or 3 fingers to apply continuous downward pressure above the puncture site.[6] Sufficient pressure is applied to stop bleeding without obscuring the distal pulses. Pressure is held for approximately 20 minutes, or until hemostasis occurs.

Mechanical compression devices (e.g. FemoStop) have the advantages of hands-free operation, less contact with blood, and controlled pressure. When bleeding is marked, the pressure is increased to initiate hemostasis and then decreased every few minutes to the lowest pressure that stops bleeding. The puncture site can be easily visualized via the transparent dome and closely observed while the pressure is slowly released. Maintaining pressure for a prolonged period (e.g. 2 hours) is not recommended because of the risk for tissue damage or nerve compression. Use of this device is contraindicated in patients with severe peripheral vascular disease or femoral artery or venous grafts.[7] Compression may be inadequate in patients who are markedly obese.

In an evaluation of vascular complications associated with manual and mechanical compression, Chlan et al.[8] found no difference in complication rates between the compression methods.

In a retrospective analysis of the three generations of the Angio-Seal device, Applegate et al.[9] found no significant differences between the three devices and manual compression. Successful closure rates were similar for diagnostic and PCI procedures; the overall success rate was greater than 98%. The vascular complication rates were similar to those associated with manual compression.

In a meta-analysis of the safety of vascular closure devices, Nikolsky et al.[10] found no significant difference in vascular complications between Angio-Seal and Perclose devices compared with mechanical compression. The VasoSeal device appeared to have a higher incidence of vascular complication compared with mechanical compression. With the rapidly changing technology and newer generation devices, along with the gain in operator experience, complication rates associated with the newer devices are lower than those associated with the early generation devices.

Table 19.2 Vascular complications associated with percutaneous coronary interventions

Complication	*Description*	*Signs and symptoms/comments*	*Management*
Hematomas	Blood collects in soft tissue	Expanding mass surrounding puncture site	Acute management includes providing hydration, applying pressure, marking area to monitor for expansion, maintaining bed rest, and serial monitoring of complete blood cell count
		Any hardened area under the skin	Anticoagulant and antiplatelet therapies may be interrupted, and blood transfusion may
		Slowly expanding hematomas, even from venous sites, can be dangerous because of their insidious nature	Hematomas usually resolve within a few weeks as the blood gradually spreads and is absorbed from the soft tissue
Pseudoaneurysms	Thrombus does not develop in the puncture site when the arterial sheath is removed, creating a communicating tract	A large painful hematoma, pulsatile mass, and a bruit or thrill in the groin	Any large or painful hematoma should be evaluated for pseudoaneurysm by using ultrasound
	Causes include inadequate compression after sheath removal and impaired hemostasis	Pedal pulses are usually unchanged because blood flow is not affected in the main artery	If the pseudoaneurysm is small (<2 cm), it may be observed and monitored clinically
		Pseudoaneurysms may rupture, leading to sudden massive swelling and severe pain	A large pseudoaneurysm may require ultrasound-guided compression or surgical intervention
		Nerve compression should be suspected when the pain is out of proportion to the size of the hematoma	Ultrasound-guided thrombin injection is another treatment option
		Nerve compression from groin hematomas may lead to quadriceps weakness that may take weeks or months to resolve	
Retroperitoneal hematoma	Retroperitoneal hematoma may occur if the arterial wall puncture is made above the inguinal ligament	Blood collecting in the retroperitoneal space may not produce obvious swelling and may not be evident on the surface	Diagnosis is confirmed by using computed tomography or abdominal ultrasound
	The hematoma extends into the retroperitoneal space, which lies deep in the abdominal cavity	Signs and symptoms include unexplained hypotension, ipsilateral flank pain, vague abdominal or back pain, or abdominal distension	Management includes hydration, transfusion, serial blood cell counts, and bed rest
	This serious complication could be fatal if not recognized early	Decreasing levels of hemoglobin and hematocrit and ecchymosis are late signs	
Arteriovenous fistula	A direct communication forms between an artery and a vein	Continuous bruit at access site, swollen tender extremity, and claudication due to limb ischemia	Ultrasound is ordered to confirm diagnosis

Contd...

Contd...

Complication	*Description*	*Signs and symptoms/comments*	*Management*
	Risk for this complication increases with multiple access attempts, punctures above or below the correct site, or impaired clotting		Most arteriovenous fistulas spontaneously close, so surgical repair is rarely required
Atheroembolism	Friable atherosclerotic plaque in the abdominal aorta is disrupted, creating potentially embolic debris	This complication may not be recognized for weeks to months after the percutaneous coronary intervention be indicated	Management is generally conservative: providing hydration, monitoring urine output and controlling hypertension
	Showers of microemboli may result in microvascular glomerular obstruction, necrotizing fasciitis, and blue toe syndrome		Surgical management (i.e. embolectomy) may be indicated
	Even small amounts of debris can have severe consequences, if embolized to the kidneys, viscera, or brain		Distal embolic protection devices are used whenever feasible in patients undergoing percutaneous coronary interventions associated with high-risk of distal embolization (e.g. saphenous vein grafts)

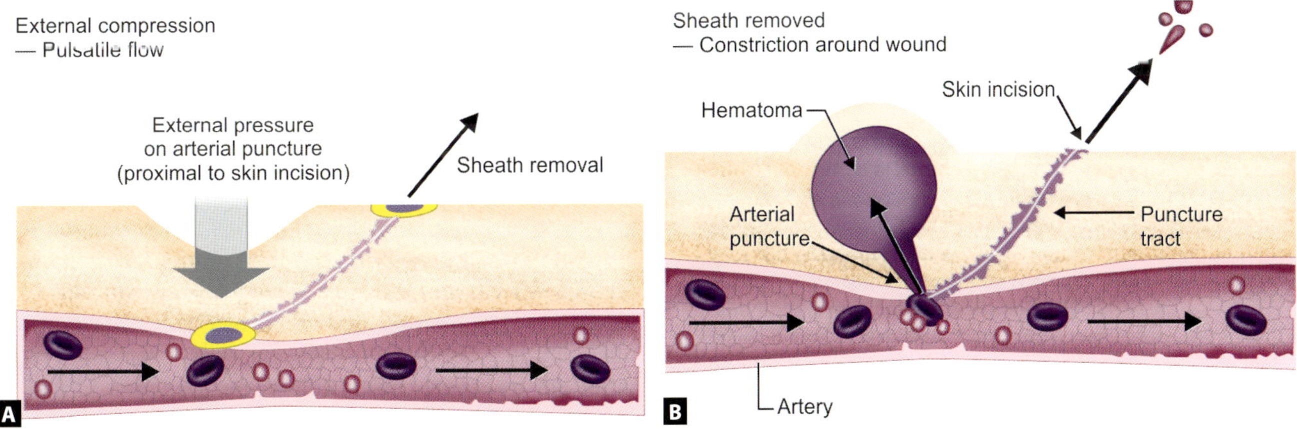

Figs 19.2A and B (A) Once the sheath is removed, external compression is applied 1–2 cm above site; (B) Effective compression was not maintained, causing a hematoma to develop

ISAR-CLOSURE Trial[11] *published in JAMA:* November 2014 was a large multicenter randomized trial that compared manual compression to closure using Femoseal or Exoseal VCD. Primary endpoint was vascular access site complications (hematoma >5 cm, pseudoaneurysm, AV fistula, access site related major bleeding, ipsilateral leg ischemia, and need for intervention or local infection at 30 days). Access site related vascular complications were observed in 6.9% of VCD patients compared to 7.9% of manual compression group. This trial proved noninferiority of VCDs compared to manual compression. Femoseal group had lower time to hemostasis and closure device failure rate compared to Exoseal device. PEVAR trial.[12] compared safety and effectiveness of percutaneous endovascular aortic aneurysm repair with use of 21 F stent graft system and 6 or 10 F suture mediated closure system. 150 patients were randomized 2:1 to percutaneous or

Table 19.3 Vascular closure devices

Category	*Description*	*Device (brand name)*
Collagen plugs	Hemostasis is achieved by delivering collagen extravascularly to the surface at the femoral artery	VasoSeal
	The collagen attracts platelets to the arterial puncture site, resulting in a seal at the site	
	Collagen reabsorbs during a 6-week period	
Absorbable anchors	The device consists of an absorbable suture material and a small collagen plug	Angio-Seal
	It creates a mechanical seal by sandwiching the arteriotomy between the suture anchor and the collagen sponge	
	The material dissolves within 90 days	
Topical hemostasis patches	Topical patches with a marine toxin, thrombin, or a biopolymer as a hemostasis agent seal the tissue tract without arteriotomy	Syvek patches
		Chilo-Seal
		Clo-Sur PAD
	This external device leaves no foreign matter	D-Stat
	Manual compression is still required	
	Longer duration of compression may be needed in patients who are hypertensive or obese	
Suture-mediated devices	The devices suture the arteriotomy site to achieve immediate hemostasis	Perclose
	Potential complications include Infection, laceration, and partial dissection	
Staple-mediated devices	Staples create a purse-string suture closure, allowing for hemostasis	StarClose
Biosealants	A liquid procoagulant mixture of thrombin and collagen is delivered to the puncture site to seal the site	Duett
	Accidental injection into the femoral artery could lead to acute leg ischemia	

open femoral closure. 6F Perclose Proglide device was used in 50 patients and 51 patients received 10F Prostar XL device. Vascular closure device use compared to open surgical femoral closure was associated with shorter procedural time, shorter time to hemostasis and trend towards decreased blood loss and groin pain.

The most frequent vascular complications were ecchymosis (37%), hematoma (20%), and oozing (15%). Vascular closure devices are alternative methods for achieving and maintaining hemostasis.

Compared with other compression methods, vascular closure devices are associated with decreased compression time, improved patient comfort, and earlier ambulation but not with significant decreases in bleeding or vascular complications.[13]

A minor annoying problem with many closure devices is persistent oozing around the closure site, particularly in patients receiving antiplatelet and anticoagulation therapy. Infection at the femoral access site is rare, but increased occurrence of infection has been noted with closure devices introduced in the tissue tract.[14] Prophylactic antibiotic therapy may be prescribed for patients at higher risk (e.g. those with diabetes) before the PCI procedure if a vascular closure will be used for hemostasis. All vascular closure devices are subject to failure and manual and/or mechanical pressure may be required if bleeding occurs despite their use.

VASCULAR CLOSURE DEVICES

Some vascular closure devices[15,16] are classified in Table 19.3.

Active Approximators

Physically close the arteriotomy with clip or suture:

- *Suture-based devices:* These percutaneously deploy a suture at arteriotomy site mimicking open surgical closure. For example, Perclose Proglide device and Prostar XL. Advantage is no restriction on activity and no contraindications to anticoagulation. Limitations are learning curve and changes in anatomy of the lumen.
- *Clip-based devices:* Starclose device deploys 4 mm nitinol clip at arteriotomy site. However, it affects MRI evaluation of adjacent area if required.

Passive Approximators

These deploy a plug, sealant or gel at arteriotomy site:

- *Collagen plugs:* Angio-Seal device uses intravascular anchor footplate to secure extravascular polyethylene glycol plug at arteriotomy site. All components are absorbable. Limitation is same access site cannot be used in 90 days. Femoseal VCD uses extravascular locking disc along with intravascular anchor plate. Another example is Vascade Device.

- *Sealant or gel-based devices:* X Seal VCD, Mynx VCD, Exoseal VCD, Fast seal VCD.
- *Compression-assist devices:* Axera 2 access system uses shallow angle arteriotomy (10–15°) to give access for procedure. After sheath removal, manual compression is easy due to shallow angle.
- *Catalyst II and III devices* have nitinol disc coated with thrombogenic material (kaolin or protamine sulfate) that aids in coagulation.
- *External hemostatic devices:* These are externally placed on the skin and achieve hemostasis by mechanical pressure or by accelerating clotting cascade, e.g. TR band or Safeguard Radial.

Bed rest guidelines vary with institutional policy, the technique used for hemostasis, the size of the sheath, and use of antiplatelet therapy after the PCI procedure. Tagney and Lackie conducted a study to determine if bed rest times could be shortened without increasing complication rates in patients after diagnostic catheterization and PCI. They found that bed rest times could be reduced from 6 hours to 3 hours without an increase in complication rates. Standard assessment of the PCI access sites includes monitoring the arterial and venous puncture sites for bleeding, hematoma, ecchymosis, localized tenderness, pulsating mass and new bruits. Assessment of peripheral circulation includes evaluation of bilateral pulses for comparison, warmth and color of the affected extremity, and capillary refill. Immobilization of the affected extremity is indicated during the period of bed rest. An extremity immobilizer may be necessary in patients who have restless leg syndrome or are unable to comply with keeping the extremity straight. Patients with brachial puncture sites are on bed or chair rest with the arm straight for a minimum of 2 hours. Using the affected arm for blood pressure checks should be avoided during the recovery period. The brachial site is monitored for bleeding, swelling, distal pulses, sensation, and motor function. Weak pulses or lack of pulses could be a sign of arterial spasm. Numbness and weakness may indicate medial nerve compromise or impaired circulation.

Patients should be reassured that the small hard lump palpable in the groin region will gradually disappear. Ecchymosis, the result of a hematoma, may take several weeks to resolve. Patients should be told that the discoloration will most likely expand and change color from dark blue to greenish yellow before disappearing. If femoral nerve compression occurred, leg weakness may persist for weeks to several months.

Patients should seek medical assistance if they have expansion of and/or pulsation in the groin swelling, new or significantly worsening discoloration, leg weakness, numbness, or pallor, redness, warmth at the access site, or pus-like drainage from the site.

Radial Approach

Benefits of the radial artery approach include decreased bleeding at the access site and earlier ambulation.[17] The arterial sheath is usually removed immediately after the PCI procedure. A specially made tourniquet (e.g. HemoBand) may be applied at the puncture site, and then pressure is gradually released until hemostasis is achieved. If such a tourniquet is not available, manual compression is adequate. After hemostasis is achieved, a pressure bandage may be applied. A wrist splint may be used to decrease episodes of wrist flexion. Patients may ambulate once sedation wears off. They are advised to avoid flexion and extension of the wrist for the remainder of the day. The radial and ulnar pulses are both monitored as part of the assessment. Loss of a radial pulse may be due to thrombosis, dissection, inappropriate suturing, or spasms. Local swelling is treated with ice and analgesics. Re-bleeding is treated with elevation of the hand of the affected extremity and local pressure. Persistent bleeding may be due to a lacerated artery. An inflatable blood pressure cuff can be used to control bleeding; however, surgical intervention may be indicated.

Patients should be advised to avoid strenuous activity the week after the PCI procedure, but they may resume walking and driving in 48 hours.

SUMMARY OF RECOMMENDATIONS[18]

- *Groin:* Need to keep affected leg still until after sheath removed; clear dressing over access site; while femoral sheath is in, head of bed (HOB) elevated less than 30°; flexible sheaths allow HOB elevation up to 60°; sheath pulled when activated clotting time is less than 180; after sheath is removed, HOB needs to be flat with patient on bed rest for 1–4 hours, depending on hemostasis method; vital signs and neurovascular assessments every 15 minutes for first 4 hours, every 30 minutes for 2 hours, then every hour until stable; perform orthostatic checks after bed rest.
- *Radial:* Sheath removed immediately and dressing applied; may receive medication to decrease arterial spasm for sheath removal; wristband applied to obtain hemostasis and arm board positioned to minimize mobility. Vital signs and neurovascular assessments every 15 minutes while wristband on. Wristband removed after 1–2 hours and pressure dressing applied (for 24 hours).

Wrist immobilized for 2–4 hours after wristband removed. Keep arm at heart level for 24 hours.

Patient can walk after sheath removal with care taken to evaluate for effects of sedation and fluid shifts before ambulation.

Back pain (most often occurs with femoral approach); may logroll with assistance; back rubs, pain medication available.

Notify staff if access site feels warm or wet; any pain (anginal, back, leg); inability to void with abdominal fullness.

Discharge Instructions

- *Femoral site:* Groin restrictions—no heavy lifting, no tub baths for 2 days
- *Radial site:* Do not drive, avoid wrist movement, do not lift more than 1 pound for 2 days; avoid strenuous arm movement for 5 days; no tub baths for 3 days.

REFERENCES

1. Schnyder G, Sawhney N, et al. Common femoral artery anatomy is influenced by demographics and comorbidity: Implications for cardiac and peripheral invasive studies. Catheter Cardiovasc Interv. 2001;53:289-95.
2. Merriweather N, Sulzbach-Hoke LM. Managing risk of complications at femoral vascular access sites in percutaneous coronary intervention. Critical Care Nurse. 2012;32(5):16-29.
3. Bridget Shoulders-Odom, MS, ACNP-BC, CCRN. Management of patients after percutaneous coronary interventions. Critical Care Nurse. 2008;28(5):26-41.
4. Trimarchi S, et al. BMC2 Registry, Retroperitoneal hematoma after percutaneous coronary intervention: A report from the BMC2 registry. JACC Interv. 2010;3:845-50.
5. Tizon- Marcos H, et al. Incidence of compartment syndrome of the arm in a large series of transradial approach for coronary procedures. Journal Interven Cardiol. 2008;21:380-4.
6. Shaffer RB. Arterial and venous sheath removal. In: Wiegand DJ, Carlson KK (Eds). AACN Procedure Manual for Critical Care, 5th edition. St Louis, MO: Elsevier Saunders; 2005. pp.602-9.
7. FemoStop plus femoral compression system [package insert]. Wilmingham, MA: Radi Medical Systems; 2004.
8. Chlan LL, Sabo J, Savik K. Effects of three groin compression methods on patient discomfort, distress, and vascular complications following a percutaneous coronary intervention procedure. Nurs Res. 2005;54(6):391-8.
9. Applegate RJ, Sacrinty M, Kutcher MA, et al. Vascular complications with newer generations of Angioseal vascular closure devices. J Interv Cardiol. 2006;19(1):67-74.
10. Nikolsky E, Mehran R, Halkin A, et al. Vascular complications associated with arteriotomy closure devices in patients undergoing percutaneous coronary procedures: a meta-analysis. J Am Coll Cardiol. 2004;44(6):1200-9.
11. Schulz-Schupke S, Helde S, Gewalt S, et al. Comparison of vascular closure devices vs manual compression after femoral artery puncture: the ISAR-CLOSURE randomized clinical trial. JAMA. 2014;312:1981-7.
12. Nelson PR, Kracjer Z, Kansal N, et al. A multicenter, randomized, controlled trial of totally percutaneous access versus open femoral exposure for endovascular aortic aneurysm repair (the PEVAR trial). J Vasc Surg. 2014;59:1181-93.
13. Safian RD, Freed MS. The Manual of Interventional Cardiology, 3rd edn. Royal Oak, MI: Physicians' Press; 2001.
14. Wong EML, Wu EB, Chan CM, et al. A review of the management of patients after percutaneous coronary intervention. Int J Clin Pract. 2006;60:582-9.
15. Weintraub JL, Ward TJ. Vascular closure device update. Endovascular Today. 2015;1:54-60.
16. Kim MC. Vascular closure devices. Cardiol Clin. 2006;24(2):277-86, vii.
17. Jolly SS, Yusuf S, et al. Radial vs femoral access for coronary angiography and intervention in patients with acute coronary syndromes (RIVAL): A randomised, parallel group multicenter trial. Lancet. 2011;377:1409-20.
18. Coronary Artery Disease and Dysrhythmias, Chapter 765.

CHAPTER

20

Bioresorbable Vascular Scaffold

Maciej Lesiak, Aleksander Araszkiewicz

Despite significant improvement in design and technology of drug-eluting stents (DES), the implantation of metallic stents has been associated with some limitations. The concept of using a permanent metallic endovascular device to restore the patency of a stenotic artery has inherited pitfalls, namely the presence of a foreign body within the artery causing vascular inflammation, late complications such as restenosis and stent thrombosis.[1,2] Furthermore by "caging" the artery, permanent implants prevent vasomotor response to physiological stimuli and accommodative positive remodeling. For this reason, the concept of bioresorbable vascular scaffold (BVS) may become a very promising alternative to DES. After implantation a scaffold maintains sufficient radial strength to prevent vessel recoil and releases the drug to inhibit the proliferation of neointima. Over time the scaffold mass and its radial strength gradually decrease, and after 2–3 years device vanishes completely, leaving the vessel covered with a healthy endothelium and normal vasomotorical function.[3] The term "scaffold" may be more appropriate for such a device than "a stent" because it implies temporary arterial support. Recently, BVS technology has been named as the fourth revolution, rendering a novel treatment named vascular restoration therapy (VRT) in interventional cardiology.[4,5] The clear feature of VRT is that vessel scaffolding is degraded evanescently, and therapeutic advantages may be derived from allowing natural vasomotor response in the vessel.[5] In addition, the underlying benefits involve decreased or eliminated risk of very late stent thrombosis, facilitated reintervention due to the complete reabsorption of the implanted scaffold, improved noninvasive imaging of the target site using computed tomography during any postintervention period, and possibly shorter time of dual antiplatelet therapy.

More than fourteen bioresorbable scaffold designs have been presented so far. Most of them are still either under preclinical evaluation or being examined in the clinical setting. Of note, three scaffolds have already gained Conformité Européenne (CE) mark certificate, and are approved in Europe: the Absorb BVS (Abbott Vascular, Santa Clara, CA) and DESolve (Elixir Medical Corporation) for coronary artery disease, and Igaki-Tamai stent (Kyoto Medical Planning Co., Ltd. Kyoto, Japan) for the treatment of peripheral vascular disease.

IGAKI-TAMAI SCAFFOLD

The Igaki-Tamai scaffold (Kyoto Medical Planning Co., Japan), was the first fully bioresorbable stent implanted in humans and was made of poly-l-lactic acid (PLLA). The first version of the scaffold had a helical zigzag design, was mounted on a standard angioplasty balloon, and was both thermal self-expanding and balloon expandable. Scaffold expansion was achieved with the use of heated contrast (up to 70°C). The device continued expanding after its implantation over a 20–30 minute period, until it reached its final dimensions.[6,7] In the first clinical study, the Igaki-Tamai stent was assessed for feasibility and safety in 50 patients who were then followed for more than 10 years.[8] The target lesion revascularization (TLR) rate was 16%, 18%, and 28% at 1, 5, and 10 years, respectively. The major adverse cardiac event (MACE) rate was 14% at 12 months and 16%, 18%, 24%, and 50% at 3, 4, 5, and 10 years, respectively. The high survival free of cardiac death (98% at 10 years) demonstrated the long-term safety of the PLLA stent.[8]

Although the short- and long-term follow-up results were encouraging, this device failed to progress, mainly due to the large guide catheters (8F) required for implantation, and the concerns that the heated contrast used for device deployment may cause vessel wall injury. The new generation Igaki-Tamai scaffold potentially overcomes these pitfalls, as it can be implanted through a 6F guide catheter without the need for a heated contrast agent. The device is currently undergoing preclinical evaluation in Germany.

ABSORB BIORESORBALE VASCULAR SCAFFOLD

Absorb BVS (Abbott Vascular, Santa Clara, CA, USA) is currently the most widely used bioresorbable scaffold. It consists of the polymer backbone composed of Poly L-lactide acid (PLLA), covered with amorphous matrix, a 1:1 mixture of everolimus and another polymer, poly-DL-lactide (PDLLA). The scaffold has a corrugated ring design and is mounted on Xience delivery catheter. Recently, a new enhanced delivery system GT1 has been introduced in Europe. Since the scaffold itself is radio-transparent the two platinum markers are placed close to proximal and distal edge of the device to allow its proper positioning. The resorption process progresses gradually, mainly due to hydrolysis, thus minimal or no inflammation can be observed.[9] The final product of this process is CO_2 and H_2O. The Scaffold is covered with everolimus, a potent antiproliferative drug, which is released at the same rate and amount as from metallic Xience V®. Absorb BVS is a thick-strut scaffold, with the average strut thickness of 157 microns. Currently three diameters (2.5, 3.0, 3.5 mm), and 5 lengths (8, 12, 18, 23 and 28 mm) are available.

Since the scaffold is radio-transparent the use of intravascular imaging such as ultrasound (IVUS) or optical coherence tomography (OCT) is recommended during the implantation. On IVUS the struts appear as parallel lines without acoustic shadowing, whereas OCT displays the struts as empty boxes (Figs 20.1A and B).

DESOLVE, NOVOLIMUS-ELUTING CORONARY SCAFFOLD

The DESolve Novolimus-Eluting Bioresorbable Coronary Scaffold (BCS) System (Elixir Medical Corporation, Sunnyvale, California) is a PLLA-based scaffold and has several differentiating characteristics. These features include: bioresorption at about 1 year while maintaining adequate vessel support; the elimination of chronic recoil; the ability to expand the scaffold without strut fracture; and unique expansion capabilities, which minimize strut malapposition.[10] The radial strength of the device is comparable with metal stent (Elixir's BMS).

The DESolve First-in-Man trial was a prospective multicenter study enrolling 16 patients eligible for treatment.[11] The principal safety endpoint was a composite of cardiac death, myocardial infarction, and clinically indicated target lesion revascularization. The principal imaging endpoint was in-scaffold late lumen loss (LLL) assessed by quantitative coronary angiography (QCA) at 6 months. Intravascular ultrasound (IVUS) and optical coherence tomography (OCT) imaging was performed at baseline and 6 months; multislice computed tomography (MSCT) was performed at 12 months to evaluate in-stent restenosis. Acute procedural success was achieved in 100% patients receiving a study device. At 12 months, there was no scaffold thrombosis and no major adverse cardiac events directly attributable to the scaffold. At 6 months, in-scaffold LLL (by QCA) was 0.19 ± 0.19 mm; neointimal volume

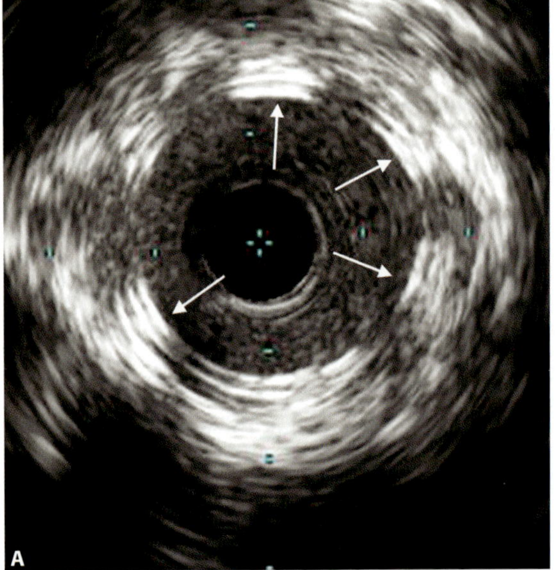

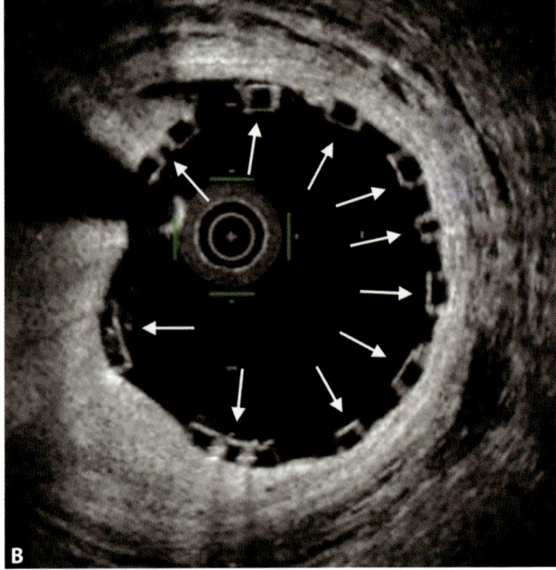

Figs 20.1A and B Intravascular imaging of Absorb bioresorbable vascular scaffold. (A) Intravascul ultrasound—parallel lines without acoustic shadowing (arrows); (B) Optical coherence tomography—empty box-like image of BVS struts (arrows)

(by IVUS) was 7.19 ± 3.56%, with no evidence of scaffold recoil or late malapposition. The positive findings were confirmed with OCT, that showed uniform, thin neointimal coverage (0.12 ± 0.04 mm). At 12 months, MSCT demonstrated excellent vessel patency.[11] The study demonstrated the feasibility and efficacy of the DESolve bioresorbable coronary scaffold. Based on this initial promising data, the DESolve NX study has recently commenced, and aims to evaluate the safety and efficacy of the device. The study is expected to include 120 patients with single *de novo* coronary artery lesions. In-scaffold LLL at 6-month follow-up is the principal endpoint. In addition, the DeSolve NX II pivotal trial has been designed to evaluate the effectiveness of the device in a broader number of patients to provide sufficient evidence for CE mark approval and is expected to start in due course.

FANTOM, SIROLIMUS-ELUTING BIORESORBABLE SCAFFOLD

A new desaminotyrosine-derived polycarbonate polymer sirolimus-eluting scaffold (Fantom, Reva Medical, San Diego, California) has thin struts (strut thickness of 125 μm) and a low crossing profile, which improves its deliverability. The base structure is covered with a thin layer of desaminotyrosine-derived polycarbonate biodegradable polymer with integrated sirolimus at a total dose of 115 μg (for the 3.0 × 18 mm scaffold). More than 80% of the total sirolimus load is eluted within the first 90 days. The Fantom scaffold is completely visible under X-ray in contrast to PLLA scaffolds. Also its appearance in intravascular imaging is different as compared to Absorb or DESolve. In OCT imaging the struts does not have a box-like image, looking more like thick-strut metal DES instead (Fig. 20.2). The tyrosine polycarbonate catabolism includes hydrolysis of the polymer to carbon dioxide and iodinated-desaminotyrosyl-tyrosine ethyl esters, which are further hydrolyzed to ethanol and iodinated-desaminotyrosyl-tyrosine. Cleavage of the latter results in tyrosine molecules and iodinated-desaminotyrosine, which are finally catabolized into carbon dioxide and water in the Krebs cycle.[12]

The Fantom scaffold is presently under clinical evaluation. First human implants of the scaffold were initiated in December 2014. In Fantom I Pilot Study patients were enrolled in Australia, Brazil, Europe and New Zealand and they will be followed for a total of five years, with primary data to be obtained at 9 and 12 months.

FANTOM II CE Trial is an ongoing study and will include 220 patients enrolled in 25 clinical sites, with primary end point of major adverse cardiac events (MACE) and late lumen loss at 6 months. Recently the early results of the study have been presented and showed an excellent acute procedural outcomes and safety of Fantom scaffold.[13]

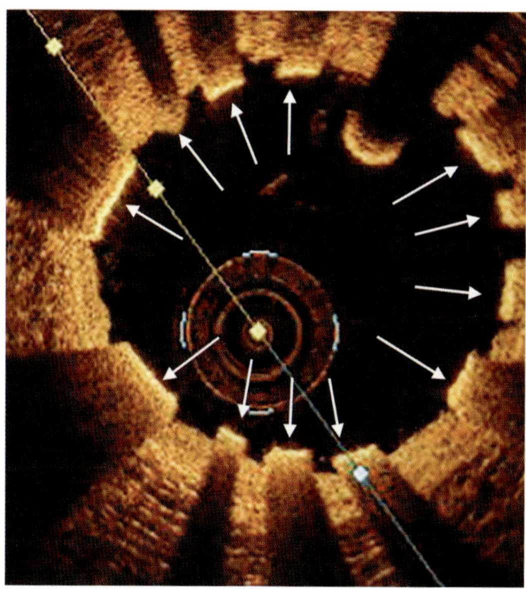

Fig. 20.2 Optical coherence tomography image of Fantom stent. Thick-struts with acoustic shadowing (arrows)

IDEAL BIOSTENT

The Ideal BioStent (Xenogenics Corp, Canton, MA, USA) is a fully bioresorbable balloon expandable scaffold. The device consists of a core backbone and a top coat.[14] The backbone is synthesized from polylactide anhydride, and a trimer of two salicylic acid molecules joined with a sebacic acid, while the top coat part is comprised of salicylate and the antiproliferative drug sirolimus. Preclinical studies have demonstrated the potential anti-inflammatory and antiplatelet properties of salicylate, which appears to reduce restenosis and promote vessel healing during the polymer's degradation.[15]

The first generation scaffold (BTI) was examined in the WHISPER study. Eleven patients were included in this prospective first-in-man trial that evaluated the safety and efficacy of the scaffold. Coronary angiography and IVUS,[15,16] performed post-procedurally and at follow-up, revealed the absence of scaffold recoil. However, IVUS and OCT showed increased neointimal formation, which was attributed to the inadequate drug dose and fast drug elution. In view of the high restenosis rate, the device was redesigned. The revised device (Ideal BioStent) has a higher drug dose, slower drug release kinetics, and an easy to use peel-away sheath.[17] The new generation Ideal scaffold is currently undergoing clinical evaluation.

MAGNESIUM METALLIC STENTS

Magnesium is the only metal that has been implemented in bioresorbable scaffold technology. A limitation of magnesium is its fragility, thus, it has been mixed with several elements such as zirconium, yttrium, and other rare earth metals to provide it with adequate radial strength.[18] An advantage of the AMS is the fact that the degradation of the magnesium alloy to inorganic salts triggers only a minor inflammatory response, and creates an electronegative charge that has been shown to have an antithrombogenic effect.[19,20] An AMS (Biotronik, Berlin, Germany) is a tubular, slotted-tube, balloon-expandable stent sculptured by laser from a tube of magnesium alloy.[21-23] The device has similar mechanical strength to other metallic stents. In the first generation AMS 1.0, the resorption process was almost completed at 2 months after implantation, resulting in late vessel recoil. To address this limitation, the scaffold was redesigned, and in the latest revision (drug-eluting AMS, DREAM 2.0) the process was prolonged up to 6 months.[24]

The efficacy of the first generation AMS was validated in the PROGRESS-AMS (Clinical Performance and Angiographic Results of Coronary Stenting) study, which was a nonrandomized, multicenter trial that included 63 patients who had *de novo* lesions with lengths of 10–15 mm and reference diameters of 3.0–3.5 mm. During a follow-up period of 4 months, there was a 23.8% clinically driven TLR incidence, associated with a high LLL (1.08 ± 0.49 mm). From 4 to 12 months, only one further patient sustained TLR, resulting in a cumulative incidence of MACE at 12 months of 26.7%.[25,26] These results were attributed to neointimal proliferation and vessel recoil caused by the premature reduction in the radial strength of the implanted devices. To overcome these limitations, the company added the antiproliferative drug paclitaxel, and changed the design of the scaffold and the composition of the magnesium alloy, thus providing the device with increased strength, and a prolongation of its resorption process. The efficacy of the new revision DREAMS (drug-eluting absorbable metallic stents) 1.0 was evaluated in the BIOSOLVE-1 trial. In this prospective multicenter FIM trial, 46 patients with a single *de novo* coronary artery lesion were implanted with 47 scaffolds. At 1-year follow-up, the MACE rate was 7% (two TLR and one MI), whereas the LLL, although improved, remained high (0.52 ± 0.39 mm).[27]

The second generation DREAMS (DREAMS 2.0 G) scaffold incorporates sirolimus elution instead of paclitaxel and possesses tantalum radiopaque end-markers. Preclinical evaluation of the device revealed reduced inflammation, and a higher endothelization rate compared with the previous revision. In BIOSOLVE-II study 121 patients treated with DREAMS 2,0 G was studied.[21] The primary end-point of the study was late lumen loss (LLL) after six months. DREAMS 2.0G demonstrates significantly improved in-segment LLL (0.27 ± 0.37 mm) compared to its precursor devices tested in the PROGRESS (0.83 ± 0.37 mm) and the BIOSOLVE-I study (0.52 ± 0.48 mm). Vasomotion of the scaffolded vessel segment was demonstrated at 6 months (80% had vasomotion ≥3% after acetylocholine or nitroglycerin test). IVUS results in a subgroup of 30 subjects demonstrate a preservation of the scaffold area with a low neo-intimal area at 6-month (neointimal hyperplasia was reduced by 73% compared to BIOSOLVE-I group). No intraluminal masses were observed in OCT at any time in a subgroup of 25 subjects. DREAMS 2G in BIOSOLVE-II demonstrates a low TLF (3.3%) and TLR (1.7%) rate at 6-month, which is comparable to other absorbable scaffolds and permanent drug eluting stents.[27] Moreover no definite or probable scaffold thrombosis was observed with DREAMS 2G nor any of its precursor devices tested in PROGRESS and BIOSOLVE-I in a total of 232 subjects.[24]

Further evaluation is however needed to confirm these positive results in clinical settings and to examine its safety and efficacy in the treatment of CAD.

BIORESORBABLE VASCULAR SCAFFOLD RATIONALE AND CLINICAL INDICATIONS

There are numerous potential advantages of BVS over metallic DES. The liberation of coronary artery from permanent scaffold re-establishes physiological vasomotion, restores vessel original geometry and preserves laminar blood flow. This in turn may limit the development of neoatherosclerosis. Contrary to metallic stents, where late luminal loss may deteriorate the early result of percutaneous coronary intervention (PCI), after deployment of BVS a late luminal gain has been observed.[3] The absence of permanent foreign material reduces the risk of late stent thrombosis, myocardial infarction, and sudden death. Preliminary data suggest that the longer the observation time, the greater the advantage of BVS over metallic stents. Thus, it is obvious that BVS should be predominantly used in young patients, particularly with long lesions or diffuse disease where multiple long stents are required. Especially patients with lesions located in mid portion of left anterior descending coronary artery, obtuse marginal branch or distal right coronary artery will benefit, since the use of BVS will allow for potential future by-pass grafting. Regardless of the lack of sufficient data it seems that the use of BVS should not be restricted only to subjects with stable coronary artery disease, since patients with acute coronary syndromes, including ST-segment elevation myocardial infarction will have the same benefit in a long run.

ABSORB BIORESORBABLE VASCULAR SCOFFOLD CLINICAL STUDIES

So far, the most widely studied bioresorbable scaffold is Absorb BVS. Two designs of the BVS have been assessed in clinical trials. The safety and feasibility of the BVS 1.0 was tested in the open-label prospective study: a bioresorbable everolimus eluting coronary stent system for patients with single *de novo* coronary artery lesions (ABSORB Cohort A trial).[28] At 6 months, the angiographic in-stent late lumen loss (LLL) was 0.44 mm with the evidence of scaffold significant recoil (–11.8%) as measured by intravascular ultrasound (IVUS).[29,30] However, vasomotion appeared to be restored, with inducible vasoconstriction and vasodilatation in the treated segment.[29] To improve the mechanical characteristics of BVS and reduce recoil, a second-generation BVS (1.1) has been introduced. BVS 1.1 has a smaller maximum circular unsupported surface area, a more uniform strut distribution, and improved stent retention.[31] The efficacy of the BVS 1.1 was assessed in the ABSORB Cohort B trial, which recruited 101 patients with single or two-vessel *de novo* disease, with all subjects receiving a 3 × 18 mm BVS.[29] At 6-month follow-up, there was only one case of target lesion revascularization (TLR), while LLL was only 0.19 ± 0.18 mm; at 2-year follow-up, LLL was 0.27 ± 0.20 mm. Although after 6-months there was significant reduction in minimal lumen area (MLA) on IVUS, as compared with the baseline measurement (6.60 ± 1.22 to 6.37 ± 1.12 mm^2, $p < 0.005$), the scaffold area was gradually increasing with longer observation time.[32,33] Multimodality imaging of the ABSORB Cohort B patients after three years revealed that in IVUS mean lumen and scaffold area remained stable between 2nd and 3rd year, whereas significant reduction in plaque area behind the struts was observed, with a trend toward adaptive restrictive remodeling of external elastic membrane.[33] Hyperechogenicity of the vessel wall, a surrogate of the bioresorption process, decreased from 23.1% to 10.4%, with a reduction of radiofrequency backscattering for dense calcium and necrotic core. The count of strut cores detected on optical coherence tomography (OCT) increased significantly, most likely reflecting the dismantling of the scaffold. Importantly, 98% of struts were covered with endothelium. At 3-year follow-up, seven cases of ischemia-driven TLR was reported. The total major adverse cardiovascular events (MACE) rate was 10.0%, with no scaffold thrombosis. More complex population has been studied in the ongoing prospective, single-arm, open-label registry ABSORB EXTEND.[34] Patients with lesions ≤28 mm in length and reference vessel diameter of 2.0–3.8 mm have been included. At one year, for the first 512 patients enrolled in the study, the composite endpoints of ischemia-driven MACE and target vessel failure were 4.3% and 4.9%, respectively. The cumulative rate of definite and probable scaffold thrombosis was 0.8%.[35]

ABSORB II trial was designed to compare an everolimus-eluting bioresorbable scaffold with an everolimus-eluting metallic stent (Xience).[36] In this single-blind, multicenter, randomized trial, 501 patients with evidence of myocardial ischemia, and one or two *de novo* native lesions in different epicardial vessels were enrolled. The patients were randomized in a 2 : 1 ratio to receive treatment with BVS or treatment with an everolimus-eluting metallic stent. The co-primary endpoints of this study were vasomotion (change in mean lumen diameter before and after nitrate administration at 3 years), and the difference between minimum lumen diameter (after nitrate administration) after the index procedure and after 3 years. Secondary endpoints were: procedural performance of the device, assessed by quantitative angiography and intravascular ultrasound; composite clinical endpoints (death, myocardial infarction, and coronary revascularization); device and procedural success; as well as angina status, assessed by the Seattle Angina Questionnaire (SAQ) and exercise testing at 6 and 12 months. The one-year results of ABSORB II were recently published in the *Lancet*.[36] Cumulative rates of first new or worsening angina, from adverse event reporting, were lower (72 patients—22% in the bioresorbable scaffold group, vs 50–30% in the metallic stent group, $p = 0.04$). Patients' performance during maximum exercise and angina status, measured by SAQ, were similar. The one-year composite, device orientated endpoint was similar for BVS and DES groups (16 patients—5%, vs five patients—3% $p = 0.35$). Three patients in the BVS group developed definite or probable scaffold thrombosis (one definite acute, one definite sub-acute, and one probable late), as compared with no patients in the metallic stent group. There were 17 cases of MACE (5%) in the BVS group, as compared with five (3%) events in the DES group. The most common adverse events were: myocardial infarction (15 cases—4%, vs two cases—1%, respectively) and clinically indicated target-lesion revascularization (four cases—1%, vs three cases—2%, respectively). In conclusion the authors stated that BVS showed similar one-year clinical outcome to the everolimus-eluting metallic stent.

Conversely, heterogeneous outcomes have been reported from registries enrolling more complex population as compared with ABSORB II Study. The results of the GHOST registry were published recently.[37] A total of 1189 patients underwent percutaneous coronary intervention with the implantation of one or more BVS in 10 high-volume European centers. In the registry patients with acute coronary syndromes, calcified lesions, chronic total occlusions, and complex bifurcation lesions were included. The primary outcome was target lesion failure (TLF), defined as the combination of cardiac death, target vessel myocardial infarction, or clinically driven target lesion revascularization. A total of 1731 BVS were implanted. Technical success was achieved in 99.7% of cases. TLF occurred in 67, out of 1189 patients, at a median of 109 (interquartile range 8–227) days after implantation. The cumulative incidence of TLF was 2.2% at 30 days and 4.4% at 6 months. The annualized rate of TLF was 10.1%. At 6 months, the rate of cardiac death was 1.0%, target vessel myocardial infarction 2.0%, TLR 2.5%, and target vessel revascularization 4.0%. The cumulative incidence of definite/probable scaffold thrombosis was 1.5% at 30 days and 2.1% at six months, with 16 of 23 cases occurring within 30 days after index PCI. Real-world outcomes of BVS in GHOST registry showed acceptable rates of TLF at six months, although the rates of early and midterm scaffold thrombosis, mostly clustered within 30 days, were not negligible. It should be noted that follow-up data were available only to 76% of patients. Complete one-year outcomes of Ghost-EU patients were presented at TCT 2015 meeting.[38] The cumulative incidence of TLF was 5.2%, TLR 4.1%, target vessel MI 2.4% and scaffold thrombosis 2.0%.

Absorb BVS has been also evaluated in the setting of acute coronary syndrome (ACS). The BVS STEMI first study was a prospective, single-arm, single-centre study, reporting data following BVS implantation in 49 STEMI patients.[39] The procedural success was 97.9%, while no patients had angiographically-visible residual thrombus at the end of the procedure. OCT analysis (performed in 31 patients) showed that mean percentage of malapposed struts per patient was 2.80 ± 3.90%. At 30-day follow-up, target-lesion failure rate was 0%, and no death or scaffold thrombosis were reported. Other interesting results in the STEMI subset come from the Prague-19 multicenter study, where 40 patients undergoing primary PCI were evaluated. The 6-month survival free from death, MI or TVR was 95%, while an OCT substudy (performed on 21 patients) demonstrated that only 1.1% of scaffold struts were malapposed.[40] In TROFI II study the arterial healing response was compared in randomized fashion, between the absorb and the metallic everolimus-eluting stent (EES) in patients with STEMI.[41] At 6 months, OCT-measured healing score (the presence of uncovered and/or malapposed stent struts and intraluminal filling defects) was lower in the Absorb arm when compared with EES arm [1.74 (2.39) vs 2.80 (4.44); difference (90% CI) -1.06 (-1.96, -0.16); P, noninferiority <0.001]. Also, device-oriented composite endpoint was also comparably low between groups (1.1% absorb vs 0% EES). One case of definite subacute stent thrombosis occurred in the absorb arm (1.1% vs 0% EES; P = ns). Gori et al. published the results of a series of 133 ACS patients with thrombotic lesions stented with BVS.[42] After one year of observation there were 4 deaths; 3 definite and 1 probable in-BVS thromboses (all in the first 6 months).

Recently three large important randomized studies have been published on BVS: ABSORB III, ABSORB Japan and ABSORB China.[43-45] ABSORB III was a large multicenter randomized trial, with 2008 patients with stable or unstable angina and up to two *de novo* lesions, with a head-to-head comparison of the Absorb BVS (1322 patients) against its metallic counterpart Xience (686 patients).[43] TLF, a primary end point of the study, was similar in both groups and occurred in 7.8% of patients who received resorbable scaffold compared with 6.1% of patients who received the conventional stent (p = 0.007 for noninferiority). Device thrombosis occurred in 1.5% of the Absorb-treated patients and 0.7% in the Xience patients, with not statistically significant difference. Absorb China, regulatory approval study enrolled 480 patients with one or two *de novo* native coronary artery lesions, randomized to either the Absorb BVS (241 patients) or Xience (239 patients). The primary end point of the study was angiographic in-segment late lumen loss at 1 year.[44] The difference was not significant (0.19 mm among Absorb patients and 0.13 mm for those treated with Xience). Of note, in-device mean lumen diameter, percent diameter stenosis, and late loss were all significantly worse with the Absorb stent. Clinically, 1-year rates of TLF (cardiac death, target vessel MI, or ischemia-driven TLR) were similar in both Absorb and Xience groups: 3.4% vs 4.2%, (p = 0.62), as well as definite/probable stent thrombosis (0.4% vs 0.0%, respectively; p = 1.00). In ABSORB Japan noninferiority, single-blind, multicenter, randomized trial patients with one or two *de novo* lesions were randomized at 38 Japanese sites in a 2:1 ratio to Absorb BVS (266 patients) vs Xience (134 patients).[45] Similarly to ABSORB III study, the primary endpoint was target lesion failure (a composite of cardiac death, target vessel myocardial infarction, or ischemia-driven target lesion revascularization) at one year. TLF at 12 months was 4.2% with BVSs and 3.8% with Xience (p noninferiority < 0.0001). Definite/probable device thrombosis occurred in both groups in 1.5%, whereas TLR was 1.1% with BVS and 1.5% Xience. Recently, a large propensity-matched all-comers population results were published to compare BVS with EES in the real-world setting.[46] The analysis of 905 matched pairs of patients treated with ABSORB BVS in the GHOST-EU registry and those treated with XIENCE EES from the XIENCE V USA registry revealed a similar 1-year clinical outcome. The incidence of device-oriented composite endpoint at 1 year was 5.8% versus 7.6%; p = 0.12, for BVS and EES respectively, with similar ischemia-driven TLR (4.6% vs 3.5%; p = 0.22). Also there were no significant difference in definite or probable device thrombosis between Absorb and Xience stent (1.8% vs 1.1% respectively; p = 0.23). Interestingly, cardiac death was significantly less likely to occur in the BVS group (0.7% vs 1.9%; p = 0.03), with a trend toward a reduction in myocardial infarction (2.4% vs 4.0%; p = 0.07).

ABSORB BIORESORBABLE VASCULAR SCAFFOLD IMPLANTATION TECHNIQUE

The polymeric nature of the scaffold caries physical limitations that should be taken into account before deployment. Due to the strict dilatation limits over-expansion can lead to strut fracture or disruption of the scaffold inside the vessel. Careful vessel sizing before BVS implantation is crucial for procedural success. As a general rule, BVS should not be implanted into lesions that cannot be adequately prepared with balloon inflations, particularly when the balloon used for predilatation cannot be fully expanded or when the result of preparation is unsatisfactory. The deployment should proceed gradually, pressurizing the delivery system in 2 ATM. increments, every 5 seconds until complete expansion of the scaffold. Upon device deployment, target pressure should be maintained for at least 30 seconds. Postdilatation with larger balloons is possible, as long as overexpansion will be not greater than 0.5 mm, as compared with scaffold nominal diameter. Upon deployment, one should aim to obtain <10% residual stenosis, full scaffold expansion and optimal strut apposition. Postdilatation with a high-pressure, non-compliant balloon is strongly recommended unless intracoronary imaging confirms full device expansion and apposition. The proper technique of implantation allows to avoid the possible complications including acute and subacute stent thrombosis.[47]

SPECIAL LESION SUBSETS

Although majority of studies on BVS enrolled patients with relatively simple lesions it seems that some advantages should be expected also in more complex anatomy. Main branch stenting in bifurcation lesion will prevent prolonged side branch jailing if BVS is used. In ostial and aorto-ostial lesions some overhang of a scaffold will not produce permanent flow turbulence, nor will it cause any problem with future access to the vessel. Nevertheless, placement of BVS in ostial lesions should be performed with special caution, since some studies found that this subset of lesions may be especially prone to MACE.[48] In-stent restenosis also may become a potential indication for the use of scaffolds. Although vessel vasomotion will not be restored BVS will provide longer, and more potent drug delivery as compared to drug-eluting balloons. Unlike DES, complete resorption of a scaffold will prevent long-term multiple metallic strut layering in a vessel lumen. Severely calcified vessel will not benefit from scaffold resorption, because positive effect of vasomotion will not appear anyway. Nevertheless, accurate lesion preparation, with optimal predilatation or the use of additional devices, like cutting or scoring balloons or even rotational atherectomy will make scaffold delivery and implantation possible in majority of cases. Even such vessels may benefit from struts' disappearance by reduction of the risk of late stent thrombosis and possible late lumen gain.

When treatment of bifurcation lesions is planned with BVS, the provisional stenting technique seems to be a logical approach. However, BVS is a fragile device, thus the proximal optimization technique, side branch (SB) fenestration, and kissing balloon inflation should be performed with caution. The bench tests showed that crossing a struts of the scaffold with 2.5 mm balloon at a pressure of 8 ATM can at most lead to a rupture of single struts, usually connectors (Fig. 20.3A).[49,50] Typical kissing, due to the size of two balloons filled with high pressure can damage the BVS (Fig. 20.3B). In cases were side branch stenting is required T or TAP techniques may

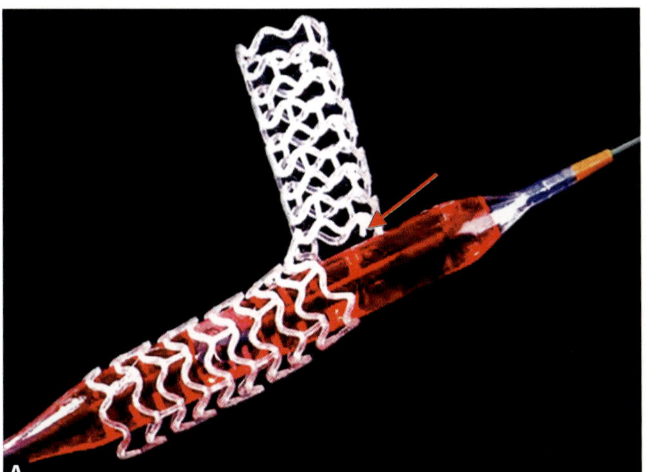

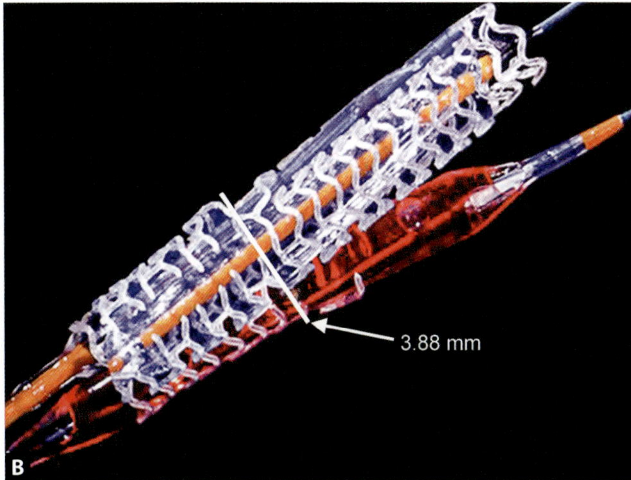

Figs 20.3A and B The bench tests of Absorb BVS. (A) Single fracture of a connector of a 3.0 × 18 mm scaffold after strut crossing with 2.5 mm balloon, at a pressure of 8 AT; (B) Major rupture of a 3.0 × 18 mm scaffold after kissing balloon postdilatation with 3.0 and 2.5 non-compliant balloon inflated up to 10 ATM

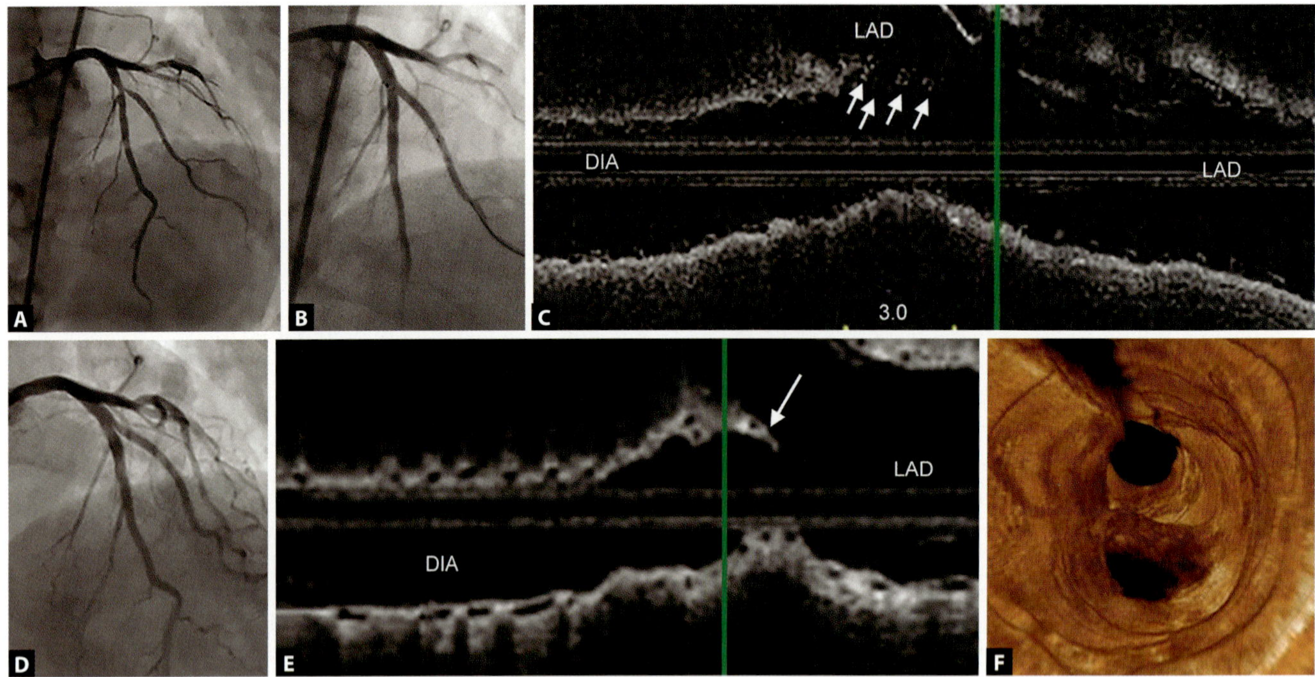

Figs 20.4A to F Bifurcation lesion of left anterior descending (LAD) and diagonal (DIA) coronary artery. (A) Baseline image; (B) After stenting with two BVS (3.0 × 18 mm and 2.8 × 18 mm) with TAP technique; (C) Longitudinal OCT OFDI image showing 3 mm long neocarina composed of two layers of struts (arrows); (D) Angiographic follow-up after 18 months; (E) OCT OFDI image showing the neocarina covered with neointima (arrow); (F) 3D OCT reconstruction of bifurcation at 18 month

be used (Figs 20.4A to F). Due to its dilatation limits main vessel scaffolds should be sized rather according to proximal than distal reference diameter. Low pressure implantation is then recommended, followed by proximal optimization technique (POT) with adequately sized short balloon. Final kissing balloon postdilatation should be performed with minimal protrusion of the side branch balloon (mini-kissing, or snuggle technique).

Chronic total occlusion (CTO) constitute a special subset of coronary lesions, with the lowest PCI success rate irrespective of the approach. Long and diffuse disease, often with extensive amount of calcium, as well as difficulty in the assessment of distal vessel diameter make the use of BVS particularly challenging. However, adequate lesion preparation after wire crossing, nitroglicerin injection to dilate the vessel lumen and utilization of intravascular imaging make the use of BVS possible. Two papers have been recently published on BVS implantation in CTO lesions. Vaquerizo et al. presented a series of 35 patients, with multislice computed tomography (MSCT) performed at baseline and at six to eight months after procedure.[51] At 6-month follow-up, no major adverse events were observed but MSCT identified two cases of scaffold reocclusion. In another paper,[52] 40 consecutive patients (78% male, mean age 59.9 ± 8.3, diabetics 30%) with CTO treated with BVS were enrolled. Patients with reference vessel diameter above 4 mm, metallic stents, excessive calcium and tortuosity were excluded. Mean J-CTO score was 1.6. Antegrade technique was used in 38 patients (85%). A total of 63 BVS were implanted with the average number of 1.6 per patient, and the scaffold length of 42.4 mm ± 21.5. High pressure postdilatation was performed in 38 patients. Procedural success was achieved in all patients with no device-related complications. At follow-up (median time 434 days), there were no deaths, one patient experienced subacute and late scaffold thrombosis (ST), another one developed symptomatic in-scaffold focal restenosis treated with repeat PCI. At control angiography, performed at the median time of 264 days in 23 patients (58%), no more restenosis or vessel reocclusion was found.

DUAL ANTIPLATELET THERAPY AFTER BIORESORBABLE VASCULAR SCAFFOLD IMPLANTATION

Currently there are no specific recommendations regarding dual antiplatelet therapy after PCI with bioresorbable scaffolds. Given the early data showing slightly increased

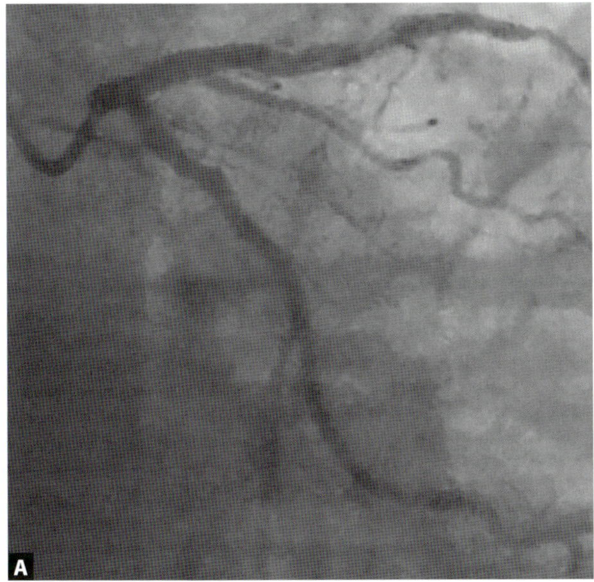

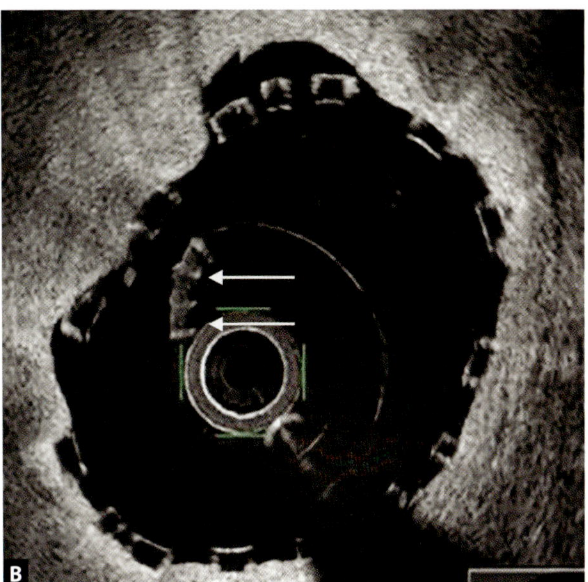

Figs 20.5A and B Left main stenting with a 3.5 x 15 mm scaffold postdilated with 4.0 noncompliant balloon up to 24 ATM. (A) Angiographic image; (B) OCT OFDI image showing struts fractures. Floating struts in the lumen of the vessel (arrows)

risk of scaffold thrombosis, especially within the first weeks after implantation, more potent antiplatelet drugs should be considered, especially after complex procedures with or suboptimal PCI result. We recommend ticagrelor or prasugrel rather than clopidogrel, particularly within the first 4–12 weeks postprocedure.[47]

DEVICE LIMITATIONS

As with any novel technology scaffolds have several limitation, many of them are not negligible. The main limitations of BVS are strut's thickness and its potential of fracture. Thick struts make the whole device bulky (crossing profile >1 mm) hampering its passage across calcified bends or not optimally prepared lesions. Due to the same reason using of 5F catheters, or support "mother-and-child" catheters is difficult. Additionally thick-strut, as compared to thin-strut stents are more thrombogenic and less forgiving in relation to suboptimal deployment (malapposition, underexpantion etc.).[53] Polymeric scaffold have restricted expansion limits. Postdilatation with a balloon diameter more than 0.5 mm bigger than the scaffold diameter may lead to strut fracture with subsequent loss of radial strength and possible vessel collapse. Ruptured strut prolapse into the lumen of the vessel may disturb the flow, which increase the risk of thrombosis (Figs 20.5A and B). The other restrictions are: limited sizes and diameters currently available, the need of slow and prolong dilatations (possible ischemia), lack of visibility on X-ray imaging, and probably the need for more potent dual antiplatelet therapy, at least until specific data are available.

FUTURE DIRECTIONS

The idea of "leaving nothing behind" after percutaneous coronary intervention is a very exiting concept in modern interventional cardiology. New generation metallic DES perform extremely well, being very effective and safe. However, after doing their great job, DES become redundant or even unwanted, as unwanted is a plaster cast on a leg after the bone is healed. If current technology meets the challenge, major limitations will be overcome, and scaffolds prove to be at least as safe and effective as current DES, than in a long run we will be facing a real breakthrough not only in cardiology, but generally in medicine.

REFERENCES

1. Lüscher TF, Steffel J, Eberli FR, Joner M, Nakazawa G, et al. Virmani R. Drug-eluting stent and coronary thrombosis. Biological mechanisms and clinical implications. Circulation. 2007;115:1051-8.
2. Nakazawa G, Otsuka F, Nakano M, Vorpahl M, Yazdani SK, Ladich E, Kolodgie FD, Finn AV, Virmani R. The pathology of neoatherosclerosis in human coronary implants bare-metal and drug-eluting stents. J Am Coll Cardiol. 2011;57: 1314-22.
3. Serruys PW, Garcia-Garcia HM, Onuma Y. From metallic cages to transient bioresorbable scaffolds: change in paradigm of coronary revascularization in the upcoming decade. Eur Heart J. 2012;33:16b 25b.

4. Strandberg E, Zeltinger J, Schulz DG, et al. Late positive remodeling and late lumen gain contribute to vascular restoration by a non-drug eluting bioresorbable scaffold: a four-year intravascular ultrasound study in normal porcine coronary arteries. Circ Cardiovasc Interv. 2012;5:39-46.
5. Onuma Y, Serruys PW. Bioresorbable scaffold: the advent of a new era in percutaneous coronary and peripheral revascularization. Circulation. 2011;123:779-97.
6. Tamai H, Igaki K, Kyo E, et al. Initial and 6-month results of biodegradable poly-l-lactic acid coronary stents in humans. Circulation. 2000;102:399-404.
7. Zhang Y, Bourantas CV, Farooq V, Muramatsu T, Diletti R, Onuma Y, et al. Bioresorbable scaffolds in the treatment of coronary artery disease. Med Devices. 2013;12:37-48.
8. Nishio S, Kosuga K, Igaki K, et al. Long-term (10 years) clinical outcomes of first-in-human biodegradable poly-l-lactic acid coronary stents: Igaki-Tamai stents. Circulation. 2012;125: 2343-53.
9. Otsuka F, Pacheco E, Perkins LE, Lane JP, Wang Q, Kamberi M, Frie M, Wang J, Sakakura K, Yahagi K, Ladich E, Rapoza RJ, et al. Long-term safety of an everolimus-eluting bioresorbable vascular scaffold and the cobalt-chromium XIENCE V stent in a porcine coronary artery model. Circ Cardiovasc Interv. 2014;7:330-42.
10. Yan J, Bhat VD. Elixir Medical's bioresorbable drug eluting stent (BDES) programme: an overview. EuroIntervention. 2009;5 Suppl. F: F80–F82.
11. Verheye S, Ormiston JA, Stewart J, Webster M, Sanidas E, Costa R, Costa JR Jr, Chamie D, Abizaid AS, Pinto I, Morrison L, Toyloy S, Bhat V, Yan J, Abizaid A. A next-generation bioresorbable coronary scaffold system: from bench to first clinical evaluation: 6- and 12-month clinical and multimodality imaging results. JACC Cardiovasc Interv. 2014;7:89-99.
12. Kochman J, Koltowski L, Abizaid A, et al. First European implantation of the new, thin-strut, sirolimus-eluting bioresorbable scaffold. Kardiol Pol. 2015;73:224.
13. Costa JR. FantomTM sirolimus eluting biresorbable scaffold. Transcatheter Cardiovascular Therapeutics, San Francisco, California, USA; 2015.
14. Jabara R, Chronos N, Robinson K. Novel bioabsorbable salicylate-based polymer as a drug-eluting stent coating. Catheter Cardiovasc Interv. 2008;72:186-94.
15. Jabara R, et al. Novel fully bioabsorbable salicylate-based sirolimus-eluting stent. EuroIntervention. 2009;5 Suppl. F: F58-64.
16. Jabara R. Poly-anhydride based on salicylic acid and adipic acid anhydride. EuroPCR; Barcelona, Spain; 2009.
17. Jabara R. Bio-mechanical properties and ABC of bioresorption of adipic acid. Presented at: PCR Focus Group on Bioresorbable Vascular Scaffolds. Rotterdam, The Netherlands; 2012.
18. Campos CM, et al. Bioresorbable drug-eluting magnesium-alloy scaffold for treatment of coronary artery disease. Int J Mol Sci. 2013;14:24492-500.
19. Anstall HB, Hayward GH, Huntsman RG, et al. The effect of magnesium on blood coagulation in human subjects. Lancet. 1959;1:814-5.
20. Rukshin V, Shah PK, Cercek B, Finkelstein A, Tsang V, Kaul S. Comparative antithrombotic effects of magnesium sulfate and the platelet glycoprotein IIb/IIIa inhibitors tirofiban and eptifibatide in a canine model of stent thrombosis. Circulation. 2002;105:1970-5.
21. Waksman, R, Pakala R, Kuchulakanti PK, Baffour R, Hellinga D, Seabron R, Tio FO, Wittchow E, Hartwig S, Harder C, et al. Safety and efficacy of bioabsorbable magnesium alloy stents in porcine coronary arteries. Catheter. Cardiovasc Interv. 2006;68:607-17; Discussion 618-09.
22. Bose, D, Eggebrecht, H, Haude M, et al. First absorbable metal stent implantation in human coronary arteries. Am Heart Hosp J. 2006;4: 128-30.
23. Bose D, Eggebrecht H, Erbel R. Absorbable metal stent in human coronary arteries: Imaging with intravascular ultrasound. Heart. 2006;92:892.
24. Haude M. Safety and clinical performance of the drug eluting absorbable metal scaffold in the treatment of subjects with de novo lesions in native coronary arteries-BIOSOLVE-II. Transcatheter Cardiovascular Therapeutics, San Francisco, California, USA; 2015.
25. Erbel R, Di Mario C, Bartunek J, Bonnier J, de Bruyne B, Eberli FR, Erne P, Haude M, Heublein B, Horrigan M, Ilsley C, Böse D, Koolen J, Lüscher TF, Weissman N, et al. PROGRESS-AMS (Clinical Performance and Angiographic Results of Coronary Stenting with Absorbable Metal Stents) Investigators. Temporary scaffolding of coronary arteries with bioabsorbable magnesium stents: A prospective, non-randomised multicentre trial. Lancet. 2007;369(9576):1869-75.
26. Waksman R, Erbel R, Di Mario C, Bartunek J, de Bruyne B, Eberli FR, Erne P, Haude M, Horrigan M, Ilsley C, Böse D, Bonnier H, Koolen J, Lüscher TF, Weissman NJ. PROGRESS-AMS (Clinical Performance Angiographic Results of Coronary Stenting with Absorbable Metal Stents) Investigators. Early- and long-term intravascular ultrasound and angiographic findings after bioabsorbable magnesium stent implantation in human coronary arteries. JACC Cardiovasc Interv. 2009;2:312-20.
27. Haude M, Erbel R, Erne P, Verheye S, Degen H, Böse D, Vermeersch P, Wijnbergen I, Weissman N, Prati F, Waksman R, Koolen J. Safety and performance of the drug-eluting absorbable metal scaffold (DREAMS) in patients with de novo coronary lesions: 12 month results of the prospective, multicentre, first-in-man BIOSOLVE-I trial. Lancet. 2013;381:836-44.
28. Ormiston JA, Serruys PW, Regar E, Dudek D, Thuesen L, Webster MW, Onuma Y, Garcia-Garcia HM, McGreevy R, et al. A bioabsorbable everolimus-eluting coronary stent system for patients with single de-novo coronary artery lesions (ABSORB): a prospective open-label trial. Lancet. 2008;371:899-907.
29. Serruys PW, Ormiston JA, Onuma Y, Regar E, Gonzalo N, Garcia-Garcia HM, Nieman K, Bruining N, Dorange C, Miquel-Hébert K, Veldhof S, Webster M, et al. A bioabsorbable everolimus-eluting coronary stent system (ABSORB): 2-year outcomes and results from multiple imaging methods. Lancet. 2009;373:897-910.
30. Onuma Y, Dudek D, Thuesen L, Webster M, Nieman K, Garcia-Garcia HM, et al. Five-year clinical and functional multislice computed tomography angiographic results after coronary implantation of the fully resorbable polymeric everolimus-eluting scaffold in patients with de novo coronary artery disease: the ABSORB cohort A trial. JACC Cardiovasc Interv. 2013;6: 999-1009.
31. Okamura T, Garg S, Gutiérrez-Chico JL, Shin ES, Onuma Y, García-García HM, Rapoza RJ, Sudhir K, Regar E, et al.

In vivo evaluation of stent strut distribution patterns in the bioabsorbable everolimus-eluting device: an OCT ad hoc analysis of the revision 1.0 and revision 1.1 stent design in the ABSORB clinical trial. EuroIntervention. 2010;5:932-8.
32. Diletti R, Farooq V, Girasis C, Bourantas C, Onuma Y, Heo JH, Gogas BD, van Geuns RJ, Regar E, de Bruyne B, Dudek D, Thuesen L, Chevalier B, McClean D, Windecker S, Whitbourn RJ, Smits P, Koolen J, Meredith I, Li X, Miquel-Hebert K, Veldhof S, Garcia-Garcia HM, Ormiston JA, et al. Clinical and intravascular imaging outcomes at 1 and 2 years after implantation of absorb everolimus eluting bioresorbable vascular scaffolds in small vessels. Late lumen enlargement: does bioresorption matter with small vessel size? Insight from the ABSORB cohort B trial. Heart. 2013;99:98-105.
33. Serruys PW, Onuma Y, Garcia-Garcia HM, Muramatsu T, van Geuns RJ, de Bruyne B, Dudek D, Thuesen L, Smits PC, Chevalier B, McClean D, Koolen J, Windecker S, Whitbourn R, Meredith I, Dorange C, Veldhof S, Hebert KM, et al. Dynamics of vessel wall changes following the implantation of the Absorb everolimus-eluting bioresorbable vascular scaffold: a multi-imaging modality study at 6, 12, 24 and 36 months. EuroIntervention. 201;9:1271-84.
34. Ishibashi Y, Onuma Y, Muramatsu T, Nakatani S, Iqbal J, Garcia-Garcia HM, Bartorelli AL, Whitbourn R, Abizaid A, et al. ABSORB EXTEND Investigators. Lessons learned from acute and late scaffold failures in the ABSORB EXTEND trial. EuroIntervention. 2014;10:449-57.
35. Abizaid A, Costa JR Jr, Bartorelli AL, Whitbourn R, van Geuns RJ, Chevalier B, Patel T, Seth A, Stuteville M, Dorange C, Cheong WF, Sudhir K, et al. The ABSORB EXTEND study: preliminary report of the twelve-month clinical outcomes in the first 512 patients enrolled. EuroIntervention. 2015;10:1396-401.
36. Serruys PW, Chevalier B, Dudek D, Cequier A, Carrié D, Iniguez A, Dominici M, van der Schaaf RJ, Haude M, Wasungu L, Veldhof S, Peng L, Staehr P, Grundeken MJ, Ishibashi Y, et al. A bioresorbable everolimus-eluting scaffold versus a metallic everolimus-eluting stent for ischaemic heart disease caused by de-novo native coronary artery lesions (ABSORB II): an interim 1-year analysis of clinical and procedural secondary outcomes from a randomised controlled trial. Lancet. 2015;385:43-54.
37. Capodanno D, Gori T, Nef H, Latib A, Mehilli J, Lesiak M, Caramanno G, Naber C, Di Mario C, Colombo A, Capranzano P, Wiebe J, Araszkiewicz A, Geraci S, Pyxaras S, Mattesini A, Naganuma T, Münzel T, et al. Percutaneous coronary intervention with everolimus-eluting bioresorbable vascular scaffolds in routine clinical practice: early and midterm outcomes from the European multicentre GHOST-EU registry. EuroIntervention. 2015;10:1144-53.
38. Capranzano P. on behalf of the GHOST-EU Investigators. The use of fully bioresorbable vascular scaffolds in real-world setting: the latest evidence. Transcatheter Cardiovascular Therapeutics, San Francisco, California, USA, 2015.
39. Diletti R, et al. Everolimus-eluting bioresorbable vascular scaffolds for treatment of patients presenting with ST-segment elevation myocardial infarction: BVS STEMI first study. Eur Heart J. 2014;35:777-86.
40. Kocka V, Malý M, Toušek P, Buděšínský T, Lisa L, Prodanov P, et al. Bioresorbable vascular scaffolds in acute ST-segment elevation myocardial infarction: a prospective multicentre study 'Prague 19'. Eur Heart J. 2014;35:787-94.
41. Sabaté M, Windecker S, Iñiguez A, Okkels-Jensen L, Cequier A, Brugaletta S, Hofma SH, Räber L, Christiansen EH, Suttorp M, Pilgrim T, Anne van Es G, Sotomi Y0, García-García HM, Onuma Y, et al. Everolimus-eluting bioresorbable stent vs. durable polymer everolimus-eluting metallic stent in patients with ST-segment elevation myocardial infarction: results of the randomized ABSORB ST-segment elevation myocardial infarction-TROFI II trial. Eur Heart J. 2016;37:229-40.
42. Gori T, Schulz E, Hink U, Kress M, Weiers N, Weissner M, Jabs A, Wenzel P, Capodanno D, et al. Clinical, Angiographic, Functional, and Imaging Outcomes 12 Months After Implantation of Drug-Eluting Bioresorbable Vascular Scaffolds in Acute Coronary Syndromes. JACC Cardiovasc Interv. 2015;8:770-7.
43. Ellis SG, Kereiakes DJ, Metzger DC, Caputo RP, Rizik DG, Teirstein PS, Litt MR, Kini A, Kabour A, Marx SO, Popma JJ, McGreevy R, Zhang Z, Simonton C, Stone GW. ABSORB III Investigators. Everolimus-Eluting Bioresorbable Scaffolds for Coronary Artery Disease. N Engl J Med. 2015;373:1905-15.
44. Gao R, Yang Y, Han Y, Huo Y, Chen J, Yu B, Su X, Li L, Kuo HC, Ying SW, Cheong WF, Zhang Y, Su X, Xu B, Popma JJ, et al. ABSORB China Investigators. Bioresorbable Vascular Scaffolds Versus Metallic Stents in Patients With Coronary Artery Disease: ABSORB China Trial. J Am Coll Cardiol. 2015;66:2298-309.
45. Kimura T, Kozuma K, Tanabe K, Nakamura S, Yamane M, Muramatsu T, Saito S, Yajima J, Hagiwara N, Mitsudo K, Popma JJ, Serruys PW, Onuma Y, Ying S, Cao S, Staehr P, Cheong WF, Kusano H, et al. ABSORB Japan Investigators. A randomized trial evaluating everolimus-eluting Absorb bioresorbable scaffolds vs. everolimus-eluting metallic stents in patients with coronary artery disease: ABSORB Japan. Eur Heart J. 2015;36:3332-42.
46. 1-Year Outcomes of Everolimus-Eluting Bioresorbable Scaffolds Versus Everolimus-Eluting Stents: A Propensity-Matched Comparison of the GHOST-EU and XIENCE V USA Registries. JACC: Cardiovascular Interventions. Available online 6 January 2016. doi:10.1016/j.jcin.2015.10.042
47. Tamburino C, Latib A, van Geuns RJ, Sabate M, Mehilli J, Gori T, Achenbach S, Alvarez MP, Nef H, Lesiak M, Di Mario C, Colombo A, Naber CK, Caramanno G, Capranzano P, Brugaletta S, Geraci S, Araszkiewicz A, Mattesini A, Pyxaras SA, Rzeszutko L, Depukat R, Diletti R, Boone E, et al. Contemporary practice and technical aspects in coronary intervention with bioresorbable scaffolds: a European perspective. EuroIntervention. 2015;11:45-52.
48. Gori T, Wiebe J, Capodanno D, Latib A, Lesiak M, Pyxaras S, Mehilli J, Caramanno G, Di Mario C, Brugaletta S, Weber J, Capranzano P, Sabaté M, Mattesini A, Geraci S, Naber C, Araszkiewicz A, Colombo A, Tamburino C, Nef H, Münzel T. Early and midterm outcomes of bioresorbable vascular scaffolds for ostial coronary lesions: insights from the GHOST-EU registry. EuroIntervention. 2015;11(5). pii: 20150614-01. doi: 10.4244/EIJY15M09_10. [Epub ahead of print]
49. Ormiston JA, Webber B, Ubod B, et al. Absorb everolimus-eluting bioresorbable scaffolds in coronary bifurcations: a bench

study of deployment, side branch dilatation and post-dilatation strategies. EuroIntervention. 2015;10:1169-77.

50. Lesiak M. BVS in bifurcations—techniques, acute and long-term outcomes. Xth meeting of European Bifurcation Club, Bordeaux; 2014.
51. Vaquerizo B, Barros A, Pujadas S, Bajo E, Estrada D, Miranda-Guardiola F, Rigla J, Jiménez M, Cinca J, et al. Bioresorbable everolimus-eluting vascular scaffold for the treatment of chronic total occlusions: CTO-ABSORB pilot study. EuroIntervention. 2015;11:555-63.
52. Lesiak M, Łanocha M, Araszkiewicz A, Siniawski A, Grygier M, Pyda M, Olasińska-Wiśniewska A, Iwanczyk S, Skorupski W, Mitkowski P, Lesiak MB, Grajek S. Percutaneous coronary intervention for chronic total coronary artery occlusion with the implantation of bioresorbable everolimus-eluting scaffolds. Poznan CTO-Absorb Pilot Registry. Eurointervention 2016, accepted.
53. Kolandaivelu K, Swaminathan R, Gibson WJ, Kolachalama VB, Nguyen-Ehrenreich KL, Giddings VL, Coleman L, Wong GK, Edelman ER. Stent Thrombogenicity Early in High-Risk Interventional Settings Is Driven by Stent Design and Deployment and Protected by Polymer-Drug Coatings. Circulation. 2011;123(13):1400-9.

CHAPTER

21

Hybrid Coronary Revascularization

Piroze M Davierwala, Omür Akhavuz

INTRODUCTION

Coronary artery bypass grafting (CABG) is considered to be the "gold standard" in patients with multivessel and/or left main coronary artery disease (CAD).[1] CABG has been proven to be superior to both, percutaneous coronary intervention (PCI) and optimal medical therapy (OMT), with regard to long-term symptom relief, major adverse cardiac or cerebrovascular events and survival benefit.[1-4] However, CABG is associated with significant surgical trauma leading to a long rehabilitation period and delayed postoperative improvement in the quality of life (QoL), chiefly because of the use of cardiopulmonary bypass (CPB) and median sternotomy.[5] Hybrid coronary revascularization (HCR) procedure is an alternative approach to multivessel CAD that combines the benefits of cardiac surgery and cardiology. HCR can be defined as minimally invasive left internal thoracic artery to left anterior descending coronary artery bypass grafting (minimally invasive direct coronary artery bypass [MIDCAB] or robotic LITA-LAD) using a sternal-sparing incision without aortic manipulation and CPB combined with PCI of the non-LAD territories.[6,7]

Patients undergoing HCR gain from the survival benefit of the LITA to LAD bypass, while the minimally invasive approach lowers the morbidity by avoiding median sternotomy, rib retraction, aortic manipulation, and cardiopulmonary bypass, and reduces the occurrence of postoperative complications associated with conventional CABG, such as atrial fibrillation, bleeding, transfusion, and infection.[8-14] The aim of the HCR procedure is to achieve complete coronary revascularization with outcomes equivalent to conventional CABG, while ensuring faster patient recovery, shorter hospital stays, and earlier return to work due to lower morbidity and mortality rates.[5]

In 1996, Angelini and colleagues reported the first HCR procedure, and several patient series using HCR have been published since then.[4] These series supported HCR as a feasible option for the treatment of selected patients with multivessel CAD involving the left main coronary artery. Moreover, in 2005, Indolfi and colleagues reported lower rates of restenosis and better clinical outcomes with the introduction of drug-eluting stents (DESs), making HCR a more sustainable and feasible option.[15,16]

Nevertheless, HCR has not been established in all hospitals because of practical and logistical reasons. For successful implementation of HCR procedures in hospitals, not only is a close cooperation between surgeons and interventional cardiologists necessary, but logistical issues such as sequencing and timing of the procedures, and the use of aggressive anticoagulant therapy after PCI also has to be considered.[7,13,17]

PROCEDURE STRATEGY: TIMING AND STAGING

The optimal timing and the sequence of revascularization in patients undergoing HCR is still controversial.[18] Three options are available.

Staged MIDCAB Prior to PCI

The PCI, as a separate procedure following CABG, not only allows for optimal antiplatelet therapy, but also enables imaging of the LITA-LAD graft to confirm its patency. Furthermore, PCI of high-risk targets can be attempted, if a patent LITA-LAD is demonstrated.[19] The staged procedure can be performed within a few days to weeks.[20] The main advantage of performing CABG first is reduction in bleeding complications associated with dual antiplatelet therapy that is mandatory after PCI. Contrarily, this strategy could become disadvantageous in the event of complications or suboptimal results following PCI, making conventional CABG necessary. Acetylsalicylic acid (ASS) is administered 4–6 hours following CABG after ruling out bleeding complications. A $P2Y_{12}$ inhibitor is started either the next day or prior to the PCI.

Staged PCI before MIDCAB

The PCI-first strategy is most commonly used in an emergency situation, when a non-LAD culprit lesion requires primary PCI.[21] Patients undergoing primary PCI of the non-LAD vessel for STEMI are best treated with a LITA-LAD bypass for residual LAD disease. Staged CABG is best delayed for a minimum of 6 months (preferably 12 months) in order to avoid risk of thrombosis of DES.[22,23] when $P2Y_{12}$ inhibitors are stopped prematurely. Moreover, judicious interruption of $P2Y_{12}$ inhibitors minimizes risk of bleeding during CABG. However, it may not be possible to wait such a long time in some instances. Therefore, patients with LAD lesions warranting earlier CABG should either undergo PCI of non-LAD lesions with bare-metal stents, which have higher restenosis rates, but lower risk of thrombosis following stoppage of $P2Y_{12}$ inhibitors 4–6 weeks after PCI or accepting a higher risk of perioperative bleeding if dual antiplatelet therapy is continued. The timing of discontinuation of $P2Y_{12}$ inhibitors prior to surgery depends on the type of drug used.[24]

Simultaneous PCI and MIDCAB

Today, the fields of interventional cardiology and cardiovascular surgery are converging and moving more towards minimally invasive procedures. Hybrid operating rooms (OR) is becoming a standard part of cardiovascular set-ups and offers the potential to transform delivery and management of cardiac care (Fig. 21.1). HCR procedure in a hybrid OR combines different modalities of treatment into a team approach. There are benefits to building this approach, which is entirely dependent on the personnel and resources

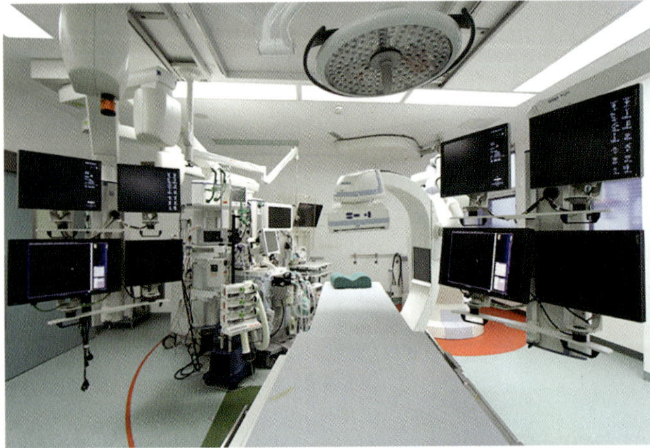

Fig. 21.1 Hybrid operating room, which includes the operating table and lights, anesthesia machine and the mobile C-arm that can be moved away from the operating table during surgery. On either side are one set of monitors each for the interventional cardiology team

available to develop and maintain such a team and facility. The hybrid OR allows for a single stage HCR procedure, which necessitates a multidisciplinary team approach involving cardiac surgeons, interventional cardiologists, anesthesiologists, nursing staff and perfusionists, who work together on the same operating table with the single goal of achieving a complete revascularization. It is accomplished by performing a MIDCAB (LITA-LAD bypass) first, immediately followed by PCI of the non-LAD vessels. It allows for immediate evaluation of the treatment by way of a completion angiogram. It increases patient convenience and reduces overall OR time and the potential risk of inter-stage morbidity and mortality. Certainly, a hybrid OR set-up is convenient but not mandatory. In hospitals where hybrid ORs are not available, it is possible to transport the patient from the surgical OR following MIDCAB to the cardiac catheterization laboratory for PCI. Intravenous heparin is utilized for anticoagulation during surgery and PCI. However, a loading dose of clopidogrel has to be administered through the nasogastric (NG) tube after PCI of non-LAD targets, which could be a potential drawback of this approach as it does increase the risk of bleeding complications. The anticoagulation guidelines for such procedures can be summarized as follows:

- ASA preprocedure
- *Intravenous heparin prior to transection of the LITA*: 100 U/kg bolus dose
- ACT to be maintained above 300 seconds during surgery and PCI
- *Clopidogrel, once LITA-LAD patency is confirmed by a check angiogram*: 600 mg through the NG tube (provided chest tube drainage is minimal)
- PCI is performed in the hybrid OR
- Heparin infusion is continued for 48 hours to maintain aPTT between 60 seconds and 80 seconds
- *ASA 6 hours postprocedure*: 500 mg per rectal or intravenously
- *Clopidogrel*: Maintenance dose 75 mg daily, started on the first postoperative day.

INDICATIONS AND CONTRAINDICATIONS FOR THE HYBRID CORONARY REVASCULARIZATION PROCEDURE

Indications

Current American and European guidelines for myocardial revascularization recommend CABG through a median sternotomy in most patients with severe multivessel CAD including the proximal LAD. They do not include hybrid procedures as yet.[25] This is chiefly due to the limited availability of outcome data and a lack of randomized trials.

Table 21.1 Suitability and contraindications for HCR procedure	
Suitability for HCR	*Contraindications to HCR*
Patient factors:	*Contraindications to MIDCAB:*
Young patients	Non-graftable LAD
Older, frail patients (>80 years)	Deep intra-myocardial LAD*
Patients with debilitating comorbidities	Inability to undergo off-pump beating heart revascularization*
Obesity	Previous surgery involving left thoracic cavity
Handicapped/disabled patients	Left subclavian artery stenosis rendering LITA use unsuitable*#
Thoracic skeletal abnormalities making sternotomy high-risk	Lack of tolerance of single lung ventilation based on FEV1 <50% of expected/1 L
Calcified/Procelain aorta	
Patient wish	
Lesion factors	*Contraindications to PCI of non-LAD lesions*
Ostial, complex or occluded LAD lesion with simple lesions of other coronary arteries	Peripheral vascular disease precluding vascular access - consider radial artery access
Distal left main disease with simple lesions of the circumflex and RCA	Vessel size <2.5 mm
Redo-revascularization for multivessel disease and LITA available for the LAD lesion	Tortuous calcified vessels precluding stent placement
	Complex disease requiring prolonged procedure time (especially single-stage HCR)
	High SYNTAX scores (>32) especially due to complex lesions involving non-LAD vessels
	Fresh thrombotic lesions
	Renal insufficiency
	Contraindication to dual antiplatelet therapy
	Other potential contraindications:
	Cardiogenic shock
	Malignant arrhythmias
	Hemodynamic instability
	Morbid obesity

Abbreviations: HCR, hybrid coronary revascularization; MIDCAB, minimally invasive direct coronary artery bypass; LAD, left anterior descending; FEV, forced expiratory volume; RCA, right coronary artery; LITA, left internal thoracic artery

*relative contraindications

#LITA use can be considered after stenting the left subclavian artery lesion

Thus, choosing a hybrid approach is usually based on an individual or heart team decision and is usually justified under the following circumstances (Table 21.1):

Multimorbid or High-risk Patients

- This is probably the most widely accepted indication for HCR and includes patients with:
  - A high risk for sternotomy such as those:
    - With skeletal anomalies like osteogeneis imperfect or severe osteoporosis
    - Who are dependent on crutches or wheel-chairs, and
    - With a history of deep sternal wound infections following a previous sternotomy
  - A reduced life expectancy such as:
    - Advanced malignancies
    - End-stage cardiomyopathy
    - Advanced liver and renal failure not amenable for transplant
  - Comorbidities that could be considered risk factors for a sternotomy and occurrence of other postoperative complications such as:
    - Diabetes
    - Severe obesity
    - Chronic obstructive pulmonary disease

- End stage peripheral vascular disease
- Porcelain aorta
- Stroke with/without paraplegia.

Primary PCI of Circumflex/RCA

Patients with acute coronary syndromes presenting with a culprit lesion in the circumflex or RCA and an additional stenosis of the LAD may undergo primary emergency PCI of the culprit lesion by the referring cardiologist. A MIDCAB procedure involving a LITA-LAD can be performed four to six weeks later. A preoperative angiogram confirming the patency of the stents should be performed prior to surgery. In the presence of an in-stent restenosis the patient can be scheduled for a conventional CABG through a median sternotomy.

Patient Preference

Some well-informed patients want to avoid a sternotomy and opt for a hybrid approach. Patients need to be informed that they might require future reinterventions including repeat target vessel revascularization or bypass surgery. Because the choice of the hybrid revascularization in these patients is not based on medical grounds, it deserves a formal discussion between the patient, interventional cardiologist and cardiac surgeon. Although HCR can be performed in most cases, there are certain situations or comorbidities when it is contraindicated, because minimally invasive coronary surgery is not possible or advisable.

Contraindications

- *Absolute contraindications:*
  - Emergency surgery with hemodynamic compromise
  - Severe pectus excavatum
  - Severe pulmonary disease.
- *Relative contraindications:*
  - Redo surgery
  - Previously operated left chest
  - Hemodynamically significant left subclavian artery stenosis
  - Hemodialysis arteriovenous fistula on the patient's left side
  - Morbid obesity
  - Severe left ventricular dysfunction.

SURGICAL TECHNIQUES

Although MIDCAB with utilization of the LITA-LAD grafting is the most common surgical procedure used for patients undergoing hybrid procedures, other options like total endoscopic coronary artery bypass grafting (TECAB) and minimally invasive coronary artery surgery (MICAS) could also be used to further reduce surgical trauma and revascularize the whole left coronary system with arterial grafts, respectively. The main aim of these procedures is to avoid a sternotomy and its associated complications, while achieving arterial revascularization of the LAD with the LITA and other target vessels with other arterial grafts if possible.

Anesthesia considerations for all the left-sided procedures are similar. Standard monitoring and temperature management techniques are applied. A 16-gauge IV catheter is inserted prior to induction of anesthesia. At least a triple lumen catheter with or without a pulmonary artery catheter is used. Defibrillator pads are positioned on the left scapula and inferior and medial to the right breast. Intubation is performed with a double lumen endotracheal tube or a single lumen endotracheal tube (ETT) and bronchial blocker to deflate the left lung. Approximately 10 cc/kg of tidal volume are used prior to and during single-lung ventilation. Tidal volume may need to be decreased as large tidal volumes can cause shifting of the mediastinum, which may cause the retractor to slip. Oxygen saturation >90% should be maintained. If the saturation begins to drop, continuous positive airway pressure of 5 cm H_2O to the deflated lung should be added. Warming blanket should be used to avoid hypothermia. Short-acting anesthetics are used to allow early extubation.

Although extracorporeal support is seldom required, it is recommended that the heart-lung machine be on standby, especially for MICAS procedures. When necessary, CPB can be established using femoro-femoral arteriovenous cannulation. The use of a cell saver is recommended, especially for MICAS procedures.

Minimally Invasive Direct Coronary Artery Bypass (MIDCAB)

This operation was initially reported in the mid-1990s and it has found a widespread application since then.[26-30] It is usually performed through a left anterolateral minithoracotomy following a 5–7 cm skin incision over the 4th or 5th intercostal spaces (ICS) in males and an inframammary incision in females. Minimal division of the pectoral muscle fibers (muscle-sparing approach) is used to decrease the likelihood of developing a lung hernia. LITA harvest is performed under direct vision with the help of a special retractor system (Fig. 21.2A). It is possible to harvest the entire length of the LITA from the subclavian vein and up to the left 5th ICS. The patient is then heparinized with 1.5 mg/kg unfractionated heparin to maintain an activated clotting time (ACT) greater than 300 seconds. A small opening in the pericardium exactly over the LAD suffices performance of the anastomosis with

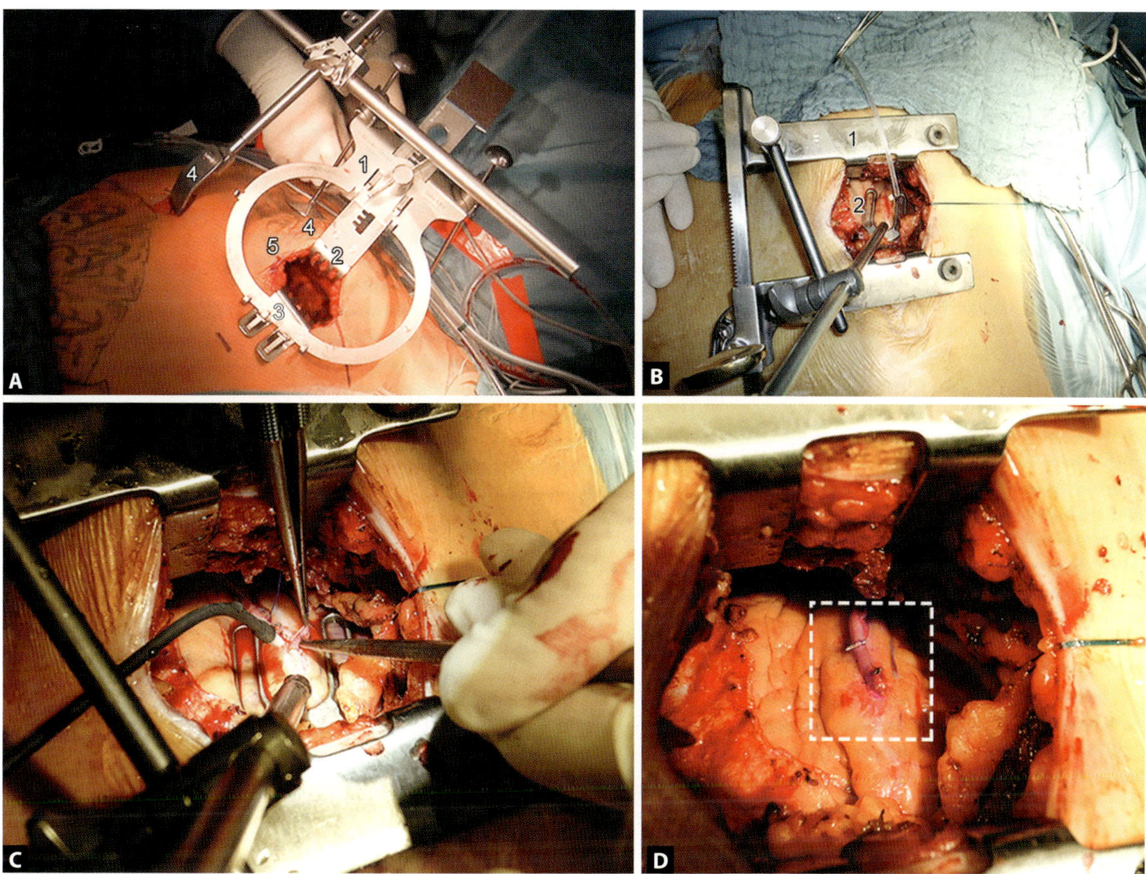

Figs 21.2A to D (A) Internal thoracic artery (ITA) harvest retractor: 1. Body 2. Upper blade to elevate the upper rib cage, which allows access to the left ITA 3. Lower blade to depress the lower rib cage, which enhances the view if the left ITA during harvest 4. Optional hook system to elevate the xiphisternum for right ITA harvest; (B) Pressure stabilizer: 1. Rib-spreader 2. Pressure stabilizer system that is attached to the rib-spreader. The 2 arms of the metallic foot, located on either side of the left anterior descending artery (LAD), stabilize a small length of the LAD for anastomosis; (C) LITA to LAD anastomosis being performed. The black plastic tube with a white tip is the mister-blower that is used to blow away the blood from the anastomotic site to improve the surgeon's visualization; (D) The completed LITA-LAD anastomosis

the LITA. Reusable pressure stabilizers are used to facilitate the anastomosis (Fig. 21.2B). Plastic shunts may be used based on surgeon preference, presence of significant retrograde coronary flow or evidence of ischemia or hemodynamic instability to maintain flow of blood to the distal LAD, while the anastomosis is being performed (Fig. 21.2C). Adequacy of the completed anastomosis (Fig. 21.2D) and graft is assessed by performing transit-time Doppler flow measurements prior to closing the patient.

Total Endoscopic Coronary Artery Bypass Grafting (TECAB)

The TECAB is an advanced form of MIDCAB developed in the late 1990s, in which CABG can be performed through three or four small holes without opening the thorax. It is an endoscopic robotic surgery performed with two robotic arms and one camera inserted into the left pleural cavity.[31] Although working through ports limits the available space to perform motions, substantially decreases the dexterity of the operator, and alters the hand-eye coordination,[32] computer-enhanced instrumentation systems have been developed to overcome these limitations. Telemanipulation enables the surgeon to work on a surgical console (input manipulator), which is away from the patient, and helps him steer the slave console (executing manipulator) located at the patient site. It consists of all the necessary electromechanical equipment needed to operate 2–3 exchangeable endoscopic instruments in addition to a high definition three-dimensional endoscopic camera. Both tactile and visual information is fed back to the master console. In this way, a virtual three-dimensional operative field is created, wherein the surgeon can manipulate steering handles with a perfect hand-eye-coordination. The introduction of telemanipulation technology to endoscopic surgery was able to address the key performance limitations of conventional endoscopic surgery, namely, reduced articulation, monocular vision, and loss of hand-eye coordination. Although the details of the operative technique are beyond the scope of this chapter, a brief summary would be appropriate. Following deflation of the left lung, the LITA harvest is performed with the help of a 30° endoscope inserted into the thorax through a camera port in the 5th ICS and two instrument arms through two 7-mm ports in the 3rd and 7th ICSs. The LITA is dissected bluntly off the chest wall moving from the lateral to the medial aspect as a pedicle, which is not detached from the chest wall until the anastomosis is finally performed in order to avoid torsion of the graft. The distal end of the graft is skeletonized to facilitate suturing of the anastomosis. The pericardiotomy is performed through a longitudinal incision in the pericardium over the probable course of the LAD. The anastomosis is performed with the help of an endostabilizer introduced under endoscopic vision by the surgeon at the operating table. After blunt dissection of the anastomotic target site, the LAD is temporarily occluded with silastic tapes placed proximal and distal to the anastomotic site. After a is performed, transection of the LITA is completed following a 5–6 mm LAD arteriotomy, and the anastomosis is performed. Graft patency can be checked by transient time Doppler flow measurements endoscopically, if a probe without a handle is available. Alternatively, intraoperative angiography has been performed using a mobile angiography unit or modern C-arm systems when TECAB operation is performed in a hybrid suite.

Minimally Invasive Coronary Artery Surgery (MICAS)

The MICAS was developed with a view to perform CABG in a less invasive manner, but at the same time with the same efficacy and safety as conventional CABG. The main goal was to accomplish complete revascularization through a closed thorax by avoiding a median sternotomy and in most cases cardiopulmonary bypass as well, which would probably reduce physical and psychological trauma experienced by patients.[33] This extended MIDCAB procedure, if you may call it so, could be used very efficiently in surgical revascularization of the left coronary system, especially with arterial grafts, while the right coronary artery could be treated with PCI, thus granting the patient the benefit of arterial grafts through a minimally invasive approach and complete revascularization through PCI of the right coronary system.

The operation is performed through a 4–6 cm incision in the left 5th ICS, more lateral than a MIDCAB incision. The pericardium is opened more extensively 1–2 cm anterior to the left phrenic nerve, extended cephalad to the level of the left atrial appendage and anterocaudally toward the diaphragmatic reflection. The LITA is harvested as done for a MIDCAB procedure. Additional conduits, preferably arterial, are harvested as well. We have recently started harvesting the right ITA through the same incision at our institution, which provides the patients with benefits of 2 ITAs (Fig. 21.2A). The proximal anastomoses could either be performed on the ascending aorta or as a Y-graft with the LITA (Fig. 21.3A), preferably prior to distal anastomoses. The positioning and stabilization of the heart for distal anastomoses is achieved with the help of specially developed positioners (Starfish NS; Medtronic, Minneapolis, Minn) and stabilizers (Octopus NS; Medtronic, Minneapolis, Minn) for minimally invasive access (Figs 21.3B and 21.3C). If exposure is poor or if the patient does not tolerate progressive mobilization of the apex despite hemodynamic support including low-dose vasopressors, femoral arterial and venous CPB (without aortic cross-clamping) is used.

Common to all left-sided procedures, a pleural chest tube is placed at the end of the procedure. Hemostasis is achieved. The left lung is reinflated, and all grafts are inspected under direct vision to rule out kinking or tension. The thoracotomy incision is closed with a single absorbable stitch around the opened ICS. Intramuscular local anesthetic like bupivacaine is administered into the ICSs above and below the site of incision. The rest of the wound is closed in layers.

Antiplatelet therapy following HCR has already been mentioned in the section on Procedure Strategy—Timing and Staging. The remaining medications such as beta-blockers, angiotensin receptor blockers and statins are the same as for conventional CABG. Use of calcium channel blockers may be recommended for patients with radial artery grafts. The patients can be discharged routinely 2–4 days, provided the postoperative course is normal. Follow-up should be performed at 6 weeks and then at 6 months, when angiography may be considered to assess patency of the grafts and stents.

RESULTS

For HCR procedures to be efficacious and safe, the results of its individual components have to be acceptable. Hence, we have first mentioned the results of minimally invasive CABG and PCI separately, followed by those of HCR.

MIDCAB

Excellent results following MIDCAB have been commonly reported with 94–98% immediate and 94% 6-month

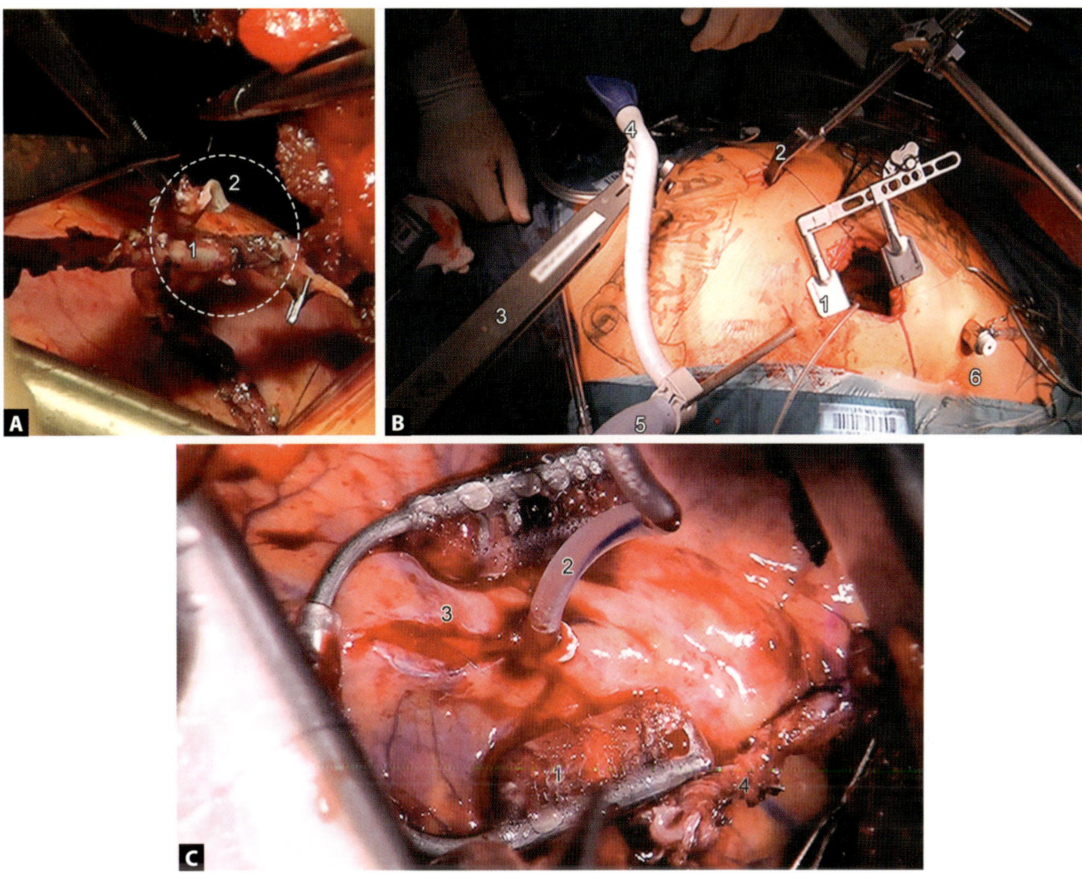

Figs 21.3A to C (A) Y-anastomosis being performed between the left and right ITAs 1. Left ITA 2. Right ITA; (B) Octopus NS stabilizer: 1. Rib-spreader 2. Optional hook system to elevate the xiphisternum for right ITA harvest 3. The metallic arm, attached to the operating table, supports the Octopus NS stabilizer 4. The mobile supporting arm of the Octopus NS stabilizer, which can be fixed by rotating the blue knob at its end 5. The Octopus NS stabilizer which consists of a long metallic arm that enters the thorax through a small port in the 7th intercostal space and the suction foot that clips onto the arm inside the thorax (6); (C) The 2 arms of the suction foot, located on either side of the left anterior descending artery (LAD), stabilize a small length of the LAD for anastomosis 1. Pods of the foot 2. Tourniquet used to occlude the LAD before opening the vessel 3. LAD

angiographic patency rates, which compare well with conventional CABG.[29,34] The mid-term results published recently by Reser et al. demonstrated an overall and MACCE-free survival of 92.4 ± 0.2% and 96.1 ± 1.7% at 24 months, respectively.[35] The 10-year results of the randomized trial comparing MIDCAB with bare metal stents for proximal LAD disease revealed no differences in the primary composite endpoint of death, MI and reintervention (47% vs 36%; p = 0.12) and hard endpoints (death and infarction) between the 2 revascularization modalities.[36] However, when a time-to-event analysis was used, the difference in event rates was statistically significant (hazard ratio [HR]: 0.65, 95% CI: 0.43 to 0.98; p = 0.04). The registry of the German Society for Thoracic and Cardiovascular Surgery reported an in-hospital mortality of <1% following MIDCAB, which compares favorably with 1.4% mortality following off-pump single-vessel and 3.6% mortality after on-pump single-vessel bypass surgery.[37] It is also lower than the 2.4% mortality reported by the STS database.[38] But a word of caution should be mentioned here. The above-mentioned results are from centers highly experienced in MIDCAB. In 2007, Holzhey and colleagues reported, that MIDCAB is technically a highly demanding procedure that should be performed by surgeons who have sufficient experience in conventional and off-pump CABG.[39] It has been shown that the complication rate of MIDCAB (viz. conversion to sternotomy, reexploration for bleeding, and reintervention on the target vessel) is significantly reduced following 100–150 MIDCAB procedures.[39] Even in the era of improved outcomes, following interventional procedures and lower in-stent restenosis rates with the use of drug-eluting stents,[40] MIDCAB, based on its very good long-term results,[41] will always remain the therapy of choice for patients with complex ostial lesions, chronic occlusions, and in-stent restenosis of the LAD.

TECAB

Initially, when TECAB was performed with CPB on an arrested heart, the reported patency rates ranged from 95% to 100% prior to discharge and 96% at the 3 month follow-up angiography.[42-45] However, the pump and ischemic times were prohibitively high. A large single center study including 100 patients also revealed that the learning curve continues beyond 100 operations, but anastomotic times of 10–30 minutes can be achieved after a long learning curve.[46] Endoscopic CABG on the beating heart is even more challenging.[42,47,48] Based on an intention-to-treat basis, the conversion rate (elective conversion to a MIDCAB procedure) in a five-center registry was 33% (37 of 117). Conversions were mostly due to calcified target vessels or the inability to locate or dissect the LAD and rarely due to other conditions such as arrhythmias or hemodynamic instability. The patency rates for completed beating-heart TECAB procedures range between 92–94%.[38] TECAB has the potential for endoscopic multivessel grafting as well.[31,49] Despite the use of advanced telemanipulator technology, its use is restricted due to the long learning curve, long operating times and poor cost-effectiveness. A more commonly applied technique is an endoscopic harvesting of both ITAs and direct coronary anastomosis via a mini-thoracotomy. This yields excellent results and very short recovery times for the patients.[49,50]

MICAS

The MICAS is not yet routinely used. However, the published series of patients show excellent results oftentimes superior to conventional or off-pump CABG.[33] Lemma and coworkers reported 137 patients operated with this technique with a 1.4% incomplete revascularization and revision for bleeding. There were no conversions to sternotomy nor were there wound complications. Only 2 deaths occurred at a mean follow-up of 26 months. A positive stress test was reported in 4.3% of patients.[51] An angiographic patency study involving 91 patients who were prospectively enrolled to undergo minimally invasive multivessel CABG revealed a 100% patency for the LIMA-LAD graft and 92% patency for all grafts.[52] It can be assumed that these operations are performed by dedicated, experienced surgeons on selected patients. Only a more widespread application of these procedures and the treatment of a broader variety of patients together with randomized studies would bring light to their significance in the future.

PCI

The efficacy of PCI in addition to medical therapy in patients with single vessel CAD has been published in several randomized controlled trials (RCT), meta-analyses, and large-scale registries.[53-56]

The Medical, Angioplasty or Surgery Study II (MASS II) trial, covering 611 patients with multivessel disease, all recruited at a single institution, is the only RCT comparing medical therapy with PCI (72% with BMS; 28% with balloon angioplasty only) and CABG. On comparison of medical therapy with PCI over a 10-year period, the rates for all-cause mortality were 31% and 24.1% ($p = 0.09$), for myocardial infarction 20.7% and 13.3% ($p < 0.01$), and for freedom from angina 43% and 59% ($p < 0.001$), respectively.[54] A meta-analysis, based on individual patient data from RCTs that were performed before the introduction of DES, reported no difference in mortality between PCI and CABG, although mortality following CABG was lower in diabetic patients and those aged 65 years or more.[55] Another meta-analysis including six randomized trials involving 6055 patients, which compared CABG with arterial grafts and PCI (balloon angioplasty, BMS and DES), reported a significant reduction in mortality (relative risk [RR] 0.73; 95% confidence interval [CI] 0.62–0.86), myocardial infarction (RR 0.58; 95% CI 0.48–0.72) and repeat revascularization (RR 0.29; 95% CI 0.21–0.41) in favor of CABG.[57] However, there was a trend towards excessive stroke rate after CABG (RR 1.36; 95% CI 0.99–1.86; $p = 0.06$). Several RCTs and meta-analyses indicate that CABG is associated with a greater risk of early stroke than PCI, which diminishes during long-term follow-up.[58,59]

HCR

The HCR could combine the beneficial effects of all the above-mentioned techniques to give the patient the best possible revascularization with the least possible trauma, especially the early risk of stroke after conventional CABG. This concept has been actually applied for almost 15 years and provides an additional approach to revascularization for patients with multivessel CAD. The general consensus is that hybrid integrated revascularization is feasible and safe.[12,60-63] Friedrich and colleagues reviewed the results of eighteen studies in literature, which included 367 patients. At 6 months the LITA stenosis rate was 2% and in-stent restenosis was 12%.[62] In 2008, our group published a survival of 92.5% (95% CI 86.5–98.4%) at 1 year and 84.8% (95% CI 73.5–94.9%) at 5 years in a large single center series.[21] Eight patients died during follow-up (208 patient-years). A total of 23 patients had an angiogram for recurrent angina. One patient had an occluded LITA bypass. Five patients showed significant in-stent-restenosis with the need for reintervention. At one year freedom from MACCE and angina was 85.5% (95% CI 76.9–94.1%) and 75.5% (95% CI 62.7–87.3%), respectively.

The short-term results have been excellent.[64] Before a new therapeutic approach is routinely used, it has to be compared to well-proven standard modalities of treatment. Several controlled studies comparing the safety, feasibility, and efficacy of HCR with off-pump CABG have been published in the last 5 years.[65-67] However, the number of patients undergoing HCR in these studies was small and hence, conclusions drawn from such studies have to be viewed with caution. A recently published meta-analysis, which included 422 patients undergoing HCR and > 5000 patients undergoing off-pump CABG, revealed no differences in in-hospital mortality (RR 0.57, 95% CI 0.13–2.59, p = 0.47) or MACCE rates (RR 0.63, 95% CI 0.24–1.64, p = 0.34) between groups. Nevertheless, HCR was associated with significantly shorter hospitalization (RR 0.55, 95% CI 0.13–0.97, p = 0.01), length of ICU stay (RR 0.45, 95% CI 0.10–0.80, p < 0.05), intubation time (RR 0.48, 95% CI 0.13–0.84, p < 0.01) and need for red blood transfusion (RR 0.67, 95% CI 0.56–0.82, p < 0.001).[68] With regard to mid-term outcomes, Shen et al. reported that mortality, myocardial infarction and stroke at 3 years after HCR were comparable to both, CABG and PCI in patients with multivessel disease.[20] However, the cumulative MACCE rate in the hybrid group (6.4%) was significantly lower than that in the PCI group (22.7%; p < 0.001), but similar to that in the CABG group (13.5%; p = 0.14). This was chiefly driven by a higher incidence of repeat revascularization in the PCI group. But interestingly, compared with the hybrid group, repeat revascularization in the PCI group was mainly concentrated in the LAD (2 vs. 10 events; p = 0.029), and PCI with DES for non-LAD offered a similar repeat revascularization rate in the hybrid and PCI groups (4 versus 8 events; p = 0.307). This clearly demonstrates the benefit of surgical revascularization of the LAD with the LITA. Although HCR appears to be an attractive option, especially in the elderly and those at a higher risk due to comorbidities[2] one must keep in mind the potentially higher rate of target vessel revascularization for non-LAD vessels, especially in diabetic patients.[69]

No RCTs comparing HCR with CABG or PCI exist, which is mandatory in the current era of evidence-based medicine. Large, multicenter RCTs are needed to compare HCR with off-pump CABG to identify patient populations that would benefit most from HCR. Furthermore, the optimal strategy or the order of revascularization should also be determined through such trials.

CONCLUSION

In summary, minimally invasive bypass surgery continues to play an increasing role in surgical revascularization. MIDCAB is still limited to patients with single-vessel disease, but has excellent long-term data to confirm the efficacy of this approach. Endoscopic bypass grafting using robotic assistance is still an evolving procedure that is applied only to selected patients, and its continued application will strongly depend on technological improvements that make the procedure technically easier and economically justifiable. MICAS is still in its infancy, but has proven to be clinically efficacious and safe. Although it matches conventional CABG clinically and angiographically in experienced hands, its wide applicability also depends on technological innovations and randomized trials that, at the least, need to prove its noninferiority, if not its superiority to conventional CABG. For now, HCR is a good option for elderly patients with multiple comorbidities or those at a high risk for sternal complications following a sternotomy. Its frequent use in low-intermediate risk patients necessitates large multicenter RCTs.

REFERENCES

1. Serruys PW, et al. Percutaneous coronary intervention versus coronary-artery bypass grafting for severe coronary artery disease. N Engl J Med. 2009:360(10):961-72.
2. Harskamp RE, et al. Comparison of hybrid coronary revascularization versus coronary artery bypass grafting in patients ≥65 years with multivessel coronary artery disease. Am J Cardiol. 2014;114(2):224-9.
3. Guyton RA. Coronary artery bypass is superior to drug-eluting stents in multivessel coronary artery disease. Ann Thorac Surg. 2006;81(6):1949-57.
4. Angelini GD, et al. Integrated left small thoracotomy and angioplasty for multivessel coronary artery revascularisation. Lancet. 1996. 347(9003):757-8.
5. Bonaros N, et al. Quality of life improvement after robotically assisted coronary artery bypass grafting. Cardiology. 2009;114(1):59-66.
6. Gilard M, et al. Same-day combined percutaneous coronary intervention and coronary artery surgery. Cardiology. 2007; 108(4):363-7.
7. Kon ZN, et al. Simultaneous hybrid coronary revascularization reduces postoperative morbidity compared with results from conventional off-pump coronary artery bypass. J Thorac Cardiovasc Surg. 2008;135(2):367-75.
8. Zimrin D, et al. A hybrid alternative for high risk left main disease. Catheter Cardiovasc Interv. 2007;69(1):123-7.
9. Boylan MJ, et al. Surgical treatment of isolated left anterior descending coronary stenosis. Comparison of left internal mammary artery and venous autograft at 18 to 20 years of follow-up. J Thorac Cardiovasc Surg. 1994;107(3):657-62.
10. Davidavicius G, et al. Hybrid revascularization strategy: a pilot study on the association of robotically enhanced minimally invasive direct coronary artery bypass surgery and fractional-flow-reserve-guided percutaneous coronary intervention. Circulation. 2005;112(9 Suppl):I317-22.
11. de Canniere D, et al. Combination of minimally invasive coronary bypass and percutaneous transluminal coronary angioplasty in the treatment of double-vessel coronary disease:

Two-year follow-up of a new hybrid procedure compared with "on-pump" double bypass grafting. Am Heart J. 2001;142(4): 563-70.
12. Katz MR, et al. Integrated coronary revascularization: percutaneous coronary intervention plus robotic totally endoscopic coronary artery bypass. Circulation. 2006;114(1 Suppl):I473-6.
13. Kiaii B, et al. Simultaneous integrated coronary artery revascularization with long-term angiographic follow-up. J Thorac Cardiovasc Surg. 2008;136(3):702-8.
14. Kappetein AP, et al. Comparison of coronary bypass surgery with drug-eluting stenting for the treatment of left main and/or three-vessel disease: 3-year follow-up of the SYNTAX trial. Eur Heart J. 2011;32(17):2125-34.
15. Vassiliades TA, Jr, et al. Integrated coronary revascularization with drug-eluting stents: immediate and seven-month outcome. J Thorac Cardiovasc Surg. 2006;131(5):956-62.
16. Indolfi C, M Pavia, IF Angelillo. Drug-eluting stents versus bare metal stents in percutaneous coronary interventions (a meta-analysis). Am J Cardiol. 2005;95(10):1146-52.
17. Reicher B, et al. Simultaneous "hybrid" percutaneous coronary intervention and minimally invasive surgical bypass grafting: feasibility, safety, and clinical outcomes. Am Heart J. 2008;155(4):661-7.
18. DeRose JJ. Current state of integrated "hybrid" coronary revascularization. Semin Thorac Cardiovasc Surg. 2009;21(3):229-36.
19. Mack MJ, DL Brown, A Sankaran. Minimally invasive coronary bypass for protected left main coronary stenosis angioplasty. Ann Thorac Surg, 1997;64(2):545-6.
20. Shen L, et al. One-stop hybrid coronary revascularization versus coronary artery bypass grafting and percutaneous coronary intervention for the treatment of multivessel coronary artery disease: 3-year follow-up results from a single institution. J Am Coll Cardiol. 2013; 61(25):2525-33.
21. Holzhey DM, et al. Minimally invasive hybrid coronary artery revascularization. Ann Thorac Surg. 2008;86(6):1856-60.
22. Bangalore S, et al. Outcomes with various drug-eluting or bare metal stents in patients with ST-segment-elevation myocardial infarction: a mixed treatment comparison analysis of trial level data from 34 068 patient-years of follow-up from randomized trials. Circ Cardiovasc Interv. 2013;6(4):378-90.
23. Bangalore S, et al. Short- and long-term outcomes with drug-eluting and bare-metal coronary stents: a mixed-treatment comparison analysis of 117 762 patient-years of follow-up from randomized trials. Circulation. 2012;125(23):2873-91.
24. Bellemain-Appaix A, et al. Association of clopidogrel pretreatment with mortality, cardiovascular events, and major bleeding among patients undergoing percutaneous coronary intervention: a systematic review and meta-analysis. JAMA. 2012;308(23):2507-16.
25. Windecker S, et al. 2014 ESC/EACTS guidelines on myocardial revascularization. EuroIntervention. 2015;10(9):1024-94.
26. Calafiore AM, et al. Left anterior descending coronary artery grafting via left anterior small thoracotomy without cardiopulmonary bypass. Ann Thorac Surg. 1996;61(6):1658-63; discussion 1664-5.
27. Cremer J, et al. Off-bypass coronary bypass grafting via minithoracotomy using mechanical epicardial stabilization. Ann Thorac Surg, 1997; 63(6 Suppl):S79-83.
28. Subramanian VA, McCabe JC, Geller CM. Minimally invasive direct coronary artery bypass grafting: two-year clinical experience. Ann Thorac Surg. 1997;64(6):1648-53; discussion 1654-5.
29. Diegeler A, et al. Angiographic results after minimally invasive coronary bypass grafting using the minimally invasive direct coronary bypass grafting (MIDCAB) approach. Eur J Cardiothorac Surg. 1999;15(5):680-4.
30. Bucerius J, et al. Endoscopic internal thoracic artery dissection leads to significant reduction of pain after minimally invasive direct coronary artery bypass graft surgery. Ann Thorac Surg. 2002;73(4):1180-4.
31. Kappert U, et al. Technique of closed chest coronary artery surgery on the beating heart. Eur J Cardiothorac Surg. 2001;20(4):765-9.
32. Falk VMJ, Guthart G, Salisbury JK, Walther T, Gummert J, Mohr FW. Dexterity enhancement in endoscopic surgery by a computer-controlled mechanical wrist. Minim Invasive Ther Allied Technol. 1999;8(4):235-42.
33. McGinn JT, Jr, et al. Minimally invasive coronary artery bypass grafting: dual-center experience in 450 consecutive patients. Circulation. 2009;120(11 Suppl):S78-84.
34. Mack MJ, et al. Results of graft patency by immediate angiography in minimally invasive coronary artery surgery. Ann Thorac Surg. 1999. 68(2):383-9; discussion 389-90.
35. Reser D, et al. Mid-Term Outcomes of Minimally Invasive Direct Coronary Artery Bypass Grafting. Thorac Cardiovasc Surg. 2015;63(4):313-8.
36. Blazek S, et al. Comparison of bare-metal stenting with minimally invasive bypass surgery for stenosis of the left anterior descending coronary artery: 10-year follow-up of a randomized trial. JACC Cardiovasc Interv. 2013;6(1):20-6.
37. Gummert JF, Funkat A, Krian A, Cardiac surgery in Germany during 2004: a report on behalf of the German Society for Thoracic and Cardiovascular Surgery. Thorac Cardiovasc Surg. 2005;53(6):391-9.
38. de Canniere D, W-GG, Cichon R, Gulielmos V, Van Praet F, Seshadri-Kreaden U, Falk V. Feasibility, safety, and efficacy of totally endoscopic coronary artery bypass grafting: multicenter European experience. The Journal of Thoracic and Cardiovascular Surgery. 2007;134(3):710-6.
39. Holzhey DM, et al. Cumulative sum failure analysis for eight surgeons performing minimally invasive direct coronary artery bypass. J Thorac Cardiovasc Surg. 2007;134(3):663-9.
40. Thiele H, et al. Randomized comparison of minimally invasive direct coronary artery bypass surgery versus sirolimus-eluting stenting in isolated proximal left anterior descending coronary artery stenosis. J Am Coll Cardiol. 2009;53(25):2324-31.
41. Holzhey DM, et al. Seven-year follow-up after minimally invasive direct coronary artery bypass: experience with more than 1300 patients. Ann Thorac Surg. 2007;83(1):108-14.
42. Falk V, et al. Total endoscopic off-pump coronary artery bypass grafting. Heart Surg Forum. 2000;3(1):29-31.
43. Damiano RJ, Jr, et al. Initial United States clinical trial of robotically assisted endoscopic coronary artery bypass grafting. J Thorac Cardiovasc Surg. 2000;119(1):77-82.
44. Reichenspurner H, et al. Use of the voice-controlled and computer-assisted surgical system ZEUS for endoscopic coronary artery bypass grafting. J Thorac Cardiovasc Surg. 1999; 118(1):11-6.

45. Kappert U, et al. Wrist-enhanced instrumentation: moving toward totally endoscopic coronary artery bypass grafting. Ann Thorac Surg. 2000;70(3):1105-8.
46. Bonatti J, et al. Effectiveness and safety of total endoscopic left internal mammary artery bypass graft to the left anterior descending artery. Am J Cardiol. 2009;104(12):1684-8.
47. Falk V, et al. Total endoscopic computer enhanced coronary artery bypass grafting. Eur J Cardiothorac Surg. 2000;17(1):38-45.
48. Falk V, et al. Endoscopic coronary artery bypass grafting on the beating heart using a computer enhanced telemanipulation system. Heart Surg Forum. 1999;2(3):199-205.
49. Srivastava S, et al. Use of bilateral internal thoracic arteries in CABG through lateral thoracotomy with robotic assistance in 150 patients. Ann Thorac Surg. 2006;81(3):800-6; discussion 806.
50. Subramanian VA, et al. Robotic assisted multivessel minimally invasive direct coronary artery bypass with port-access stabilization and cardiac positioning: paving the way for outpatient coronary surgery? Ann Thorac Surg. 2005;79(5):1590-6.
51. Lemma M, Athanasiou T, Contino M. Minimally invasive cardiac surgery-coronary artery bypass graft. Multimed Man Cardiothorac Surg. 2013. 2013:mmt007.
52. Ruel M, et al. Results of the Minimally Invasive Coronary Artery Bypass Grafting Angiographic Patency Study. J Thorac Cardiovasc Surg. 2014;147(1):203-8.
53. Boden WE, et al. Optimal medical therapy with or without PCI for stable coronary disease. N Engl J Med. 2007;356(15):1503-16.
54. Hueb W, et al. Ten-year follow-up survival of the Medicine, Angioplasty, or Surgery Study (MASS II): a randomized controlled clinical trial of 3 therapeutic strategies for multivessel coronary artery disease. Circulation. 2010;122(10):949-57.
55. Hlatky MA, et al. Coronary artery bypass surgery compared with percutaneous coronary interventions for multivessel disease: a collaborative analysis of individual patient data from ten randomised trials. Lancet. 2009;373(9670):1190-7.
56. Hannan EL, et al. Comparative outcomes for patients who do and do not undergo percutaneous coronary intervention for stable coronary artery disease in New York. Circulation. 2012;125(15):1870-9.
57. Sipahi I, et al. Coronary artery bypass grafting vs percutaneous coronary intervention and long-term mortality and morbidity in multivessel disease: meta-analysis of randomized clinical trials of the arterial grafting and stenting era. JAMA Intern Med. 2014;174(2):223-30.
58. Bravata DM, et al. Systematic review: the comparative effectiveness of percutaneous coronary interventions and coronary artery bypass graft surgery. Ann Intern Med. 2007;147(10):703-16.
59. Farkouh ME, et al. Strategies for multivessel revascularization in patients with diabetes. N Engl J Med. 2012;367(25):2375-84.
60. Bonatti J, et al. Treatment of double vessel coronary artery disease by totally endoscopic bypass surgery and drug-eluting stent placement in one simultaneous hybrid session. Heart Surg Forum. 2005;8(4):E284-6.
61. Bonatti J, et al. Robotic totally endoscopic coronary artery bypass and catheter based coronary intervention in one operative session. Ann Thorac Surg. 2005;79(6):2138-41.
62. Friedrich GJ, Bonatti J. Hybrid coronary artery revascularization—review and update 2007. Heart Surg Forum. 2007;10(4):E292-6.
63. Wittwer T, et al. Follow-up experience with coronary hybrid-revascularisation. Thorac Cardiovasc Surg. 2000;48(6):356-9.
64. Halkos ME, et al. Clinical and angiographic results after hybrid coronary revascularization. Ann Thorac Surg. 2014;97(2):484-90.
65. Bachinsky WB, et al. Comparative study of same sitting hybrid coronary artery revascularization versus off-pump coronary artery bypass in multivessel coronary artery disease. J Interv Cardiol. 2012;25(5):460-8.
66. Halkos ME, et al. Hybrid coronary revascularization versus off-pump coronary artery bypass for the treatment of left main coronary stenosis. Ann Thorac Surg. 2011;92(6):2155-60.
67. Halkos ME, et al. Hybrid coronary revascularization versus off-pump coronary artery bypass grafting for the treatment of multivessel coronary artery disease. Ann Thorac Surg. 2011;92(5):1695-701; discussion 1701-2.
68. Hu FB, LQ Cui, Short-term clinical outcomes after hybrid coronary revascularization versus off-pump coronary artery bypass for the treatment of multivessel or left main coronary artery disease: a meta-analysis. Coron Artery Dis. 2015;26(6):526-34.
69. Repossini A, et al. Hybrid coronary revascularization in 100 patients with multivessel coronary disease. Ann Thorac Surg. 2014;98(2):574-80; discussion 580-1.

CHAPTER

22

Difficult Situations in Coronary Angioplasty

Lalita Nemani

PART 1: ANOMALOUS CORONARY ORIGIN

"The best tools won't automatically produce high-end graphics; it is limited by imagination"

INTRODUCTION

Anomalous origin of coronary artery (AOCA) are rare congenital abnormalities recognized as potential cause of sudden death in the young and accelerated atherosclerosis in the adult. Diagnostic difficulties and their unseen natural/unnatural history have generated great interest to the cardiologists.[1] They are the most frequent cause of inconclusive angiograms, prolonged procedural and fluoroscopy time, high contrast load and incomplete percutaneous interventions.[2] A tight stenosis in the ectopic vessel can irk any interventional cardiologist at first sight. A combo of experience and dedicated hardware is essential for single stage angioplasty. The experience to intervene is limited to anecdotal cases reports and a few series.[3-5] A present, there is no reliable estimate of the likelihood of success with angioplasty and stenting of such vessels. The purpose of this text is to resolve the conundrum "a diseased AOCA is better bypassed than recanalized by wire".

DEFINITION

The coronary arteries are the only branches arising from ascending aorta and are two in number. Coronary arteries arise more or less perpendicular to the aortic wall. The ostia are located in the middle of the sinus, just above the free leaflet margin of the aortic leaflet and below the sinotubular junction. The right coronary artery arises from the right anterior facing sinus and follows the right atrioventricular groove and posterior interventricular groove. The left coronary artery arising from posteriorly positioned left sinus bifurcates into LAD and LCX after a variable length of 2–40 mm and track anterior interventricular groove and left atrioventricular groove respectively (Fig. 22.1).

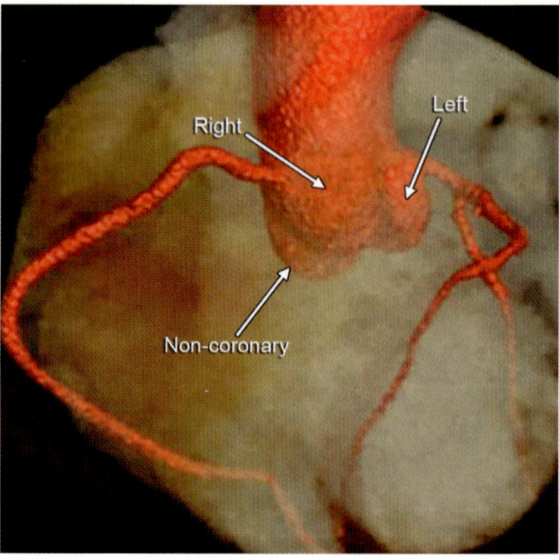

Fig. 22.1 Computed tomography (CT) with 3D reconstruction in LAO 40° view shows the normal aortic root, the relative disposition of cusps in relation to each other and the origin of coronaries

The left anterior descending, circumflex, and right coronary arteries are considered to be essential elementary units of coronary anatomy to support entire myocardium in normal heart. Anomalous origin of coronary artery (AOCA) is defined as a deviation from this normal anatomical pattern.[6,7] Significant benign variants are the major obstacle of all times to stamp what exactly is an anomalous coronary.

CLASSIFICATION

Origin of coronary artery (OCA) can be classified according to the coronary artery involved and the site of origin (Fig. 22.2).

AOCA		
AORCA • Right sinus • Left sinus • Posterior sinus • Aortic origin • Extra-aortic origin	AOLCA • Left sinus • Right sinus • Posterior sinus • Aortic origin • Extra-aortic origin	SCA • Right sinus • Left sinus

Fig. 22.2 A simplified classification of anomalous origin of coronary arteries

Abbreviations: AORCA, anomalous origin of right coronary artery; AOLCA, anomalous origin of left coronary artery; SCA, single coronary artery

EPIDEMIOLOGY

The incidence of AOCA is 0.1–0.3% from angiographic studies.[8] Anomalous origin of right coronary artery (AORCA) is 6–8 times more common than that of left coronary artery (AOLCA). The frequency of different patterns of AOCA as reported in literature is mentioned in Table 22.1.[9-12]

Anomalous origin of coronary artery (AOCA) is associated with sudden death in the young, especially in athletes <30 years of age.[13-16] Anatomical features of these anomalous coronaries that predispose to ischemia are—acute angle take off, narrow slit like orifice, proximal intramural course and compression between the great arteries. The aberrant course also affects blood flow and predisposes to atherosclerosis. Risk of sudden death exists with any coronary anomaly with interarterial course.[17,18] AOCA with anterior (prepulmonic), posterior (retro-aortic) or intraconal (intraseptal) course is generally considered benign (Fig. 22.3).[18,19]

DIAGNOSIS

The diagnosis of coronary anomaly requires a high index of suspicion as no symptom or sign is specific for its presence. The clinical spectrum at presentation ranges from asymptomatic nature to angina, dyspnea, syncope, heart failure, myocardial infarction (MI) and sudden death.[20-24]

Transthoracic echocardiography (TTE) can give information about the location of the ostium in relation to the sinotubular junction (STJ), and can identify interarterial , intramural and intraseptal course of AOCA.[18,25,26]

- 2D and color Doppler parasternal long axis (PLAX) view and/or modified apical views demonstrate origin of the AAOCA in relation to the STJ.
- 2D parasternal short axis (PSAX) and modified PSAX can demonstrate origin and course of the coronary arteries and color flow may show the relation to the aorta and pulmonary trunk (Fig. 22.4).

Table 22.1 The incidence of anomalous origin of coronary arteries according to series and cases in literature (coronary angiogram based)

Type of anomaly		*Incidence (%) and (% of AORCA)*
Benign (80%)	Anomalous RCA	0.09–0.25 (3)
	Anomalous Circumflex from right sinus	0.1–0.3 (30–40)
	Separate origin of LAD and LCx from left sinus	0.4 (30)
	LCx from posterior sinus	<0.01 (<0.3)
	Absent LCx	0.003 (0.2)
Clinically significant (20%)	LMCA from right sinus	0.02 (1)
	LAD from right sinus	0.03 (2)
	RCA from left sinus	0.02–0.17 (10)
	Single coronary artery	0.044–0.23
	LMCA from pulmonary artery	<0.01(<1)
	LAD/RCA from PA	<0.01(<1)
	Coronary fistulas	50% of AOCA

Abbreviations: LAD, left anterior descending artery; LCx, left circumflex; LMCA, left main coronary artery; AOCA, anomalous origin of coronary artery

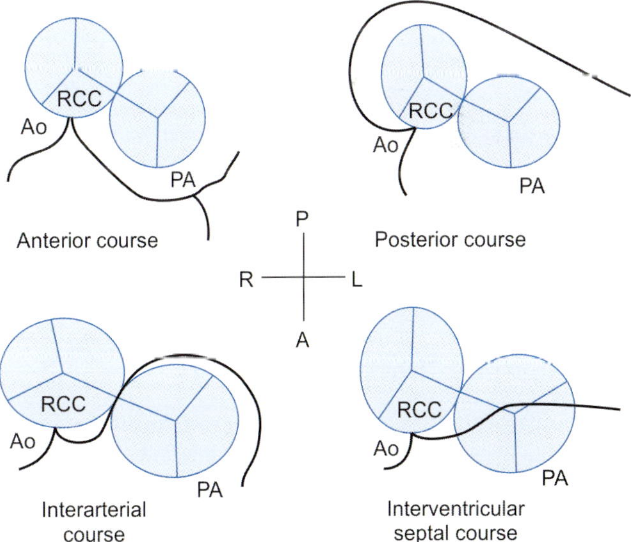

Fig. 22.3 Among the four common courses for an AOCA arising from the opposite sinus, the interarterial course between the aorta and the pulmonary artery is malignant. Anterior (Prepulmonic), posterior (Retroaortic) and septal are the benign courses

Abbreviations: Ao, aorta; PA, pulmonary artery; RCC, right coronary cusp

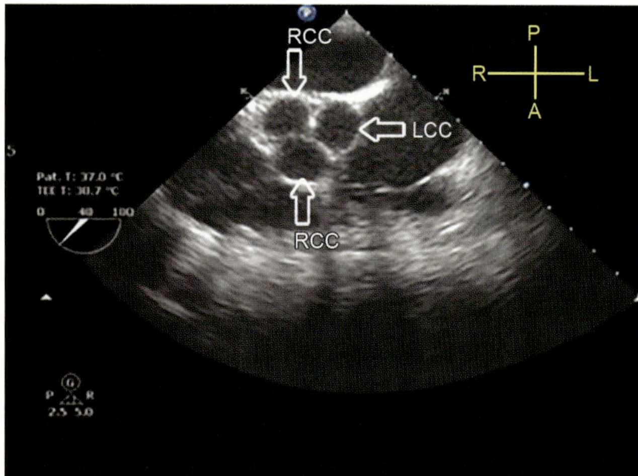

Fig. 22.4 Transesophageal echocardiography of aortic root in short-axis view showing relative normal position of cusps
Abbreviations: LCC, left coronary cusp; RCC, right coronary cusp

The TTE may suffice in pediatric population for initial screening but not in the adult where TEE (transesophageal echo) may be slightly superior. However, a second diagnostic modality is definitely required for confirmation in either case.

Coronary angiography is the standard investigation for the diagnosis of these anomalous vessels. Additional imaging modalities in the form of cardiac magnetic imaging or ultrafast CT angiography[27-30] is required to delineate the morphology of the ostium and risk stratification based on the initial course of the coronary artery anomalies (CAA).

ANGIOGRAPHIC PROFILING OF ANOMALOUS CORONARIES

Optimal knowledge of the best projections for visualization of normal coronary ostia would ease the identification of abnormal ostia (Table 22.2).

Angiographic Profiling of AORCA

The anomaly should be suspected whenever the RCA ostium is not precisely cannulated with routine maneuvers. A systemic approach is mandatory before withdrawal of the first catheter. Jim et al's 3 step approach[2] acts as a guide to cannulate the anomalous RCA ostium speedily. This consists of a right sinus injection followed by left coronary sinus injection, and finally the aortography to delineate the anomalous ostium. Routine angiographic views such as LAO-cranial/caudal and RAO are usually sufficient.

- A long horizontal proximal segment in LAO projection of RCA which is seen in a non-selective injection with diagnostic right Judkins catheter suggests an anomalous origin of RCA arising either from parent sinus, non-coronary sinus or left sinus. The exact sinus of origin can be confirmed in an RAO projection (Figs 22.5 and 22.6).[31]
- Anteriorly displaced RCA (anterior one-third of right sinus) is the most common anomaly and can be selectively imaged[32] with Judkins Right or Amplatz Left (AL1), in the 30° right anterior oblique projection with the catheter pointing anterior (to the right) (Figs 22.7A to D).
- Anomalous RCA from left sinus appear as radiopaque dot during RAO ventriculography (end on view anterior to aorta).[33]
- High takeoff RCAs can be imaged sub selectively by a right sinus angiogram with conventional right diagnostic catheters (Fig. 22.8).[32]

Anomalous Circumflex

An anomalous circumflex artery should be suspected when one sees a long left main and a presumed small/trivial/blocked circumflex on angiogram.[22,33] The missing circumflex invariable will be found to arise from right coronary cusp or proximal RCA. The retroaortic course can be seen on RAO projection as circumflex moves leftward and behind the aorta. The RAO projection during left ventriculography, aortography, or coronary angiography, will visualize the artery on end and appear as a radiopaque "dot" posterior to the aorta.[33] The key observation for the anomalous circumflex is a "dot" behind the aorta seen in the RAO view (Figs 22.9A and B).

Anomalous LAD (Dual LAD Type IV to VI)

Dual LAD is a rare and complicated coronary anomaly. The first report on types I–IV dual LAD was in 1983 by Spindola-Franco et al.[34] New types were detected and identified as type V dual LAD in 2010 (Manchanda et al.[35]) and type VI dual LAD in 2011 (Maroney and Klein.[36] The first three types of dual LAD arise from the left sinus while the next three arise from the left sinus (Table 22.3). Type IV is the rarest and deadliest with reported incidence of 0.01–0.7% in patients undergoing cardiac catheterization.[37] A familiarity with this anomaly avoid surgical trauma and un-necessary stenting in cases of interarterial course.[38]

The anomaly is suspected by visualization of a relatively short LAD and absence of collaterals and an avascular area in the distribution of the left coronary artery.[37,38] LAD is identified by the presence of septal branches arising from it (Figs 22.10A and B).

Anomalous Origin of Left Main Coronary Artery from Right Sinus

When not visualized in the left sinus, the LM should be suspected to arise from the right sinus. ALMCA can be

Table 22.2 Best angiographic projections for visualization of normal coronary ostium

Coronary artery	*Angiographic projection*	*Angiographic image*	
Left main		A: LAO caudal	B: AP caudal
• Ostium	Spider view		
• Shaft	AP caudal		
• Distal	Plain AP		
LAD		C: LAO cranial	D: AP cranial
• Ostio proximal LAD	LAO caudal AP caudal		
• Mid and distal LAD/ diagonals	AP cranial RAO cranial		
• Diagonals	LAO cranial		
Cx		E: RAO caudal	F: RAO caudal
• Ostial	AP caudal		
• Proximal	RAO caudal		
• Distal obtuse marginal	RAO cranial		
• Dominant LCx distal	LAO cranial		
RCA		G: Plain LAO	H: Plain RAO
• Ostium	LAO caudal/LAO		
• Proximal	LAO/LAO caudal		
• Mid RCA	LAO/Lateral/RAO		
• Distal RCA	AP cranial/LAO caudal		
• Crux	AP cranial		
• PDA/PLVB	AP cranial/LAO cranial		

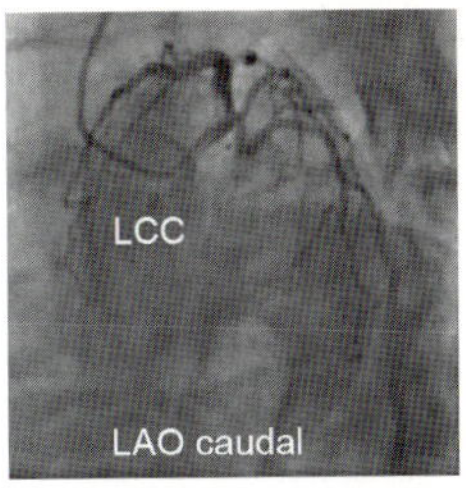

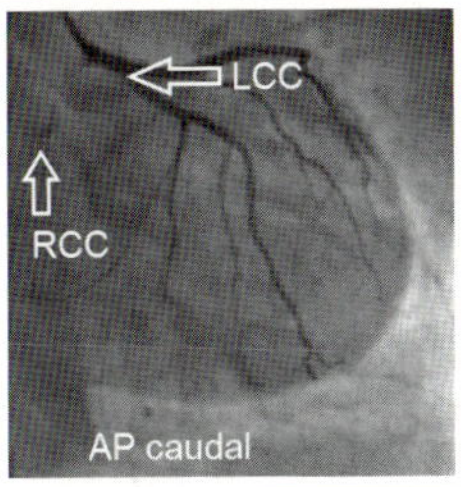

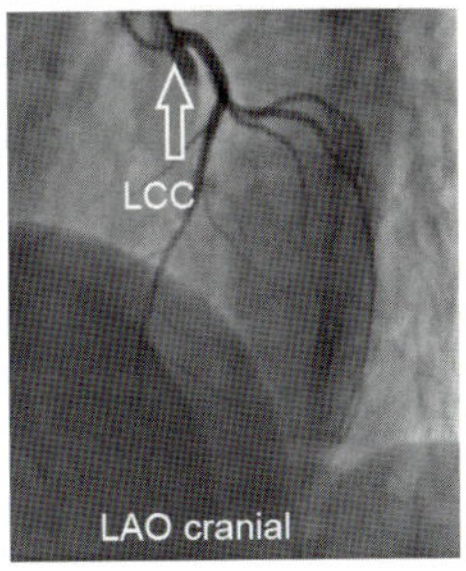

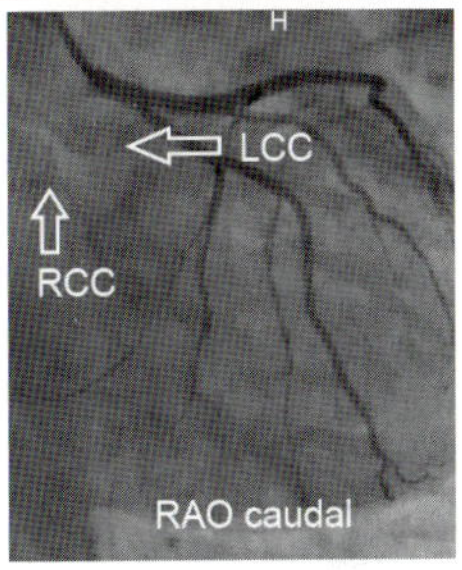

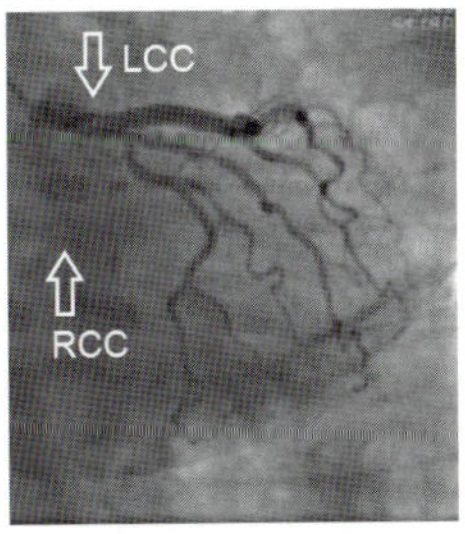

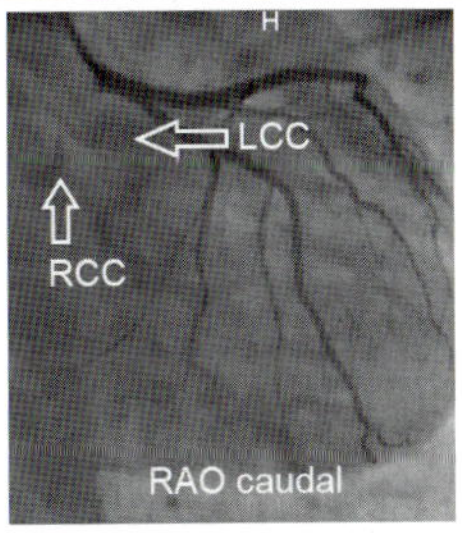

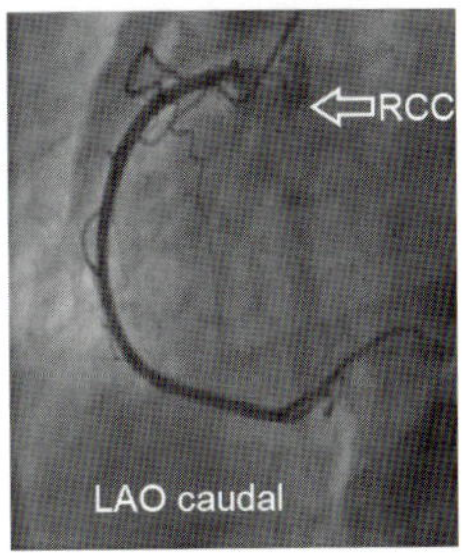

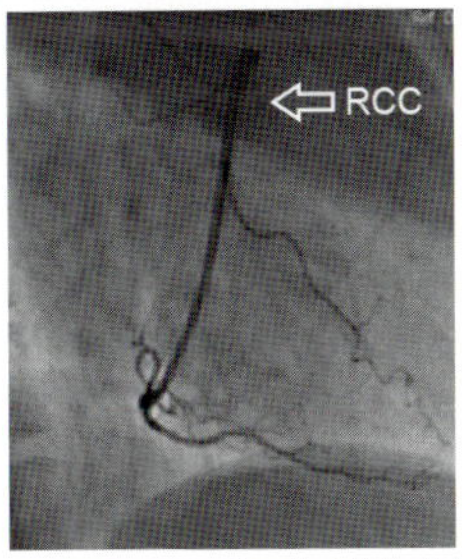

Abbreviations: AP, anteroposterior; Cx, circumflex; LAD, left anterior descending artery; LAO, left anterior oblique; LCC, left coronary cusp; LCx, left circumflex; PDA, posterior descending artery; PLVB, posterior left ventricular branch; RAO, right anterior oblique; RCA, right coronary artery; RCC, right coronary cusp

diagnosed by the Dot and eye technique on angiography described by Serota H et al. (Figs 22.11A to D).[39]

- *Septal LM:* During RAO coronary angiography, the ALMCA and the circumflex coronary artery form an ellipse (downward loop/bottom of the eye), with the LMCA forming the inferior portion and the circumflex artery forming the superior portion. Septal perforating arteries branching from the LMCA help identify this anomaly.
- *Anterior course:* In RAO view, the ALMCA forms the superior portion and circumflex forms the inferior portion of the eye (upward loop/top of the eye).

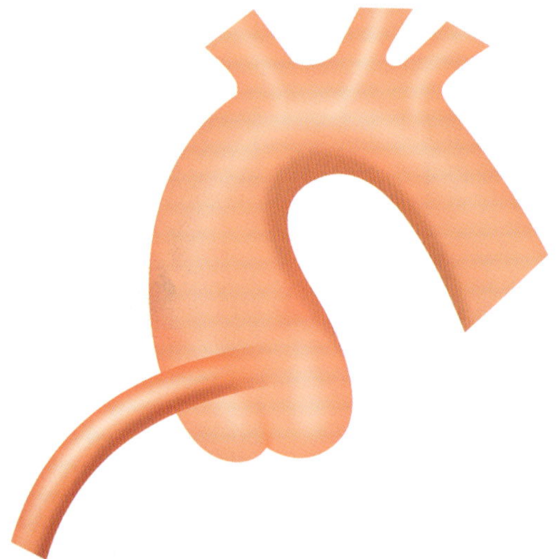

Fig. 22.5 Suspicion of anomalous origin of right coronary artery from right coronary in routine coronary angiogram: A long horizontal proximal portion of the coronary tangential to aortic sinus is the indication

- *Retroaortic course:* In RAO view, ALMCA appears as dot behind the aortic root
- *Interarterial course:* In RAO view, ALMCA appears as a dot (end on view) anterior to the aortic root.

Some suggest keeping a wedge catheter in pulmonary artery or contrast injection in PA to delineate the course of anomalous coronaries. These are all things of past, as now MDCT/CT coronary angiography can resolves these issues efficiently. However, knowledge of these is useful when alone in the desert (Figs 22.12A and B).

PERCUTANEOUS INTERVENTION IN AOCA: TECHNICAL CHALLENGES

The anomalous coronaries are a challenge to even the most experienced interventionalist. Improper visualization during CAG, inability to obtain a co-axial engagement of catheter during angioplasty difficulty in the advancement of the balloon or the stent are the major hurdles posed by the aberrant vessels in percutaneous intervention. For successful

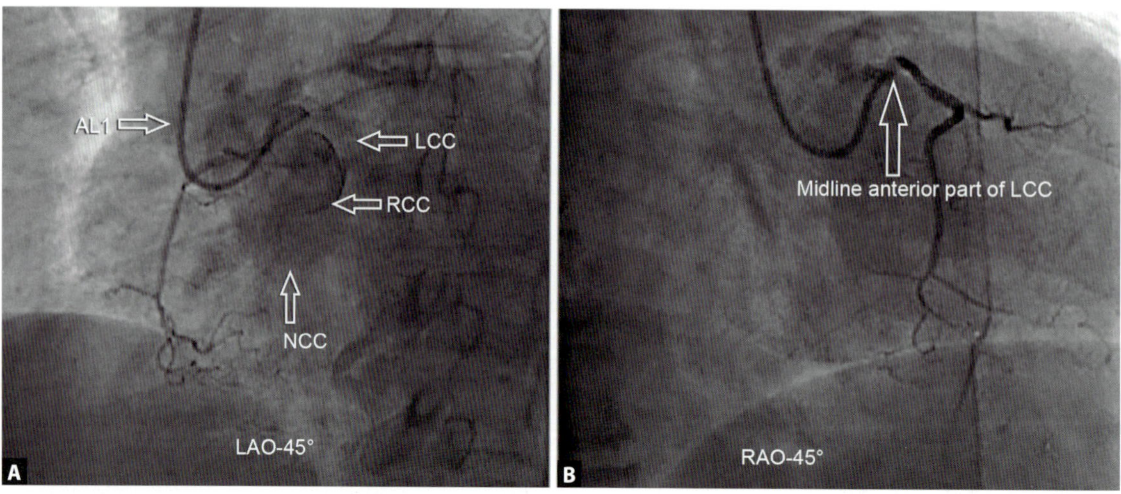

Figs 22.6A and B AORCA from left sinus. Diagnostic coronary angiogram illustrating the effortless hooking of AORCA (Type D) in LAO-45° (A) and RAO-45° (B)

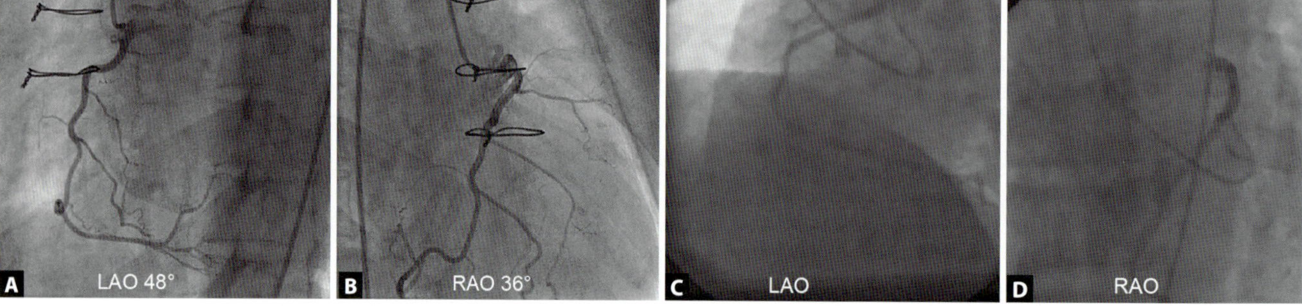

Figs 22.7A to D Anteriorly displaced AORCA. Optitorque 5 Fr diagnostic catheter shows non-selective high origin of AORCA from right sinus (AORCA type RC) in LAO view (A) and RAO view (B); (C) Amplatzer 2 diagnostic for selective hooking in LAO 40–60° showing high and close to mid line origin of RCA; (D) RAO hooking with AL2 showing high and anterior RCA (AORCA type RA)

PCI, adequate knowledge about the ostium and anatomical course is required.

The ostia of anomalous coronary arteries are difficult to cannulate with routine guide catheters owing to their juxta commissural location and initial tangential course. Choosing appropriate guiding catheter and skilful planned maneuvering is the crux of successful angioplasty.

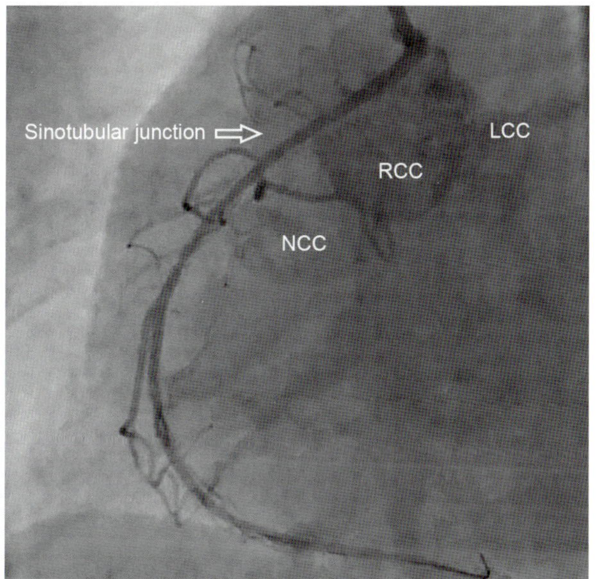

Fig. 22.8 High take off RCA. Selective cannulation of AORCA from post wall of aorta using Amplatzer left guide catheter

Sudden cardiac death is mostly related to interarterial or intramyocardial course [**M**] but the anatomy of origin and proximal course [**O** and **P**] are most important for intervention. Selective cannulation and stabilization of guide are decided by the configuration of O and P. A reliable 3D definition of coronary sinus configuration, morphometry and location of ostium and proximal course of the coronary are major determinants for guide selection and success of PCI in anomalous coronary artery[40] irrespective of distal bed [DB]. However, stenting of cases with interarterial course is shunned as it invited fatal complications (Fig. 22.13).[41]

GUIDE CATHETER SELECTION

Successful PCI of AORCA relies on optimal guiding catheter seating and back-up support. Rahman and others[42] are the first to provide solution for catheter selection based on patient's image data, but these are only for the coronaries with normal origin and shape. There are no standard guidelines for selection of appropriate hardware and neither can there be one, as each case is unique in itself. Experience helps in choosing the guide, but the operator should be ready to switch over to another catheter if the primary approach does not yield results.

Guide Catheter Selection for AORCA[3-5]

The guide catheter selection for PCI of AORCA is as nonspecific as its classification for location. Classification of AORCA as proposed by Nemani L et al. and Sarkar et al. act

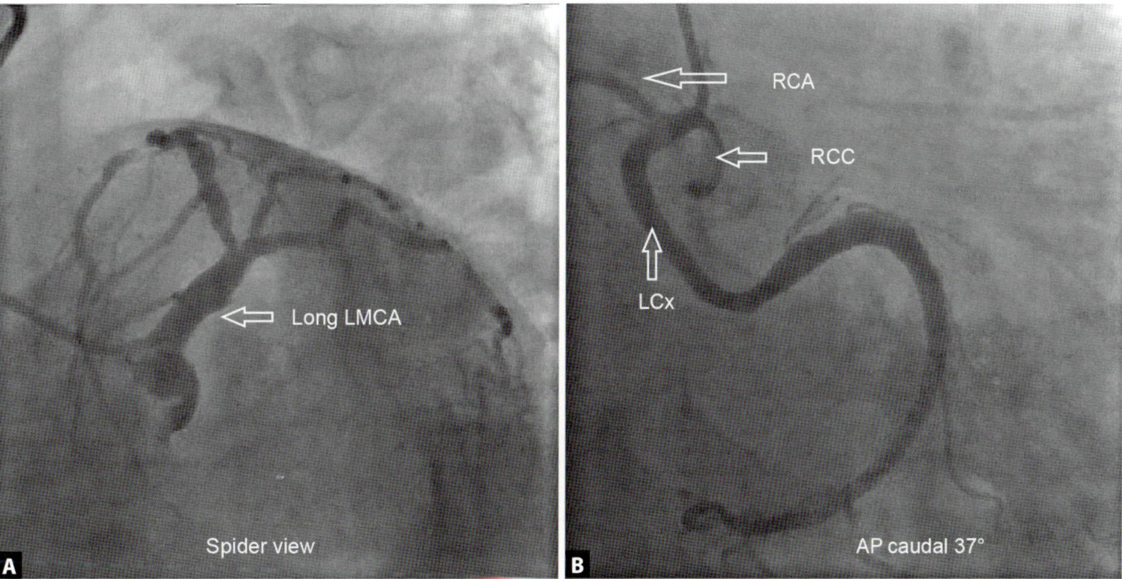

Figs 22.9A and B (A) Spider view showing long left main with small trivial/blocked circumflex; (B) AP caudal projection showing anomalous circumflex arising from proximal RCA in right sinus

Table 22.3 Classification of dual LAD

Types	*Short LAD*		*Long LAD*	
	Origin	*Course*	*Origin*	*Course*
I	Proximal LAD	Proximal IVG	Short LAD	Epicardial course on the left ventricle
II	Proximal LAD	Proximal IVG	Short LAD	Epicardial course on the left ventricle
III	Proximal LAD	Proximal IVG	Short LAD	Intramyocardial course in the septum
IV	LMCA/LSOV	Proximal IVG	RCA or RCS	Epicardial course on the right ventricle or intramyocardial course within the septal crest
V	LSOV	Proximal IVG	RCS	Epicardial course on the right ventricle or intramyocardial course within the septal crest
VI	LMCA	Proximal IVG	RCA	Underneath the RVOT in the area of the interventricular septum origin course origin course type

Abbreviations: IVG, interventricular groove; LAD, left anterior descending artery; LMCA, left main coronary artery; LSOV, left sinus of Valsalva; RCA, right coronary artery; RCS, right coronary sinus

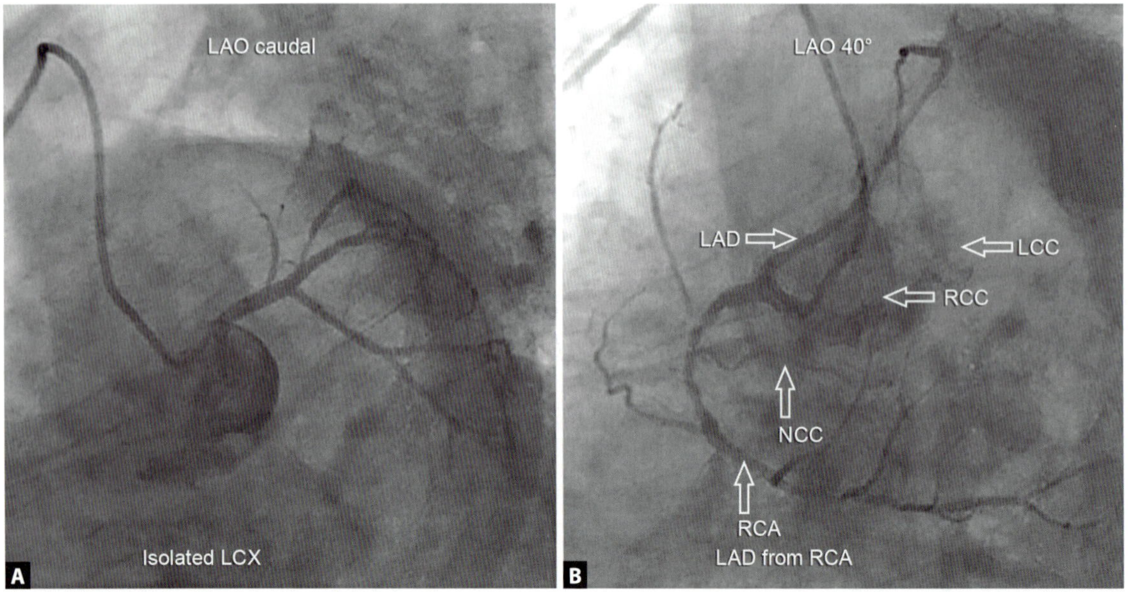

Figs 22.10A and B Anomalous LAD from right sinus: (A) LAO caudal view showing isolated LCx and relatively avascular LAD territory; (B) Anomalous LAD from right sinus demonstrated with non-selecting hooking with Optitorque diagnostic catheter in LAO. Retroaortic course (benign). This course can be well perceived by keeping Swan-Ganz catheter in pulmonary artery in AP and lateral projections

as benchmarks for selection of guide (Figs 22.14 and 22.15). AORCA from right sinus is easy to diagnose but more difficult to cannulate as there are no default catheters. The site of origin and immediate angle between the proximal part and site of origin are crucial to choose a particular guide catheter. Suggested catheters of choice based on consensus and experience are mentioned below (Tables 22.4 and 22.5).

- Anteriorly displaced RCA from right sinus can be effectively hooked with Judkins Right with clockwise rotation from default position. Many a time the procedure is successfully completed with the catheter hooking off ostium with only wire support (use of buddy wire enhances guide support) (Fig. 22.16).
- AORCA from left sinus originates anterior, superior, adjacent, or directly from the left main coronary, but practically never posterior to the left main coronary. The Judkins left catheter is designed to engage an ostium in the left sinus, hence with slight modifications cannulation of the anomalous RCA in a coaxial fashion can be accomplished (Figs 22.17 and 22.18).[29]

Figs 22.11A to D Four courses of the anomalous LMCA from the right sinus as described by Serota et al. (A) Septal course; (B) Anterior (prepulmonic) course; (C) Posterior (Retro aortic) course; (D) Interarterial course

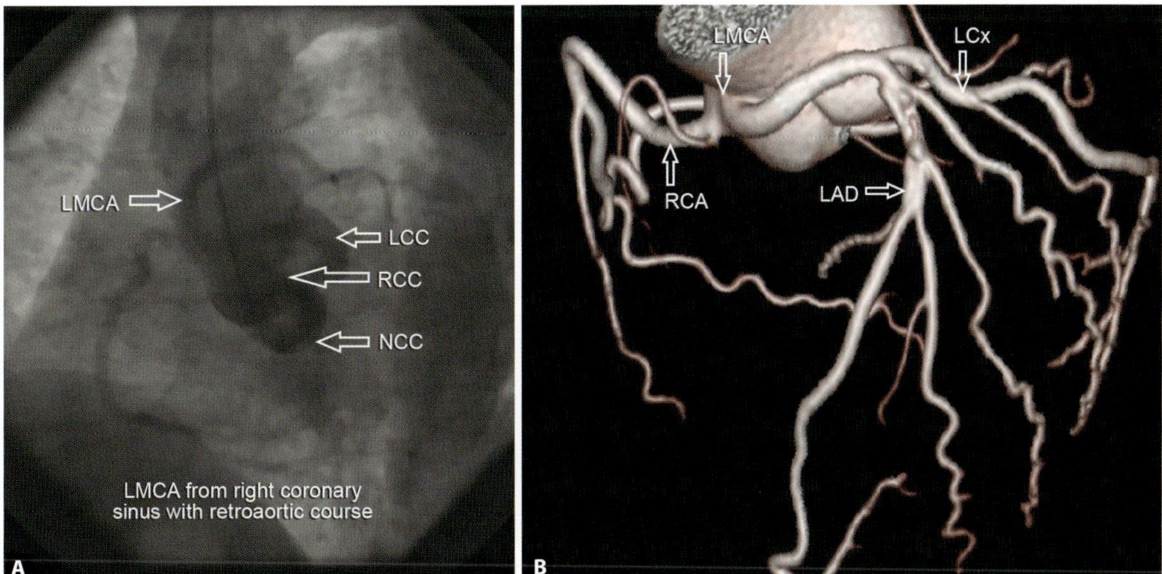

Figs 22.12A and B LMCA from right sinus with retroaortic course. (A) Angiographic view; (B) CT angiographic view

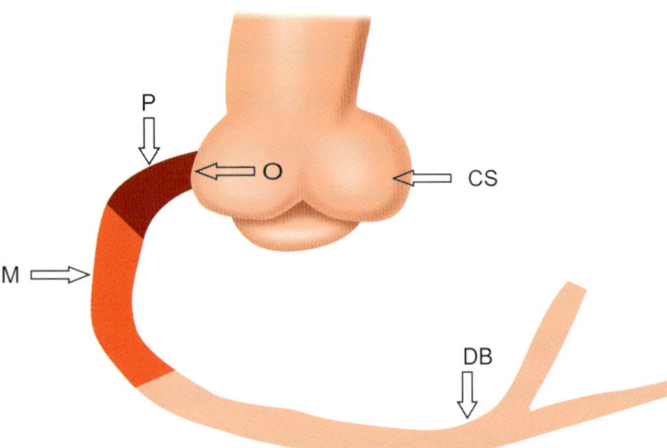

Fig. 22.13 AORCA anatomy in relation to PCI. The site of origin and the angle between proximal part of coronary artery and site of origin (sinus or aortic wall) are extremely important for intervention. These two features decide the selection of a particular guide for PCI

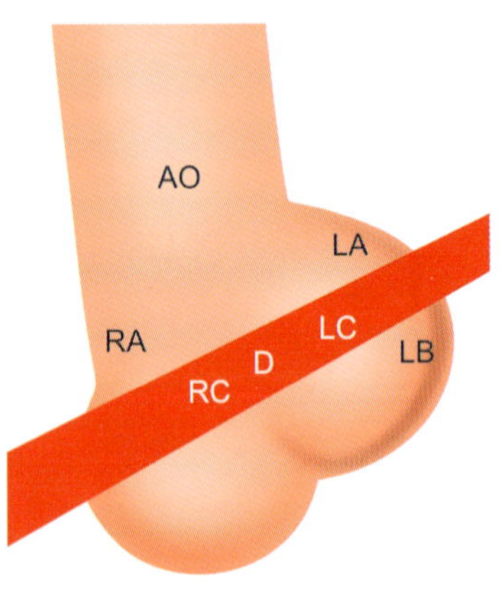

Hypothetical anomalous origin of AORCA in IAO cranial. Origin from right coronary sinus are labeled as high take off (RA), low take off (RB) anterior or posterior to normal origin but not from midline of aorta (RC). Origin from left coronary sinus are classified as LA, and LC respectively. Origin either from RCS or LCS in the midline are labeled D. Origin from noncoronary sinus/posterior sinus called P

Fig. 22.14 Nemani I et al. Classification of AORCA

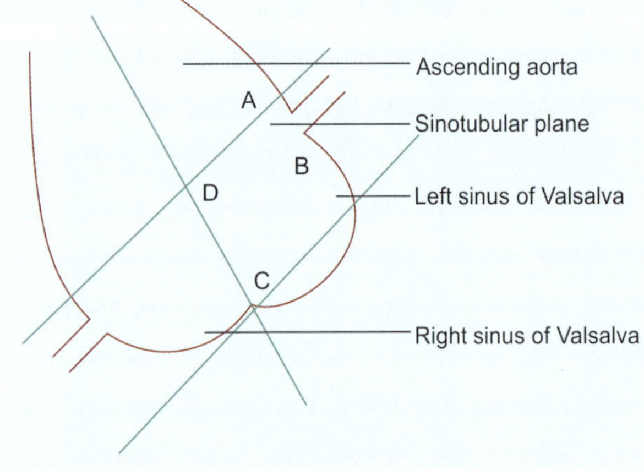

Fig. 22.15 Sarkar's classification of AORCA from left sinus

Guide Catheter Selection for AOLCA

The choice of catheter is usually based upon the angle and the take off of the anomalous vessel and the operator preference. Though surgical intervention is class I recommendation, level of evidence B in the ACC/AHA guidelines for the management of adults with congenital heart disease for anomalous LCA, a few studies have demonstrated the feasibility of PCI, especially in the situation of acute coronary syndrome (Table 22.6).

Single Coronary Artery

A rare anomaly where a single ostium of aortic origin supplies the entire heart. It has been classified angiographically by Lipton[43] and Yamanaka and Hobbs[8] based on ostial location, anatomical distribution and course of the trunk (Table 22.7).

Stenting has become an increasing attractive option to surgery for single coronary which lacks malignant features and may become inevitable in the situation of acute coronary syndrome. There are only a few case reports owing to rarity of the condition and technical challenges in the procedure. Suggested hardware has been mentioned in Table 22.8.

Anomalous Origin of the Right Coronary Artery from the Left Anterior Descending Coronary Artery

This is a subgroup of single coronary artery, is relatively rare and more benign than other types of anomalous origin of the right coronary artery (RCA).[56-59] A variant RCA may originate from mid left anterior descending coronary artery (LAD) coursed via a conal branch. A few case reports have been described but they usually are of no clinical significance.

Word of Caution

Coronary angioplasty with stenting may be a feasible therapeutic option for a single anomalous coronary artery. PCI could prove catastrophic with a flow limiting dissection or thrombus. Operator should be aware of the potential risk of complications and the limitations of the procedure.

ANCILLARY HARDWARE AND TECHNIQUES

Access

Both radial and femoral are equally effective and decision should be left to the operator.[4,5,59]

Guidewire

The tortuous course of these vessels makes wiring a difficult task, thereby increasing the risk of perforation. One should

Table 22.4 Guide catheter selection for PCI of AORCA

Classification	*Location of ostium*	*Guide catheter of choice*	*Comment*
Right sinus	High origin (RA)	Upward take—Amplatzer left (AL1 or AL2)	Nemani L, et al.[5]
	Low origin (RB)	Horizontal take—Judkin's Right (JR)	
	Middle (same level) origin (RC)	Down slant—Multipurpose (MP)/ Amplatzer right (AR1)	
Left sinus	High origin—above left ostium (LA)	Usually displaced Anteriorly—Judkin's right (JR)	The JL catheter is pushed deep into the left sinus to form a U. The larger curve prevents the catheter from engaging the LCA and allows for selective cannulation of the anomalous RCA
Most commonly arises anterior and cephalad to left ostium	Low origin—below left ostium (LB)		The undersized JL 3.0 or 3.5 is advanced with a clockwise twist so that the catheter inverts itself, pointing up with the secondary curve resting on the left coronary cusp
	Adjacent/Midline to left ostium (LC)		Leya catheter is a modification of the AL-1 consisting of a right angled deviation of the tip
Noncoronary sinus (P)—very rare Existence was doubted[illegible]	Incidence: 0.003%	Anterior displaced—Judkin's right (JR)/Amplatzer right (AR1 or AR2)	Word of caution—confirm it by echo or 3DCT as all these posterior RCA are not from non-coronary sinus but usually arising posteriorly from the right sinus just adjacent to the commissural line
Aortic origin (A)	High take off RCA—1–4 cm above STJ	Posterior displaced—Judkin's right	Extreme caudal turn to reach the right AV groove. Unrecognized ostium pose problem for surgeon during aortic clamping

Table 22.5 Guide catheter of choice for AORCA from left sinus according to Sarkar et al.

Classification	*Description*	*Guide catheter of choice*
Type A	Origin from the aorta above the sinotubular junction	Judkin's left (JL)
Type B	Origin just below the ostium of the left coronary artery forward curve	Judkin's left (JL)
Type C	Origin below the sinotubular plane between the midline and the left coronary artery	Voda left (VL)
Type D	Origin along the midline	Amplatzer (AL1 or 2)

start with a floppy or soft tip wire[59] and hydrophilic in case of extreme tortousity.

Tips and Tricks

Many a times, the procedure would require hooking off ostium. In such case, use of microcatheter, buddy wire and anchoring balloon techniques can be used to enhance guide support and deep engagement without dissection. Two wires-two vessel angioplasty technique[59] is extremely useful in successful angioplasty of anomalous LCx and single coronary artery.

Figs 22.16A and B Successful PCI of AORCA high and anterior from right sinus (RA) using Judkin's right guide catheter. (A) LAO 48° view; (B) AP cranial 35° view

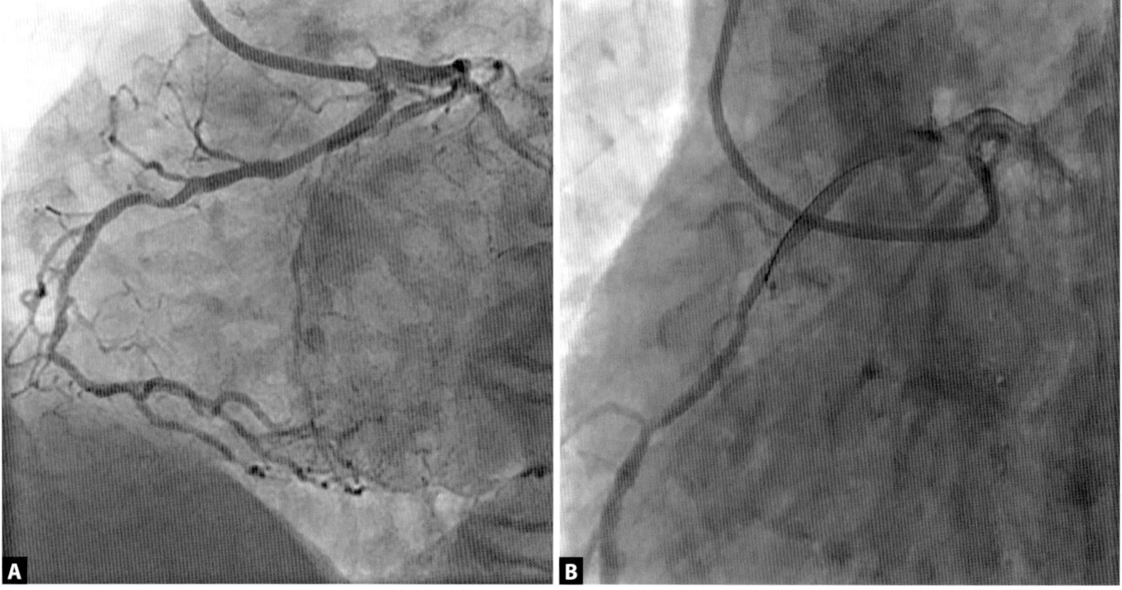

Figs 22.17A and B PCI of AORCA from left sinus. (A) The hooking of AORCA from LCS (type-LB) by using EBU-3.0 in LAO view; (B) The hooking of AORCA from LCS (type-LA) using JL-4.0 in LAO wherein the curve is further modified by pushing deep into LCS to facilitate easier cannulation

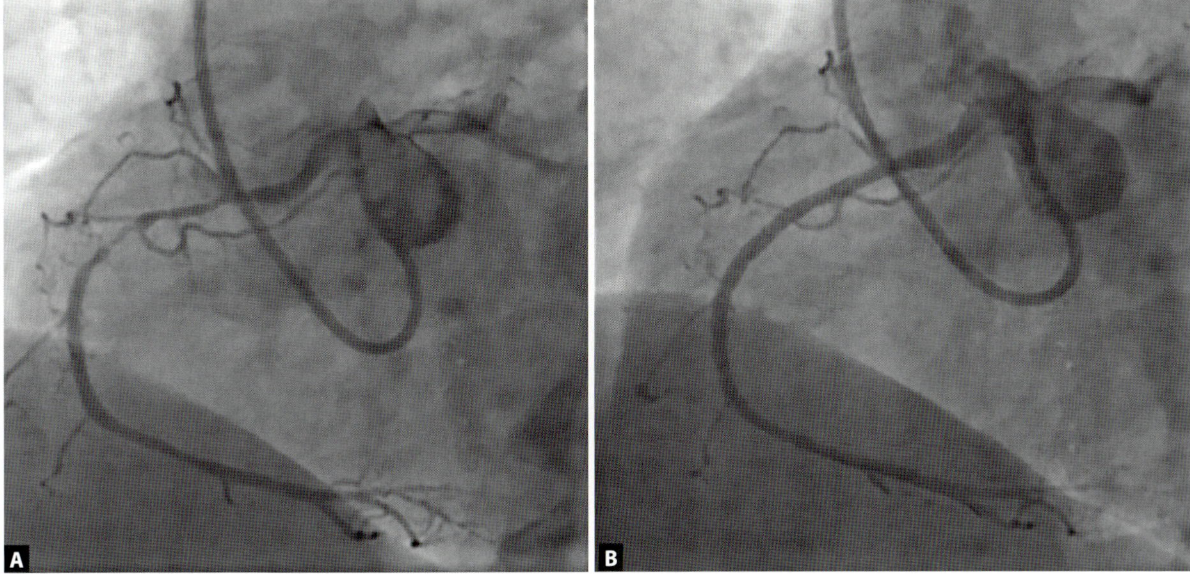

Figs 22.18A and B PCI of AORCA from left sinus (Type D) using Amplatzer (AL2). (A) Mid 80% stenosis in RCA in LAO view before stenting; (B) After successfully stenting

Table 22.6 Guide catheter of choice for AOLCA

Ostium location	*Guide catheter of choice*	*Access site*
Anomalous LCx[43,44]		
• Right aortic sinus	Amplatzer right catheter/ Judkins right	Femoral or radial
• Proximal RCA	Judkin's right catheter/ Amplatzer right	Radial/ femoral
• Distal RCA	Judkin's right catheter	
LM from right sinus		
• Interarterial	AL1 (Schrale et al.)	Femoral
• Retro aortic	RJ - OKA Mach 1 (Routoulas et al.)	Femoral
LAD from RCS/RCA (Isolated/Dual LAD type IV-VI)		
• Interarterial	JR4 (Hershey J et al., Kang et. al.)	Femoral
• Retro aortic	ECR 4 (Vijayvergiya et al.)	Femoral
• AV groove	AR2 (Gupta et al.)	Femoral

Table 22.7 Angiographic types of isolated single coronary artery (modified Lipton classification)

Ostial location
• R- Right sinus of Valsalva
• L-Left sinus of Valsalva
Anatomical distribution
• I-The solitary dominant vessel follows the course of either a normal right or left coronary artery (RI or LI)
• II- One coronary artery arises from the proximal part of the normally located other coronary artery (RII or LII)
• III- LAD and LCx arise separately from common trunk originating from the right sinus of Valsalva (RIII)
Course of the transverse trunk
• Anterior to the great vessels
• Between the aorta and pulmonary arteries
• P- Posterior to the great vessels
• S- Septal type": A part of the route passes through interventricular septum
• "Combined type": Combination of diverse routes

Table 22.8 Suggested guide catheters for PCI of single coronary artery

Types	*Guide catheter of choice*	*References*
LIPTON L-I A	LAD- Judkin's left 3.5 LAUNCHER 6F Extra back-up (EBU) guide was used for CX	Ozeren, et al.[44] Mishra, et al.[45] Quintal, et al.[46] Devi Dutta S[47]
LIPTON R-IC	6 French short-Amplatz left 0.75 (SAL 0.75) guiding catheter (Vector, Medtronic Inc).	Ohta, et al.[48]
LIPTON R-II P	Judkin's right –RCA	B Akdeniz, et al.[49]
LIPTON R-III C	RCA- Judkin's right/AL1 LCX-Amplatzer	Ohta, et al Chan CNS, et al.[50]
LIPTON R-IIIB	LAD- Left bypass	Ref[51-55]
LIPTON R-IIIP	RCA- right amplatzer	Ref[51-55]

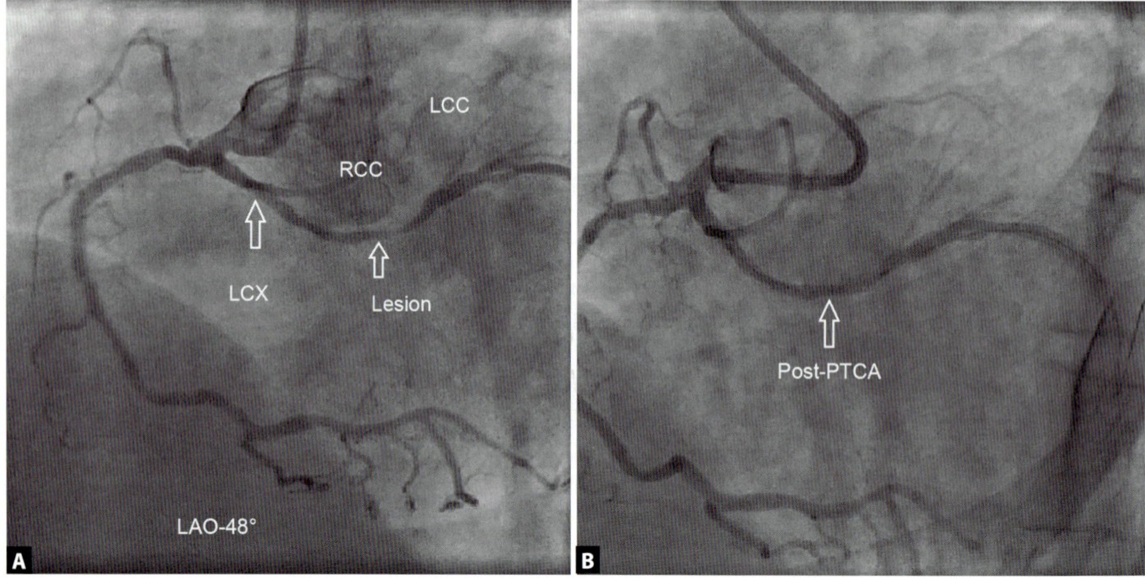

Figs 22.19A and B (A) Anomalous circumflex from proximal RCA in LAO view hooked with Judkin's right. Showing 80–90% stenosis in the mid-segment; (B) Direct, successfully stented with single guidewire help

CONCLUSION

Coronary artery of anomalous origin is rare and each case poses a challenge due to lack of state-of-art angioplasty in such vessel. A good understanding of the exact anatomy preceding PCI reduces complications, procedural time and radiation, failed attempt and the need of rescue bypass graft. The limitation of routine CAG should be overcoming by CT or MRI when needed. Unlike normal coronary where in fact, Judkin's himself said that "no points are earned for coronary catheterization—the catheters know where to go if not thwarted by the operator",[60] selecting hooking of ectopic ostium, keeping up with ectopic ostium and its unusual proximal bend and tortuous course needs a good imagination because guide catheter alone will not do.

REFERENCES

1. Barriales-Villa R, et al. Congenital coronary artery anomalies. Rev Esp Cardiol. 2006;59(4):360-70.
2. Jim MH, Siu CW, Ho HH, Miu R, Lam YM, Lam L, Chan RH, Lee SW. Anomalous origin of right coronary artery from the left coronary sinus: incidence, characteristics, and a systematic approach for rapid diagnosis. J Interv Cardiol. 2005;18(2):101-6.
3. Sarkar K, Sharma SK, Kini AS. Catheter selection for coronary angiography and intervention in anomalous right coronary arteries. J Interv Cardiol. 2009;22:234-9.
4. Uthayakumaran K, Subban V, Lakshmanan A, et al. Coronary intervention in anomalous origin of the right coronary artery (ARCA) from the left sinus of valsalva (LSOV): a single center experience. Indian Heart J. 2014;66:430-4.
5. Nemani L, Jyotsna M, Barik R, Krishna VKS. Tools and techniques for angioplasty of anomalous origin of right coronary artery. Journal of Indian College of Cardiology. 2015;5(3):189-97.
6. Angelini P. Normal and anomalous coronary arteries: definitions and classification. Am Heart J. 1989;117(2):418-34.
7. Angelini P. Coronary artery anomalies--current clinical issues: definitions, classification, incidence, clinical relevance, and treatment guidelines. Circulation. 2007;115:1296-305.
8. Yamanaka O, Hobbs RE. Coronary artery anomalies in 126,595 patients undergoing coronary arteriography. Cathet Cardiovasc Diagn. 1990;21:28e40.
9. Namgung J, Kim JA. The prevalence of coronary anomalies in a single centre of Korea: origination, course, and termination anomalies of aberrant coronary arteries detected by ECG gated cardiac MDCT. BMC Cardiovasc Disord. 2014;14:48.
10. Chaitman BR, Lesperance J, Saltiel J, Bourassa MG. Clinical, angiographic, and hemodynamic findings in patientswith anomalous origin of the coronary arteries. Circulation. 1976;53:122-31.
11. Giuliani ER, Gersh BJ, McGoon MD, Hayes DL, Schaff HV (Eds). Mayo Clinic Practice of Cardiology, 3rd edition. St. Louis. MO; Mosby; 1998. pp.1815-35.
12. Lipton MJ, Barry WH, Obrez I, Silverman JF, Wexler L. Isolated single coronary artery: diagnosis, angiographic classification, and clinical significance. Radiology. 1979;130:39-47.
13. Brothers J, Gaynor JW, Paridon S, et al. Anomalous aortic origin of a coronary artery with an interarterial course: understanding current management strategies in children and young adults. Pediatr Cardiol. 2009;30:911-21.
14. Eckart RE, Scoville SL, Campbell CL, et al. Sudden death in young adults: a 25-year review of autopsies in military recruits. Ann Intern Med. 2004;141:829-34.
15. Sharma V, Burkhart HM, Dearani JA, et al. Surgical unroofing of anomalous aortic origin of a coronary artery: a single-center experience. Ann Thorac Surg. 2014;98:941-5.
16. Taylor AJ, Rogan KM, Virmani R, et al. Sudden cardiac death associated with isolated congenital coronary artery anomalies. J Am Coll Cardiol. 1992;20:640-7.
17. Virmani R, Burke AP, Farb A. Sudden cardiac death. Cardiovasc Pathol 2001;10:275-82.
18. Frommelt PC, Berger S, Pelech AN, et al. Prospective identification of anomalous origin of left coronary artery from the right sinus of Valsalva using transthoracic echocardiography: importance of color Doppler flow mapping. Pediatr Cardiol. 2001;22:327-32.
19. Lytrivi ID, Wong AH, Ko HH, et al. Echocardiographic diagnosis of clinically silent congenital coronary artery anomalies. Int J Cardiol. 2008;126:386-93.
20. Angelini P. Normal and anomalous coronary arteries: definitions and classification. Am Heart J. 1989;117:418-34.
21. Angelini P, Villason S, Chan AV, Diez JG. Normal and anomalous coronary arteries in humans. In: Angelini P (Ed). Coronary artery anomalies: a comprehensive approach. Philadelphia: Lippincott, Williams & Willkins; 1999. pp.27-150.
22. Angelini P, Velasco JA, Flamm S. Coronary anomalies: incidence, patho-physiology and clinical relevance. Circulation. 2002;105:2449-54.
23. Barriales-Villa R, Morís C, López-Muñiz A, Hernández LC, San Román L, Barriales V, et al. Anomalías congénitas de las arterias coronarias en el adulto descritas en 31 años de estudios coronariográficos en el Principado de Asturias: principales características angiográficas clínicas. Rev Esp Cardiol. 2001;54:269-81.
24. Kragel AH, Roberts WC. Anomalous origin of either the right or left main coronary artery from the aorta with subsequent coursing between aorta and pulmonary trunk: analysis of 32 necropsy cases. Am J Cardiol. 1988;62:771-7.
25. Cohen MS, Herlong RJ, Silverman NH, et al. Echocardiographic imaging of anomalous origin of the coronary arteries. Cardiol Young. 2010;20:26-34.
26. Walsh R, Nielsen JC, Ko HH, et al. Imaging congenital coronary artery anomalies. Pediatr Radiol. 2011;41:1526-35.
27. Gharib AM, Ho VB, Rosing DR, Herzka DA, Stuber M, Arai AE, Pettigrew RI. Coronary artery anomalies and variants: technical feasibility of assessment with coronary MR angiography at 3 T. Radiology. 2008;247:220-7.
28. Ten Kate GJ, Weustink AC, de Feyter PJ. Coronary artery anomalies detected by MSCT-coronary angiography in the adult. Neth Heart J. 2008;16:369-75.

29. Mikolich JR. Cardiac magnetic resonance imaging and coronary computed tomography angiography in the diagnosis of anomalous coronary artery. J Am Coll Cardiol. 2009;53:456.
30. Kang JW, Seo JB, Chae EJ, et al. Coronary artery anomalies: classification and electrocardiogram-gated multidetector computed tomographic findings. Semin Ultrasound CT MR. 2008;29:182-94.
31. Richard KM, Ralph AB, David CC, Simon HS, Guiding catheter selection for right coronary artery angioplasty. 1990;19:58-67.
32. Kaluski E, Solanki P, Sanchez-Ross M, et al. Anteriorly displaced right coronary artery in acute myocardial infarction: What should every cardiologist know? Cardiovasc Revascul Med. 2011;12(1):59-64.
33. Kern M. Anomalous coronary artery angiography made simple. Cath Lab Digest. 2013;21(12).
34. Spindola-Franco H, Grose R, Solomon N. Dual left anterior descending coronary artery: angiographic description of important variants and surgical implications. Am Heart J. 1983;105:445-55.
35. Manchanda A, Qureshi A, Brofferio A, Go D, Shirani J. Novel variant of dual left anterior descending coronary artery. J Cardiovasc Comput Tomogr. 2010;4:139-41.
36. Maroney J, Klein LW. Report of a new anomaly of the left anterior descendingartery: type VI dual LAD. Catheter Cardiovasc Inter2011; (September) http://dx.doi.org/10.1002/ccd.23219 .
37. Kosar F. An unusual case of double anterior descending artery originating from the left and right coronary arteries. Heart Vessels. 2006;21:385-7.
38. Kheirkhah J, Sadeghipour P, Kouchaki A. An anomalous origin of left anterior descending coronary artery from right coronary artery in a patient with acute coronary syndrome. Tehran Heart Cent. 2011;6(4):217-9.
39. Serota H, Barth CW, Seuc CA, Vandormael M, Aguirre F, Kern MJ. Rapid identification of the course of anomalous coronary arteries: the "dot and eye" method. Am J Cardiol. 1990;65:891-8.
40. Nguyen, Thanh M, et al. Stenting of atherosclerotic stenoses in anomalously arising coronary arteries. The Journal of Invasive Cardiology. 2004;16(5):283-6.
41. Jaffe Ronen, et al. Primary stenting of an anomalous left main coronary artery with an interarterial course during cardiac arrest imaging with CT angiography. Circulation: Cardiovascular Imaging. 2009;2(4):351-2.
42. Rahman SU, Wesarg S, Völker W. Patient specific optimal catheter selection for right coronary artery, Proceedings of SPIE Medical Imaging 2011, Florida, USA.
43. Lipton MJ, Barry WH, Obrez I, Silverman JF, Wexler L. Isolated single coronary artery: diagnosis, angiographic classification, and clinical significance. Radiology. 1979;130:39-47.
44. Ozeren A, Ates I, Karabag T. Successful stenting of all three branches in a patient with single anomalous coronary artery arising from the left sinus of valsalva: A case report. International Journal of Case Reports and Images. 2012;3(7):19-22.
45. Mishra TK, Mishra CK, Das B. Percutaneous coronary intervention in a patient with single coronary artery. Indian Heart Journal. 2014;66(3):382-5. doi:10.1016/j.ihj.2014.03.011.
46. Quintal R, Nguyen T, Glancy LD. Successful percutaneous coronary angioplasty via solitary ostium in the aorta (single coronary artery) J Invasive Cardiol. 2003;8:446-7. [PubMed]
47. Devidutta S1, Sharma G, Jagia P Coronary stenting in a patient with single coronary artery and double-vessel disease. J Invasive Cardiol. 2013;25(7):E147-50.
48. Ohta H, Sumiyoshi M, Suwa S, et al. Primary coronary angioplasty with stenting for acute coronary syndrome in patients with isolated single coronary artery: A report of 2 cases. JPN Heart J. 2003;44:759-65.
49. Akdeniz B, Gölddeli Ö, Güneri S, Baris N. Percutaneous coronary intervention in a patient with a single right coronary artery: A case report and review of the literature. Int J Angiol. 2007; 16(2):66-8.
50. Chan CN, Berland J, Cribier A, Letac B. Angioplasty of the right coronary artery with origin of all three coronary arteries from a single ostium in the right sinus of Valsalva. Am Heart J. 1993;126:985-7.
51. Baljepally RM, Pollock SH, Magram MY. Transluminal angioplasty of a single coronary artery anomaly during acute myocardial infarction - a case report. Angiology. 1993;44: 981-4.
52. Grenadier E, Beyar R, Amikam S, Markiewicz W. Two-vessel PTCA of single anomalous coronary artery. Am Heart J. 1992;123:220-2.
53. Lawton J, McGrath J, Jones JS, Dehmer GJ. Treatment of coronary artery disease in an anomalous coronary artery by placement of an intracoronary stent. Cathet Cardiovasc Diagn. 1997;41: 185-8.
54. Zweiker R, Luha O, Klein WW. Rescue percutaneous transluminal coronary angioplasty in a patient with a single coronary artery arising from the right Sinus Valsalva: Previously unreported scenario and review of literature. J Intern Med. 2002;252: 84-7.
55. Nath A, Kennett JD, Politte LL, Sanfelippo JF, Alpert MA. Anomalous right coronary artery arising from the midportion of the left anterior descending coronary artery—case reports. Angiology. 1987;38:142-6.
56. Hughes MM. Anomalous origin of the right coronary artery from the left anterior descending coronary artery. Cathet Cardiovasc Diagn. 1997;42:308-9.
57. Amasyali B, Kursakliogluk H, Kose S, Iyisoy A, Kilic A, Isik E. Single coronary artery with anomalous origin of the right coronary artery from the left anterior descending artery with a unique proximal course. JPN Heart J. 2004;45:521-5.
58. Biffani G, Lioy E, Loschiavo P, Parma A. Single coronary artery, anomalous origin of the right coronary artery from the left anterior descending artery. Eur Heart J. 1991;12: 1326-9.
59. Abdou SM, Wu CJ. Treatment of aortocoronary dissection complicating anomalous origin right coronary artery and chronic total intervention with intravascular ultrasound guided stenting. Catheter Cardiovasc Interv. 2011;78:914-9.
60. Judkins MP. Percutaneous transfemoral selective coronary angiography. Radiol Clin North Am. 1968;6(3):467-92.

PART 2: CALCIFIC CORONARIES

"By failing to prepare, you are preparing to fail"
–Benjamin Franklin

BACKGROUND

"Clots, calcification and chronic total occlusion are the bane for intervention cardiologist". Calcification in the coronary artery (CAC) indicates the advanced stage of coronary artery disease. CAC invites more adverse events in natural history, intervention and surgery.[1-6] Percutaneous coronary intervention (PCI) in calcified coronaries poses a unique challenge. A high rate of procedural failure is unavoidable. Despite the committed attempt to yield a calcified plaque, it results in inadequate dilatation and its related family of problems like dissection, perforation, stent under-expansion, no reflow or slow flow due to distal embolization, stent thrombosis and restenosis.[6,7] Although plaque modification by modern devices and the use of drug-eluting stents have modestly improved outcomes in calcified vessels, adverse event rates are still high.[6-9] Innovation in plaque modifying devices will key to future improvement in dealing with heavily calcified lesion in coronary artery as the surgeons would continue to struggle for a beauty spot to connect graft but with worse outcome.[5,10]

DEFINITION OF CAC

Calcification in the coronary artery calcium (CAC) in vivo by fluoroscopy was first detected in 1950s[11] and an association between the CAC and the risk of cardiovascular events was first described in 1980.[12] Calcification on angiography is defined as the readily apparent densities noted within the vascular wall at the site of the stenosis with or without positive remodelling. Angiographic CAC is often classified into 3 groups: none or mild, moderate, and severe. Severe calcification is most commonly defined as radiopacities in the wall of coronary artery under fluoroscope in still images without contrast opacification (Fig. 22.20). The dense calcification of arterial wall is usually concentric. Moderate calcification is seen as radiopacities only in scenes or loops, i.e. with cardiac motion but without contrast opacification.[13,14] Committee on Vascular Lesions, American Heart Association (AHA) 1995 has labelled calcified coronary as type V—significant calcification is type Vb and little calcium is type Vc.[15]

EPIDEMIOLOGY

The male gender and elderly have more predilections for calcific lesions in coronary artery. More than 90% of men and >67% of women older than 70 years of age have significant calcific coronary artery.[9,16] The prevalence of CAC in patients undergoing PCI ranges from 17% in randomized trials to 35% in real-world populations. In ACUITY and HORIZONS-AMI trials, moderate or severe calcification was noted in 29.4% undergoing PCI. The incidence of moderate to dense CAC in patients undergoing PCI for non-ST elevation acute coronary syndrome (NSTEACS) and ST elevation myocardial infarction (STEMI) were approximately 27% and 38% respectively.[17]

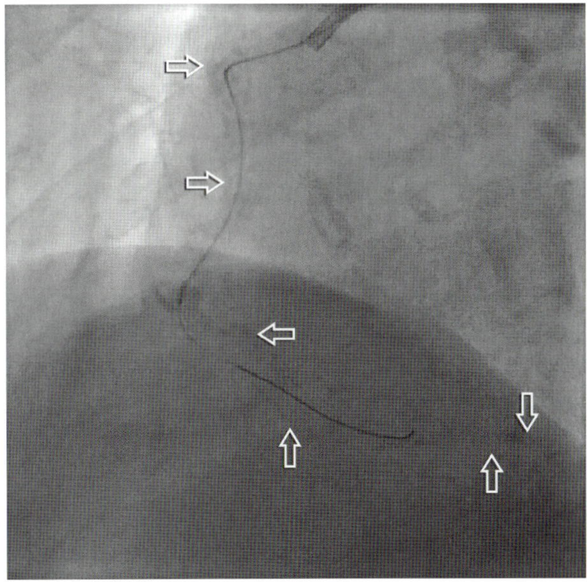

Fig. 22.20 Fluoroscope during coronary intervention shows dense calcification in right coronary artery in its entire length which is apparent in still image without contrast injection, marked by arrows

PATHOPHYSIOLOGY AND RISK FACTORS

The two types of CAC are intimal and medial calcification. Intimal calcification is predominantly atherosclerotic, while medial calcification is associated with advanced age, diabetes, and chronic kidney disease.[18,19] Both are associated with increased risk for adverse events. The extent of CAC correlates with plaque burden and severity of stenosis but there may be positive remodeling of vessel in early stages.[20] Microcalcifications in the fibrous cap predispose to plaque rupture due to the incremental shearing stress.[21] Calcific nodules disrupt the fibrous cap and promote thrombosis. The repeated cycles of plaque rupture and healing result in the development of obstructive fibrocalcific lesions, commonly seen in patients with stable angina and sudden cardiac death due to acute coronary syndrome.[22] Sometimes, the dense underlying calcification poses indomitable challenge during PCI even in ACS.

DETECTION OF CORONARY CALCIFICATION

Conventional coronary angiogram (CAG), computed tomography (CT), intravascular ultrasound (IVUS) and optical coherence tomography (OCT) are the methods for detection and quantification of coronary calcium. The angiographic visualization or perception of coronary calcification and its severity is dealt in the definition. The different diagnostic modalities and their advantages or disadvantages are mentioned in Table 22.9.

PERCUTANEOUS INTERVENTION IN CALCIFIED ARTERIES

Interventional cardiologist would face more calcific coronary lesion in future because of the aging population.[30,31] PCI in a calcified lesion is deterrent due to significant adverse events during and following intervention in both acute coronary syndrome and chronic CAD. Of note, the 1-year follow-up result of pivotal ORBIT II[32] study shines a new hope.

Table 22.9 Diagnostic modalities for detection of coronary calcium (CAC)

Diagnostic modality	*Comment*
CT Angiogram	The best for screening CAC High sensitivity and specificity Reasonable for cardiovascular risk assessment in either asymptomatic or symptomatic patient[23,24]
Conventional coronary angiogram	Low-moderate sensitivity High specificity (high positive predictive value) for detection of CAC[25]
Intravascular ultrasound (IVUS)	90–100% sensitive 99–100% specific[26] Calcified plaque appears as bright echo with acoustic shadowing[27] Location and extent of calcification can be graded (color code) *Superficial calcium:* Intimal-luminal interface *Deep calcium:* Medial-adventitial border (or closer to the adventitial than lumen), Both superficial and deep
Optical coherence tomography (OCT)	Calcification appears as low-intensity and low attenuation areas with sharp borders[28] Sensitivity of 95–100% Specificity of 97–100% Resolution is higher Assess calcium thickness and measure calcium volume[29]

Optimal Assessment of Lesion

The crux to select the optimal strategy for calcified lesions is the accurate assessment of the lesion morphology. IVUS or OCT or both may supplement angiography during procedure. Both the tests inform better than coronary angiogram regarding the extent and density of calcification, response of calcific plaque to plaque medication tools and complication. Calcification increases the diameter of vessels with less than 50% stenosis but larger chunk of calcium shrinks the vessel diameter. The fact should be borne in mind while selecting and sizing the devices.

Vascular Access and Arterial Sheath

Assessment of calcific lesion, lesion preparation and delivery of stent in the target lesion need a **3D** protocol consisting of **D**iscipline (experience), **D**evices (dedicated hardware) and **D**aringness. A 6 Fr guide catheter is the minimum that is required.[33] Transfemoral approach is wide accepted. Despite the initial hiccups, transradial has gained momentum and has almost replaced transfemoral approach. The backup support is mainly a mechanics of the catheter than the approach.[34,35] PCI of calcified lesions can be safely and effectively done via transradial approach using 6 Fr, 7 Fr or sheath-less hydrophilic guide catheter.

Guide Catheter

A good backup support is imperative. In the left coronary, good guiding catheter support can be achieved with a guide with passive back-up. Usually extra backup (EBU; Medtronic), XB (Cordis) or Voda (Boston Scientific) is sufficient. Some cases may need Amplatzer guide. In the right coronary artery, excellent support can be achieved with the left Amplatzer family of catheters in cases which right Judkin's guide fails.

Active Backup Maneuvers

Anchor wire or balloon technique is frequently used to improve support for forward advancement of the hardware.

- *Anchor wire technique:* If there is a reasonable sized side branch proximal to the occlusion, a second wire in the side branch supports the guide (Fig. 22.21).
- *Anchor balloon technique:* A balloon over a second wire is parked in the side branch proximal to the occlusion with low inflation to support a stable position of the guiding

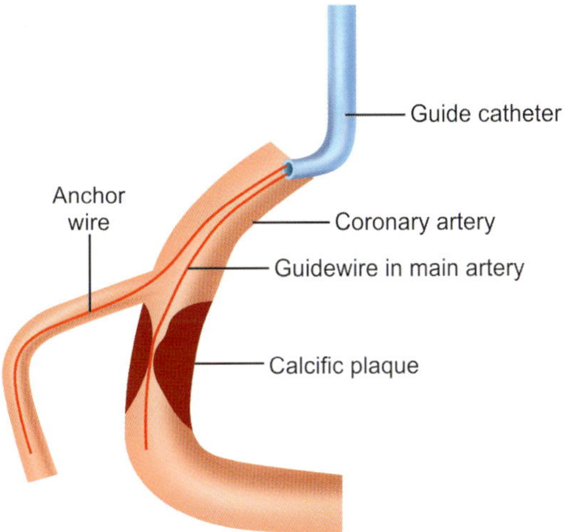

Fig. 22.21 Anchor wire technique

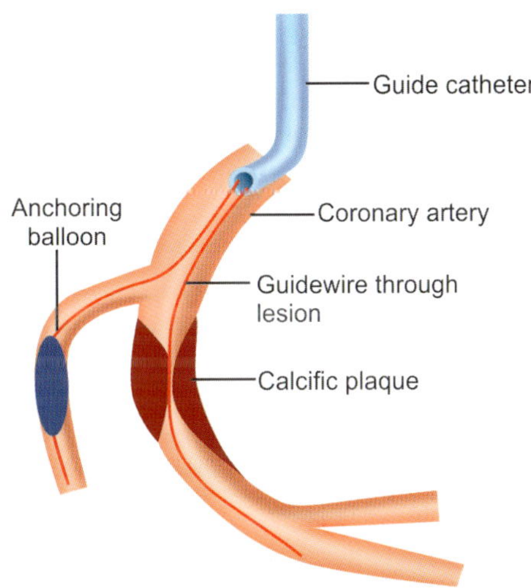

Fig. 22.22 Anchor balloon technique

catheter. The guide is pushed over the balloon shaft to enable deeper engagement, with an eye for dissection during maneuvering (Fig. 22.22).

Guidewire

The guidewire of choice is not strict. The two groups of wires usually used for calcified lesion are polymer-coated and coil wires. It is ideal to start with a soft tip wire and later changing to harder and stiffer wire if needed.

- *Polymer coated wires:* Hydrophilic, and thus have better penetrability. However, they are limited by the risk of subluminal plane entry and false lumen, long dissections or perforations in inexperienced hand.
- *Coil wires:* They are known for their torquability and pushability. Torquability is more with stiffer wires, and so are the chances of creating false channel.
  - *Tapered tip wires (e.g. Conquest or Crossit)*: Greater chances of entering microchannels.
  - *Stiffer coil wires (Crossit 300–400/Miracle 9, 12 g/ Persuader)*: Increased penetration at the cost of false lumen.

Preparation of Lesion

Two types of devices are used to yield the lesion:

1. *Plaque modification devices/Atherotomy devices:* Used for mild to moderate calcified lesions.
   - Simple/cutting or scoring balloon
   - FX MiniRail.
2. *Debulking devices/Atherectomy devices:* For densely calcified lesions
   - Rotational atherectomy
   - Excimer laser
   - Orbital atherectomy.

CUTTING BALLOON ANGIOPLASTY

Cutting balloon (CB) is a non-compliant balloon catheter with 3–4 microsurgical blades or atherotomes mounted longitudinally on its outer surface.[36] The atherotomes (microsurgical blades), are 3–5 times sharper than conventional surgical blades, measure 10 or 15 mm in length by 0.011–0.013" in height by 0.004–0.006" in width, and are mounted along the length of the cutting balloon. When the balloon is inflated, the blades align radially and deliver longitudinal incisions in the plaque and vessel. Balloon sizes of 2.00–3.25 mm are provided with 3 atherotomes; those of 3.50–4.00 mm have 4 atherotomes. The cutting balloon was first designed by Barath et al.[37] and at present the Flexitome Cutting Balloon (Boston Scientific Corp., Natick, Massachusetts) is available in market (Figs 22.23A to D).

Mechanism of Action

Cutting and scoring balloons do not remove calcium. They improve vessel compliance by creating discrete incisions in the atherosclerotic plaque. This controlled cutting and scoring of the plaque enables greater lesion expansion and reducing recoil while preventing uncontrolled dissections. In contrast to conventional balloon, there is limited vessel injury and stretch.

Procedural Tips

Cutting balloon can be delivered over any guidewire through a 6–7 F sheath. A 6 Fr sheath suffices for a balloon size of 3.25 mm or less, the rest require larger sheaths. Sizing the CB

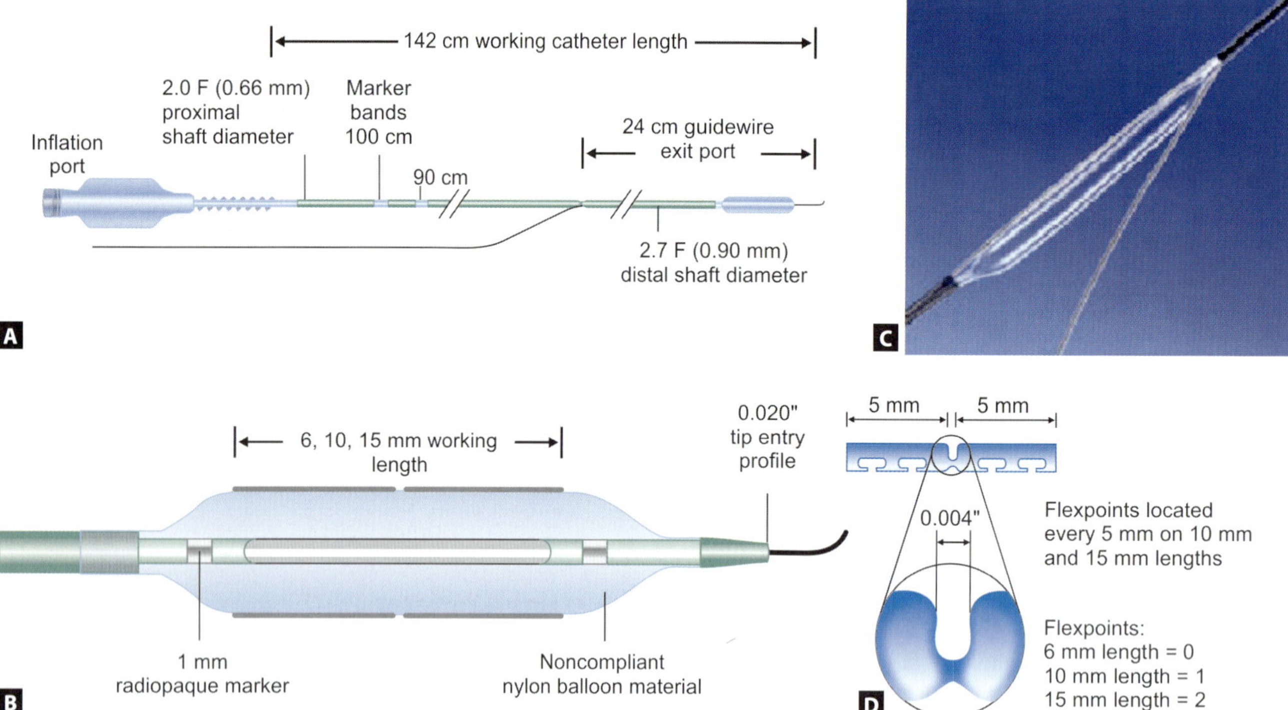

Figs 22.23A to D Flexitome cutting balloon device: (A) Monorail system; (B) Cutting balloon; (C) 3d image; (D) Cross-section of balloon showing atherotomes arrangement

Source: Boston Scientific Corp., Natick, Massachusetts

is the most critical step and ideally the balloon-to-artery ratio should be 1:1. Slow inflation (nominal pressure of 4–6 atm for 60–90 sec) and deflation is recommended. Higher pressures of 10–12 atm may be required in eccentric lesions.

Efficacy

Randomized controlled trials of CBA versus simple balloon angioplasty[38-41] have shown similar restenosis rate and major adverse cardiac events (MACE) with CBA as with simple balloon angioplasty. However, myocardial infarction and vessel perforation were more common with CBA.

Indications

Cutting balloon angioplasty is safe and yields acceptable result in mild calcific lesions as an adjunct to simple balloon angioplasty.[42] It is favored in ISR, bifurcations, aorta-ostial lesions and saphenous vein graft lesions and has received ESC approval for use in ISR.

Present Role in Treatment of Calcific Coronaries

The CBA is useful only in mild calcification to prepare the lesion before stent deployment. It fails to find a place in routine cathlabs for the treatment of calcific coronary lesions due to its bulky nature. It is reserved for difficult situations where controlled dilatation is expected to yield better results than plain balloon dilatation. In recent years, CBA is regaining momentum as ROTACUT prior to DES implantations. Small studies have shown it to be superior to the conventional approach with RA and a plain balloon in terms of optimal stent expansion.[43] However, randomized trials are required to confirm.

The FX MiniRail

The FX MiniRail™ catheter (Abbott Laboratories Inc., Abbott Park, Illinois) is a scoring balloon of unique design (Fig. 22.24). It has an integral wire positioned external to a dilating balloon, and a short, 12-mm guidewire lumen distal to the balloon. When the device is threaded over the guidewire, the steerable guidewire remains outside of the balloon. The balloon inflates against the external wires which prevent slippage, and introduce high focal stresses longitudinally along the luminal surface of the lesion at low inflation pressures. This is a low profile, 6 F guide compatible system. The distal guidewire lumen facilitates rapid, single operator exchanges.[44]

Present role in calcific lesion angioplasty: This is no longer used in treatment of CAC as no benefit has been demonstrated. It may have some role in in-stent restenosis.

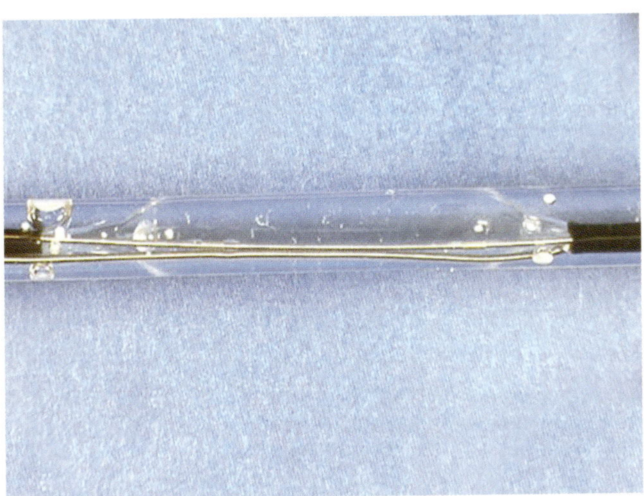

Fig. 22.24 FX MiniRail RX PTCA Catheter represents an innovative approach to dilatation. Its unique, dual-wire design concentrates stress along the two wires to create expansion planes at low inflation pressures, facilitating dilatation of challenging lesions like calcific lesion, very tight lesion and in-stent restenosis
Source: Abbott Laboratories Inc., Abbott Park, Illinois

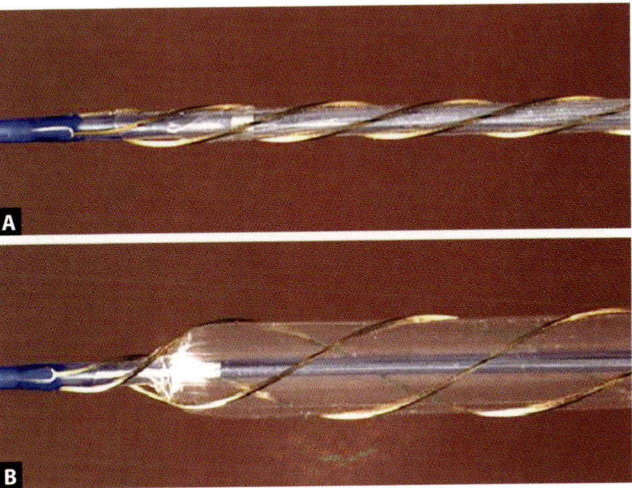

Figs 22.25A and B The Angiosculpt™ scoring balloon catheter (AngioScore, Fremont, CA) showing three rectangular scoring wires that spiral around the longitudinal axis of a semi-compliant balloon. (A) Deflated balloon; (B) Inflated balloon

The Angiosculpt

The Angiosculpt™ scoring balloon catheter (AngioScore, Fremont, CA) is a modified version of the cutting balloon technique.[45,46] It has three rectangular scoring wires that spiral around the longitudinal axis of a semi-compliant balloon (Figs 22.25A and B). Balloon inflation focuses uniform radial forces along the edges of the nitinol element, thus scoring the plaque in a more precise manner. Angiosculpt balloons are lower profile (2.7F), and 0.014" system compatible with 6F guiding catheters. It is more flexible given the spiral arrangement of scoring wires with two radiopaque markers at the working ends of the scoring balloon. It is capable of creating more scoring marks per millimeter (mm) of plaque. It is designed to achieve higher nominal and burst pressures (as high as 20 atm) suited for calcified and circumferential plaque.

Present Role

It has been used successfully in treating fibro-calcific, bifurcation and ostial lesions. In mild-to-moderate calcific lesions, it can be lesion preparation prior to stenting. However, its fame has faded after the introduction of debulking devices and newer generation of coronary stents.

PLAIN BALLOON ANGIOPLASTY

Plain balloon angioplasty in non-compliant calcific lesions is associated with more complications.[47-51] Acute luminal gain is not satisfactory predisposing to high restenosis rates (Figs 22.26A to D). The resulted decrease in vascular compliance is in the explanation for higher rates of dissection, and acute vessel closure.

Present Role in Calcific Lesion Angioplasty

It could be the procedure of choice in less calcific vessel angioplasty. Procedural success varies from 74% to 92%. The issues with plain balloon preparation prior to stenting are mentioned in Table 22.10.

Bare Metal Stents or Drug-eluting Stents

Drug-eluting stents (DES) is superior to bare metal stents (BMS) in calcified lesions. Less neointimal hyperplasia after DES implantation reduces angiographic late loss, restenosis, and repeat revascularization.[47-51] Moreover, similar rates of stent thrombosis are seen with DES and BMS in calcified lesions, with comparable rates of death and MI.[52-55] Greater rates of restenosis and repeat revascularization in DES-treated calcified compared with non-calcified lesions[56] could be explained by under expansion and laceration induced aggressive neointimal formation.

Atherectomy Devices

"The cardinal indication for plaque modification is the calcific lesion, which in the absence of plaque modification confers an

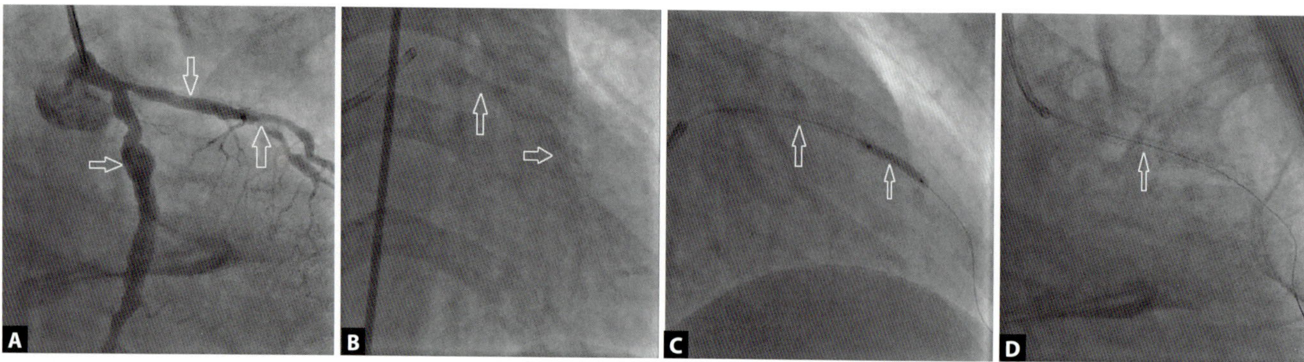

Figs 22.26A to D (A) RAO-Coronary angiogram of LAD in RAO-caudal view with significant focal stenosis in mid-LAD with dense calcium in proximal and mid-LAD. Mild to moderate calcification of LCx with positive remodeling of apparent as marked by yellow arrow; (B) Calcification LAD is apparent under fluoroscope; (C) Balloon dilatation of LAD as preparation to stent; (D) Mild persistent under expansion of stent after noncompliant balloon dilatation post-stenting

Table 22.10 Problems encountered are in plain angioplasty and their solutions

Problem encountered	*Recommended maneuver*
Balloon may slip while dilating	Use a longer balloon, keep tug on balloon
Balloon inflations fails	Plan Rota before second attempt
Coronary dissection	Stent only when dissection is flow limiting. Consider rota before bail-out stenting

increased risk of procedural failure, stent under deployment, restenosis and other major adverse cardiovascular events."

Moussa I et al

DIRECTIONAL ATHERECTOMY

Directional atherectomy (DA) is used to excise atherosclerotic plaque with an instrumented directional coronary atherectomy (DCA) catheter.

Description of Device

The original DCA catheter, "The Atherocath" is equipped with a rotating cutter affixed to an elastic drive shaft, encased in a cylindrical stainless steel housing (Figs 22.27A and B).

Mechanism of Action

The cutter contacts the plaque through a small window located in the housing. An inflated balloon (lower pressures than balloon angioplasty <50 psi) located opposite the cutting window holds the catheter in place and pushes the plaque into the cutting window. During the procedure, the cutter begins on the proximal side of the window and is advanced across the occlusion distally, shaving away at the plaque and pushing the debris into the collecting chamber of the nose cone.

Present Role

Directional coronary atherectomy became the first of the "new" percutaneous, catheter-based devices approved for the treatment of coronary disease was quickly and enthusiastically embraced by the interventional community. The CAVEAT and CCAT[57,58] showed unexpected poor performance with DCA though BOAT[59] was encouraging. A high incidence of perforation (1%), death and MI were described. DCA suffered a major blow after introduction of coronary stents. DA is now history as the only device (Flexicut by Abbott vascular) had been withdrawn. Five modified generations of the original device have been described but none succeeded. Though FDA approved it in 1990, it failed to find its place in present day cath lab due to its bulky nature and increased risk of complications.

ROTATIONAL ATHERECTOMY

The year 2012 marks the 25th anniversary of the introduction of rotational atherectomy (RA) in the treatment of obstructive coronary artery disease.

Mechanism of Action

Rotational atherectomy (RA) is consigned to prepare severely calcified plaque. In 1980, David Auth invented this device and presently it is popularized as Rotablator (SCIMED) by Boston scientific corporation. It works on the principle of differential cutting. RA ablates non-compliant tissue (i.e. calcified or fibrotic lesions) and spares elastic tissue (i.e. non-calcified or non-fibrotic vessels). "Rota leaks elastic but bites

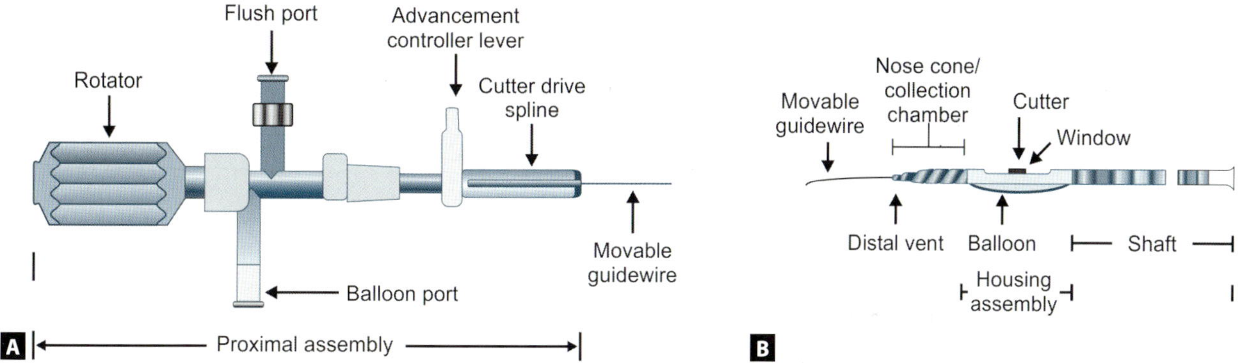

Figs 22.27A and B (A) Sketch diagram of the original Atherocath; (B) The cutter

inelastic calcific plaque". The orthogonal displacement of burr facilitates easy forward movement and avoids injury to rota wire and vessel wall. The plaque content is pulverized to microparticles (5–10 μm) and removed from microcirculation by reticuloendothelial system.

Indication

It is indicated in severe calcific lesion.[2] RA facilitates procedural success in PCI of complex lesions (ACC/AHA types B2 and C),[60,61] including chronic total occlusions,[62,63] ostial lesions[64,65] and bifurcation lesions. The long-term follows up result of RA is favorable in cases of chronic total occlusions,[66] bifurcation lesions[67,68] and side branch ostia, alone or in combination with the main vessel stenting.[69]

Contraindication

A large plaque or thrombus burden is a contraindication like in saphenous vein grafts and acute coronary syndrome.

Bare Metal Stents or Drug-eluting Stents

Acute luminal gain is lost due to restenosis when BMS is used after rota.[70,71] Therefore, DES is preferred after ablation for better long-term outcomes.[72] The ROTAXUS trial (Rotational Atherectomy Prior to Taxus Stent Treatment for Complex Native Coronary Artery Disease) was performed to determine whether lesion preparation with RA before paclitaxel-eluting stent (PES) implantation provides benefits compared with PES with balloon pre-dilation alone in calcified lesions.[73] Prepare with RA followed by stent in this study shows better immediate outcomes (92.5% versus 83.3%; p = 0.03). However, despite an early acute lumen gain advantage with RA, 9-month angiographic follow-up revealed higher late loss in the RA group. Rates of restenosis, TLR, definite stent thrombosis, and MACE were not significantly different between the groups.

Present Role

Over the past decade, rotational atherectomy has fallen out of favor primarily due to improved stent delivery systems enabling interventionalist to successfully stent lesions that would previously not be amenable to stenting (including those that are calcified). In recent times, the use of this device has been revisited with a focus on its role in modifying calcified lesions prior to deployment of drug-eluting stents (Figs 22.28A to D).

In the current practice, RA is used to prepare calcified lesions before stent implantation (Class IIa, Level of Evidence: C).[74] Reasonable experience, improvement in technique, smaller size burr and proper guiding catheters and fewer catheter exchanges limit complications. Transradial arterial access is also acceptable. Additional studies are required to determine the extent of calcification that necessitates RA before stenting. Table 22.11 shows the tips and tricks in successful rotablation and Table 22.12 mentions the recommended guide catheter for the burr size selected.

EXCIMER LASER CORONARY ATHERECTOMY

Laser energy to debulk the atheromatous plaque was introduced in 1980s and received FDA approval in 1992. The application of laser energy to the vessel results in photochemical, photomechanical, photothermic interactions that produce gas vapor and acoustic shock waves within the plaque to debulk it (Figs 22.29A to C). However, the initial lasers resulted in deep vascular and mechanical injury and are no longer used.

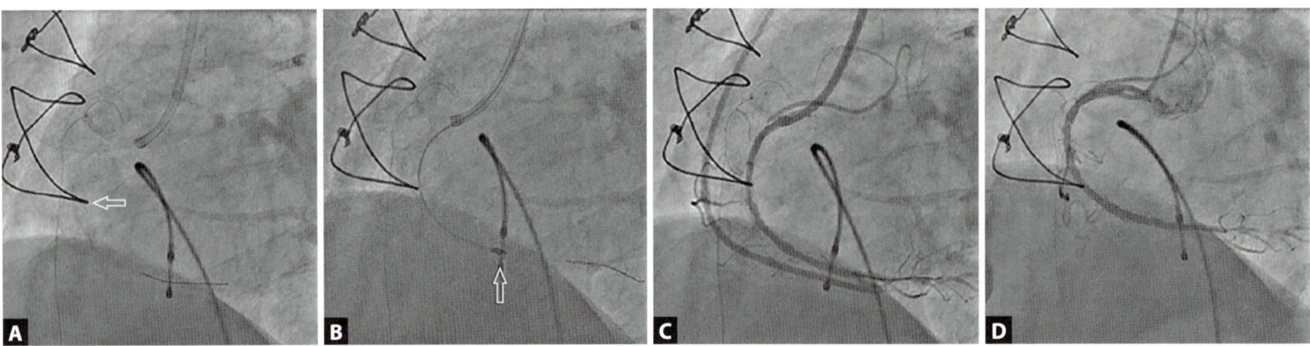

Figs 22.28A to D (A) Densely calcified right coronary artery apparent under fluoroscope with still image; (B) Rota burr marked by yellow arrow; (C) Result of rota ablation; (D) Final result of after stenting

Table 22.11 Rotablation: Tips and tricks

Rotablator assembly	Ensure flush system pressure bag > 200 mm Hg turned to full capacity Weeping of saline through seals of advancer is normal Always verify that driveshaft is correctly locked and connected to advancer
Rotablator wire	If a rota wire does not cross the lesion, a conventional wire and microcatheter are used to exchange for rota wire Beware of wire loops Be careful of wire tips When the brake is defeated, wire rotation has to be fixed with a wire clip and tip of rota wire seen on the screen
Dynaglide	Not recommended for advancement as rotational speed does not fall when resistance is met
Burr advancement	Relieve driveshaft and wire tension
Wire bias (divergence from central axis of vessel)	Respect possibility of neo-lumen perforation especially with tortuosity
Optimum conditions for rotational atherectomy technique	Single burr with burr to artery ratio of 0.5–0.6 Pecking motion instead of forceful advancement Rotational speed—140,000–150,000 Short abrasion runs of 15–20 sec Deceleration > 5,000 rpm should be avoided

Table 22.12 Guide catheter requirement for intended RA burr size

Rotablator burr size	*Large lumen guide size*
1.25 mm	5/6 Fr
1.50 mm	6 Fr
1.75 mm	7 Fr
2.00 mm	8 Fr
2.15 mm	8 Fr
2.25 mm	9 Fr
2.38 mm	9 Fr
2.50 mm	9 Fr

Excimer Laser (acronym for excited dimer, where in halogen gas is used as excited medium) with fibro-optic ultraviolet laser light delivery has proved of incremental safety. While the older generation devices operated in the infrared field (λ = 2090 nm), excimer laser coronary atherectomy (ECLA) operates in the ultraviolet field (λ = 308 nm), which minimizes vapor bubble formation.

Mechanism of Action

Excimer laser coronary atherectomy works by photoablation (vaporization) of tissue.[75] It is applied using a catheter that contains optical fibers and transmits pulses of ultraviolet light at

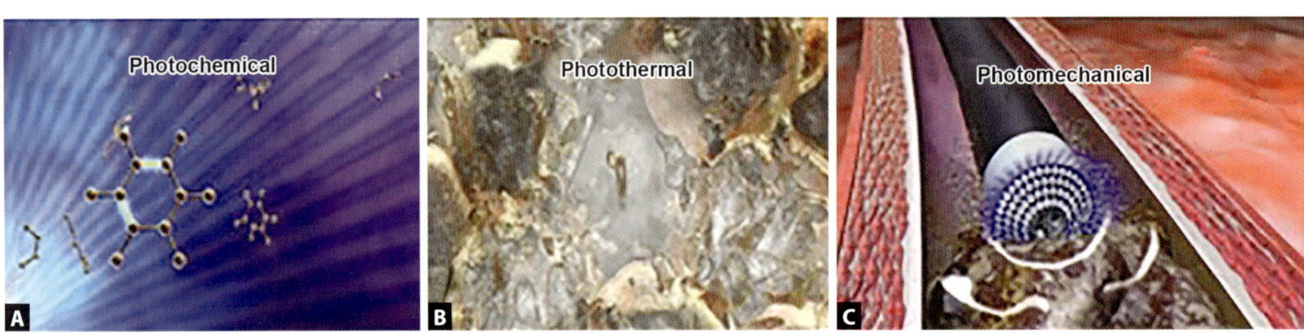

Figs 22.29A to C Mechanism of action of Laser on coronary plaque

308 nm from a Laser system to the target coronary obstruction. The ultraviolet pulses penetrate into 50 μm of tissue and cause photothermal and photochemical dissociation of carbon-carbon bonds in the cells contained within the coronary lesion. Photothermal energy generates molecular vibrations leading to the repeated breakdown of cells. This action causes water vaporization and a subsequent vapor bubble at the tip of the catheter, which amplifies plaque ablation through a photomechanical effect. The degradation particles are tiny, <10 μm (red blood cell size) and are wash out into the microcirculation. The magnitude and degree of photoablation depends on the energy and pulse repetition settings controlled at the Laser console. ELCA can vaporize plaque in complex coronary anatomy containing fibrous tissue, calcium, soft atheroma, or thrombus.

Procedural Details

The Spectranetics CVX-300 ELCA system (Spectranetics, Colorado Springs, Colorado) consists of the generator console, the Laser catheter and the activating pedal (Figs 22.30A to C). The catheter is available in 0.9-mm, 1.4-mm, 1.7-mm, and 2.0-mm diameters with specifications as provided in Table 22.13.

Ideally, the ELCA catheter size should be two-thirds of the size of the target vessel. The lesion is crossed with a coronary guidewire and the Laser catheter is then slowly advanced across the lesion. The Laser catheter provides energy during advancement and retraction of the catheter hence both should be performed slowly to optimize energy delivery. Continuous saline injection (though a pressured saline bag connected via Tuohy Borst adapter) in the guide catheter while lasing should be performed. This minimizes complications by reducing the temperature and uncontrolled photomechanical damage in the coronary artery.

Clinical Studies

In nonrandomized studies, ELCA failed to demonstrate any dramatic improvement in outcome when compared to plain old balloon angioplasty (POBA) like rotational atherectomy alone. The Amsterdam-Rotterdam trial (AMRO), failed to demonstrate the superiority of ELCA over balloon angioplasty in lesions >10 mm in length, with comparable 6-month procedural success and complication rates.[76] The ERBAC (Excimer Laser, Rotational Atherectomy, and Balloon Angioplasty Comparison) study, comparing ELCA, rotablator, and balloon angioplasty in 620 patients with type B and C lesions, demonstrated procedural success of 84% with balloon angioplasty, 88% with ELCA, and 93% with rotablator, and clinical adverse event rates of 45%, 49%, and 53%, respectively.[77] In the ELCA group of ERBAC trial, 18.5% of lesions could not be crossed by the laser catheter and required crossover to POBA. ELCA might have a major role in ISR due to stent under-expansion. ELCA can be used to vaporize/modify the calcific-fibrotic plaque behind the stent which can be further dilated by a noncompliant balloon and ensure optimal stent deployment. The use of ELCA to treat stent under expansion was demonstrated in Ellement registry by Latib and colleagues.[78] The use of ELCA became limited to treatment of under expanded stent lesions.

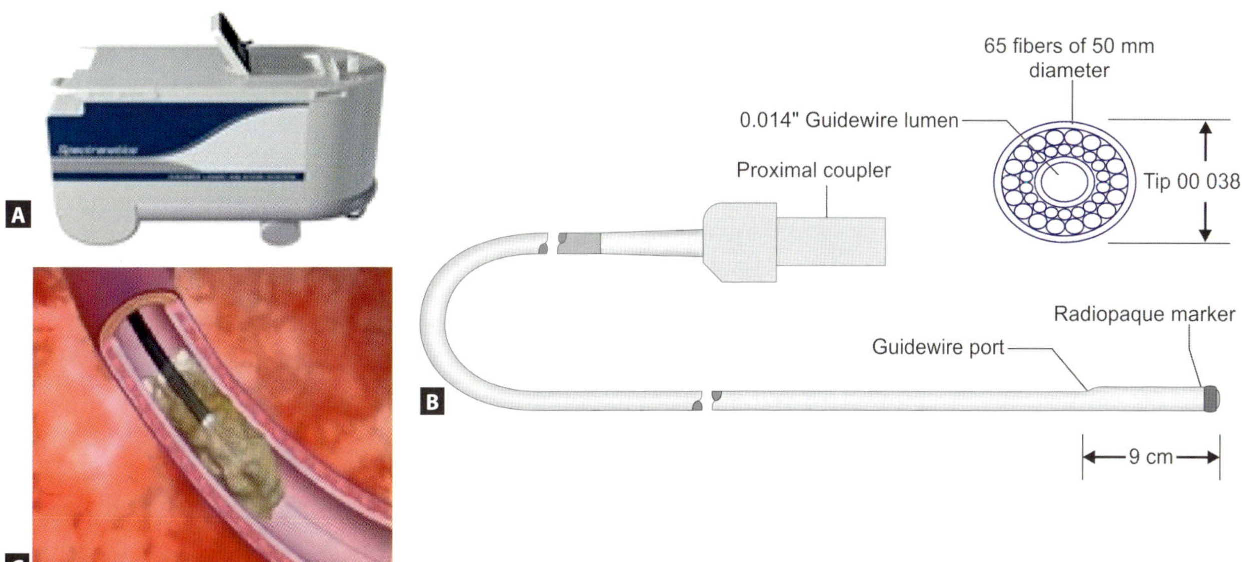

Figs 22.30A to C Spectranetics CVX-300 ELCA system (Spectranetics, Colorado Springs, Colorado)

Table 22.13 Technical specifications of the Spectranetics excimer Laser coronary atherectomy catheter system

Laser catheter	*0.99 mm*	*1.4 mm*	*1.7 mm*	*2.0 mm*	*0.9 mm OTW catheter*
Guide catheter compatibility	6 Fr	7 Fr	7 Fr	8 Fr	6 Fr
Minimum vessel diameter	1.5 mm	2.2 mm	2.5 mm	3.0 mm	1.5 mm
Fluence (mJ/mm^2)	30–60	30–60	30–60	30–60	30–60
Repetition rate (Hz)	25–40	25–40	25–40	25–40	25–40

These results were in part due to first-generation devices used without a developed saline flush technique during the Laser procedure. With the advent of the 0.9-mm Laser catheter and its higher fiber density, energy settings, and ablative power, subsequent registries have challenged this limited use. Bilodeau et al.[79] studied the use of the 0.9-mm Laser catheter in a prospective registry of 100 complex lesions, one-third of which had failed previous balloon angioplasty, one-third of which were CTOs, and 80% of which were calcified lesions. The investigators demonstrated a high Laser success rate of 92%, allowing for adjunctive therapy such as balloons and bare-metal stents in 93% of lesions.

Present Role of ELCA

The 2011 ACC/AHA/SCAI PCI guidelines recommend ELCA in fibrotic or moderately calcified lesions that cannot be crossed or dilated with conventional balloon angioplasty (class IIb).

Future Role

Laser may prove to be the preferred atherectomy device in vessels with up to moderate calcification, especially in the clinical setting of acute coronary syndrome, where there is thrombus-laden plaque and the potential for distal embolization. It may also have a special role in the treatment of STEMI, even in patients with hemodynamic instability and cardiogenic shock. Excimer Laser's unique properties permit dissolution of thrombus and plaque to particulate material (size of red blood cells), rapid clearance of thrombus and restoration of TIMI flow within the infarct-related artery with limited distal embolization. This helps to assess the true length of the lesion and favor shorter stent implantation. The stent is deployed in a less thrombotic milieu and reduce the incidence of malapposition and stent thrombosis. High-energy Laser parameters have been demonstrated in in vitro studies to decrease platelet aggregation and this antiplatelet effect could prove to be of additional benefit.[80]

Trials validating the safety and efficacy of Laser in AMI include CARMEL and Extended FAMILI. The CARMEL trial[81] enrolled 151 patients with AMI, including patients with cardiogenic shock, failed thrombolytic therapy, and occluded saphenous vein grafts (SVGs). The trial demonstrated Laser angiographic and procedural success rates of 97%, 95%, and 92%, respectively. The Extended FAMILI registry[82] studied the effects of excimer Laser in 100 AMI patients with respect to myocardial perfusion and ST-segment resolution and demonstrated an impressive rate of 92% in TIMI myocardial perfusion grade 2 and 3. Results from larger randomized studies evaluating the strategies of Laser/stenting in AMI (TAAMI study and GREECE study) may through more light on the role of ELCA in acute MI.

ORBITAL ATHERECTOMY SYSTEM

DIAMONDBACK 360® Coronary Orbital Atherectomy System (OAS; Cardiovascular Systems, Inc., St. Paul, Minnesota) was approved in October 21, 2013, by the US FDA in the treatment of calcified coronary lesions.

Mechanism of Action

The orbital atherectomy system (OAS) works on the principle of optimal use of centrifugal forces and differential sanding wherein the plaque is ablation and the healthy tissue is flexed away, similar to RA.

Device Description

The system consists of a diamond-coated crown (Figs 22.31A to C), which orbits over the atherectomy guide wire in an elliptical path. The Viper guidewire is included in the system. The crown is available in 1.25-mm and 1.5-mm sizes, with a maximum orbit that is influenced by the rotational speed of the crown (1.82 mm and 2.16 mm for each, respectively). Position of the crown within the vessel is controlled via a control handle.

Procedural Details

The OAS is passes over the viper guidewire across the lesion. A Viper Slide lubricant is continuously infused in addition to saline to provide lubrication, cooling, and

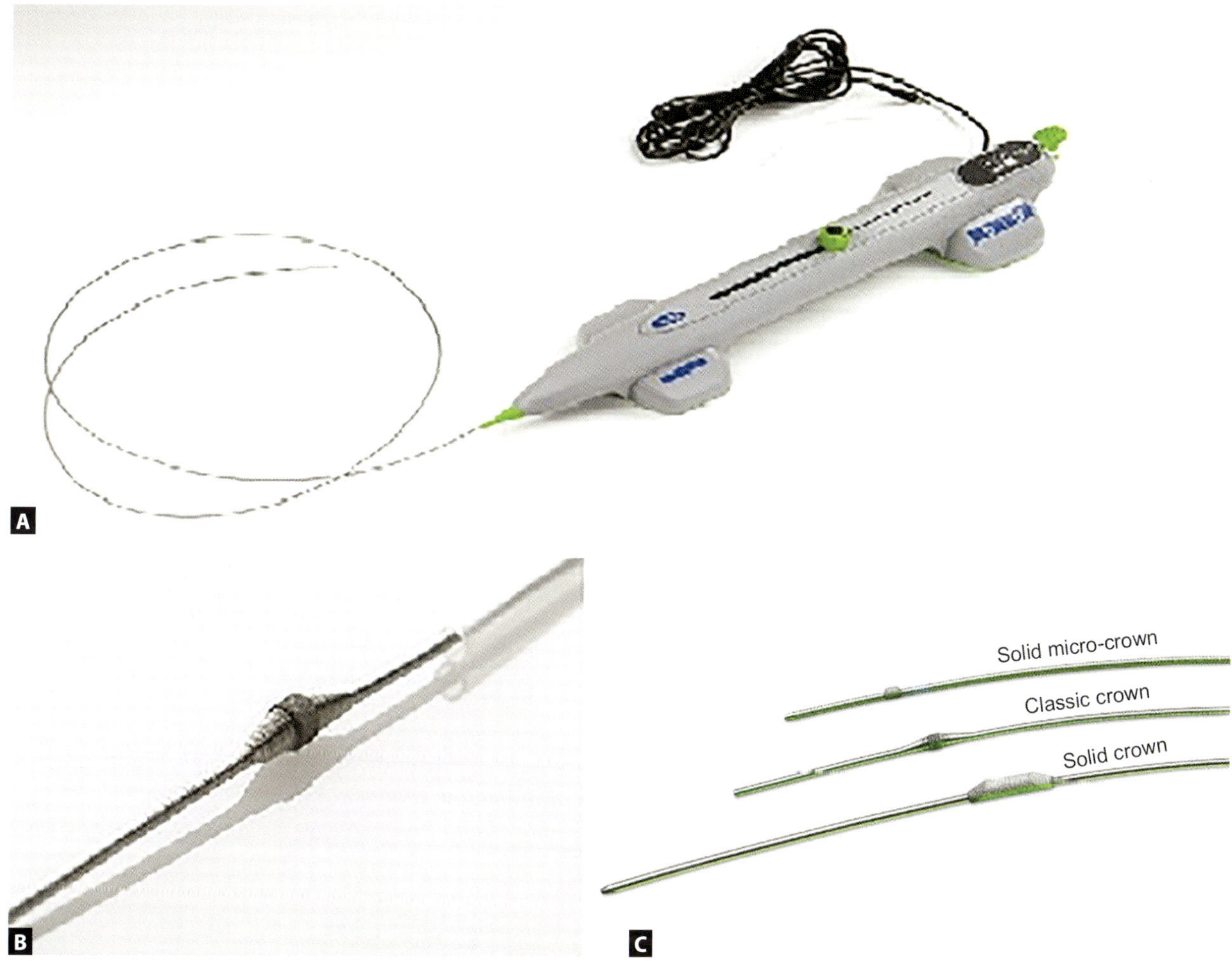

Figs 22.31A to C OAS system. (A) DIAMONDBACK 360® Coronary Orbital Atherectomy System (OAS; Cardiovascular Systems, Inc., St. Paul, Minnesota); (B) The elliptical crown; (C) Different crowns available

flush of microparticle. As the crown rotates and orbit increases, centrifugal force presses the crown against the lesion, reducing arterial calcium.[81] Unlike in RA, minuscule (<2 microns) particulates are produced which do not require embolic protection. Continuous blood flow while orbiting minimizes the risk of thermal injury to the vessel (advantage over RA).

Indication

Severely calcified coronary artery lesions either de novo or after coronary artery bypass grafting (CABG), where percutaneous transluminal coronary angioplasty (PTCA) is indicated.

Clinical Studies

ORBIT-I was the first to demonstrate the use of the OAS in calcific lesion. It was a non-randomized trial[83] of 50 patients and showed significant benefits in the form of reduction in the percentage of diameter stenosis from 85.6% to 40%. The success in this trial fuelled the ORBIT-II trial,[32,84] wherein 443 patients with severely calcified lesions were studied. Result showed dissection in 3.4%, perforation in 1.8%, slow or no reflow in 0.9%, and 1.8% abrupt closure. The composite of Q- and non–Q-wave MI were seen in 9.3% of patient's in-hospital. All of these complications are well within the range of those seen in trials of rotational or Laser atherectomy. The primary efficacy endpoint (stent delivery with residual stenosis <50%

and freedom from 30-day MACE) was appreciated by 88.9% of patients, and the primary safety endpoint of freedom from 30-day MACE was appreciated by 89.6% of patients. This drew the attention of FDA for positive verdict for future use of the DIAMONDBACK 360® Coronary Orbital Atherectomy System.

Contraindications

- Lesion where the Viper Wire guidewire cannot pass across the coronary lesion.
- Lesion is within a bypass graft or stent.
- Inappropriate candidate for bypass surgery, angioplasty, or atherectomy therapy.
- Angiographic evidence of thrombus, or has only one open vessel, or has angiographic evidence of significant dissection at the treatment site.
- Women who are pregnant or children.

Tips and Tricks

Orbital atherectomy system (OAS) is ideal for moderate to severe calcified vessels 2–4 mm.

- Consider placing a transvenous pacemaker for the RCA or dominant LCX, or in high-risk patients.
- Limit spin time (each run) to 30 seconds. Longer lesions require additional runs, not longer runs. The rest time between each run should be equal to or longer than the run time.
- Avoid use of the Viper wire in small branches. The radiopaque portion of the wire should be kept at least 0.5 cm distal to the most distal target.
- Avoid closing the hemostatic valve on the Y connector too tightly.
- Keep the crown tip at least 5 mm proximal to the lesion when starting and finishing a run and avoid orbital atherectomy with ostial lesions.
- Use the "pecking" motion for advancement of crown. Advance the knob a maximum of 1 cm/second and do not end the run in the middle of a lesion. Never force the crown through the lesion. Increase the rotation speed after the initial low-speed run passes through the lesion without audible, high-pitched resistance from the device.[83]

Present Role

Orbital atherectomy system (OAS) treatment is an effective method to modify calcified coronary lesion compliance to facilitate optimal stent placement. The Diamondback 360 Coronary Orbital Atherectomy System is the first FDA approved novel technology to treat severely calcified lesions with relative cost benefits.

Strategy for Intervention in Calcified Lesions

Management strategy should be planned after thorough evaluation of lesion by angiography supplemented with IVUS/OCT. Decision would depend on the vessel size and distribution of calcium.[85] The following strategy is proposed based on experience and evidence based studies.

Vessel Size <2.5 mm

Avoid implanting a stent except for rescue situation as rates of restenosis are high. Plan for a rota with 1.25/1.5 burr and complete the procedure with POBA (low pressure balloon for longer dilatation times).

Vessel Size >2.5 mm

- *Superficial calcification:* If mild calcium (arc of calcium is <90°), cutting balloon is generally sufficient. However, dissections are common. Avoid immediate stenting as stent under-explanation is common. Preferable do a high pressure balloon dilatation and then implant the stent for optimal results. If the calcium is significant (arc >180°), Rota/orbital atherectomy should be the first choice and end with optimal stent deployment.
- *Deep calcification:* Balloon angioplasty is usually sufficient to dilate the lesion followed by optimal stenting.

SUCCESSFUL ROTA (FIGS 22.32 TO 22.34)

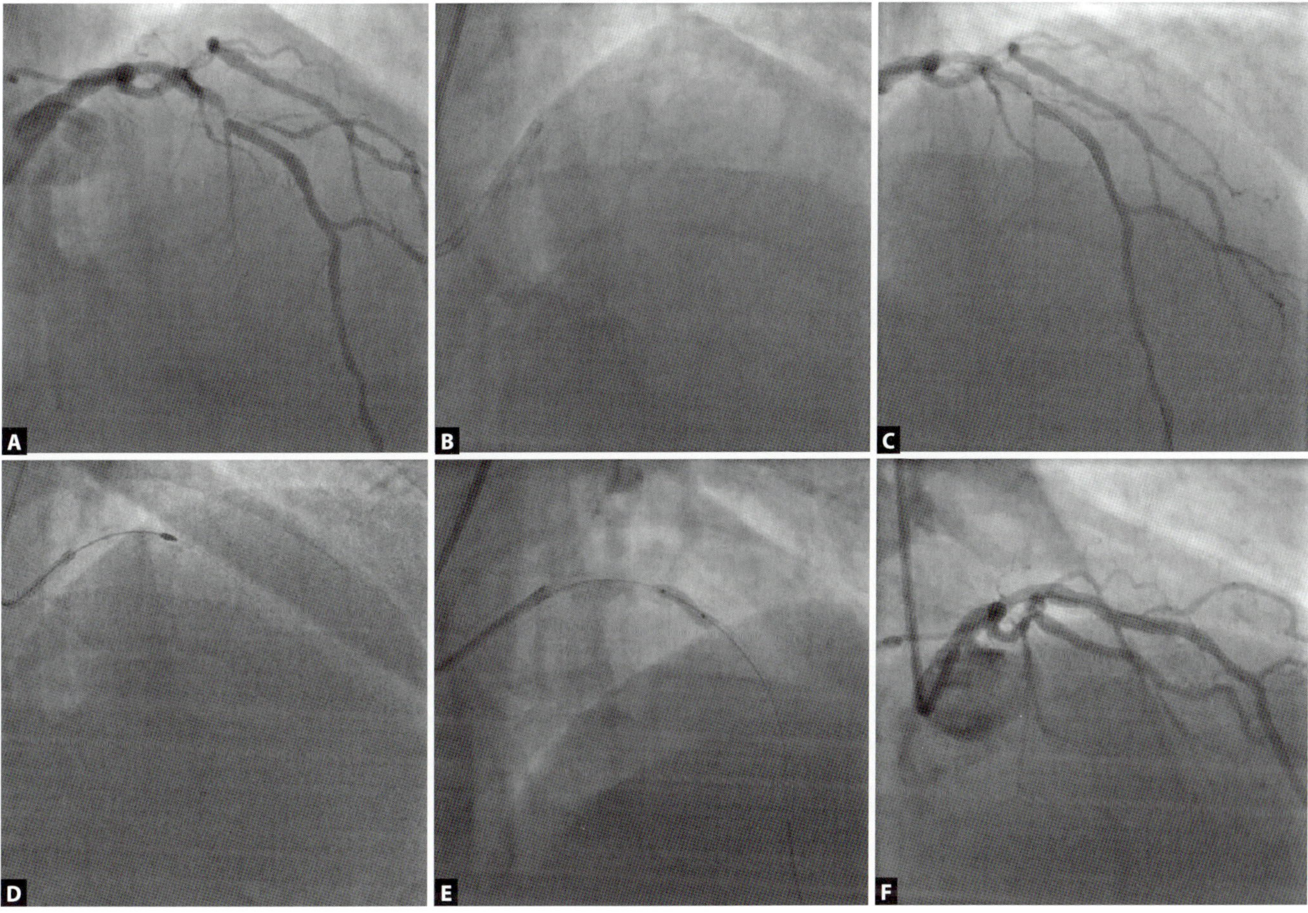

Figs 22.32A to F (A) RAO cranial view showing tight focal stenosis in proximal LAD; (B) RAO cranial view showing severe calcium in proximal LAD; (C) Lesion crossed with choice floppy guidewire and exchanged with rota wire over a microcatheter; (D) Rota with 1.5 burr done; (E) Lesion dilated with 2.0 × 10 balloon at 10 atm; (F) Final result after stenting with

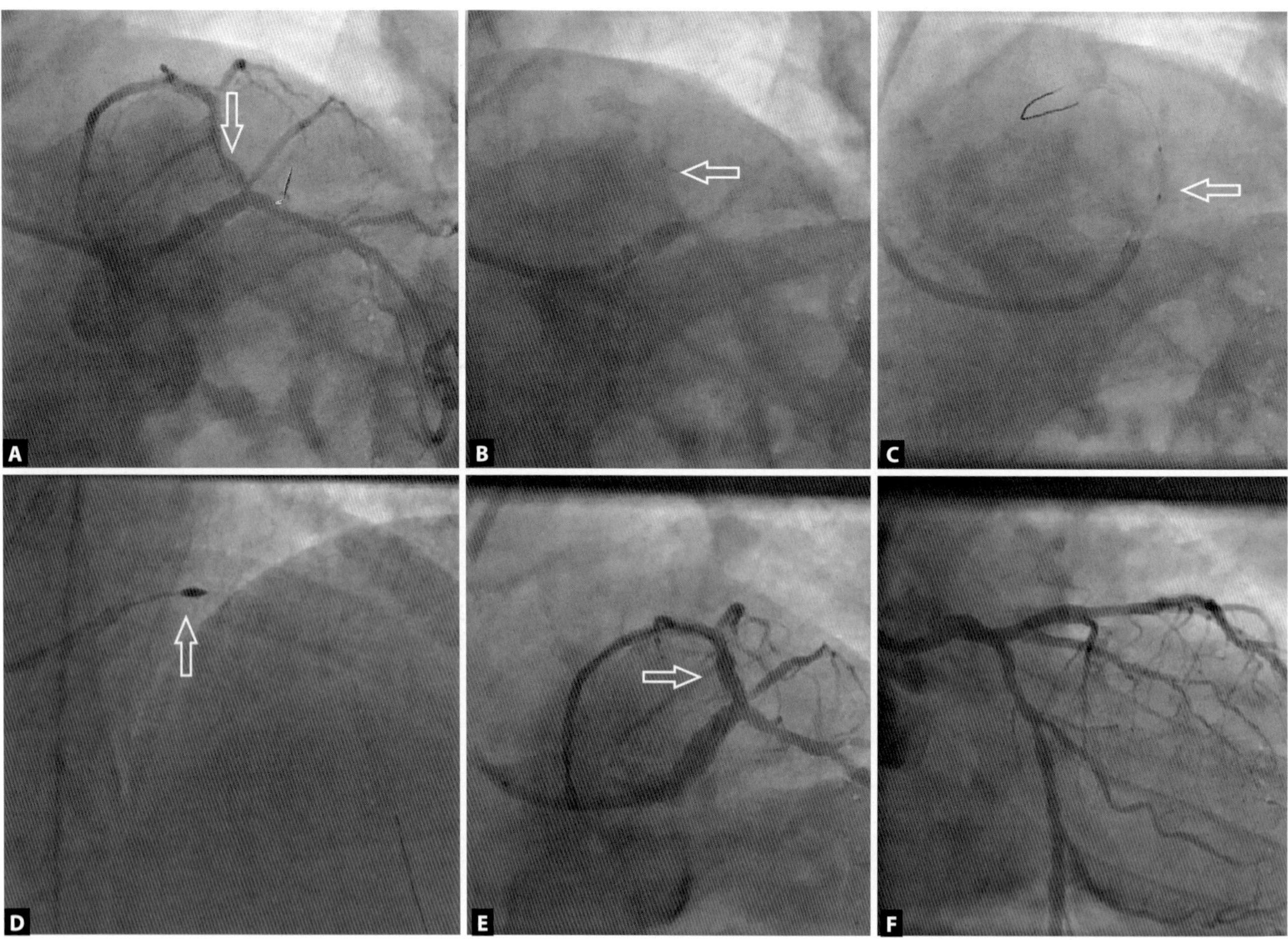

Figs 22.33A to F (A) LAO caudal view showing significant disease in ostio-proximal LAD and stent in mid LAD; (B) LAO caudal view showing significant calcium in ostio-proximal LAD; (C) Dog-bone effect. Failed balloon dilatation; (D) Rota with 1.25 burr; (E) Stent implanted in ostio-proximal LAD; (F) Final result in RAO caudal view

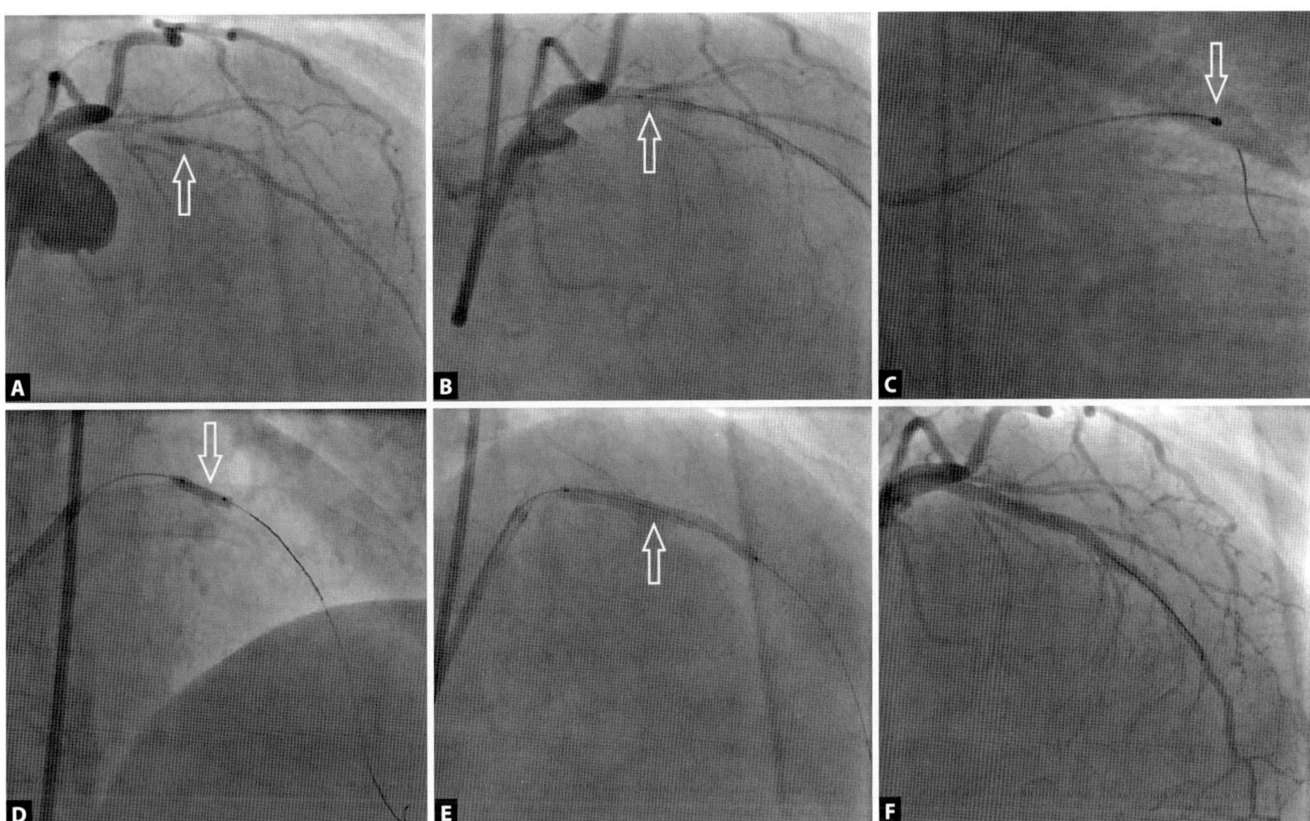

Figs 22.34A to F (A) AP cranial view showing diffuse long segment significant disease in proximal LAD with calcium; (B) Microcatheter (arrow) used to exchange rota wire over choice floppy guidewire; (C) Rota done with 1.25 burr; (D) Balloon dilatation with 2 × 10 balloon; (E) Stent implanted in proximal LAD; (F) Final result showing good result with TIMI-III flow in LAD in AP cranial view

FAILED ROTA (FIGS 22.35 AND 22.36)

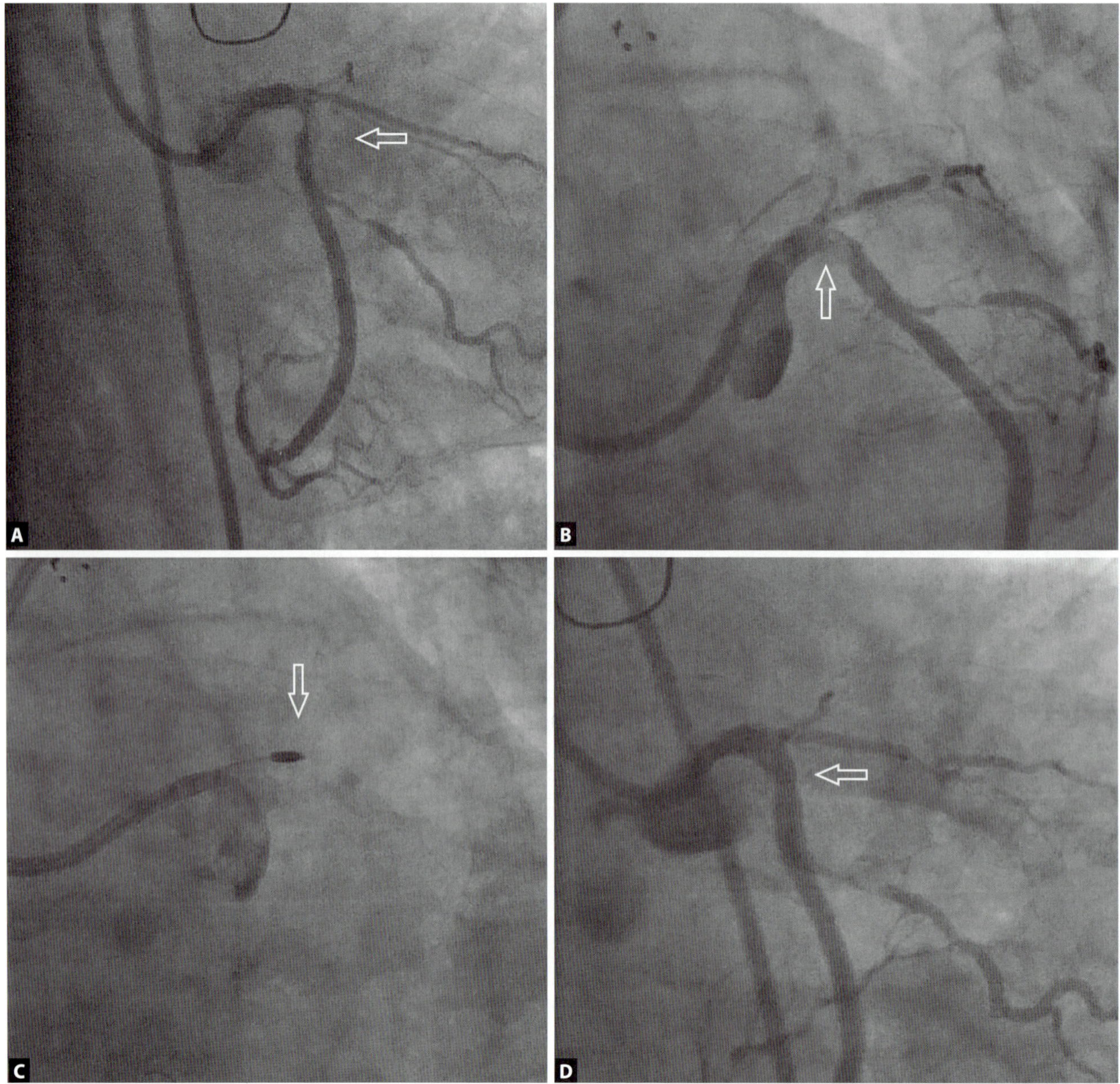

Figs 22.35A to D (A) RAO caudal view showing focal tight stenosis in ostial LCx post-CABG status with severe calcium; (B) LAO caudal view demonstrating the lesion with calcium; (C) Rota wire crossed the lesion, but burr could not be negotiated through the ostium due to the bend; (D) Lesion stented after balloon dilatation with suboptimal result

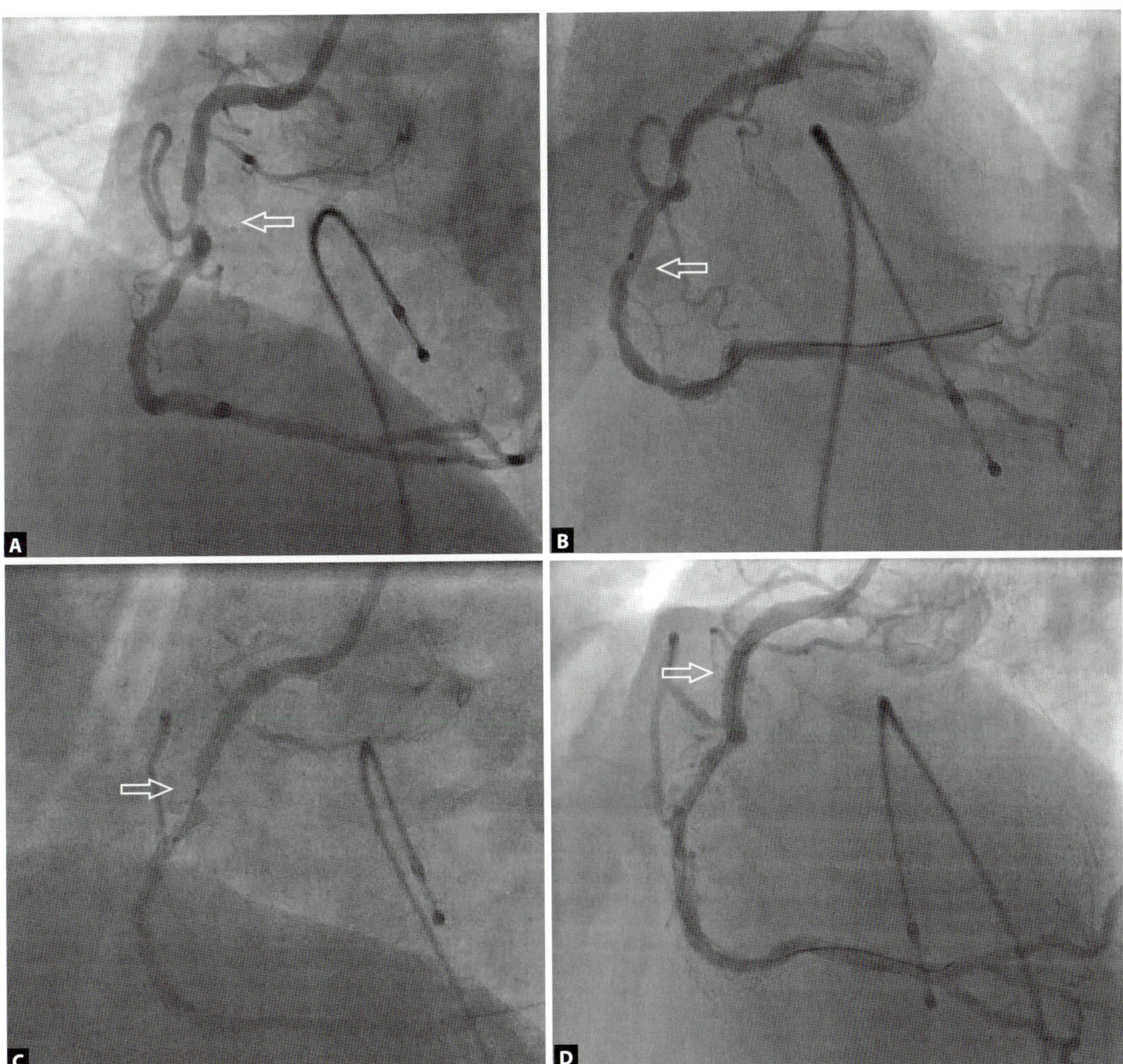

Figs 22.36A to D (A) LAO view of RCA showing mid focal 90% stenosis with significant calcium. Rota was planned after initial attempt of balloon dilatation and stenting; (B) Rota wire could be negotiated with great difficulty over a microcatheter through the tortuosity, but sufficient support was not attained; (C) Rota burr could not be passed as wire failed to give support. Serial balloon dilatations done on buddy wire support; (D) Final result after stenting

CONCLUSION

Each calcific lesion has a different look and touch. Significantly calcified lesions pose a challenge to the intervention cardiologist. Severely calcified lesions respond poorly to plain balloon angioplasty. Stents implantation in such lesions leads to incomplete and asymmetrical stent expansion in the most of cases with resultant stent thrombosis and ISR. Adequate plaque modification prior to implantation of drug-eluting stents is the key in intervening calcific lesion. RA is the most reliable modality for plaque modification in cases of dense circumferential calcium. In less severe calcification or stent under expansion, other modalities can be used. The debulking tools are in continuous process of innovation. Orbital atherectomy and BVS[86] are the two promising hopes.

REFERENCES

1. Bourantas CV, Zhang YJ, Garg S, Iqbal J, Valgimigli M, Windecker S, et al. Prognostic implications of coronary calcification in patients with obstructive coronary artery disease treated by percutaneous coronary intervention: a patient-level pooled analysis of 7 contemporary stent trials. Heart. 2014;100(15): 1158-64.
2. Bangalore S, Vlachos HA, Selzer F, Wilensky RL, Kip KE, Williams DO, Faxon DP. Percutaneous coronary intervention of moderate to severe calcified coronary lesions: insights from the National Heart, Lung, and Blood Institute Dynamic Registry. Catheter Cardiovasc Interv. 2011;77:22-8.
3. Xu Y, Mintz GS, Tam A, McPherson JA, Iniguez A, Fajadet J, et al. Prevalence, distribution, predictors, and outcomes of patients with calcified nodules in native coronary arteries: a 3-vessel intravascular ultrasound analysis from Providing Regional Observations to Study Predictors of Events in the Coronary Tree (PROSPECT). Circulation. 2012;126:537-45.
4. Madhavan MV, Tarigopula M, Mintz GS, Maehara A, Stone GW, Genereux P. Coronary artery calcification: pathogenesis and prognostic implications. J Am Coll Cardiol. 2014; 63:1703-14.
5. Bourantas CV, Zhang YJ, Garg S, Mack M, Dawkins KD, Kappetein AP, et al. Prognostic implications of severe coronary calcification in patients undergoing coronary artery bypass surgery: an analysis of the SYNTAX study. Catheter Cardiovasc Interv. 2015;85(2): 199-206.
6. Sakuragi S, Ichikawa K, Yamada K, Tanimoto M, Miki T, Otsuka H, et al. An increase in the coronary calcification score is associated with an increased risk of heart failure in patients without a history of coronary artery disease. J Cardio. 2016;67(4): 358-64.
7. Bhatt P, Parikh P, Patel A, Chag M, Chandaranan A, Parikh R, et al. "Long-term safety and performance of the orbital atherectomy system for treating calcified coronary artery lesions: 5-Year follow-up in the ORBIT I trial." Cardiovas Revascul Med. 2015;16(4):213-6.
8. Vliegenthart R, Oudkerk M, Hofman A, et al. Coronary calcification improves cardiovascular risk prediction in the elderly. Circulation. 2005;112:572-7.
9. Généreux P, Madhavan MV, Mintz GS, et al. Ischemic outcomes after coronary intervention of calcified vessels in acute coronary syndromes: pooled analysis from the HORIZONS-AMI (Harmonizing Outcomes With Revascularization and Stents in Acute Myocardial Infarction) and ACUITY (Acute Catheterization and Urgent Intervention triage Strategy) Trials. J Am Coll Cardiol. 2014;63(18):1845-54.
10. Ertelt K, Généreux P, Mintz GS, Reiss GR, Kirtane AJ, Madhavan MV, et al. Impact of the severity of coronary artery calcification on clinical events in patients undergoing coronary artery bypass grafting (from the Acute Catheterization and Urgent Intervention Triage Strategy Trial). Am J Cardiol. 2013;112(11):1730-7.
11. Blankenhorn Dh, Stern D. Calcification of the coronary arteries. Am J Roentgenol Radium Ther Nucl Med. 1959;81:772.
12. Margolis JR, Chen JT, Kong Y, et al. The diagnostic and prognostic significance of coronary artery calcification. A report of 800 cases. Radiology. 1980;137:609.
13. Modified from Ryan TJ, Faxon DP, Gunnar RP, et al. Guidelines for percutaneous transluminal coronary angioplasty: a report of the American College of Cardiology/American Heart Association Task Force on Assessment of Diagnostic and Therapeutic Cardiovascular Procedures (Subcommittee on Percutaneous Transluminal Coronary Angioplasty). J Am Coll Cardiol. 1988;12:529-45.
14. Modified from Krone R, Shaw R, Klein L, et al. Evaluation of the American College of Cardiology/American Heart Association and the Society for Coronary Angiography and Interventions lesion classification system in the current "stent era" of coronary interventions (from the ACC National Cardiovascular Data Registry). Am J Cardiol. 2003;92:389-94.
15. Stary HC, Chandler AB, Dinsmore RE, Fuster V, Glagov S, Insull W Jr, et al. A definition of advanced types of atherosclerotic lesions and a histological classification of atherosclerosis. A report from the Committee on Vascular Lesions of the Council on Arteriosclerosis, American Heart Association. Arterioscler Thromb Vasc Biol. 1995;15(9):1512-31.
16. Goel M, Wong ND, Eisenberg H, et al. Risk factor correlates of coronary calcium as evaluated by ultrafast computed tomography. AmmJ Cardiol. 1992;70:977-80.
17. Wong ND, Kouwabunpat D, Vo AN, et al. Coronary calcium and atherosclerosis by ultrafast computed tomography in asymptomatic men and women: relation to age and risk factors. Am Heart J. 1994;127:422-30.
18. Demer LL, Tintut Y. Vascular calcification: pathobiology of a multifaceted disease. Circulation. 2008;117:2938-48.
19. Johnson RC, Leopold JA, Loscalzo J. Vascular calcification: pathobiological mechanisms and clinical implications. Circ Res. 2006;99:1044-59.
20. Sangiorgi G, Rumberger JA, Severson A, et al. Arterial calcification and not lumen stenosis is highly correlated with atherosclerotic plaque burden in humans: a histologic study of 723 coronary artery segments using nondecalcifying methodology. J Am Coll Cardiol. 1998;31:126-33.
21. Kelly-Arnold A, Maldonado N, Laudier D, et al. Revised microcalcification hypothesis for fibrous cap rupture in human coronary arteries. Proc Natl Acad Sci USA. 2013;110:10741-6.
22. Burke AP, Weber DK, Kolodgie FD, et al. Pathophysiology of calcium deposition in coronary arteries. Herz. 2001;26: 239-44.

23. Greenland P, Alpert JS, Beller GA, et al. 2010 ACCF/AHA guideline for assessment of cardiovascular risk in asymptomatic adults: a report of the American College of Cardiology Foundation/American Heart Association Task Force on Practice Guidelines. J Am Coll Cardiol. 2010;56:e50-103.
24. Al-Mallah MH, Qureshi W, Lin Fy, Achenbach S, Berman DS, Budoff MJ, et al. Does coronary CT angiography improve risk stratification over coronary calcium scoring in symptomatic patients with suspected coronary artery disease? Results from the prospective multicenter international CONFIRM registry. Eur Heart J Cardiovasc Imaging. 2014;15(3):267-74.
25. Agatston AS, Janowitz WR, Hildner FJ, et al. Quantification of coronary artery calcium using ultrafast computed tomography. J Am Coll Cardiol. 1990;15:827-32.
26. Mintz GS, Popma JJ, Pichard AD, et al. Patterns of calcification in coronary artery disease. A statistical analysis of intravascular ultrasound and coronary angiography in 1155 lesions. Circulation. 1995;91:1959-65.
27. Friedrich GJ, Moes NY, Muhlberger VA, et al. Detection of intralesional calcium by intracoronary ultrasound depends on the histologic pattern. Am Heart J. 1994;128:435-41.
28. Kawasaki M, Bouma BE, Bressner J, et al. Diagnostic accuracy of optical coherence tomography and integrated backscatter intravascular ultrasound images for tissue characterization of human coronary plaques. J Am Coll Cardiol. 2006;48:81-8.
29. Kume T, Okura H, Kawamoto T, et al. Assessment of the coronary calcification by optical coherence tomography. EuroIntervention. 2011;6:768-72.
30. Pershad A, Buchbinder M. Management of calcified lesions in 2004. Int J Cardiovasc Intervent. 2005;7:199-204.
31. Rajani R, Lindblom M, Dixon G, Khawaja MZ, Holmbery S, de Belder A, et al. Evolving trends in percutaneous coronary intervention. Br J Cardiol. 2011;18.2:73-6.
32. Chambers JW, Feldman RL, Himmelstein SI, et al. Pivotal trial to evaluate the safety and efficacy of the orbital atherectomy system in treating de novo, severely calcified coronary lesions (ORBIT II). J Am Coll Cardiol Intv. 2014;7(5):510-8.
33. Kim JS, Choong WG, Kwang-Soo C. Management of calcified lesions. Chapter 12. TRI manual By TRI Working Group; 2010.
34. Ikari Y, Masuda N, Matsukage T, Ogata N, Nakazawa G, Tanabe T, Morino Y. Backup force of guiding catheters for the right coronary artery in transfemoral and transradial interventions. J Invasive Cardiol. 2009;21:570-4.
35. Ikari Y, Nagaoka M, Kim JY, Morino Y, Tanabe T. The physics of guiding catheters for the left coronary artery in transfemoral and transradial interventions. J Invasive Cardiol. 2005;17:636-41.
36. Ajani AE, Kim HS, Castagna M, et al. Clinical utility of the cutting balloon. J Invas Cardiol. 2001;13:554-7
37. Barath P, Fishbein MC, Vari S, Forrester JS. Cutting balloon: A novel approach to percutaneous angioplasty. Am J Cardiol. 1991; 68:1249-51.
38. Vaquerizo B, Serra A, Miranda F, et al. Aggressive plaque modification with rotational atherectomy and/or cutting balloon before drug-eluting stent implantation for the treatment of calcified coronary lesions. J Interv Cardiol. 2010;23:240-8.
39. De Ribamar Costa J Jr., Mintz GS, Carlier SG, et al. Nonrandomized comparison of coronary stenting under intravascular ultrasound guidance of direct stenting without predilation versus conventional predilation with a semi-compliant balloon versus predilation with a new scoring balloon. Am J Cardiol. 2007;100:812-7.
40. Grenadier E, Kerner A, Gershony G, Makhoul N, Rougin A. Optimizing plaque modification in complex lesions utilizing the angiosculpt device: acute and long term results from a two-center registry. Accessed September 3, 2013.
41. Bittl JA, Chew DP, Topol EJ, Kong DF, Califf RM. Meta-analysis of randomized trials of percutaneous transluminal coronary angioplasty versus atherectomy, cutting balloon atherotomy, or laser angioplasty. J Am Coll Cardiol. 2004;43:936-42.
42. Bernardo Saulo, PA, and Arthur C. Lee, MD, Santa Clara Valley Medical Center, San Jose, California, Volume 10 - Issue 3 - March, 2002; Cathlab digest.
43. Fumichi S, Tobaru T, Asano R, et al. Rotational atherectomy followed by cutting balloon plaque modification before drug-eluting stent implantation in calcified coronary lesions. J Am Coll Cardiol. 2012;59(13s1):E81.
44. Vitrella, Giancarlo, et al. FX MiniRAIL™ Catheter Usage for Treatment of De Novo Complex Coronary Lesions: Results from the "OFFAR". J Interven Cardiol. 2006;19(3):250-7.
45. Mishra S, Bahl VK. Coronary hardware Part 3-balloon angioplasty catheters. Indian Heart J. 2010;62:335-41.
46. de Ribamar Costa J, Jr Mintz GS, Carlier SG, et al. Nonrandomized comparison of coronary stenting under intravascular ultrasound guidance of direct stenting without predilation versus conventional predilation with a semi-compliant balloon versus predilation with a new scoring balloon. American Journal of Cardiology. 2007;100:812-7.
47. Tan K, Sulke N, Taub N, Sowton E. Clinical and lesion morphologic determinants of coronary angioplasty success and complications: current experience. J Am Coll Cardiol. 1995;25:855-65.
48. Fitzgerald PJ, Ports TA, Yock PG. Contribution of localized calcium deposits to dissection after angioplasty. An observational study using intravascular ultrasound. Circulation. 1992;86:64-70.
49. Richardson PD, Davies MJ, Born GV. Influence of plaque configuration and stress distribution on fissuring of coronary atherosclerotic plaques. Lancet. 1989;2:941-4.
50. Hoffmann R, Mintz GS, Popma JJ, et al. Treatment of calcified coronary lesions with Palmaz-Schatz stents. An intravascular ultrasound study. Eur Heart J. 1998;19:1224-31.
51. Kawaguchi R, Tsurugaya H, Hoshizaki H, et al. Impact of lesion calcification on clinical and angiographic outcome after sirolimus eluting stent implantation in real-world patients. Cardiovasc Revasc Med. 2008;9:2-8.
52. Moussa I, Ellis SG, Jones M, et al. Impact of coronary culprit lesion calcium in patients undergoing paclitaxel-eluting stent implantation (a TAXUS-IV sub study). Am J Cardiol. 2005;96:1242-7.
53. Seo A, Fujii T, Inoue T, et al. Initial and long-term outcomes of sirolimus-eluting stents for calcified lesions compared with bare-metal stents. Int Heart J. 2007;48:137-47.
54. Khattab AA, Otto A, Hochadel M, et al. Drug-eluting stents versus bare metal stents following rotational atherectomy for heavily calcified coronary lesions: late angiographic and clinical follow-up results. J Interv Cardiol. 2007;20:100-6.
55. Shimada Y, Kataoka T, Courtney BK, et al. Influence of plaque calcium on neointimal hyperplasia following bare metal and

drugeluting stent implantation. Catheter Cardiovasc Interv. 2006;67:866-9.
56. Onuma Y, Tanimoto S, Ruygrok P, et al. Efficacy of everolimus eluting stent implantation in patients with calcified coronary culprit lesions: two-year angiographic and three-year clinical results from the SPIRIT II study. Catheter Cardiovasc Interv. 2010;76:634-42.
57. Topol EJ, Leya F, Pinkerton CA, et al. A comparison of directional atherectomy with coronary angioplasty in patients with coronary artery disease. The CAVEAT Study Group. N Engl J Med. 1993;329:221-7.
58. Adelman AG, Cohen EA, Kimball BP, et al. A comparison of directional atherectomy with balloon angioplasty for lesions of the left anterior descending coronary artery. N Engl J Med. 1993;329:228-33.
59. Baim DS, Cutlip DE, Sharma SK, et al. Final results of the Balloon vs. Optimal Atherectomy Trial (BOAT). Circulation. 1998;97: 322-31.
60. Levin TN, Holloway S, Feldman T. Acute and late clinical outcome after rotational atherectomy for complex coronary disease. Cathet Cardiovasc Diagn. 1998;45:122-30.
61. Reifart N, Vandormael M, Krajcar M, et al. Randomized comparison of angioplasty of complex coronary lesions at a single center. Excimer Laser, Rotational Atherectomy, and Balloon Angioplasty Comparison (ERBAC) study. Circulation. 1997;96:91-8.
62. Gruberg L, Mehran R, Dangas G, et al. Effect of plaque debulking and stenting on short- and long-term outcomes after revascularization of chronic total occlusions. J Am Coll Cardiol. 2000;35:151-6.
63. Pagnotta P, Briguori C, Mango R, et al. Rotational atherectomy in resistant chronic total occlusions. Catheter Cardiovasc Interv. 2010;76:366-71.
64. Tan RP, Kini A, Shalouh E, Marmur JD, Sharma SK. Optimal treatment of nonaorto ostial coronary lesions in large vessels: acute and long-term results. Catheter Cardiovasc Interv. 2001;54:283-8.
65. Koller PT, Freed M, Grines CL, O'Neill WW. Success, complications, and restenosis following rotational and transluminal extraction atherectomy of ostial stenoses. Cathet Cardiovasc Diagn. 1994;31:255-60.
66. Tsuchikane E, Suzuki T, Asakura Y, et al. Debulking of chronic coronary total occlusions with rotational or directional atherectomy before stenting: final results of DOCTORS study. Int J Cardiol. 2008;125:397-403.
67. Tsuchikane E, Aizawa T, Tamai H, et al. Pre-drug-eluting stent debulking of bifurcated coronary lesions. J Am Coll Cardiol. 2007;50:1941-5.
68. Nageh T, Kulkarni NM, Thomas MR. High-speed rotational atherectomy in the treatment of bifurcation-type coronary lesions. Cardiology. 2001;95:198-205.
69. Ito H, Piel S, Das P, et al. Long-term outcomes of plaque debulking with rotational atherectomy in side-branch ostial lesions to treat bifurcation coronary disease. J Invasive Cardiol. 2009;21: 598-601.
70. Moussa I, Di Mario C, Moses J, et al. Coronary stenting after rotational atherectomy in calcified and complex lesions. Angiographic and clinical follow-up results. Circulation. 1997;96:128-36.
71. Kobayashi Y, De Gregorio J, Kobayashi N, et al. Lower restenosis rate with stenting following aggressive versus less aggressive rotational atherectomy. Catheter Cardiovasc Interv. 1999; 46:406-14.
72. Kuriyama N, Kobayashi Y, Yamaguchi M, Shibata Y. Usefulness of rotational atherectomy in preventing polymer damage of everolimus-eluting stent in calcified coronary artery. J Am Coll Cardiol Intv. 2011;4:588-9.
73. Abdel-Wahab M, Richardt G, Joachim Büttner H, et al. High-speed rotational atherectomy before paclitaxel-eluting stent implantation in complex calcified coronary lesions: the randomized ROTAXUS (Rotational Atherectomy Prior to Taxus Stent Treatment for Complex Native Coronary Artery Disease) trial. J Am Coll Cardiol Intv. 2013;6:10-9.
74. Levine GN, Bates ER, Blankenship JC, et al. 2011 ACCF/AHA/SCAI guideline for percutaneous coronary intervention: a report of the American College of Cardiology Foundation/American Heart Association Task Force on Practice Guidelines and the Society for Cardiovascular Angiography and Interventions. J Am Coll Cardiol. 2011;58(24):e44-122.
75. Topaz O. Plaque removal and thrombus dissolution with the photoacoustic energy of pulsed-wave lasers-biotissue interactions and their clinical manifestations. Cardiology. 1996;87:384-91.
76. Appelman YE, Piek JJ, Strikwerda S, et al. Randomised trial of excimer laser angioplasty versus balloon angioplasty for treatment of obstructive coronary artery disease. Lancet. 1996;347:79-84.
77. Reifart N, Vandormael M, Krajcar M, et al. Randomized comparison of angioplasty of complex coronary lesions at a single center. Excimer laser, Rotational atherectomy, and Balloon Angioplasty Comparison (ERBAC) Study. Circulation. 1997;96:91-8
78. Latib A, Takagi K, Chizzola G, et al. Excimer Laser LEsion modification to expand non-dilatable stents: the ELLEMENT registry. Cardiovasc Revasc Med. 2014;15:8-12.
79. Bilodeau L, Fretz EB, Taeymans Y, et al. Novel use of a high-energy excimer laser catheter for calcified and complex coronary artery lesions. Cathet Cardiovasc Interv. 2004;62:155-61.
80. Topaz O, Minisi AJ, Bernardo NL, et al. Alterations of platelet aggregation kinetics with ultraviolet laser emission: the "stunned platelet" phenomenon. Thromb Haemost. 2001;86:1087-93.
81. Topaz O, Ebersole D, Das T, et al; CARMEL multicenter trial. Excimer laser angioplasty in acute myocardial infarction (the CARMEL multicenter trial). Am J Cardiol. 2004;93:694-701.
82. Dave R. Extended FAMILI. Presented at: Transcatheter Cardiovascular Therapeutics meeting; 2006; Washington, DC.
83. Trayer T, Sanghvi K. Complex coronary intervention using coronary orbital atherectomy (Diamondback 360°) via a transradial approach. Cathlab Digest. 2014;22(2).
84. Parikh K, Chandra P, Choksi N, Khanna P, Chambers J. Safety and feasibility of orbital atherectomy for the treatment of calcified coronary lesions: the ORBIT I trial. Catheter Cardiovasc Interv. 2013;81:1134-9.
85. Takahiko Suzuki. Toyohashi Heart Center. Angioplasty for Calcified Lesions. *cct.gr.jp/2003/books/bookspdf/suzuki07.pdf.*
86. Basavarajaiah S, Naganuma T, Latib A, Colombo A. Can bioabsorbable scaffolds be used in calcified lesions? Catheter Cardiovasc Interv. 2014;84(1):48-52.

CHAPTER

23 Contrast-induced Nephropathy

Aditya Kapoor, Pritika Gaur

INTRODUCTION AND DIAGNOSTIC CRITERIA

Contrast-induced nephropathy (CIN), or contrast-induced acute kidney injury (CI-AKI), is the term given to iatrogenic renal dysfunction following intravascular (intravenous or intra-arterial) administration of iodinated radiographic contrast media, occurring in the absence of any other identifiable cause. It is often implicated as the third leading cause of hospital-acquired acute renal failure (ARF) and is reported to be responsible for 10–12% of all cases of in-hospital ARF.[1,2]

The currently accepted diagnostic criteria for CIN are:[1,3,4]

- An absolute increase of serum creatinine (SCr) by ≥0.5 mg/dL or
- A relative increase in SCr by ≥25% from baseline or
- A decrease in estimated glomerular filtration rate (eGFR) to 30–60 mL/min

The British Cardiovascular Intervention Society, The Royal College of Radiologists and the Renal Association have also proposed the *Improving Global Outcomes (KDIGO) definition of CI-AKI* to standardize the nomenclature used to define AKI and stage its severity. CIN is defined if one of the following criteria is met:

- SCr rises by ≥26 µmol/L within 48 hours or
- SCr rises ≥1.5 fold from the baseline value, which is known or presumed to have occurred within one week or
- Urine output is <0.5 mL/kg/hour for >6 consecutive hours.

If a baseline SCr is not available within 1 week the lowest Cr value recorded within 3 months of the episode of AKI can be used. While SCr has traditionally been used to diagnose CIN, it has limited sensitivity in diagnosing subtle impairment of renal function. Moreover it is not a real-time biomarker of renal function and is affected by numerous variables including gender, age, muscle mass and nutritional status. *Measurement of glomerular filtration rate (GFR)* is a more accurate estimate of renal function. It can help identify mild renal impairment which can be associated with reduction in GFR despite apparently 'normal' Cr levels, since normal serum levels are often maintained even when GFR is reduced by ~50%. However, direct measurement of GFR by inulin clearance and other methods is impractical in the clinical setting. *Hence estimation of GFR (eGFR)* using Cockcroft and Gault formula, the Modification of Diet in Renal Disease Study (MDRD) equation or the chronic kidney disease epidemiology collaboration (CKD-EPI) are better methods to assess the GFR.[5-7] Patients with eGFR >60 are at a low risk for developing CIN while the risk is very high for those with eGFR <30 mL/min.

Serum Cystatin Ca, a renal function marker, is a protein secreted by nucleated cells and is freely filtered by the glomerulus. It increases earlier than SCr after administration of radiocontrast and is unaffected by the same confounding factors as SCr making it a more sensitive indicator of detecting reductions in GFR. *Serum or urine neutrophil gelatinase-associated lipocalin (NGAL)* levels have also been found to be useful for early diagnosis (within 4 hours) as well as for and prognostication of AKI. However, more data are required before these markers are recommended to routinely diagnose CIN.

CLINICAL FEATURES, MANAGEMENT AND PROGNOSIS

The decline in renal function is usually transient and self-limited, with the increase in SCr peaking on the 3rd–5th day and returning to baseline within 2 weeks in the majority of the patients. Since the renal impairment is nonoliguric and the patient often asymptomatic, it may go undetected if renal function is not monitored routinely following administration of contrast media (especially among high-risk patients). Occasionally, the renal dysfunction may be more marked, leading to oliguria and decline of urine output within 24–48 hours, peaking of SCr in 5–10 days with normalization in 2–3 weeks. In some cases (~1%), the renal impairment is more persistent necessitating dialysis.

The management of CIN is similar for other causes of acute renal failure and involves monitoring of electrolytes, fluid balance, body weight and nutrition, in close consultation with a nephrologist. What is more important is the identification of high risk patients who are likely to develop CIN and proper institution of preventive strategies (as outlined in subsequent sections).

The alterations in renal function in CIN, although mild are known to be associated with adverse *short- and long-term clinical outcomes*, especially in patients with pre-existing renal disease. Occurrence of AKI following cardiac catheterization procedures is reported to be associated with an inhospital mortality of 20% and 1-year mortality of up to 66%.[8,9] The minority of patients of CIN who need dialysis have the highest inhospital (~30%) and 2 year mortality rates (~70–80%)[10,11] Whether CIN is itself a cause of the increase in mortality or is simply a marker of underlying risk/comorbidity is unclear and the direct link between CIN and adverse cardiovascular outcomes is not yet established. What is important is to employ preventive measures in all patients undergoing radiocontrast administration to reduce the incidence of CIN.

INCIDENCE AND PREDISPOSING FACTORS

There is a large discrepancy in the documented incidence of CIN because of the wide ranging definitions used to characterize CIN, the inherent limitations of using SCr as a diagnostic criteria and heterogeneity of studies with differences in patient populations, types and volume of contrast used and varying preventive strategies. It is also underestimated since patients are often asymptomatic and the renal impairment may go undetected. The reported incidence of CIN in patients with normal pre-existing renal function is 1–2% [12,13]

Important predisposing factors which have been identified to be associated with development of CIN include pre-existing renal impairment, diabetes mellitus, advanced age, intravascular volume depletion, congestive heart failure, type, volume and route of contrast administration, concomitant use of other nephrotoxic drugs, sepsis, anemia and peri-procedural drop in hematocrit. (Table 23.1) *Of these, pre-existing renal impairment* is one of the most important risk factor for development of CIN. Studies have reported baseline creatinine to be an independent predictor of CIN, with reported incidence rates of 14.8–55% in patients with underlying renal dysfunction.[8,10,14] Risk can be further stratified according to the National Kidney Foundation Kidney Disease Quality Initiative (KDOQI) classification based on estimated glomerular filtration rate (eGFR), with values <60 mL/min/1.73 m^2 considered to be a cut-off for increased risk of CIN.[15] A pooled analysis of patients receiving intravenous contrast demonstrated a 0.6% incidence of CIN in patients with GFR >40 mL/min, vs 4.6% and 7.8% in those with GFR <40 mL/min and GFR <30 mL/min respectively.[16] The risk of CIN in patients with eGFR <30 is reported to be ~30–40% and the risk of need for dialysis approximately 2–8%.[2,17]

Table 23.1 Risk factors for contrast-induced hephropathy

Nonmodifiable	*Modifiable*
Age	Contrast dose, type and route of administration
Renal failure	Volume depletion, dehydration
Diabetes	Low hematocrit
Hypotension	Nephrotoxic drug use
Sepsis	

The incidence of CIN in *diabetic patients* has been reported to be 5.7–29.4%.[12,18,19] Although some studies have reported that diabetes mellitus in the absence of underlying renal failure does not predispose to CIN, coexisting chronic kidney disease and diabetes exponentially increase the risk for CIN compared with that for chronic kidney disease alone. Occurrence of CIN is common in patients with diabetes and pre-existing renal impairment (serum creatinine >1.5 mg/dL or GFR <60 mL/min/1.73 m^2), especially in those with diabetic nephropathy. Amongst diabetics with pre-existing renal impairment, nearly 1 in 3 patients have a chance of developing CIN and at any given degree of baseline GFR, diabetes doubles the risk of developing CIN compared with nondiabetic patients.[20,21]

The route, volume and type of contrast administration (intravenous or intra-arterial) and the underlying patient subset (advanced age, associated comorbid conditions, e.g. chronic severe hypertension, diabetes and atherosclerotic vascular disease) also influence whether a particular patient develops CIN. Compared with the intra-arterial route, the intravenous route needs lesser amounts of contrast and since the agent gets diluted in the circulation before reaching the renal vasculature, the chances of athero-embolization are negligible. *Amongst all diagnostic or therapeutic procedures involving contrast administration*, the highest rates of CIN are reported in those undergoing coronary angiography and percutaneous coronary interventions, highlighting the importance of CIN for the practicing cardiologist.[8,10]

The causal link between *intravenous* iodinated contrast material and CIN has recently come into question based on various studies wherein it has been suggested that the nephrotoxicity of intravenous contrast material was perhaps extrapolated largely from studies involving intra-arterial injection of radiocontrast.[22,23] McDonald et al. reported a retrospective analysis on the causal association of intravenous radiocontrast with CIN amongst 157,140 scans in 53,439 patients undergoing abdominal, pelvic, and thoracic CT scans from 2000 to 2010. Even after propensity score adjustment for risk factors, the *incidence of CIN was not significantly different between those administered intravenous contrast and those who did not receive contrast.* When the patients were grouped on basis of SCr levels into low (<1.5 mg/dL), medium (1.5–2.0 mg/dL) and high-risk (>2.0 mg/dL), the incidence of CIN still remained the same. The study concluded that further prospective randomized trials be performed to assess whether administration of intravenous contrast material is indeed nephrotoxic.[24]

DEVELOPMENT OF CLINICAL SCORES FOR RISK STRATIFICATION

Since the individual contribution of each risk factor to the development of CIN is difficult to quantify, risk scores have been developed to predict the occurrence of CIN and identify patients with higher chance to develop CIN. However most of these scores have been derived from patients undergoing coronary angiography (i.e. intra-arterial injection of contrast) and hence their ability to predict risk in the setting of contrast administered via the intravenous route is not well studied. Bartholomew et al. used 8 variables to create a risk score (creatinine clearance <60 mL/min, use of intra-aortic balloon pump, urgent coronary procedure, diabetes mellitus, congestive heart failure, hypertension, peripheral vascular disease, and volume of contrast) and defined CIN as ≥1 mg/dL rise in Scr following the procedure.[25] Mehran et al. have developed a risk score including 3 additional variables (age, hypotension and anemia) and used a cut-off of change in SCr ≥25% or ≥0.5 mg/dL at 48 hours to define CIN.[26] Using these scores in clinical practice especially in patients with a high propensity to develop CIN can appropriately risk stratify them and enable institution of adequate preventive strategies.

PATHOPHYSIOLOGY OF CONTRAST-INDUCED NEPHROPATHY

The pathophysiology of CIN remains incompletely understood. Although various mechanisms have been postulated to explain the genesis of CIN, the most likely reason is prolonged vasoconstriction and impaired autoregulation secondary to contrast media exposure leading to renal medullary hypoxia. The immediate response following contrast media administration is a biphasic change in renal vascular hemodynamics: first a rapid, short lasting renal vasodilatation with an increase in renal blood flow followed by prolonged vasoconstriction. This leads to increase in intra-renal vascular resistance and reduction in renal blood flow.[27] These hemodynamic changes produce a decrease in GFR and renal medullary ischemia due to:

- *Reduction in oxygen supply*: Under normal physiological conditions, despite high oxygen consumption in the renal medulla, its outer portion is oxygen deficient due to its distance from the vasa recta. Locally vasoactive compounds such as prostaglandins, nitric oxide (NO) and adenosine help increase the regional blood flow in the renal medulla and adjust it to the available, albeit limited, O_2 supply.[28] Any interference in these mechanisms as happens after administration of contrast worsens the oxygen supply leading to renal medullary hypoxia.
- *Enhanced medullary oxygen consumption*: Contrast media also induce an osmotic diuresis that increases fluid delivery and consequent tubular reabsorption in the ascending limb of Henle's loops, thereby increasing energy need and O_2 consumption: the result will be a worsening of medullary hypoxia.[29,30] Histopathologic changes consistent with 'osmotic nephrosis' have also been reported in biopsy specimens of kidneys exposure to radiocontrast.
- In addition, formation of reactive oxygen species (ROS) secondary to medullary hypoxia and resultant alterations in nitric oxide metabolism, endothelin and adenosine cause direct tubular and vascular endothelial injury leading to apoptosis and cell death, renal vasoconstriction and fall in renal perfusion.
- Direct cytotoxicity due to contrast media and interference with the Na+/Ca^{2+} exchanger leading to intracellular Ca^{2+} overload are also important contributory factors.
- Under physiological conditions, the renal vasculature maintains low viscosity of the blood flowing through the vasa recta to counteract the high vascular resistance. Contrast media lead to altered rheology of blood due to formation of echinocytes and stomatocytes which reduces red cell deformability and increase in whole blood viscosity and resistance to renal vascular flow.

PREVENTION STRATEGIES

Risk Assessment

The risk of CIN is higher in patients with concomitant morbidities (as defined above) and it is essential that all patients should be assessed for risk and renal parameters measured and monitored, if required. Baseline SCr levels should be measured in all such patients before angiography and creatinine clearance rate or eGFR estimated to accurately identify those patients who are at increased risk for CIN (eGFR <60 mL/min/1.73 m^2). Some authors recommend that only eGFR and not SCr be used to assess renal function in stable outpatients. Alternative imaging methods which do not necessitate contrast medium injection may be considered in patients with high risk and assessment should be done whether the potential benefits from the contrast study outweigh the increased risk of CI-AKI.

Monitoring of SCr levels is recommended only for patients at risk; although the optimum time for remeasurement after contrast administration is not clear, it should be usually performed within 48–96 hours. If SCr increases by 0.25–0.50 mg/dL or ≥25% above baseline, then levels should continue to be monitored. A nephrology consult may be required in patients in whom the SCr levels do not return to baseline within 1 week of the index procedure. In all patients (and especially those with underlying risk factors), steps should be taken to minimize precipitating factors such as hypotension, volume depletion, anemia, heart failure symptoms, and administration of nephrotoxic medications.

Given the multiple number of postulated mechanisms for the pathogenesis of CIN, various prophylactic measures, targeting renal vasoconstriction and hypoxia-induced oxidative stress have been tried. A brief outline is presented below:

Hydration

Prehydration and correction of hypovolemia are very important in all patients before any diagnostic or therapeutic procedures requiring intravascular injection of contrast media. Intravenous hydration before and after administration of iodinated contrast, remains the mainstay for prevention of CIN, especially in patients with an eGFR <60 mL/min/1.73 m^2. Although no large randomized controlled trial has directly compared volume expansion vs no volume expansion, there is general consensus that adequate volume expansion helps prevent the occurrence of CIN. Various postulated mechanisms of benefit include augmentation of intravascular volume, dilution of the contrast load, vasodilation, suppression of renin-angiotensin-aldosterone axis and release of antidiuretic hormone with resultant promotion of diuresis.

- Prehydration with 0.45% saline started 12 hours before and continued 12 hr pos-angiography was reported superior to hydration with 0.45% saline plus mannitol or saline plus furosemide (CIN 11% vs 28% vs 40%; p = 0.05) in preventing CIN in high risk patients with chronic renal insufficiency undergoing cardiac angiography.[31]
- The PRINCE trial also reported a modest benefit of forced diuresis (using intravenous 0.45% saline, mannitol, and furosemide) compared to control (0.45% saline plus placebo) in prevention of CIN, provided a high urine flow rate can be achieved.[32]

Different strengths of saline solution: Although some studies have reported comparable efficacy of half isotonic (0.45%) or isotonic (0.9%) sodium chloride administered 12 hours prior to and after contrast in reducing the incidence of CIN, others have reported that 0.45% saline was not as effective as 0.9% saline.[33,34]

Comparison of *intravenous versus oral saline hydration* has also revealed conflicting results, with one study failing to demonstrate a significant difference, while the other reported that intravenous hydration was superior.[35,36]

Role of sodium bicarbonate ($NaHCO_3$): The benefits of $NaHCO_3$ include (a) alkalinization of urine which alters the local redox potential and reduces the viscosity of the contrast agents, thus minimizing their nephrotoxicity and (b) providing intravenous hydration.

- Multiple single-center, prospective trials have evaluated the use of isotonic $NaHCO_3$ infusions with mixed results, with smaller, nonblinded studies reporting some benefit.[37-39] Merten et al. reported the superiority of hydration with isotonic sodium bicarbonate (154 mEq/L) started 1 hour before and continued for 6 hour after radiocontrast administration as compared to hydration with sodium chloride (incidence of CIN 1.7% vs 13.6%, p = 0.02).[40] The benefit of hydration with $NaHCO_3$ over NaCl (6 hours before and after contrast) was also reported by Ozcan et al. in patients with mild baseline renal insufficiency (CIN rates 4.5% vs 13.6%, p = 0.036).[41] However other studies reported that both $NaHCO_3$ and NaCl were comparable and *the mode of hydration was perhaps not important if a low-toxicity contrast agent was used.*[38,39,42]
- A meta-analysis of 3609 patients (in 19 trials) by Jang et al. concluded that despite significant substantial heterogeneity amongst studies, $NaHCO_3$-based regimes were superior to NaCl-based ones (odds ratio 0.56; 95% CI 0.36–0.86; p = 0.008).[43]
- A review of various trials of $NaHCO_3$ (comprising of 3563 patients) by Zoungas et al. identified substantial heterogeneity amongst trials but concluded that earlier reports may have overestimated the magnitude of benefit and hydration with $NaHCO_3$ was not reported to have any significant effect on the risk for dialysis, heart failure, and total mortality.[44]

The European Renal Best Practice guidelines state that volume expansion with *either* isotonic NaCl or $NaHCO_3$ solutions, is preferred to no volume expansion, in patients at increased risk for CIN.[45] *The CIN Consensus Working Panel* recommendations suggest that in patients kept nil orally or those with potential for hypovolemia, adequate intravenous volume expansion with isotonic crystalloid (1.0–1.5 mL/kg/hr) administered for 3–12 hours before and continued for 6–24 hours after the procedure helps prevent CIN.[46] *The Canadian Association of Radiologists Consensus Guidelines for Prevention of CIN (Update 2012)* recommends that fluid volume loading is the most important preventive measure and $NaHCO_3$ or NaCl solution should be considered for all patients with GFR <60 mL/min who receive intra-arterial contrast and is patients with GFR <45 mL/min in patients who receive intravenous contrast. However, caution needs to be exercised in patients with heart failure where excessive fluid administration may be counter-productive. Oral volume expansion is currently not recommended as a preventive strategy.

Issues Related to Contrast

- Dose
- Contrast types, route of administration, osmolality.

Dose

Volume of contrast media administered during the procedure is one of the most important *modifiable* factors in the development of CIN. The use of large doses and multiple injections (within 72 hours) is directly related to the risk of development of CIN. Every 100 mL of contrast medium increases likelihood of CIN by 12%. As a general guideline, minimizing the dose of contrast (<3–5 mL/kg or approximately 100 mL) and using automated injectors can help reduce the amount of contrast administered and therefore the incidence of CIN. In patients who develop CIN or are at high risk, repeated procedures should be avoided and further exposure to radiocontrast should be delayed until renal function has fully recovered. Recommended formulae for radiocontrast dose calculation

- *Cigarroa's formula*: 5 mL contrast/kg/SCr (mg/dL) with maximum dose <300 mL.[47]
- *Laskey's formula*: Contrast volume/eGFR ratio (cut-off ~3.7 for PCI (145). At ratio <2, risk of CIN is almost negligible.[48]
- Ratio of grams of iodine in the contrast to eGFR (cut-off <1-1.42 reduce the risk of CIN.[49]

Although primarily validated and used for patients undergoing coronary angioplasty, these can be used as a rough guide and extrapolated for use in other interventional procedures as well. The interventional cardiologist/radiologist also needs to be aware of other techniques which can help in minimizing the dose. These include diluting the contrast with normal saline (e.g. up to 1:3–1:5), bolus chase and biplane angiography to obtain multiple views with a single injection and accurate catheter positioning, especially during peripheral imaging of extremities using DSA.

Contrast Types (Table 23.2)

Iodinated radiocontrast media have varying osmolalities and viscosities. Osmolality is determined by the ratio of iodine atoms to osmotically active particles and a close relation exists between the osmolality and viscosity of contrast media. *High-osmolar ionic contrast media* (HOCM, e.g. diatrizoate) have an osmolality ~5–8 times the osmolality of plasma (1500–1800 mOsm/kg). *Nonionic low-osmolar contrast media* (LOCM e.g. iohexol) have an osmolality of 600–850 mOsm/kg which is approximately 2–3 times the osmolality of plasma. *Nonionic isoosmolar contrast media* (IOCM, e.g. iodixanol) have an osmolality similar to that of plasma (~290 mOsm/kg). The IOCM despite their lower osmolality have an increased viscosity and dimeric IOCM have about twice the viscosity as compared to monomeric LOCM.

Table 23.2 Various types of contrast agents with their generic and brand names

High osmolar	Diatrizoate
Low osmolar	Ioxaglate (Hexabrix)
	Iohexol (Omnipaque)
	Iopamidol (Isovue 370)
	Iopromide (Ultravist)
	Ioversol (Optiray)
	Iomeprol (Iomeron)
Iso-osmolar	Iodixanol (Visipaque)

Route of administration:

- The incidence of CIN following *intravenous* use of IOCM or LOCM has been reported to be not significantly different, especially amongst patients without underlying risk factors.
- On the other hand, *intra-arterial administration* of IOCM (iodixanol) is associated with a lower risk of CIN particularly in high-risk diabetic patients undergoing coronary or aortofemoral angiography. However other studies evaluating intra-arterial use have either reported no significant difference between IOCM vs LOCM or a higher incidence of CIN in those receiving IOCM. The greater nephrotoxicity could perhaps be due to the higher viscosity of the IOCM (iodixanol) compared with LOCM.
- In a meta-analysis comparing IOCM (iodixanol) with LOCM, Heinrech et al. reported no significant difference in the incidence of CIN, especially after *intravenous* administration or in patients without pre-existing renal insufficiency.[50] However, in those with *renal insufficiency and procedures requiring intra-arterial contrast*, IOCM were associated with a lower risk for CIN.
- *Message*: There is some evidence to suggest that IOCM (iodixanol) is associated with lower rates of CIN than LOCM, especially in those with pre-existing renal impairment with and without diabetes. The use of *IOCM may particularly be beneficial in patients with renal insufficiency and diabetes who are receiving intra-arterial contrast.*

Low-osmolar vs high-osmolar contrast agents:

- Initial randomized trials of ionic vs nonionic contrast showed no significant difference in CIN, although subset analysis did suggest that amongst patients with pre-existing renal dysfunction, non-ionic LOCM were more nephroprotective.
- Comparison of iohexol (LOCM) vs diatrizoate (HOCM) in patients undergoing angiography revealed that the incidence of CIN was 2 times more common in the HOCM group (7% vs 3%, $p < 0.002$) and this was especially evident in those with baseline renal insufficiency with or without diabetes.[51]
- A meta-analysis of 31 randomized trials comparing LOCM vs HOCM by Barrett et al. reported that the pooled odds of rise in SCr > 0.5 mg/dL was 0.61 (95% confidence interval [CI], 0.48–0.77) for LOCM; this nephroprotective effect was only significant in patients with pre-existing renal impairment (OR 0.5; CI, 0.36–0.68).[52]
- *Message*: In patients with existing renal impairment, LOCM are superior to HOCM to prevent CIN. Presently LOCM have largely replaced HOCM due to fewer side effects and better tolerability.

Iso-osmolar versus low osmolar agents:

- The efficacy of IOCM in reducing AKI compared with that of LOCM has been debated. While some studies and meta-analyses have shown no significant difference in the rates of CIN between IOCM and LOCM, others have shown contrasting results. Retrospective analysis of 20,242 patients by Davenport et al. reported that LOCM predispose to CIN only in patients with eGFR <30 mL/min/1.73 m^2 while in patients with baseline eGFR >45 mL/min/1.73 m^2 both were comparable.[53]
- Various trials have studied the role of ISOM vs LOCM in high risk patients (including renal insufficiency with/without diabetes). The RECOVER [iodixanol vs ioxaglate39] and NEPHRIC (iodixanol vs iohexol) trials reported the superiority of IOCM over LOCM for prevention of CIN.[54,55] However the ICON (iodixanol vs ioxaglate) and CARE (iodixanol vs iopamide) trials did not find any significant difference between the two groups.[56,57]
- Some LOCM are more likely to cause CI-AKI. Studies have shown that of all, LOCM, only iohexol has been associated with *a significantly increased risk of developing CIN* the incidence of CIN with *iohexol compared with* other LOCM (iopamidol) or IOCM (iodixanol) has been reported to be 25%, 13.5% and 11%, respectively; $p < 0.05$).[58,59]
- A meta-analysis of 2727 patients undergoing cardiac angiography in 16 double-blind randomized trials comparing the incidence CIN in patients receiving IOCM (iodixanol) versus LOCM revealed that the *CIN was significantly less common with IOCM group* amongst all patient groups (1.4% vs 3.5%, $p < 0.001$) as well as in those with renal impairment (2.8% vs 8.4%, $p < 0.001$) and with coexisting renal insufficiency and diabetes mellitus.[60]
- *Based on these initial data, the* American College of Cardiology/American Heart Association's revised 2007 guidelines for the management of patients with unstable angina/non-ST elevation myocardial infarction, accorded IOCM a class IA recommendation for coronary angiography in patients with chronic kidney disease.
- *However the latest meta-analysis* of comparison of renal safety of IOCM (iodixanol) versus LOCM by Reed et al. comprising of 16 trials including 2,763 subjects revealed that there was no difference in the incidence of CI-AKI in two groups (RR: 0.79, 95% CI: 0.56–1.12, $p = 0.19$).[61] Comparing individual agents, IOCM (iodixanol) was superior to the LOCM (ioxaglate and iohexol) but similar in efficacy to other LOCM (iopamidol, iopromide, iomeprol, and ioversol). Hence the propensity to develop CIN following contrast may be in fact governed by the underlying physicochemical properties of different agents. Therefore the *2009 ACC/AHA guidelines for percutaneous coronary interventions revised the recommendations* for patients with chronic renal insufficiency stating that either IOCM (level of evidence A) or LOCM (other than ioxaglate and iohexol, level of evidence B) may be used.

Other Measures with Unproven Benefit

N-acetylcysteine

The rationale of using N-acetylcysteine (NAC) for prevention of CIN is based on the fact that it is an antioxidant and free radical scavenger that leads to vasodilation through nitric oxide-mediated pathways. Since the bioavailability of oral NAC is low (5–10%), studies have also assessed the role of IV NAC in prevention of CIN. The commonly used dose regimes are 600–1200 mg orally twice daily on the day before the procedure and the day of the procedure while or intravenous (150 mg/kg in 500 mL NS over 30 minutes prior and 50 mg/kg in 500 mL NS over 4 hours after contrast administration). It is unclear whether NAC is useful in preventing CIN since small studies and various meta-analysis have reported conflicting results.

- The meta-analysis by Trivedi et al. evaluated high-dose oral or IV NAC for the prevention of CIN (≥1200 mg daily or a single periprocedural dose >600 mg (within 4 hours of contrast exposure) and reported an odds ratio of 0.46 (95% confidence interval [CI], 0.33–0.63) for the occurrence of CIN. The analysis concluded that *high-dose NAC reduced the incidence of CIN.*[62]
- A later pooled analysis, Loomba et al. however reported that although NAC (600 mg) prevented CIN in patients undergoing coronary angiography, there was no significant benefit in terms of pre- and post-procedure SCr levels, need for dialysis and all-cause mortality. The authors concluded that the *dose and route of administration of NAC does not have any significant effect on clinical outcomes after angiography.*[63]

- A structured review and meta-analysis of various NAC trials by O'Sullivan et al. also revealed similar results; *NAC did not reduce the incidence of CIN* (pooled OR 1.05; 95% confidence interval [CI] 0.38–2.88; p = 0.92) *or the mean SCr levels* (pooled weighted mean difference, 4.38; 95% CI 10.40–1.65; p = 0.15).[64]
- Combining the results of 10 NAC trials involving 1916 patients, Sun et al. reported a *nonsignificant trend towards benefit in patients treated with intravenous NAC* (summary risk ratio 0.68, 95% CI, 0.46–1.02). The analysis summarized that there was significant heterogeneity in NAC effect across studies and the efficacy of NAC on clinical endpoints such as dialysis, hospital stay and mortality was not convincing.[65]
- *Message*: Based on these data, currently not enough evidence exists to recommend NAC for the prevention of CIN in patients undergoing angiography.

It also needs to be borne in mind that NAC may lower SCr levels without affecting renal function; in contrast serum cystatin C levels, which are a more accurate measure of GFR, are unaffected by NAC. Studies have shown that in patients with renal insufficiency undergoing contrast CT, administration of NAC was reported to reduce the incidence of CIN as defined by changes in SCr levels. However, when CIN was defined using cystatin C levels, there was no benefit of NAC.[66]

Dopamine has also been studied as a preventive strategy for CIN based on its renal vasodilatory effects and ability to enhance GFR and renal blood flow. While few studies found dopamine to be effective in preventing CIN, especially in those with elevated baseline SCr (>2 mg/dL), others found it to have no effect.[67-70] *Fenoldopam*, a selective, dopamine-1 receptor agonist which causes systemic and renal arteriolar vasodilatation was initially shown to reduce the incidence of CIN in small observational studies. However subsequent randomized trials have shown contrasting results with some reporting a trend toward reduced incidence of CIN, and others reporting no benefit.[71,72] *Current evidence does not support the use of dopamine or fenoldopam to prevent CIN.* Since adenosine is involved in the pathogenesis of CIN, it was hypothesized that adenosine A1-receptor antagonist, *theophylline*, may help prevent CIN by countering the reduction in renal blood flow and GFR following contrast administration. Although several nonrandomized and randomized studies have been conducted, overall data are inconsistent. While oral (200 mg od) as well as intravenous (165 mg) theophylline have been reported to reduce the incidence of CIN, other studies failed to demonstrate any benefit of theophylline compared with placebo in preventing CIN.[70,73-75] Meta analysis of theophylline trials have revealed considerable heterogeneity among the studies with different dosing schedules of theophylline, varying hydration protocols and types of contrast, making it *difficult to recommend it as a conclusive measure for prevention of CIN.*

Hemofiltration or hemodialysis to remove the contrast media without depleting intravascular volume has also been used to counter the adverse effects of CIN. Studies in patients with CRF on dialysis, observed that high-flux hemodialysis and hemodiafiltration effectively remove radiocontrast as compared to low-flux hemodialysis and hemofiltration. Schindler et al.[76] Continuous venovenous hemofiltration has also been reported to be beneficial for prevention of CIN in patients with severe chronic renal insufficiency. However whether this actually prevents CIN is questionable and prophylactic hemodialysis does not diminish the rates of CIN.[77] The European Renal Best Practice guidelines do not recommend prophylactic intermittent hemodialysis or hemofiltration to prevent CIN.

The fact that intracellular Ca+ overload and alterations in calcium metabolism are observed in CIN, studies have also investigated the role of *calcium channel antagonists* in preventing CIN. While some studies have reported benefit of agents like nitrendipine, others have failed to demonstrate any favorable effect using nitrendipine and nifedipine. Other agents which have been tried for prevention of CIN include *prostaglandin E1, atrial natriuretic peptide, ascorbic acid, furosemide, nebivolol, tocopherol, Trimetazidine, recombinant human erythropoietin and statins* but none of them is currently recommended for routine use.

WITHHOLDING VARIOUS DRUGS

- *Potentially nephrotoxic medications* such as nonsteroidal anti-inflammatory drugs and aminoglycosides should be withheld or avoided.
- *Metformin*: Although metformin is not nephrotoxic it is exclusively excreted via the kidneys and lactic acidosis has been reported in patients on metformin who develop CIN following administration of contrast. According to the American College of Radiology guidelines, metformin should be withheld for 48 hours prior to contrast administration in *all* patients with *eGFR <45 mL/min* and in those with *eGFR ≥45 mL/min and liver dysfunction, heart failure and sepsis.*
- Whether *angiotensin-converting enzyme (ACE) inhibitors and ARBs* contribute to increased risk of developing CIN is controversial. While few studies have reported an increased risk of CIN in patients receiving ACEI/ARBs, others have reported either no increase in risk or in fact, reduced risk of development of CIN in such patients. according to the Kidney Disease Improving Global Outcomes (KDIGO) guidelines for Acute Kidney Injury Work Group, the effectiveness of withholding ACEI and ARB in patients at high risk for CIN undergoing angiography is not well established. An individualized

decision needs to be taken for each case, considering the risk versus benefit of continuing or withholding ACEI/ARB especially in high risk patients.

CONCLUSION

Contrast-induced nephropathy (CIN) is an important cause of hospital-acquired renal dysfunction following the use of iodinated contrast media failure, especially in patients with a associated risk factors. The most important predisposing factors include pre-existing renal insufficiency and diabetes. The development of an adequate prophylaxis strategy has been limited by the lack of an effective understanding of the exact pathophysiology of CIN. Of all reported preventive measures, maintaining adequate periprocedural hydration, limiting the amount of contrast use and using IOCM or LOCM agents (esepcially in those with renal impairment) are the most important. With an increasing number of referrals for cardiac catheterization and radiology studies in an aging patient population with higher comorbidities, the incidence of CIN is likely to increase. Since the patients often are asymptomatic, physicians need to be aware of the likelihood of occurrence of CIN in patients with risk factors and to monitor renal function in this group. Future research needs to be directed towards accurately identifying high risk patients and testing newer therapies in adequately powered and well designed randomized clinical trials.

REFERENCES

1. Gleeson TG, Bulugahapitiya S, Contrast-induced nephropathy. American Journal of Roentgenology. 2004;183(6):1673-89.
2. Mccullough P, Sandberg K. Epidemiology of contrast induced nephropathy. Rev Cardiovasc Med. 2003:4(suppl 5):S3-S9
3. Kolonko A, Kokot F, Wiecek A. Contrast-associated nephropathy—old clinical problem and new therapeutic perspectives. Nephrol Dial Transplant. 1998;13(3):803-6.
4. Rabbani AB, Nallamothu BK. Contrast-induced nephropathy risk assessment in real world practice. Am J Med. 2011;124: 1127-8.
5. Cockcroft DW, Gault MH. Prediction of creatinine clearance from serum creatinine, Nephron. 1976;16(1):31-41.
6. Levey AS, Bosch JP, Lewis JB, Greene T, Rogers N, Roth D. A more accurate method to estimate glomerular filtration rate from serum creatinine: a new prediction equation, Annals of Internal Medicine. 1999;130(6):461-70.
7. Levey AS, Stevens LA, Schmid CH, et al. A new equation to estimate glomerular filtration rate. Annals of Internal Medicine. 2009;150(9):604-12.
8. Rihal CS, Textor SC, Grill DE, et al. Incidence and prognostic importance of acute renal failure after percutaneous coronary intervention. Circulation. 2002;105:2259-64.
9. Best PJ, Lennon R, Ting HH, et al. The impact of renal insufficiency on clinical outcomes in patients undergoing percutaneous coronary interventions. J Am Coll Cardiol. 2002;39:1113-9.
10. McCullough PA, Wolyn R, Rocher LL, et al. Acute renal failure after coronary intervention: Incidence, risk factors, and relationship to mortality. Am J Med. 1997;103:368-75.
11. Gruberg L, Mintz GS, Mehran R, et al. The prognostic implications of further renal function deterioration within 48 h of interventional coronary procedures in patients with pre-existent chronic renal insufficiency. J Am Coll Cardiol. 2000;36:1542.
12. Parfrey PS, Griffiths SM, Barrett BJ, et al. Contrast material induced renal failure in patients with diabetes mellitus, renal insufficiency, or both. A prospective controlled study. N Engl J Med. 1989;320:143-9.
13. Rich MW, Crecelius CA. Incidence, risk factors, and clinical course of acute renal insufficiency after cardiac catheterization in patients 70 years of age or older. A prospective study. Arch Intern Med. 1990;150:1237-42.
14. Rudnick MR, Goldfarb S, Wexler L, et al. Nephrotoxicity of ionic and nonionic contrast media in 1196 patients: A randomized trial. The Iohexol Cooperative Study. Kidney Int. 1995; 47:254-61.
15. McCullough PA, Adam A, Becker CR, et al. Risk prediction of contrast-induced nephropathy. Am J Cardiol. 2006;98:27K-36K.
16. Thomsen HS, Morcos SK. Risk of contrast-medium-induced nephropathy in high-risk patients undergoing MDCT—a pooled analysis of two randomized trials. Eur Radiol. 2009;19:891-7.
17. Goldfarb S, McCullough PA, McDermott J, Gay SB. Contrast-induced acute kidney injury: specialty-specific protocols for interventional radiology, diagnostic computed tomography radiology, and interventional cardiology. Mayo Clin Proc. 2009;84(2):170-9.
18. Bagshaw SM, Culleton BF. Contrast-induced nephropathy: Epidemiology and prevention. Minerva Cardioangiol. 2006;54:109-29.
19. Mehran R, Nikolsky E. Contrast-induced nephropathy: definition, epidemiology, and patients at risk. Kidney International. Supplement. 2006. pp. S11-S15.
20. Hardiek KJ, Katholi RE, Robbs RS, Katholi CE. Renal effects of contrast media in diabetic patients undergoing diagnostic or interventional coronary angiography. Journal of Diabetes and its Complications. 2008;22(3):171-7.
21. Barrett BJ, Parfrey PS, Vavasour HM, McDonald J, Kent G, Hefferton D, et al. Contrast nephropathy in patients with impaired renal function; high versus low osmolar media. Kidney Int. 1992;41:1274-933
22. McDonald JS, McDonald RJ, Comin J, et al. Frequency of acute kidney injury following intravenous contrast medium administration: a systematic review and meta-analysis. Radiology. 2013;267(1)119-28.
23. Rao QA, Newhouse JH. Risk of nephropathy after intravenous administration of contrast material: a critical literature analysis, Radiology. 2006;239(2):392-7.
24. McDonald RJ, McDonald JS, Bida JP, et al. Intravenous contrast material-induced nephropathy: causal or coincident phenomenon? Radiology. 2013;267(1):106-18.
25. Bartholomew BA, Harjai KJ, Dukkipati S, et al. Impact of nephropathy after percutaneous coronary intervention and a method for risk stratification. Am J Cardiol. 2004;93:1515-9.
26. Mehran R, Aymong ED, Nikolsky E, et al. A simple risk score for prediction of contrast-induced nephropathy after percutaneous coronary intervention: Development and initial validation. J Am Coll Cardiol. 2004;44:1393-9.

27. Murphy SW, Barrett BJ, Parfrey PS. Contrast nephropathy. Journal of the American Society of Nephrology. 2000;11(1): 177-82.
28. Heyman SN, Rosen S, Rosenberger C. Renal parenchymal hypoxia, hypoxia adaptation, and the pathogenesis of radiocontrast nephropathy. Clinical Journal of the American Society of Nephrology. 2008;3(1):288-96.
29. Bucher AM, deCecco CN, Schoepfetal UJ. Is contrast medium osmolality a causal factor for contrast-induced nephropathy? BioMed Research International, vol. 2014, Article ID 931413, 8 pages, 2014.
30. Andreucci M, Faga T, Pisani A, Sabbatini M, Michael A. Pathogenesis of acute renal failure induced by iodinated radiographic contrast media. Austin Journal of Nephrology and Hypertension. 2014;1(1):1-6.
31. Solomon R, Werner C, Mann D, et al. Effects of saline, mannitol, and furosemide to prevent acute decreases in renal function induced by radiocontrast agents. N Engl J Med. 1994;331: 1416-20.
32. Stevens MA, McCullough PA, Tobin KJ, et al. A prospective randomized trial of prevention measures in patients at high risk for contrast nephropathy: results of the PRINCE Study. Prevention of Radiocontrast Induced Nephropathy Clinical Evaluation. J Am Coll Cardiol. 1999;33:403-11.
33. Solomon RJ, Natarajan MK, Doucet S, et al. Cardiac Angiography in Renally Impaired Patients (CARE) study: a randomized double-blind trial of contrast-induced nephropathy in patients with chronic kidney disease. Circulation. 2007;115:3189-96.
34. Mueller C, Buerkle G, Buettner HJ, et al. Prevention of contrast media-associated nephropathy: randomized comparison of 2 hydration regimens in 1620 patients undergoing coronary angioplasty. Arch Intern Med. 2002;162:329-36.
35. Taylor AJ, Hotchkiss D, Morse RW, et al. PREPARED: Preparation for angiography in renal dysfunction: A randomized trial of inpatient vs outpatient hydration protocols for cardiac catheterization in mild-to-moderate renal dysfunction. Chest. 1998;114:1570-4.
36. Trivedi HS, Moore H, Nasr S, et al. A randomized prospective trial to assess the role of saline hydration on the development of contrast nephrotoxicity. Nephron Clin Pract. 2003;93:C29-C34.
37. Motohiro M, Kamihata H, Tsujimoto S, et al. A new protocol using sodium bicarbonate for the prevention of contrast-induced nephropathy in patients undergoing coronary angiography. Am J Cardiol. 2011;107:1604-8.
38. Adolph E, Holdt-Lehmann B, Chatterjee T, et al. Renal Insufficiency Following Radiocontrast Exposure Trial (REINFORCE): a randomized comparison of sodium bicarbonate versus sodium chloride hydration for the prevention of contrast-induced nephropathy. Coron Artery Dis. 2008;19:413-9.
39. Brar SS, Shen AY, Jorgensen MB, et al. Sodium bicarbonate vs sodium chloride for the prevention of contrast medium-induced nephropathy in patients undergoing coronary angiography: a randomized trial. JAMA. 2008;300:1038-46.
40. Merten GJ, Burgess WP, Gray LV, et al. Prevention of contrast induced nephropathy with sodium bicarbonate: A randomized controlled trial. JAMA. 2004;291:2328-34.
41. Ozcan EE, Guneri S, Akdeniz B, Akylldlz IZ, Senaslan O, Baris N, et al. Sodium bicarbonate, N-acetylcysteine, and saline for prevention of radiocontrast-induced nephropathy. A comparison of 3 regimens for protecting contrast-induced nephropathy in patients undergoing coronary procedures. A single-center prospective controlled trial. Am Heart J. 2007;154:539-44.
42. Vasheghani-Farahani A, Sadigh G, Kassaian SE, Khatami SM, Fotouhi A, Razavi SA. Sodium bicarbonate plus isotonic saline versus saline for prevention of contrast-induced nephropathy in patients undergoing coronary angiography: a randomized controlled trial. Am J Kidney Dis. 2009;54:610-8.
43. Jang JS, Jin HY, Seo JS, Yang TH, Kim DK, Kim TH et al. Sodium bicarbonate therapy for the prevention of contrast-induced acute kidney injury: a systematic review and meta-analysis. Circ J. 2012;76:2255-65.
44. Zoungas S, Ninomiya T, Huxley R, Cass A, Perkovic V, et al. Systematic Review: Sodium Bicarbonate Treatment Regimens for the Prevention of Contrast-Induced Nephropathy. Annals of Internal Medicine. 2009;151:631-W207.
45. Fliser D, Laville M, Covic A, et al. A European Renal BestPractice (ERBP) position statement on the Kidney Disease Improving Global Outcomes (KDIGO) Clinical Practice Guidelines on Acute Kidney Injury: part 1: definitions, conservative management and contrast-induced nephropathy. Nephrology Dialysis Transplantation. 2012;27(12):4263-72.
46. Stacul F, Adam A, Becker CR, et al. Strategies to reduce the risk of contrast-induced nephropathy. Am J Cardiol. 2006;98: 59K-77K.
47. Cigarroa RG, Lange RA, Williams RH, Hillis D. Dosing of contrastmaterial to prevent contrastnephropathy in patients with renal disease. The American Journal of Medicine. 1989;86:649-52.
48. Laskey WK, Jenkins C, Selzer F, et al. Volume-to-creatinine clearance ratio: a pharmacokinetically based risk factor for prediction of early creatinine increase after percutaneous coronary intervention. Journal of the American College of Cardiology. 2007;50(7):584-90.
49. Keaney JJ, Hannon CM, Murray PT. Contrast-induced acute kidney injury: how much contrast is safe? Nephrology Dialysis Transplantation. 2013;28 (6):1376-83.
50. Heinrich MC, Haberle L, Muller V, Bautz W, Uder M. Nephrotoxicity of iso-osmolar iodixanol compared with nonionic low-osmolar contrast media: meta-analysis of randomized controlled trials. Radiology. 2009;250:68-86.
51. Rudnick MR, Goldfarb S, Wexler L, et al. Nephrotoxicity of ionic and nonionic contrast media in 1196 patients: A randomized trial. The Iohexol Cooperative Study. Kidney Int. 1995;47:254-61.
52. Barrett BJ, Carlisle EJ. Metaanalysis of the relative nephrotoxicity of high- and low-osmolality iodinated contrast media. Radiology. 1993;188:171-8.
53. Davenport MS, Khalatbari S, Cohan RH, Dillman JR, Myles JD, Ellis JH. Contrastmaterial-induced nephrotoxicity and intravenous low-osmolality iodinated contrast material: risk stratification by using estimated glomerular filtration rate. Radiology. 2013;268(3):719-28.
54. Jo SH, Youn TJ, Koo BK, Park JS, Kang HJ, Cho YS, Chung WY, Joo GW, Chae IH, Choi DJ, Oh BH, Lee MM, Park YB, Kim HS. Renal toxicity evaluation and comparison between visipaque (iodixanol) and hexabrix (ioxaglate) in patients with renal insufficiency undergoing coronary angiography: the RECOVER study: a randomized controlled trial. J Am Coll Cardiol. 2006;48(5):924-30.

55. Aspelin P, Aubry P, Fransson SG, Strasser R, Willenbrock R, Berg KJ. Nephrotoxic effects in high-risk patients undergoing angiography. Nephrotoxicity in High-Risk Patients Study of Iso-Osmolar and Low-Osmolar Non-Ionic Contrast Media Study Investigators. N Engl J Med. 2003;348(6):491-9.
56. Mehran R. ICON—A prospective, randomized, placebo-controlled trial of ioxaglate versus iodixanol in patients at increased risk for contrast nephropathy. Proceedings of Transcatheter Cardiovascular Therapeutics. 2006;3:10.
57. Solomon RJ, Natarajan MK, Doucet S, Sharma SK, Staniloae CS, Katholi RE, Gelormini JL, Labinaz M, Moreyra AE. Cardiac Angiography in Renally Impaired Patients (CARE) study: a randomized double-blind trial of contrast-induced nephropathy in patients with chronic kidney disease. Investigators of the CARE Study. Circulation. 2007;115(25):3189-96.
58. Solomon R. The role of osmolality in the incidence of contrast-induced nephropathy: a systematic review of angiographic contrast media in high risk patients. Kidney Int. 2005;68:2256-63.
59. Sharma SK, Kini A. Effect of nonionic radiocontrast agents on the occurrence of contrast-induced nephropathy in patients with mild-moderate chronic renal insufficiency: pooled analysis of the randomized trials. Catheter Cardiovasc Interv. 2005;65: 386-93.
60. McCullough PA, Bertrand ME, Brinker JA, et al. A meta-analysis of the renal safety of isosmolar iodixanol compared with low-osmolar contrast media. J Am Coll Cardiol. 2006;48:692-9.
61. Reed M, Meier P, Tamhane UU, Welch KB, Moscucci M, Gurm HS. The relative renal safety of iodixanol compared with low-osmolar contrast media: a meta-analysis of randomized controlled trials. JACC Cardiovasc Interv. 2009;2(7):645-54.
62. Trivedi H, Daram S, Szabo A, Bartorelli AL, Marenzi G. High-dose N-acetylcysteine for the prevention of contrast-induced nephropathy. Am J Med. 2009;122(9):874.e9-15.
63. Loomba RS, Shah PH, Aggarwal S, Arora RR. Role of N-Acetylcysteine to Prevent Contrast-Induced Nephropathy: A Meta-analysis. Am J Ther, 2013.
64. O'Sullivan S, Healy DA, Moloney MC, Grace PA, Walsh SR. The role of N-acetylcysteine in the prevention of contrast-induced nephropathy in patients undergoing peripheral angiography: a structured review and meta-analysis. Angiology. 2013;64(8): 576-82.
65. Sun Z, Fu Q, Cao L, Jin W, Cheng L, Li Z. Intravenous N-acetylcysteine for prevention of contrast-induced nephropathy: a meta analysis of randomized controlled trials. PLoS One. 2013;8(1):e55124.
66. Hoffmann U, Fischereder M, Krüger B, Drobnik W, Krömer BK. The value of N-acetylcysteine in the prevention of radiocontrast agent-induced nephropathy seems questionable. J Am Soc Nephrol. 2004;15(2):407-10
67. Kapoor A, Sinha N, Sharma RK, et al. Use of dopamine in prevention of contrast induced acute renal failure—A randomized study. Int J Cardiol. 1996;53:233-6.
68. Hans SS, Hans BA, Dhillon R, et al. Effect of dopamine on renal function after arteriography in patients with pre-existing renal insufficiency. Am Surg. 1998;64:432-6.
69. Gare M, Haviv YS, Ben-Yehuda A, et al. The renal effect of low-dose dopamine in high-risk patients undergoing coronary angiography. J Am Coll Cardiol. 1999;34:1682-8.
70. Abizaid AS, Clark CE, Mintz GS, et al. Effects of dopamine and aminophylline on contrast-induced acute renal failure after coronary angioplasty in patients with preexisting renal insufficiency. Am J Cardiol. 1999;83:260-3, A265.
71. Tumlin JA, Wang A, Murray PT, et al. Fenoldopam mesylate blocks reductions in renal plasma flow after radiocontrast dye infusion: A pilot trial in the prevention of contrast nephropathy. Am Heart J. 2002;143:894-903.
72. Allaqaband S, Tumuluri R, Malik AM, et al. Prospective randomized study of N-acetylcysteine, fenoldopam, and saline for prevention of radiocontrast-induced nephropathy. Catheter Cardiovasc Interv. 2002;57:279-83.
73. Huber W, Ilgmann K, Page M, et al. Effect of theophylline on contrast material-nephropathy in patients with chronic renal insufficiency: Controlled, randomized, double-blinded study. Radiology. 2002;223:772-9.
74. Kapoor A, Kumar S, Gulati S, et al. The role of theophylline in contrast-induced nephropathy: A case-control study. Nephrol Dial Transplant. 2002;17:1936-41.
75. Erley CM, Duda SH, Rehfuss D, et al. Prevention of radiocontrast-media-induced nephropathy in patients with pre-existing renal insufficiency by hydration in combination with the adenosine antagonist theophylline. Nephrol Dial Transplant. 1999;14: 1146-9.
76. Schindler R, Stahl C, Venz S, Ludat K, Krause W, Frei U. Removal of contrast media by different extracorporeal treatments. Nephrology Dialysis Transplantation. 2001;(16,7):1471-4.
77. Lehnert T, Keller E, Gondolf K, Schäffner T, Pavenstädt H, Schollmeyer P. Effect of haemodialysis after contrast medium administration in patients with renal insufficiency. Nephrology Dialysis Transplantation. 1998;13(2)358-62.

CHAPTER

24

Rehabilitation after Percutaneous Transluminal Coronary Angioplasty

Rajendra G Bahaley

INTRODUCTION

Cardiovascular disease (CVD) is the most common cause of death worldwide. Today, the cardiologists approach to the patient with acute myocardial infarction (MI) has changed dramatically. The infarct is often interrupted by thrombolysis and/or coronary interventions that leave the heart relatively undamaged and able to withstand further ischaemic stresses.

The exponential growth in percutaneous transluminal coronary angioplasty (PTCA) since its first clinical application in 1977 by Andreas Gruentzig has been dramatic. Currently, more than one million coronary angioplasty and stent implantation procedures are performed annually.

We know percutaneous coronary intervention (PCI) is only focal treatment of systemic problem. It is usually done, only to flow limiting lesions, and all physiologically insignificant lesions (<70%) are left alone to be taken care of by medical management and lifestyle modification.

Success is not only in achieving angiographic TIMI 3 flow but is also in the follow up and it starts from the point the patient is wheeled out from Cath Lab. Target should be to treat the lesion and also to provide wholesome patient care. Currently, the annual risk of major cardiac event following PCI is 5–7%. Cardiac rehabilitation (CR) can assist these patients symptomatically as well as physically and mentally in coping with their coronary disease.

In this chapter, we will mainly focus on rehabilitation of patients who have undergone revascularization by PTCA and secondary prevention (SP).

CARDIAC REHABILITATION DEFINITION

A broader definition embrace those of the World Health Organization (WHO) and European Society of Cardiology (ESC) and includes the intentions of the United States (US) Public Health Service as follows, "CR is the coordinated sum of interventions required to ensure the best physical, psychological and social conditions so that patients with chronic or post-acute CVD may, by their own efforts, preserve or resume optimal functioning in society and, through improved health behaviors, slow or reverse progression of disease".[1] It is a complex intervention that may involve a variety of therapies, including risk factor education, psychological input and drug therapy. None the less, international clinical guidelines consistently identify exercise therapy as a central element of CR.[1-4]

Cardiac rehabilitation program (CRP) has become an integral part of the standard of care in modern cardiology. Its scope has shifted from the emphasis on exercise therapy to comprehensive secondary prevention strategies managing risk factors and nutritional, psychological, behavioral and social factors that can affect patient outcomes.

EVIDENCE BASE

There is ample evidence attesting to the benefits of CR.[5] CR promotes recovery, enables patients to achieve and maintain better health and reduces the risk of death in people who have heart disease. A combination of exercise, psychological interventions and education appears to be the most effective form of rehabilitation.[6]

Benefits of Cardiac Rehabilitation

- Improvement in exercise tolerance
- Improvement in psychosocial well-being
- Improvement in blood lipid levels
- Reduction in symptoms
- Reduction in cigarette smoking/tobacco use
- Reduction of stress
- Reduction in blood pressure
- Better control of diabetes
- Reduction in morbidity and mortality.

Importance

Patients, who undergo an angioplasty and possibly the placement of stents, have a much higher chance of survival if they receive structured follow-up care such as CRP. Randal Thomas and team gathered data from Mayo Clinic register on patients who had been treated with PCI.[7] After analyzing 14 years' worth data the authors found that mortality from all causes was reduced by 46% in angioplasty patients who took part in CR.

The PCI, although a vital procedure, is not a heart disease cure. CRPs are effective at improving recovery, quality of life and long-term survival because they help the lifestyle and medication therapies that have been shown to slow or even reverse the progression of atherosclerosis.

Indication

In a recent presidential advisory from the American Heart Association (AHA), Baledy and co-authors[8] made a clear and compelling case for the importance of CRP as SP centers. Given the significant benefits that cardiac rehabilitation (RC)/ secondary prevention (SP) programs bring CVD prevention, every recent major evidence-based guideline from the AHA and the American College of Cardiology (ACC) foundation about the management and prevention of Coronary Heart Disease (CHD) provides a Class I recommendation for the referral to CR/SP programs for those patients with recent myocardial infarction (MI) or acute coronary syndrome (ACS), chronic stable angina, heart failure, or after coronary artery bypass grafting (CABG) or PTCA. CR/SP is also indicated for those patients after valve surgery or cardiac transplantation.

Components of Cardiac Rehabilitation

Traditionally, CR is divided into three phases.[9] All phases of CR aim to facilitate recovery and to prevent further CVD.

Phase I or inpatient phase is initiated while the patient is still in the hospital. Because of the shorter hospital stay with modern cardiology, it is limited to early mobilization to make self care possible by discharge and counseling about the nature of illness or interventions, to reassure the patient about further progress, need for continued medication, risk factors management, exercise prescription and follow up planning. It is delivered on individual basis or to groups of patients. Evidence shows that when SP treatments are started in the hospital, patients are more likely to adhere to those treatments in the long-term, and more likely to remain free from recurrent cardiovascular (CV) events.[10]

Phase II is a supervised ambulatory outpatient program which consist of outpatient monitored exercise and aggressive risk factor reduction. It is conducted during convalescence. Ideally it should start within the first few days after discharge from the hospital. Ambulatory CR usually ends within 2–12 weeks. They vary widely in content. Almost all contain an element of group exercise which is conducted by health professional. An educational and supportive element is inevitably delivered together with exercise. Sessions may be offered once, twice or thrice per week. Best practice ambulatory programs are conducted by a multidisciplinary team. However, it is recognized that a CRP can be conducted by one appropriately trained health professional provided there is adequate external medical and other support.

Phase III is lifetime maintenance phase in which physical fitness and additional risk factor reduction are emphasized. Individual studies and meta-analysis have reported benefits in terms of reduced mortality, recurrent events and readmissions.

Now, healthcare has incorporated an additional focus on the continuum of care—the provision of care is not only during but also after CVD event.[11]

The AHA, the ACC foundation and the American Association of Cardiovascular and Pulmonary Rehabilitation (AACVPR) have outlined the core components of contemporary CR and SP programs and produced guidelines for detection, management and prevention of CVD. These core components include patient assessment, exercise training, physical activity counseling, tobacco cessation, nutritional counseling, weight management, aggressive coronary risk-factor management and psychological counseling.[12-14] Other subjects discussed during CR visits include sexual dysfunction, alcohol consumption and stress management. Patient care should be individualized to provide the most effective and efficient care.

EDUCATION AND COUNSELING

For the patient, the time following hospitalization for a CVD event and/or PTCA is filled with concerns, questions and confusion. Exercise training (ET) has traditionally been the primary focus of CR. However, education and counseling have been considered as important as ET in facilitating recovery from cardiac events. ET, education and counseling are now universally recognized as integral components of comprehensive CR/SP. To facilitate a return to normal living, patients require guidelines about resuming driving, sexual activity, work and other activities. Information and advice about lifestyle change are necessary for SP of CVD. Motivation to adhere to advice and prescribed medication is strongly influenced by patients' understanding of the disease, the acute event and the need for risk factor modification.

Education and counseling of inpatients is undertaken on an individual basis and at some hospitals, in groups as well. The quality of intervention rather than characteristics of the patients may determine the effectiveness of education and counseling program. For example, educational strategies may be unsuccessful because the information given was too much or too general.[15] Further, educational counseling maybe ineffective because contradictory information and advice are often given by different health professionals.[16,17] Clarification is therefore required to reduce confusion. Moreover, information needs to be repeated and reinforced. The teaching ability of the educator and the manner in which information is delivered are critical to patients' acceptance of the material. Knowledge gained is considered by patients to be a major benefit from CRPs.

Education and counseling involve teaching patients and their families to understand the illness and its management. Understanding the factors that may have caused it may also help them assume a large degree of responsibility for their care.

Instructional aides (physical, printed and audiovisual) are very useful as part of educational process. It is important to stress that CHD is a chronic health problem and that there is 'no cure', but that some medical intervention and modification of lifestyle maybe necessary to alleviate symptoms and reduce the risk of future problems. Advice should be realistic practical and accurate.[18] It should be based on evidence and imparted in clear unambiguous ways.

OBJECTIVES

CR/SP programs are in fact, risk factor intervention programs. Effective management of lifestyle and associated risk factors is the basic objective of CR.

It includes intervention strategies for the following modifiable CVD risk factors:

- Tobacco use
- Hypertension
- Diabetes
- Hyperlipidemia
- Obesity
- Physical inactivity
- Psychological concerns.

Tobacco Cessation

Tobacco consumption is one of the most preventable causes of CVD. Smoking and tobacco cessation is the most cost effective of all the lifestyle modifications recommended to prevent CVD. The overall mortality risk of smokers who quit decreases by 50% in the first couple of years and tends to approach that of nonsmokers in approximately 5–15 years of cessation of smoking.[19]

In post-PCI patient smoking increases incidence of death 1.75 times and Q wave MI 2 times. If patients quit smoking risk of reinfarction, sudden death and mortality decreases by 50%. Goal is to achieve complete cessation and no exposure to environmental tobacco smoke. Many tools are used for tobacco cessation. They include pharmacologic assistance (nicotine substitutes, bupropion), counselling, education and group support.[20] Strong advice from physician to stop smoking is important. Evidence suggests that interventions to stop smoking/tobacco cessations are more likely to be effective if they are initiated in hospital when patients are more highly motivated rather than after discharge from hospital.[15,21,22]

Hypertension Management

High blood pressure is very prevalent among patients referred to CR. A decrease in systolic blood pressure by 10 mm Hg can decrease cardiovascular mortality by 20–40% and a reduction of diastolic blood pressure by 5–6 mm Hg results in a reduction of stroke by 42% and CHD events by 15%.[23,24] Understanding of the disease and its treatment certainly improves patients' compliance and reduces the risk associated with high blood pressure.[25]

The effectiveness of antihypertensive drugs in lowering blood pressure is well established. Further, beneficial effects upon blood pressure in cardiac patients have been reported from two multifactorial interventions including exercise training.[26,27]

A meta-analysis of studies conducted showed that 1 kg fall in weight achieved a 1.6 mm Hg reduction in mean systolic blood pressure and a fall of 1.33 mm Hg in mean diastolic blood pressure.[28] The reduction was more prominent when the blood pressure was higher.

A reduction in alcohol consumption alone achieved a reduction of 4.8 mm Hg and 3.3 mm Hg in systolic and diastolic blood pressure respectively, and together with a reduction of weight of 7.5 kg, systolic and diastolic blood pressure were reduced by 10.2 mm Hg and 7.5 mm Hg respectively.[29] Similarly, reduced sodium intake has been shown to be effective in reducing blood pressure.[30]

Education and behavioral interventions for weight reduction, physical activity and moderation of dietary sodium and alcohol consumption are recommended as definitive or adjunctive therapy for hypertension. The goal for secondary prevention should be 120/80 mm Hg.

Diabetes Management

Many patients referred for CR have diabetes. These patients have a particularly high cardiovascular risk profile. The majority will have another associated risk factor (smoking, hypertension, hypercholesterolemia, overweight, obesity). Therapeutic education is very important tool that helps improve diabetes control. CRP can help achieve better glycemic control. This has been shown to reduce cardiovascular morbidity and mortality.[31] The goal of diabetes management is to maintain glycosylated haemoglobin (HbA1c) concentration of <7.

Weight loss and exercise have been shown to improve the insulin resistance associated with type 2 diabetes.

The benefits of exercise for a patient with type 2 diabetes are substantial.[32] Regular exercise improves blood glucose control, improves sensitivity to insulin, decreases dose of insulin or oral hypoglycemic agents, decreases plasma insulin level, improves glucose tolerance and lowers HbA1c levels. It reduces the risk of CVD and its complications, and improves overall health and wellness in these patients.

Exercise can prevent or delay the onset of type 2 diabetes in patients with prediabetes.[33]

Lipid Control

The evidence of cholesterol reduction in patients with CHD involved in CRP is exceptionally strong. Hypercholesterolemia is the risk factor with the highest percentage of attributable risk post MI.[34] Yusuf et al. showed that every 1 mmol/L (38.7 mg/dL) decline in LDL cholesterol results in a 21% decrease in cardiovascular event.[35]

A controlled study of extremely intensive and dietary restriction, stress management, exercise and social support produced significantly reduced total cholesterol levels and dietary fat intake in the intervention group at 1 year.[36]

Many aspects of CR will contribute to improve patients' lipid profile. These include physical exercise, nutritional counselling and weight management.

Pharmacologic treatment is often added to therapeutic lifestyle changes to achieve cholesterol targets-Total cholesterol <150 mg/dL, LDL <70 mg/dL, TG <170 mg/dL, HDL >40 mg/dL.

Weight Management

The negative effects of overweight and obesity on physical activity and the incidence of hypertension, increased cholesterol and diabetes have been confirmed in many studies. Patients are instructed on their specific weight issues and on methods that can help achieve a healthy body weight through a combination of decreased calorie intake and increased calorie expenditure.[37]

The goal of weight management is body mass index (BMI) of 18.5–24.5 kg/m^2 and waist circumference of <40 inches in men and <35 inches in women. The initial goal of weight loss therapy should be to reduce body weight by approximately 10% from baseline.

Considerable weight loss occurred amongst the dedicated subjects enrolled in a study of one year intervention including a low fat vegetarian diet, group discussion for social support, stress management and exercise.[36]

According to a review of 21 studies involving obese patients, a mean weight loss of 7–9 kg was achieved immediately after treatment, with weight loss being related to the length of the program rather than technique used.[38] While weight gain is common after interventions cease.

Nutritional Counseling

Apart from providing essential nutrients to the body, eating and drinking are pleasurable experiences, a fact that seems to be forgotten by many of those giving advice.

Dietary modifications often require major change in the patient's normal eating habits, and it is important that factual information is presented objectively and consistently, in a way that can be readily understood by the patient and his family. For most it is better to emphasize an alteration in general eating habits, rather than the necessity of adhering to specific dietary plan. Involvement of the patient's family is very important.

The aim of nutritional counseling in CR is to help patients understand the impact of food on one's health and make healthy food choices. For that reason, baseline daily calorie intake and dietary information are gathered by dietician. Recommendations are given to patients tailored on their individual diet profile. General dietary recommendations for cardiac patients include a reduced intake of saturated fats (<7% of total calories) and cholesterol (<200 mg/day), an increased intake of polyunsaturated and monounsaturated fats, an adequate repartition of calorie sources (about 50–60% of total calories for carbohydrates, 15–20% for proteins and <30% for fat) and an increased fibre intake (about 20–30 g/day). Based on recent studies, there has been specific recommendations for patients with heart disease that emphasize moderation and plant-based food.[14]

Physical Inactivity

Sedentary lifestyle contributes to significantly increased risk of CVD. Low cardiorespiratory fitness (CRF)[39,40] and accumulated sitting time[41,42] have been associated with increased risk of CVD and all cause mortality. It is clear that the relationship between CVD risk and level of physical activity (PA) and CRF are inverse, graded and most importantly, modifiable.[43] Health professionals should view increasing PA and CRF, as well as reducing overall sitting time as important goals within CVD risk reduction program.

Physical Activity

Regular PA has been shown to have many CV benefits including weight loss, blood pressure reduction, glycemic control and lipid profile improvements. A meta-analysis of 11 exercise rehabilitation randomized trials showed that regular exercise was associated with a significant 28% reduction in all-cause mortality and a possible 24% reduction in recurrent MI.[44] There seems to be a dose-response relation between PA and health in general and CHD in particular. A meta-analysis by Sattlemair et al. found that "some PA is better than none" and "additional benefits occur with more PA".[45]

Most guidelines recommend that exercise should be performed for a minimum of 30 minutes per day at least 5 days per week and preferably daily, should involve moderately intensive (target heart rate of 60–75% of the average maximum heart rate or the perception of moderate exercise 12–14 on the Borg scale) aerobic activity such as brisk walking, jogging, cycling, swimming, etc. and should be supplemented by an increase in daily lifestyle activities.[46-48]

EXERCISE TRAINING

The term 'exercise training' (ET) applies to a program of repeated exercise undertaken at a guided or prescribed intensity and frequency over a period of time, usually several weeks.

The scientific data clearly established that ET results in improvements in exercise tolerance. Appropriately prescribed and conducted ET is therefore a key component of CR. Meyers et al. showed that improvement of one metabolic equivalent (MET) in functional capacity imparts a 12% reduction in all-cause mortality.[39] Jolly et al. showed that abnormal heart rate recovery which is a predictor of mortality, can be normalized by ET with improvement in mortality.[49]

Three mechanisms could potentially explain an improvement in myocardial perfusion after comprehensive CR including ET: (1) direct regression of atherosclerotic lesions, (2) formation of collateral vessels and (3) a change in dynamics of epicardial flow via flow-mediated or endogenous stimuli of the vessel. After 4 weeks of ET, there was a 29% increase in coronary artery flow reserve in comparison to the non exercise controlled group.[50]

Exercise protocols should include not only endurance but also resistance training as improvement in muscle strength could benefit patients' performance of activities of daily living. Nearly all forms of exercise require a combination of dynamic and isometric contractions to one extent or another. When performed properly, resistance exercise enhances muscular strength and endurance, and has been shown to provide not only CV benefits, but favourable metabolic adaptations and benefits to bone health as well. Thus, appropriately guided resistance exercise is widely used tool as a compliment to aerobic exercise in CRP. Resistance training exercises maybe started 2-3 weeks following the PTCA.

Post-PTCA patients can begin ET as outpatients almost immediately after hospital discharge. CR/SP staff should stress to patients who have undergone PTCA, the importance of adherence to preventive medication.

EXERCISE PRESCRIPTION

The explicit principles of exercise prescription including frequency, intensity, duration and exercise mode, absolute and relative contraindications to exercise, guidelines for terminating exercise, as outlined by the American College of Sports Medicine (ACSM)[51] and the AACVPR,[52] should be specifically tailored to each individual patient.

Exercise prescription methodology after PTCA is similar in MI and CABG patients. Compared to patients who have undergone primary PTCA for an acute MI, patients who undergo elective PTCA may be able to progress at a faster rate because they have not recently sustained myocardial damage.

INTENSITY OF EXERCISE TRAINING

Low to moderate intensity ET is recommended for all CRP. Low levels of ET are considered safe and require lesser supervision than higher levels of ET. Categorization of exercise intensity (low, moderate, high) maybe by symptoms, perceived exertion by Borg's scale[53] or by heart rate. As one of the aims of reconditioning through ET is to lead to a more active long term lifestyle, it is preferable that the activity is enjoyable and acceptable. Low to moderate levels of ET coupled with regular physical activity at home approaches that of high intensity ET as a mode of enhancing physical working capacity.

It is possible for patients to monitor their own exercise levels, based either upon heart rate or perceived exertion.

Frequency and Duration of Exercise Session

Currently most authorities recommend supervised exercise of moderate or high intensity 2–3 times a week. Duration of each exercise session should be 45–60 minutes.

Group CR, including exercise, should be offered to all patients with CVD.

Risk Stratification

If a low or moderate intensity exercise program is undertaken, technological risk stratification is not required. Determining the clinical state of the patient in terms of presence or absence of shortness of breath, the recent presence or absence of heart failure and other clinical indicator of the size of infarction or impairment of ventricular function is sufficient.[54-58] This pattern of risk stratification removes much of the cost applicable to technological investigation without any apparent increase in hazard for the patients.

A stress test and/or echocardiogram may be undertaken to assess residual ischemia or ventricular function in individual patients. This is a clinical decision. Such tests are not necessary part of CR.

Conducting Exercise Program

Many thousands of patients have passed through low to moderate intensity exercise programs without mishap. The adequacy and safety of such low cost, low equipment program is widely accepted.[54,59-63] These types of program are recommended by the WHO Expert Advisory Committee for both basic and intermediate CR facilities.[54] CR exercise programs should be established in all sizable hospitals treating cardiac patients and in other appropriate facilities to facilitate patient access.

Content of Exercise Classes

Low to moderate intensity ET is recommended for most patients. Exercise session should be started with a warm-up period of light calisthenics and stretching of major muscle groups. It is desirable to take patients through a series of activities before starting dynamic exercise or strength training exercise. The main aerobic activity maybe largely based upon walking, which may be maintained for 20–30 minutes and/or light circuit training with rest in between. A record of exercise intensity, duration, heart rate or perceived exertion should be charted for each patient at each attendance.

A cool down period with gradually lessening levels of activity, followed by a period of rest, relaxation and breathing exercise, is commonly practised and appreciated by patients. A total duration of low to moderate intensity ET should be between 45 minutes and 60 minutes, including rest between activities. For high intensity exercise, usually continuous, the exercise time is usually 20–30 minutes. Patients monitoring in programs of high intensity exercise commonly includes at least occasional or intermittent electrocardiographic strips or telemetry. Because most CRPs offer low to moderate intensity ET, it is unnecessary to undertake electrographic monitoring. Patients are encouraged to be active in the group to a level where they are just aware of breathing (low intensity exercise) or aware of some breathlessness without sweating (moderate intensity exercise). Patients are observed to assure that they do not exceed these limits. They are also warned to cease activity and report staff, should unsteadiness, fatigue, muscle strain, significant breathlessness, chest pain or other symptoms develop. Observation of each patient by the staff and the patient's own perception of the rate of exertion maybe coupled with intermittent brief counting of heart rate. In many programs, patients are trained to measure the heart rate themselves. Patients with physically demanding work or leisure time activity may achieve added benefit from the high intensity exercise program.

Home Exercise Programs

A home exercise program is recommended for those patients who are unable to attend a group exercise program. Such patients require guidance regarding exercise, education and behavior change as well as support. Simple verbal and written instructions to such patients are required together with discussion about activity and behavior while in hospital (inpatient rehabilitation) and as a part of discharge planning. Ideally patients receiving a home based program should attend at least one group of exercise sessions for guidance. They should learn self-monitoring based on observation of heart rate during activities or recognition of symptoms to the level of awareness of breathing (Borg scale 10–12).[53] They should be advised to continue activity at that level on daily basis preferably for half an hour each day. Home exercise programs generally involve daily walking at low or moderate intensity as well as other physical activities with gradual progression to achieve an increase in muscular strength for exercise of daily living.

ALCOHOL CONSUMPTION

Moderate alcohol consumption (1–2 drinks/day) is associated with a reduced CV and all-cause mortality compared with both abstinence and heavy drinking.[64] The pattern and amount of alcohol intake appears to be more important than the type. Possible explanations for moderate alcohol consumption benefits include: HDL increased by stimulating the hepatic production of apo A-I and A-II, fibrinogen levels reduction, fibrinolysis stimulation, inflammation reduction and inhibition of platelet activation.[65-69]

SEXUAL COUNSELING

Sexual activity is an important component of quality of life. It is therefore important to provide sexual counseling to patients during CR sessions.[70] The sexual needs of an individual cannot be ignored. Sexual dysfunction is common in patients with CVD. This is due to the side effects of medication (beta-blockers in particular), the coexistence of other risk factors (diabetes, dyslipidemia, smoking, and hypertension) and psychological factors (depression, anxiety and the fear of triggering heart attack during intercourse, etc). Therefore, brief education and counseling is helpful in facilitating the successful resumption of sexual activity.

MANAGEMENT OF PSYCHOSOCIAL AND PROFESSIONAL ISSUES/STRESS

Patients with heart disease are often confronted with psychological and social problems that can affect both morbidity and mortality. Depression, anxiety, and denial occur in up to 20% of patients following MI.[71] The INTERHEART study quite clearly demonstrated that stress was the third most important risk factor for coronary events, following lipids and smoking, and accounts for approximately 30% of the population's attributable risk of acute MI.[33] Psychosocial stress affects CVD process through the increase in blood pressure, blood glucose, lipid levels and body weight. It also promotes the progression of atherosclerosis, inflammation and endothelial dysfunction.[72]

Recovering from PTCA and adjusting to subsequent life changes is a challenge for most cardiac patients and their families.[73] Several psychosocial factors, including depression, anxiety, and social isolation, can impede recovery.[74,75]

Cardiac rehabilitation reduces both anxiety and depression in coronary patients.[76,71] Predischarge counseling is useful in improving the morale and aiding a successful return to home and work.

Cardiac rehabilitation is an important therapeutic tool for distressed cardiac patients as many CRPs also offer stress management workshops to help patients identify, avoid and deal with stressful situations.[77]

Exercise training has been associated with reduction in stress and its related mortality.[78,79] Besides ET, many CR centres offer other stress reduction techniques training including meditation, relaxation breathing, yoga, etc.

Because PTCA patients have not usually experienced the crisis of acute cardiac events such as MI or CABG, they frequently deny any psychological difficulties or the need for rehabilitation program.[80] They need to be included in CR/SP as psychological intervention enhances the recovery process as evidenced by increased adherence to recommendations and decreased morbidity and mortality.

Stress management programs assist the patient to identify stressors, or to recognize characteristic emotional and physical responses to stress, to decrease levels of general arousal and to develop effective coping strategies. Through the use of various techniques including relaxation therapy, meditation, anxiety management and biofeedback, the patient is taught to reduce stressful reactions by altering stress inducing perceptions of situations.

SUMMARY

Cardiac rehabilitation has evolved from simple exercise program towards comprehensive SP. As studies demonstrate physiological benefits, improved mortality and cost efficacy, rehabilitation and SP have become a standard of care for patients with CVD. It is time for CR programs to become SP centres and to expand the scope of patients cared for in CR/SP. The importance of SP needs to be stressed in all patients who have undergone PTCA, as these patients believe that coronary atherosclerosis has been cured and SP and behavior modification are not necessary.

The PTCA should be combined with aggressive lifestyle intervention, including exercise. Referral of patients following PTCA to CR/SP is a Class I recommendation.[81]

REFERENCES

1. Fletcher GF, Balady GJ, Amsterdam EA, et al. Exercise standards for testing and training: a statement for healthcare professionals from the American Heart Association. Circulation. 2001; 104:1694-740.
2. Wenger NK, Froelicher ES, Smith LK, et al. Cardiac rehabilitation as secondary prevention. Agency for Health Care Policy and Research and National Heart, Lung, and Blood Institute. Clin Pract Guide. 1995;17:1-23.
3. Cardiac Rehabilitation. SIGN Publication No. 57. Edinburgh, United Kingdom: Scottish Intercollegiate Guidelines Network; 2002. Available at: *http://www.show.scot.nhs.uk/sign/guidelines/fulltext/57/index.html*. Accessed June 11, 2003.
4. Stone JA, Cyr C, Friesen M, et al. Canadian guidelines for cardiac rehabilitation and atherosclerotic heart disease prevention: a summary. Can J Cardiol. 2001;17(Suppl B):3B-30B.
5. Ades PA. Cardiac rehabilitation and secondary prevention of coronary heart disease. New England Journal of Medicine. 2001;345:892-902.
6. NHS centre for reviews and dissemination. Cardiac rehabilitation. Effective Health Care. 1998;4:1-12.
7. Goel K, Lennon RJ, Tilbury RT, Squires RW, Thomas RJ. Impact of cardiac rehabilitation on mortality and cardiovascular event. Circulation 2011; DOI: 10.1161/CIRCULATIONAHA.110.983536.
8. Balady GJ, Ades PA, Bittner VA, et al. Referral, enrolment, and delivery of cardiac rehabilitation /secondary prevention programs at clinical centres and beyond: a presidential advisory from the American Heart Association. Circulation. 2011;124:2951-960.
9. Squires RW, Gau GT, Miller TD, et al. Cardiovascular rehabilitation: status. Mayo Clin Proc. 1990;65:731-55.
10. Fonarow GC, Gawlinski A, Moughrabi S, Tillisch JH. Improved treatment of coronary heart disease by implementation of a Cardiac Hospitalalization Artherosclerosis Management Program (CHAMP). Am F Cardiol. 2001;84:819-22.
11. Aston G. Creating a cardiac care continuum. Hospitals and health networks. Am Hospital Assoc. 2010;84:32,34,36.
12. Thomas RJ, King M, Lui K, et al. AACVPR/ACC/AHA 2007 performance measures on cardiac rehabilitation for referral to and delivery of cardiac rehabilitation/secondary prevention services. J Cardiopulm Rehabil Prev. 2007; 27:260-90.
13. AHA; ACC; National Heart, Lung, and Blood Institute, et al. AHA/ACC guidelines for secondary prevention for patients with coronary and other atherosclerotic vascular disease: 2006 update endorsed by the National Heart, Lung, and Blood Institute. J Am Coll Cardiol. 2006; 47:2130-9.

14. Balady GJ, Williams MA, Ades PA, et al. Core components of cardiac rehabilitation/secondary prevention programs: 2007 update: a scientific statement from the American Heart Association Exercise, Cardiac Rehabilitation, and Prevention Committee, the Council on Clinical Cardiology; the Councils on Cardiovascular Nursing, Epidemiology and Prevention, and Nutrition, Physical Activity, and Metabolism; and the American Association of Cardiovascular and Pulmonary Rehabilitation. Circulation. 2007; 115:2675-82.
15. Sivarajan ES, Newton KM, Almes MJ, Kempf TM, Mansfield LW, Bruce RA. Limited effects of outpatient teaching and counselling after myocardial infarction: a controlled study. Heart Lung. 1983;12:65-73.
16. Report on attitudes of health care providers towards cardiac rehabilitation and secondary prevention services. Melbourne: Heart Research Centre; 1999.
17. Worcester MC. Processes and patterns of recovery following myocardial infarction. PhD thesis. Melbourne. 1979.
18. Thompson DR, Lewin RJP. Management of the post-myocardial infarction patient: rehabilitation and cardiac neurosis. Heart. 2000; 84:101-5.
19. Mohiuddin SM, Mooss AN, Hunter CB, et al. Intensive smoking cessation intervention reduces mortality in high-risk smokers with cardiovascular disease. Chest. 2007;131:446-52.
20. Brennan A. Efficacy of cardiac rehabilitation 2: Smoking and behaviour modification. Br J Nurs. 1997;6:737-40.
21. Taylor CB, Housten-Miller N, Killen JD, DeBusk RF. Smoking cessation after acute myocardial infarction: Effects of a nursemanaged intervention. Ann Intern Med. 1990;113:118-23.
22. Burt A, Illingworth D, Shaw TRD, Thornley P, White P, Turner R. Stopping smoking after myocardial infarction. Lancet. 1974;1:34.
23. Hedner T, Hansson L, Jern S. What is happening to blood pressure? Blood Press. 1996;5:132-3.
24. Zanchetti A. What blood pressure levels should be treated? Clin Investig. 1992;70:S2-6.
25. Aldana SG, Whitmer WR, Greenlaw R, et al. Cardiovascular risk reductions associated with aggressive lifestyle modification and cardiac rehabilitation. Heart Lung. 2003;32:374-82.
26. Kallio V, Hamalainen H, Hakkila J, Luurila OJ. Reduction in sudden deaths by a multifactorial intervention programme after acute myocardial infarction. Lancet. 1979;2:1091-4.
27. Haskell WL, Alderman EL, Fair JM, Maron DJ, Mackey SF, Superko HR, et al. Effects of intensive multiple risk factor reduction on coronary atherosclerosis and clinical cardiac events in men and women with coronary artery disease: the Stanford Coronary Risk Intervention Project (SCRIP). Circulation.
28. Staessen J, Fagard R, Amery A. The relationship between body weight and blood pressure. J Human Hypertension. 1988;2:207-17.
29. Puddey I, Parker M, Beilin LJ, Vandongen R, Masarei JRL. Effects of alcohol and caloric restrictions on blood pressure and serum lipids in overweight men. Hypertension. 1992;20:533-41.
30. Midgley JP, Matthew AG, Greenwood CMT, Logan AG. Effect of reduced dietary sodium on blood pressure. A meta-analysis of randomized controlled trials. JAMA. 1996;275:1590-7.
31. Banzer JA, Maguire TE, Kennedy CM, et al. Results of cardiac rehabilitation in patients with diabetes mellitus. Am J Cardiol. 2004;93:81-4.
32. Colberg SR, Albright AL, Blissmer BJ, et al. American College of Sports Medicine and the American Diabetes Association joint position statement. Exercise and type 2 diabetes. Med Sci Sports Exerc. 2010;42:2282-303.
33. Knowler WC, Barrett-Connor E, Fowler SE, et al. Reuction in the incidence of type 2 diabetes with lifestyle intervention or metformin. NEJM. 2002; 346:393-403.
34. Yusuf S, Hawken S, Ounpuu S, et al. Effect of potentially modifiable risk factors associated with myocardial infarction in 52 countries (the INTERHEART study): case-control study. Lancet. 2004;364:937-52.
35. Yusuf S, Lonn E, Bosch J. Lipid lowering for primary prevention. Lancet. 2009;373:1152-5.
36. Ornish D, Brown SE, Scherwitz LW, Billings JH, Armstrong WT, Ports TA, et al. Can lifestyle changes reverse coronary artery disease? The Lifestyle Heart Trial. Lancet. 1990;336:129-33.
37. Allison TG. Improving weight loss in cardiac rehabilitation. Circulation. 2009;119:2650-2.
38. Brownell KD, Jeffery RW. Improving long-term weight loss: pushing the limits of treatment. Behav Ther. 1987;18:353-74.
39. Myers J, Prakash M, Froelicher V, et al. Exercise capacity and mortality among men referred for exercise training. NEJM. 2002;346:793-801.
40. Blair SN, Kohl HW 3rd, Paffenbarger RS Jr, et al. Physical fitness and all cause mortality. A prospective study of healthy men and women. JAMA. 1989;262:2395-401.
41. Katzmarzyk P, Church T, Craig C, et al. Sitting time and mortality from all causes, cardiovascular disease, and cancer. Med Sci Sports Exerc. 2009; 41:998-1005.
42. Stamatakis E, Hamer M, Dunstan D. Screen based entertainment time, all cause mortality, and cardiovascular events: population based study with ongoing mortality and hospital events follow-up. F Am Coll Cardiol. 2011;57:292-9.
43. Paffenbarger RS, Kampert JB, Le IM, et al. Changes in physical activity and other lifeway patterns influencing longevity. MedSci Sports Excer. 1994;26:857-65.
44. Clark AM, Hartling L, Vandermeer B, et al. Meta-analysis: secondary prevention programs for patients with coronary artery disease. Ann Intern Med. 2005;143:659-72.
45. Sattelmair J, Pertman J, Ding EL, et al. Dose response between physical activity and risk of coronary heart disease: a meta-analysis. Circulation. 2011;124:789-95.
46. Smith SC Jr, Benjamin EJ, Bonow RO, et al. AHA/ACCF secondary prevention and risk reduction therapy for patients with coronary and other atherosclerotic vascular disease: 2011 update: a guideline from the American Heart Association and American College of Cardiology Foundation. Circulation. 2011;124:2 458-73.
47. Artinian NT, Fletcher GF, Mozaffarian D, et al. Interventions to promote physical activity and dietary lifestyle changes for cardiovascular risk factor reduction in adults: a scientific statement from the American Heart Association. Circulation. 2010;122:406-41.
48. Graham I, Atar D, Borch-Johnsen K, et al. European guidelines on cardiovascular disease prevention in clinical practice: full text. Fourth Joint Task Force of the European Society of Cardiology and other societies on cardiovascular disease prevention in clinical practice (constituted by representatives

of nine societies and by invited experts). Eur J Cardiovasc Prev Rehabil. 2007;14:S1-113.
49. Jolly MA, Brennan DM, Cho L. Impact of exercise on heart rate recovery. Circulation. 2011;124:1520-6.
50. Hambrecht R, Fiehen E, Weigl C, et al. Regular physical exercise corrects endothelial dysfunction and improves exercise capacity in patients with chronic heart failure. Circulation. 1998;98: 2709-15.
51. American College of Sports Medicine: Guidelines for Exercise Testing and Prescription, 6th edn. Baltimore, Lippincott Williams & Wilkins, 2000.
52. American Association of Cardiovascular and Pulmonary Rehabilitation: Guidelines for Cardiac Rehabilitation Programs, 4th edn. Champaign, III, Human Kinetics, 2003.
53. Borg G. Perceived exertion as an indicator of somatic stress. Scand J Rehabil Med. 1970;2:92-8.
54. World Health Organisation Expert Committee. Rehabilitation after cardiovascular diseases, with special emphasis on developing countries. Technical report series number 831. Geneva: World Health Organization; 1993.
55. Moss AJ, Goldstein RE, Hall WJ, Bigger JT, Fleiss JL, Greenberg H, et al. Detection and significance of myocardial ischemia in stable patients after recovery from an acute coronary event. Multicenter Myocardial Ischemia Research Group. JAMA. 1993;269:2379-85.
56. Myers MG, Baigrie RS, Chariat ML, Morgan CD. Are routine non-invasive tests useful in prediction of outcome after myocardial infarction in elderly people? Lancet. 1993;342:1069-72.
57. Cleempoel H, Vainsel H, Bernard R, Dramaix M, Lenaers A, VanKuyk M, et al. Predictors of early death after acute myocardial infarction: two months follow-up. Eur Heart J. 1986;7:305-11.
58. Fubini A, Cecchi E, Bobbio M, Spinnler MT, Bergerine S, DiLeo M, et al. Value of exercise stress test, radionuclide angiography and coronary angiography in predicting new coronary events in asymptomatic patients after a first episode of myocardial infarction. Int J Cardiol. 1992;34:319-25.
59. Report on 1996 survey of Victorian cardiac rehabilitation programs. Melbourne: Heart Research Centre; 1999.
60. Hare DL, Fitzgerald H, Darcy F, Race E, Goble AJ. Cardiac rehabilitation based on group light exercise and discussion: an Australian hospital model. J Cardiopulm Rehabil. 1995;15: 186-92.
61. Worcester MC. Cardiac rehabilitation programmes in Australian hospitals. Canberra: National Heart Foundation of Australia; 1986.
62. Briffa T, Bunker S, Catford M, Humphries J, Inder K, O'Meara N, Whitelum D, Worcester M. 1992 survey of cardiac rehabilitation programs in Australian hospitals. Proceedings of the 3rd Annual Scientific Meeting of the Australian Cardiac Rehabilitation Association. Brisbane; 1993.
63. Minimal standards for outpatient (phase 2) cardiac rehabilitation and cardiac rehabilitation policy statements. Canberra: National Heart Foundation of Australia; 1994.
64. Di Castelnuovo A, Costanzo S, Bagnardi V, et al. Alcohol dosing and total mortality in men and women: an updated meta-analysis of 34 prospective studies. Arch Intern Med. 2006;166:2437-45.
65. Suh I, Shaten BJ, Cutler JA, et al. Alcohol use and mortality from coronary heart disease: the role of high-density lipoprotein cholesterol. The Multiple Risk Factor Intervention Trial Research Group. Ann Intern Med. 1992;116:881-7.
66. Folsom AR, Wu KK, Davis CE, et al. Population correlates of plasma fibrinogen and factor VII, putative cardiovascular risk factors. Atherosclerosis. 1991;91:191-205.
67. Mukamal KJ, Jadhav PP, D'Agostino RB, et al. Alcohol consumption and hemostatic factors: analysis of the Framingham Offspring cohort. Circulation. 2001;104:1367-73.
68. Albert MA, Glynn RJ, Ridker PM. Alcohol consumption and plasma concentration of C-reactive protein. Circulation. 2003;107:443-7.
69. Lacoste L, Hung J, Lam JY. Acute and delayed antithrombotic effects of alcohol in humans. Am J Cardiol. 2001;87:82-5.
70. Mitchell ME. Sexual counselling in cardiac rehabilitation. J Rehabil. 1982;48:15-8.
71. Milani RV, Lavie CJ, Cassidy MM. Effects of cardiac rehabilitation and exercise training programs on depression in patients after major coronary events. Am Heart J. 1996;132:726-32.
72. Ranjit N, Diez-Roux AV, Shea S, et al. Psychosocial factors and inflammation in the multi-ethnic study of atherosclerosis. Arch Intern Med. 2007;167:174-81.
73. Milani RV, Lavie CJ. Impact of cardiac rehabilitation on depression and its associated mortality. Am J Med. 2007;120:799-806.
74. Lavie CJ, Milani RV. Cardiac rehabilitation and exercise training in secondary coronary heart disease prevention. Prog Cardiovasc Dis. 2011;53:397-403.
75. Hughes JW, Bon-Wilson A, Eichenauer K, Feltz G. Behavioral medicine for patients with heart disease-the case of depression and cardiac rehabilitation. US Cardiol. 2010;7:55-60.
76. Kugler J, Seelbach H, Kruskemper GM. Effects of rehabilitation exercise on anxiety and depression in coronary patients: a meta-analysis. British Journal of Clinical Psychology. 1994;33:401-10.
77. Collins JA, Rice VH. Effects of relaxation intervention in phase II cardiac rehabilitation: replication and extension. Heart Lung. 1997;26:31-44.
78. Gaw-Ens B, Laing GP. Risk factor reduction behaviours in coronary angioplasty and myocardial infarction patients. Can J Cardiovasc Nurs. 1994;5:4-12.
79. Kolman L, Shin N, Krishnan SM, et al. Psychological distress in cardiac rehabilitation participants. F Cadiopulm Rehabil Prev. 2011;31:81-6.
80. Barth J, Schneider S, von Kanel R. Lack of social support in the etiology and prognosis of coronary heart disease: a systematic review and meta-analysis. Psychosom Med. 2010;72:229-38.
81. King III SB, Smith SC, Hirschfield JW, et al. 2007 focused update of the ACC/AHA/SCAI. 2005 guideline update for percutaneous coronary intervention. Circulation. 2008;117:261-95.

CHAPTER

25 Outcomes of Coronary Angioplasty

Chandrashekhar V Patil

Percutaneous coronary intenvention (PCI) has become one of the most frequently performed interventions in medicine[1] and its progress over years has resulted in steady decline in periprocedural adverse events. Various risk models[2] like Syntax score are developed to assess short-term (in-hospital or 30-day) and medium-to-long-term (≥1 year) outcomes.

Coronary revascularization by PCI has been performed for more than 38 years. Major adverse coronary events (MACE) from PCI include death, the risks of emergent coronary artery bypass grafting (CABG), future vessel closure or stent thrombosis, and subsequent restenosis. These events have decreased since the initial series of balloon angioplasty published in 1978.[3] Although, the first publication reported that 14% of patients required urgent or emergent CABG, modern rates have fallen to 0.4%.[3] This reduction in rates of PCI-induced CABG relates to combination of clinical experience, modern antithrombotic medications, and the development of coronary stents. Procedure related myocardial infarction (MI) (definition and prognostic implications of these infarcts remain debated) occurs during PCI by a variety of mechanisms including direct vessel injury, side branch compromise, thrombus formation, and distal embolization. Their incidence has decreased over the past 35 years. The first balloon angioplasty report published in 1979,[3] noted that 5–10% of patients had a procedure-related MI, whereas a recent randomized trial published in 2010[4] found a rate of less than 1%.

Abrupt vessel closure after balloon angioplasty occurred in approximately 8% of cases,[5] and very early experiences with stents showed a 16% subacute closure rates.[6] But development of dual antiplatelet therapy and refinement of scaffold design and implantation techniques have reduced its frequency to 0.4% over 30 months.[7] A similar trend also exists for restenosis. After the first series of coronary stent implantation described in 1987, clinical trials by 1994 had demonstrated improvements, although restenosis remained significant either with balloon dilatation or stenting (32% vs 22% in Benestent study at 7 months; 42% vs 32% in STRESS study at 6 months). Modern technology has reduced restenosis further by 5-to 10-fold, as demonstrated by a 2010 trial,[4] with 3–4% target-lesion and 5% target-vessel revascularization using everolimus or zotarolimus drug-eluting stents. We will discuss outcomes of PCI according to different clinical situations.

STABLE CORONARY ARTERY DISEASE PCI VERSUS MEDICAL TREATMENT

The indications for revascularization in patients with stable coronary artery disease (SCAD) are persistence of symptoms despite optimal medical treatment and improvement of prognosis.[8] Hence, revascularization and medical therapy should be considered as complementary, rather than competitive treatment strategies.

The efficacy of PCI in addition to medical therapy in patients with SCAD has been addressed in several randomized studies, large-scale registries and meta-analysis. The Medical, Angioplasty or Surgery Study II (MASS II) trial, a single center study, involving 611 patients with multivessel disease, is the only randomized controlled trail (RCT) comparing medical treatment with PCI (72% with BMS and 28% with balloon angioplasty) and with CABG. Over 10 years, comparing medical therapy with PCI, the respective rates for all-cause mortality were 31% and 24.1% ($p = 0.09$), for MI 20.7% and 13.3% ($p = 0.01$), and for freedom from angina 43% and 59% ($p < 0.001$).[9]

The COURAGE[10] trial included 2287 patients with stable angina, who had objective evidence of ischemia and significant CAD, randomizing them to medical therapy alone or medical therapy plus PCI with bare metal stents. At a median follow-up of 4.6 years, there were no significant differences between the PCI and medical therapy groups in the composite of death, MI and stroke. Freedom from angina was significantly greater in the PCI group at 3 years but the advantage was eroded by 5 years, by which time 21%

of the PCI group and 33% of the medical therapy group had received additional revascularization (p <0.001). The majority of patients (70%) had no or mild ischemia at baseline and patients with left main disease were excluded. Thus, severity of ischemia in this trial was moderate and most patients had normal LV function.[11]

The benefits have been demonstrated in patients with moderate to large amount of ischemia noted on stress myocardial perfusion imaging in the nuclear substudy[12] of COURAGE trial. The reduction in ischemic burden was marked in PCI group (78% versus 52%) in patients with moderate to severe ischemia, involving ≥10% of myocardium. The event-free survival at 5-year follow-up was directly related to the amount of residual ischemia of the left ventricle: 100% if 0% residual ischemia, 84.4% for 1 to 5%, 77.7% for 5 to 10%, and 60.7% for ≥ 10% ischemic myocardium.

In the FAME-2 trial,[13] patients with stable angina and at least one functionally significant stenosis with invasive FFR ≤ 0.80 were randomly assigned to medical therapy or FFR-guided PCI. The trial was planned to include 1632 patients but the data safety monitoring board stopped the study prematurely after enrolment of 888 patients. Final analysis showed an incidence of the primary endpoint of 4.3% in the PCI group and 12.7% in the medical therapy group (p < 0.001), but without a difference in rates of death or MI between the two groups. Interpretation of FAME-2 is complicated, in that the decision for urgent revascularization may have been influenced by the open nature of the trial. Only 50% of the patients undergoing urgent revascularization displayed objective evidence of ischemia.

Most meta-analyses comparing a strategy of PCI against initial medical therapy found no evidence in favor of an invasive strategy, in terms of survival or myocardial infarction.[14-17] Two reported a small survival benefit for PCI over medical therapy, al though this might have been influenced by the inclusion of a subset of patients who had a recent myocardial infarction (within 4 weeks).

The major limitation of the previous comparisons is the lack of use of drug-eluting stents (DES). Several meta-analyses of RCTs comparing early-generation DES with bare-metal stents reported similar rates of death and nonfatal myocardial infarction, but a 50–70% relative risk reduction in the need for repeat target vessel revascularization (TVR) with DES.[17,18] New-generation DES, with thin strut platforms, biocompatible durable or biodegradable polymers and better antiproliferative agents, have further improved efficacy and safety compared with early-generation DES and BMS compared with early-generation DES, repeat revascularization was reduced by 10–20% with newer generation.[19-22]

Compared with BMS and early-generation DES, new-generation DES have improved safety outcomes including death, MI and stent thrombosis. Several studies have reported an approximately half the risk of definite or probable stent thrombosis, than with early-generation DES, particularly during the late phase,[21-24] and some studies reported a lower risk of stent thrombosis than with bare metal stents (BMS).[18,24] A comparison of DES and BMS, embracing 76 RCTs and 117,762 patient-years of follow-up, death rate was not different but a lower risk (20–35%) of myocardial infarction with DES (except paclitaxel-eluting stents) than with BMS. In a patient-level pooled analysis of 26 RCTs in 557 women, there was a lower incidence of the composite of death or myocardial infarction in female patients treated with new-generation DES (9.2%) compared with both early-generation DES (10.9%) and BMS (12.8%; p < 0.001) at 3 years.[22] Similarly, the incidence of definite or probable stent thrombosis was lowest with new-generation DES (1.1%) followed by BMS (1.3%), and early-generation DES (2.1%; p < 0.01).

STABLE CORONARY ARTERY DISEASE PCI VERSUS CABG

Coronary artery bypass grafting (CABG) results in more complete revascularization than PCI,[25] and the placement of bypass grafts on the mid-coronary vessel makes the complexity of proximal lesions less relevant for the procedure, especially when there are chronic proximal occlusions. Several randomized controlled trials in the 80s have compared PCI with CABG as revascularization techniques for patients with multivessel disease. The early studies[26-30] RITA I, EAST, CABRI, GABI and BARI showed no significant difference in survival free of Q-wave MI at 3–5 years, but those who underwent CABG had lower repeat revascularization rate as compared to PTCA (e.g. 8% versus 54% in BARI). Importantly, diabetics who were treated with insulin or oral hypoglycemic medications had a significantly better five-year survival with CABG than with PTCA in BARI (80.6% versus 65.5%).

The use of intracoronary stents improved the durability and safety of PTCA. Coronary stenting decreases angiographic and clinical restenosis rates because large initial gain exceeds late loss (greater neo-intimal proliferation with stents as compared to POBA). In the 1990s, 4 trials[9,31-33] compared bypass surgery to PCI with bare-metal stents (BMS). The ARTS, ERACI II, SOS and MASS II trials examined the hypothesis that a reduction in restenosis would improve the gap between PCI and CABG. In pooled analysis of these four trials,[34] at five years, the cumulative incidence of death, MI and stroke was similar in patients randomized to PCI with stenting versus CABG (16.6% versus 16.9%, respectively). Repeat revascularization was more frequent after PCI as compared to CABG (29.0% versus 7.9%). The diabetic patients[35] and patients older than 65 year, demonstrated significant mortality benefit with CABG.

The restenosis caused by neointimal hyperplasia in bare metal stents have been significantly reduced by the development of drugeluting stents (DES). Repeat-revascularization rates have decreased from >50% in the PTCA era to ~30% with bare metal stents and now approximately 20% with DES.[36-38]

The SYNTAX trial[36] randomized 1,800 patients with three-vessel or left main coronary artery disease to undergo CABG or PCI using Taxus paclitaxel-eluting stent (Boston Scientific, USA). Three-year follow-up data showed MACCE rates of 28% versus 20.2% for the PCI group vs. the CABG group respectively, the difference predominantly driven by repeat revascularization (19.7% versus 10.7%, p<0.001). Stroke rate, although significantly lower in the PCI arm at 1 year, was no longer statistically significant by 3 years (2% versus 3.4%, p = 0.07). Based on anatomic complexity of their coronary artery disease, this study risk stratified patients with a "SYNTAX score" given to each patient, with higher scores reflecting more severe and complex disease burden (*www.syntaxscore.com*). Three-year event rates were similar between two treatment groups for patients with low SYNTAX scores (0–22). There were significantly higher MACCE rates for patients with intermediate SYNTAX scores (23-32), 27.4% for PTCA and 18.9% for CABG (p = 0.02). Among patients with high SYNTAX scores (>33, indicating the most complex disease), those in the PCI group had significantly higher event rates at 3 years than those in the CABG group (34.1% versus 19.5%; p<0.001). This study included 452 patients with diabetes. In patients without diabetes, there was significant survival advantage for CABG if the SYNTAX score was > 33 (2.2% versus 6.1% mortality, CABG versus PCI respectively, p = 0.04) at one-year follow-up. This difference favoring CABG was more pronounced in patients with diabetes and high Syntax score (4.1% versus 13.5%).

CABG was considered as the gold standard for patients of left main disease for decades. It was thought that two important features mitigate against the success of PCI in LM lesions (a) up to 80% of LM disease involves the bifurcation, which is known to be at higher risk of restenosis and (b) up to 80% of LM patients also have multi-vessel disease, where CABG offers a survival advantage. PCI provides at least equivalent results to CABG for lower-severity LM lesions at up to five years of follow-up. The SYNTAX trial included a pre-specified subgroup of 705 patients with predominant distal LM disease, who were randomly assigned to CABG or PCI. The primary endpoint of one-year MACCE was comparable for both revascularization strategies (CABG 13.7% versus PCI 15.8%; p = 0.39).[39] At five years' follow-up, rates of death and myocardial infarction were not significantly different, whereas CABG was associated with a higher rate of stroke (4.3% versus 1.5%; p = 0.03) and a lower risk of repeat revascularization (15.5% versus 26.7%; p < 0.001) with no significant difference in the overall MACCE rates.[40] MACCE rates were comparable for PCI and CABG in the lower (0–22) and intermediate (23–32) SYNTAX score tertiles. In patients with SYNTAX scores >32, CABG was associated with numerically lower mortality (14.1% versus 20.9%; p = 0.11) and a significantly reduced need for repeat revascularization (11.6% versus 34.1%; p < 0.001) albeit at a numerically higher risk of stroke (4.9% versus 1.6%; p = 0.13). A meta-analysis[41] assessed the 1-year outcomes of 1611 patients of left main revascularization. Whilst there was no significant difference in mortality or myocardial infarction, the CABG group showed a higher rate of stroke (1.7% versus 0.1%; p < 0.01) but a lower rate of TVR (5.4% versus 11.4%; p < 0.001).

The FREEDOM trial is the only adequately powered, randomized study of 1900 patients with mean SYNTAX score of 26 ± 9 comparing CABG against PCI with use of early-generation DES (94%) in diabetic patients undergoing elective revascularization for multi-vessel disease without LM coronary stenosis.[42] The primary outcome of death from any cause, non-fatal MI, or stroke was lower in the CABG than the PCI group, with divergence of the curves starting at 2 years. This difference was driven by a reduction of all-cause mortality (p = 0.049) and by a markedly lower rate of MI favoring the CABG group (p < 0.001). Conversely, rates of stroke were doubled in the CABG group (p = 0.03). Hence, taking available evidence into consideration, CABG is the revascularization modality of choice among diabetic patients with multi-vessel CAD; however, PCI can be considered as a treatment alternative among diabetic patients with multi-vessel disease and low SYNTAX score (≤ 22).

NON-ST ELEVATION ACUTE CORONARY SYNDROME

Non-ST-segment elevation acute coronary syndrome (NSTE-ACS) is the most frequent manifestation of acute coronary syndrome, and mortality and morbidity remain equivalent to those of patients with ST-segment elevation myocardial infarction (STEMI) during long-term follow-up. The key objectives of revascularization are symptom relief and improvement of prognosis. In patients at high immediate- and long-term risk for death and cardiovascular events, in whom an early invasive strategy may reduce that risk. Patients in cardiogenic shock, or after resuscitation, should undergo immediate angiography (within 2 hours) because of the high likelihood of critical CAD followed by revascularization.

A meta-analysis, covering seven trials with up-to-date adjunctive medication, showed a significant reduction in risk for all-cause mortality (RR = 0.75; 95% CI 0.63–0.90; p < 0.001) and myocardial infarction (RR = 0.83; 95% CI 0.72–0.96; p = 0.012), for an early invasive versus conservative approach at 2 years without excess of early hazard (death and myocardial infarction at 1 month).[43] A further meta-analysis of eight RCTs showed a significant lower incidence of death, myocardial infarction, or rehospitalization for ACS (OR = 0.78; 95% CI 0.61–0.98) for the invasive strategy at 1 year.[44] The benefit was carried mainly by improved outcomes in high-risk (biomarker-positive) patients. In a gender-specific sub-analysis, a similar benefit was found in biomarker-positive women, compared with biomarker-positive men. Importantly, biomarker-negative women tended to have a higher event rate with an early invasive strategy, indicating that early invasive procedures should be avoided in low-risk, troponin-negative, female patients.

The primary high risk criteria[2] indicating need for early invasive treatment are dynamic ST-T changes, relevant rise and fall in troponin and Grace score > 140. The secondary criteria include diabetes mellitus, renal insufficiency (GFR < 60 mL/min), reduced LV function (EF < 40%), early postinfarction angina, intermediate Grace score, recent PCI and prior CABG.

The timing of invasive evaluation should be based on patient risk profile. Patients at very high risk (refractory angina, cardiogenic shock, severe heart failure and life-threatening ventricular arrhythmia) should be considered for urgent coronary angiography (in less than 2 hours). In patients at high risk, with at least one primary high-risk criterion, an early invasive strategy within 24 hours appears to be the reasonable strategy. In lower-risk subsets, with a GRACE risk score of < 140 but with at least one secondary high-risk criterion, the invasive evaluation can be delayed without increased risk, but should be performed within 72 hours of admission. In other low-risk patients without recurrent symptoms, a noninvasive assessment of inducible ischemia should be performed before hospital discharge.

An early invasive strategy (within 0.5–14 hours), as opposed to a delayed invasive strategy (within 21–86 hours), was tested in several RCTs. In a meta-analysis of three recent trials, early catheterization, followed by coronary intervention on the first day of hospitalization, was shown to be safe and superior in terms of shorter hospital stay (28%)[45] and lower risk of recurrent ACS (41%). Similar findings were reported in another recent meta-analysis.[46]

The recent studies suggest a benefit from an invasive strategy within 24 hours in patients with a high-risk clinical profile. The Timing of Intervention in Patients with Acute Coronary Syndromes (TIMACS) trial revealed a significant 38% lower incidence of death, MI, and stroke at 6 months in high-risk patients (GRACE score > 140), with an early (≤24 hours), as compared with a delayed (≥36 hours) strategy.[47] No significant difference was observed in patients with a low-to intermediate-risk profile (GRACE score ≤140). Notably, there was no safety concern. There are no specific RCTs comparing PCI with CABG in patients with NSTE-ACS. In all trials, the decision on whether to perform CABG or PCI was left to the investigator's discretion. Culprit-lesion PCI is usually the first choice in most patients with NSTE-ACS and multivessel disease; however, there are no prospective studies comparing culprit-lesion PCI with early CABG.

The NSTE-ACS subset comprises up to 50% of patients included in most stent trials particularly those with an all-comer design. There is no particular safety concern in NSTE-ACS as new-generation DES has shown superior safety and efficacy in both SCAD and STEMI patients. Accordingly, new-generation DES is preferred over BMS as the default option.[48]

ST ELEVATION MYOCARDIAL INFARCTION

Primary PCI[49,50] is the recommended reperfusion therapy over fibrinolysis if performed by an experienced team in a timely fashion. Primary PCI is indicated for patients with severe acute heart failure or cardiogenic shock[51] due to STEMI independent from time delay of symptom onset. The radial approach should be the preferred method of access, as it has been shown to reduce the incidence of acute bleeding events and was associated with lower mortality in the subset of STEMI patients that were enrolled in the RIVAL trial.[52-54]

Stenting should be preferred over balloon angioplasty in the setting of primary PCI,[55,56] as it reduces the risk of abrupt closure, re-infarction, and repeat revascularization. Early-generation DES has not been associated with an increased risk of death, MI and stent thrombosis during long-term follow-up.[57] However, there have been concerns over an increased risk of very late stent thrombosis, owing to delayed arterial healing of stents implanted into lesions with large necrotic core.[58,59] Recent studies have demonstrated the superiority of new-generation everolimus-eluting stents in reducing major acute vascular events in STEMI patients, as compared with early-generation sirolimus-eluting stents.[60] Two dedicated trials directly compared new-generation DES with BMS among STEMI patients undergoing primary PCI. The EXAMINATION trial in 1504 STEMI patients reported no significant differences for the primary endpoint of all-cause death, re-infarction and any revascularization, in patients assigned to everolimus-eluting stents, compared with those assigned to BMS, (11.9% versus 14.2%, respectively, difference-2.3%; p = 0.19) at 1 year.[61] However, everolimus-eluting stents were associated with a lower risk of revascularization of the target lesion and definite stent thrombosis (0.5% versus 1.9%; p = 0.02). The COMFORTABLE AMI trial, examining patients assigned to either BMS or to biolimus-eluting stents, reported that the latter showed a lower risk of the composite primary endpoint of cardiac death, target-vessel myocardial infarction, and target-lesion revascularization (4.3% versus 8.7%; HR 0.49; p = 0.004) as well as a lower risk of target-vessel myocardial infarction and a trend towards a lower risk of definite stent thrombosis (0.9% versus 2.1%; p = 0.10).[62] Results were maintained through 2 years of follow-up and a pooled analysis of both trials confirmed a lower risk of stent thrombosis and re-infarction with DES than with BMS.[63] In conclusion, these findings suggest that new-generation DES are more effective and potentially safer than BMS during primary PCI in STEMI.

Thrombus aspiration is a useful adjunct during primary PCI, to further improve myocardial reperfusion by prevention of distal embolization of thrombotic material and plaque debris. Individual RCTs and meta-analyses have shown that the use of manual aspiration thrombectomy during primary PCI is beneficial to improve reperfusion and reduce the rate of MACE including mortality.[64-69] In the largest randomized trial to date, the TASTE study, the primary endpoint of all-cause mortality occurred in 2.8% of patients in the thrombus aspiration group and in 3.0% in the PCI-only group (p = 0.63) at 30 days.[70] However, events were evaluated at short-term follow-up, and there was a trend towards a reduction of events including stent thrombosis (0.2% versus 0.5%, p = 0.06) and re-infarction (0.5% versus 0.9%, p = 0.06) in favor of thrombus aspiration. These results suggest that thrombus aspiration is not essential in routine patients, but in selected cases of large thrombus burden, it is beneficial to improve TIMI flow and reduce stent thrombosis.

Staged revascularization of nonculprit lesions should be considered in STEMI patients with multivessel disease in case of symptoms or ischemia within days to weeks after primary PCI.[71] Immediate revascularization of significant nonculprit lesions during the same procedure[72] as primary PCI of the culprit vessel may be considered in selected patients.

POST-CABG PATIENTS

Post-CABG coronary ischemia may be due to progression of native vessel disease or bypass graft disease. Repeat revascularization in these patients is indicated in the presence of significant symptoms despite optimum medical treatment, and in asymptomatic patients with objective evidence of myocardial ischemia (>10% LV). The survival of patients with patent LIMA to LAD and ischemia in the territories of the circumflex and right coronary arteries does not appear to be influenced by revascularization when compared with medical treatment alone.[73] Early post-CABG graft failure is reported in up to 12% of grafts (left IMA 7%; SVG 8%) as evaluated by intraoperative angiographic control,[74] but only a minority, around 3%, are clinically apparent. In early postoperative graft failure, emergency PCI may limit the extent of myocardial infarction compared with re-do surgery.[75] The target for PCI is IMA graft or the body of the native vessel, while the anastomosis or acutely occluded SVG should be avoided due to concerns over perforation and embolization. Re-do CABG should be favored if anatomy is not feasible for PCI, or if several grafts are occluded. Early mortality is in the range of 9–15% in this group of patients, without any difference between the two revascularization arms.[75]

PCI in patients with previous CABG has worse short- and long-term outcomes than in patients without prior CABG. Re-do CABG has a two-to four-fold increased mortality compared with first-time CABG.[76] There are limited data comparing the efficacy of re-do CABG versus PCI in patients with previous CABG. In the AWESOME RCT and registry, in-hospital mortality was higher with re-do CABG than with PCI.[77] More recent observational data have shown similar long-term results in patients treated by PCI and re-do CABG, with a higher revascularization rate for the PCI patients.[78,79] Because of the higher procedural mortality with re-do CABG and the similar long-term outcome, PCI is the preferred revascularization strategy in patients with patent LIMA and favorable anatomy. CABG is preferred for patients with multiple occluded bypass grafts and native vessels, reduced LV systolic function, and absence of patent LIMA. The IMA is the conduit of choice for revascularization during re-do CABG.[80] PCI of native artery should be the preferred approach provided the native vessel is not totally occluded. If PCI in the native vessel fails, PCI in the diseased SVG remains an option.

PCI for SVGs is associated with an increased risk of distal coronary embolization due to friable atheroma in SVGs, resulting in more periprocedural MI.[81] A pooled analysis of five RCTs reported that GP IIb/IIIa inhibitors are less effective for interventions in SVGs than in native vessels.[82] Several approaches have been evaluated to prevent distal embolization of particulate debris, including distal and proximal occlusion, filter devices or mesh-covered stents.[83] As opposed to occlusive devices, distal filter devices offer the advantage of maintaining antegrade perfusion and the feasibility for contrast injections. Combined data from comparative studies between devices, support the use of distal embolic protection during SVG PCI.[84,85] The only independent predictor of 30-day MACE was plaque volume and not the type of protection device used[86] in the RCT comparing different distal protection devices in SVG PCI. Implantation of DES in SVG lesions is associated with lower risk of repeat revascularization than with BMS.[87-95] In the Swedish SCAAR registry of 3063 procedures including BMS and DES in SVG lesions, the incidence of death was lower among patients who received DES.[87] However, in the randomized ISAR-CABG trial,[93] no differences in terms of death, MI, or stent thrombosis were observed. Long-term results of early generation DES in SVG lesions are satisfactory up to 7 years, with no excess risk of stent thrombosis and lower rate of restenosis than with BMS.[92,94] Patients undergoing PCI of SVGs have impaired long-term clinical outcomes[96] compared with PCI of native coronary vessels.

SPECIAL SITUATIONS: STENT THROMBOSIS AND RESTENOSIS

Even though stent thrombosis is very rare, it has devastating clinical consequences. Since stent implantation is usually done in proximal to mid-location in large main vessels, stent thrombosis usually presents as a large myocardial infarction and patients should undergo emergency primary PCI.[97] Due to the rarity of this complication, the interventional treatment of choice remains unsettled but the use of thrombus aspiration and intracoronary IIb/IIIa platelet inhibitors is frequently advised. Aggressive, high-pressure balloon dilation with noncompliant balloon should be used to correct predisposing stent-related mechanical problems.[98] In this difficult setting, it has been suggested that intracoronary imaging should be used to correct mechanical problems and optimize final results.[98,99] While optical coherence tomography (OCT) provides superior resolution to intravascular ultrasound (IVUS) imaging and is able to identify red thrombus, limited penetration may interfere with imaging of the underlying structures.[90] Some patients with very late stent thrombosis actually have neo-atherosclerosis as the underlying substrate, and this can only be recognized with intracoronary imaging with OCT.[98] Repeat stenting in patients with stent thrombosis is controversial and should be avoided when satisfactory results are obtained with balloon dilation, a new stent may be required to treat edge dissections and adjacent lesions or to optimize final results.[99] Correction of underlying predisposing thrombogenic milieu remains important during these interventions.[96]

Adequate platelet inhibition is of great importance in minimizing the risk of stent thrombosis, as well as its recurrence. Therefore, in patients with stent thrombosis, care should be taken to select the most appropriate $P2Y_{12}$ inhibitor and ensure the compliance by adequate patient education. There is no evidence to suggest that platelet function testing is effective in guiding the type of $P2Y_{12}$ inhibitor in this setting. Since both prasugrel and ticagrelor lower the risk of primary ST,[100] these agents should be preferred over clopidogrel, if bleeding risk is not excessive. The duration of treatment should be at least 12 months after the acute event and potentially longer if well- tolerated. In cases where these new agents are contraindicated, doubling the dose of clopidogrel may be reasonable.[101]

Symptomatic or documented ischemia related to restenosis should be treated by repeat revascularization and repeat PCI remains the treatment of choice for these patients if technically feasible. Initially balloon angioplasty was frequently used in this setting, with good initial results but high rates of recurrence.[102,103] Bare-metal stents provided better early results in patients with in-stent restenosis but produced unfavorable late outcomes and were therefore reserved for patients with large vessels or postballoon suboptimal results.[102,103] Ablative techniques like rotational atherectomy and laser have failed to improve results in such patients. Even though, brachytherapy was effective for in-stent restenosis, it never achieved widespread use, mainly due to feasibility issues and increased stent thrombosis rates. Currently DES implantation is the gold standard in patients with BMS or DES in-stent restenosis. In this scenario, the results with DES are superior to those obtained with balloon, BMS or brachytherapy.[102-106] Drug-coated balloons (DCB) are also effective in these patients and particularly when more than two stent layers are already present in the vessel. Drug-coated balloons are superior to balloon angioplasty and BMS and give results similar to early-generation DES in patients with BMS or DES in-stent restenosis.[107-112] The use of intracoronary imaging provides insight into the underlying mechanisms of in-stent restenosis. The presence of an under-expanded stent should be corrected during the repeat procedure. In patients with associated multivessel disease, complex lesions like chronic total occlusions and recurrent episodes of diffuse in-stent restenosis, CABG should be considered before a new PCI attempt.

BIORESORBABLE STENTS

Completely bioresorbable stents, which dissolve after fulfilling their support function in the lesion site of the coronary vessel, have been an ultimate aim since the introduction of the metallic stents. Having a metal frame embedded in artery has long-term disadvantages; notably, incomplete healing, endothelial dysfunction, prevention of late favorable remodeling and difficult future imaging and re-intervention. Current stent platforms are based on two technologies: the manufacturing of drug-eluting, bioresorbable, polymer-based stents and drug-eluting, resorbable, metallic (magnesium) stents. The resorption process of the stent platforms takes from several months to 2 years, depending on polymer composition. Bioresorbable stents have been shown to dissolve completely over time, to restore the vasomotion of treated segments, and to result in positive remodeling with late lumen enlargement. In a patient level, pooled meta-analysis of four randomized trials[113] in which 3389 patients were randomly assigned to everolimus-eluting Absorb BVS and Xience metallic stents. The one-year relative rates of patient-oriented and device-oriented composite endpoints did not differ significantly between two groups. Target vessel-related myocardial infarction was increased with BVS compared with CoCr-EES, due in part to nonsignificant increases in periprocedural MI and device thrombosis with

BVS (RR 2.09[0.92-4.75], p=0.08). In small series of patients with relatively simple lesions, early results are promising and appear to be similar to new-generation DES.[114-116] However, confirmation in large-scale RCTs is required to establish the role for these devices in coronary interventions.

DRUG-COATED BALLOONS

The drug-coated balloons work on the concept that, with highly lipophilic drugs, even short contact times between the balloon surface and the vessel wall are sufficient for effective antiproliferative drug delivery. Three RCTs, PAC-COCATH-I and PAC- COCATH-II,[117,118] and PEPCAD-II,[119] using a paclitaxel-coated balloon, have targeted post BMS in-stent restenosis, while three others have targeted post DES in-stent restenosis.[120-122] Although, drug-coated balloons without additional stent implantation may represent an attractive option for patients with post-DES restenosis, it is not known whether they are as safe and effective as new-generation limus eluting DES.

In the randomized PEPCAD III study, the combination of a drug-coated balloon with cobalt chromium BMS was inferior to a sirolimus-eluting stent for de novo indications.[123] Also in patients with STEMI, DEB-AMI trial[124] showed that drug-coated balloons followed by BMS implantation were inferior to paclitaxel-eluting stents. A recent angiographic study[125] suggested that drug-coated balloons serve as an alternative to paclitaxel-eluting stents for the treatment of lesions in small coronary vessels; however, the role of drug-coated balloons in this setting has not been evaluated against more effective, new-generation limus eluting DES. There are various types of drug-coated balloons approved for use, with paclitaxel as the sole active drug. Most of the differences among available DEB are related to the drug carrier. Although specifically designed comparative studies are lacking, one cannot assume a class effect for all drug-coated balloons.[126]

So, in conclusion, over last 38 years, the outcomes of PCI has significantly improved, still there is a scope for improvement, especially in chronic total occlusions, post-CABG patients and diabetic subset.

REFERENCES

1. Stefanini GG, Holmes DR Jr. Drug-eluting coronary-artery stents. N Engl Med. 2013;368(3):254-65.
2. Windecker S, Kolh P, Alfonso F, et al. 2014 ESC/EACTS Guidelines on myocardial revascularization: Eur Heart J. 2014;35(37):2541-619.
3. Gruentzig AR, Senning A, Siegenthaler WE. Nonoperative dilatation of coronary-artery stenosis: percutaneous transluminal coronary angioplasty. N Eng J Med. 1979;301:61-8.
4. Serruys PW, Silber S, Garg S, et al. Comparison of Zotarolimus-eluting and everolimus-eluting coronary stents. 2010;363:136-46.
5. Lincoff AM, Popma JJ, Ellis SG, et al. Abrupt vessel closure complicating coronary angioplasty: clinical, angiographic and therapeutic profile. J Am Coll Cardiol. 1992;19:926-35.
6. Ruygrok PN, Serruys PW. Intracoronary stenting. From concept to custom. Circulation. 1996:94:882-90.
7. Mauri L, Kereiakes DJ, Yeh RW, et al. DAPT Study Investigators. Twelve or 30 months of dual anti-platelet therapy after drug-eluting stents. N Engl J Med. 2014;371:2155-66.
8. Montalescot G, Sechtem U, Achenbach S, et al. 2013 ESC guidelines on the management of stable coronary artery disease: The Task Force on the management of stable coronary artery disease of the European Society of Cardiology. Eur Heart J. 2013;34(38):2949-3003.
9. Hueb W, Lopes N, Gersh BJ, et al. Ten-year follow-up survival of the Medicine, Angioplasty, or Surgery Study (MASS II): a randomized controlled clinical trial of 3 therapeutic strategies for multivessel coronary artery disease. Circulation. 2010; 122(10):949-57.
10. Boden WE, O'Rourke RA, Teo KK, et al. Optimal medical therapy with or without PCI for stable coronary disease. N Engl J Med. 2007;356(15):1503-16.
11. Shaw LJ, Weintraub WS, Maron DJ, et al. Baseline stress myocardial perfusion imaging results and outcomes in patients with stable ischemic heart disease randomized to optimal medical therapy with or without percutaneous coronary intervention. Am Heart J. 2012;164(2):243-50.
12. Shaw LJ, Berman DS, Mancini GB, et al. Optimal medical therapy with and without percutaneous coronary intervention to reduce ischemic burden: results from COURAGE trial nuclear substudy. Circulation. 2008;117:1283-91.
13. De Bruyne B, Pijls NH, Kalesan B, et al. Fractional flow reserve-guided PCI vs. medical therapy in stable coronary disease. N Engl J Med. 2012;367(11):991-1001.
14. Bucher HC, Hengstler P, Schindler C, Guyatt GH. Percutaneous transluminal coronary angioplasty vs. medical treatment for non-acute coronary heart disease: meta-analysis of randomised controlled trials. BMJ. 2000;321(7253):73-7.
15. Katritsis DG, Ioannidis JP. Percutaneous coronary intervention vs. conservative therapy in nonacute coronary artery disease: a meta-analysis. Circulation. 2005;111(22):2906-12.
16. Stergiopoulos K, Brown DL. Initial coronary stent implantation with medical therapy vs. medical therapy alone for stable coronary artery disease: meta-analysis of randomized controlled trials. Arch Intern Med. 2012;172(4):312-9.
17. Bangalore S, Kumar S, Fusaro M, et al. Short- and long-term outcomes with drug-eluting and bare-metal coronary stents: a mixed-treatment comparison analysis of 117 762 patient-years of follow-up from randomized trials. Circulation. 2012;125(23): 2873-91.
18. Stettler C, Wandel S, Allemann S, Kastrati A, Morice MC, Schomig A, Pfisterer ME, Stone GW, Leon MB, de Lezo JS, Goy JJ, Park SJ, Sabate M, Suttorp MJ, Kelbaek H, Spaulding C, Menichelli M, Vermeersch P, Dirksen MT, Cervinka P, Petronio AS, Nordmann AJ, Diem P, Meier B, Zwahlen M, Reichenbach S, Trelle S, Windecker S, Juni P. Outcomes associated with drug-eluting and bare-metal stents: a collaborative network meta-analysis. Lancet. 2007;370(9591):937-48.
19. Dangas GD, Serruys PW, Kereiakes DJ, et al. Meta-analysis of everolimus-eluting vs. paclitaxel-eluting stents in coronary

artery disease: final 3-year results of the SPIRIT clinical trials program (Clinical Evaluation of the Xience V Everolimus Eluting Coronary Stent System in the Treatment of Patients with De Novo Native Coronary Artery Lesions). JACC Cardiovasc Interv. 2013;6(9):914-22.
20. Baber U, Mehran R, Sharma SK, et al. Impact of the everolimus-eluting stent on stent thrombosis: a meta-analysis of 13 randomized trials. J Am Coll Cardiol. 2011;58(15):1569-77.
21. Stefanini GG, Byrne RA, Serruys PW, et al. Biodegradable polymer drug-eluting stents reduce the risk of stent thrombosis at 4 years in patients undergoing percutaneous coronary intervention: a pooled analysis of individual patient data from the ISAR-TEST 3, ISAR-TEST 4, and LEADERS randomized trials. Eur Heart J. 2012; 33(10):1214-22.
22. Stefanini GG, Baber U, Windecker S, et al. Safety and efficacy of drug-eluting stents in women: a patient-level pooled analysis of randomised trials. Lancet. 2013;382(9908):1879-88.
23. Stefanini GG, Kalesan B, Serruys PW, et al. Long-term clinical outcomes of biodegradable polymer biolimus-eluting stents vs. durable polymer sirolimus-eluting stents in patients with coronary artery disease (LEADERS): 4 year follow-up of a randomised non-inferiority trial. Lancet. 2011;378(9807):1940-8.
24. Palmerini T, Biondi-Zoccai G, Della Riva D, et al. Stent thrombosis with drug-eluting and bare-metal stents: evidence from a comprehensive network meta-analysis. Lancet. 2012;379(9824):1393-1402.
25. Shaw LJ, Berman DS, Mancini GB, et al. Optimal medical therapy with and without percutaneous coronary intervention to reduce ischemic burden : results from COURAGE trial nuclear substudy. Circulation. 2008;117:1283-91.
26. Coronary angioplasty vs. coronary artery bypass surgery: the Randomized Intervention Treatment of Angina (RITA) trial. Lancet. 1993;341(8845):573-80.
27. Hamm CW, Reimers J, Ischinger T, et al. A randomized study of coronary angioplasty compared with bypass surgery in patients with symptomatic multivessel coronary disease. German Angioplasty Bypass Surgery Investigation (GABI). N Engl J Med. 1994;331(16):1037-43.
28. King SB 3rd, Lembo NJ, Weintraub WS, et al. A randomized trial comparing coronary angioplasty with coronary bypass surgery. Emory Angioplasty vs. Surgery Trial (EAST). N Engl J Med. 1994;331(16):1044-50.
29. First-year results of CABRI (Coronary Angioplasty vs. Bypass Revascularisation Investigation). CABRI Trial Participants. Lancet. 1995;346(8984):1179-84.
30. Comparison of coronary bypass surgery with angioplasty in patients with multivessel disease. The Bypass Angioplasty Revascularization Investigation (BARI) Investigators. N Engl J Med. 1996;335(4):217-25.
31. Rodriguez A, Bernardi V, Navia J, et al. Argentine Randomized Study: Coronary Angioplasty with Stenting vs. Coronary Bypass Surgery in patients with Multiple-Vessel Disease (ERACI II): 30-day and one-year follow-up results. ERACI II Investigators. J Am Coll Cardiol. 2001;37(1):51-8.
32. Serruys PW, Unger F, Sousa JE, Jatene A, et al. Comparison of coronary-artery bypass surgery and stenting for the treatment of multivessel disease. N Engl J Med. 2001;344(15):1117-24.
33. Coronary artery bypass surgery vs. percutaneous coronary intervention with stent implantation in patients with multivessel coronary artery disease (the Stent or Surgery trial): a randomised controlled trial. Lancet. 2002;360(9338):965-70.
34. Daemen J, Boersma E, Flather M, et al. Long term safety and efficacy of percutaneous coronary intervention with stenting and coronary artery bypass surgery for multivessel coronary artery disease: a meta-analysis with 5-year patient-level data from the ARTS, ERACI II, MASS II, and SoS trials. Circulation. 2008;118:1146-54.
35. Hlatky MA, Boothroyd DB, Bravata DM, et al. Coronary artery bypass surgery compared with percutaneous coronary intervention for multivessel disease: a collaborative analysis of individual patient data from ten randomized trials. Lancet, 2009;373:1190-7.
36. Serruys PW, Morice MC, Kappetein AP, et al. Percutaneous coronary intervention vs. coronary-artery bypass grafting for severe coronary artery disease. N Engl J Med. 2009;360(10): 961-72.
37. Boudriot E, Thiele H, Walther T, et al. Randomized comparison of percutaneous coronary intervention with sirolimus-eluting stents vs. coronary artery bypass grafting in unprotected left main stem stenosis. J Am Coll Cardiol. 2011;57(5):538-45.
38. Park SJ, Kim YH, Park DW, Yun SC, Ahn JM, Song HG, Lee JY, Kim WJ, Kang SJ, Lee SW, Lee CW, Park SW, Chung CH, Lee JW, Lim DS, Rha SW, Lee SG, Gwon HC, Kim HS, Chae IH, Jang Y, Jeong MH, Tahk SJ, Seung KB. Randomized trial of stents vs. bypass surgery for left main coronary artery disease. N Engl J Med. 2011;364(18):1718-27.
39. Morice MC, Serruys PW, Kappetein AP, et al. Outcomes in patients with de novo left main disease treated with either percutaneous coronary intervention using paclitaxel-eluting stents or coronary artery bypass graft treatment in the Synergy between Percutaneous Coronary Intervention with TAXUS and Cardiac Surgery (SYNTAX) trial. Circulation. 2010;121(24): 2645-53.
40. Morice MC, Serruys PW, Kappetein AP, et al. Five-Year Outcomes in Patients with Left Main Disease Treated with either Percutaneous Coronary Intervention or Coronary Artery Bypass Grafting in the SYNTAX Trial. Circulation. 2014;129:2388-94.
41. Capodanno D, Stone GW, Morice MC, et al. Percutaneous coronary intervention vs. coronary artery bypass graft surgery in left main coronary artery disease: a meta-analysis of randomized clinical data. J Am Coll Cardiol. 2011;58(14):1426-32.
42. Farkouh ME, Domanski M, Sleeper LA, Siami FS, Dangas G, Mack M, Yang M, Cohen DJ, Rosenberg Y, Solomon SD, Desai AS, Gersh BJ, Magnuson EA, Lansky A, Boineau R, Weinberger J, Ramanathan K, Sousa JE, Rankin J, Bhargava B, Buse J, Hueb W, Smith CR, Muratov V, Bansilal S, King S 3rd, Bertrand M, Fuster V, Investigators FT. Strategies for multivessel revascularization in patients with diabetes. N Engl J Med. 2012;367(25):2375-84.
43. Bavry AA, Kumbhani DJ, Rassi AN, et al. Benefit of early invasive therapy in acute coronary syndromes: a meta-analysis of contemporary randomized clinical trials. J Am Coll Cardiol. 2006;48(7):1319-25.
44. O'Donoghue M, Boden WE, Braunwald E, et al. Early invasive vs. conservative treatment strategies in women and men with unstable angina and non-ST-segment elevation myocardial infarction: a meta-analysis. JAMA. 2008;300(1):71-80.

45. Katritsis DG, Siontis GC, Kastrati A, et al. Optimal timing of coronary angiography and potential intervention in non-ST-elevation acute coronary syndromes. Eur Heart J. 2011;32(1): 32-40.
46. Navarese EP, Gurbel PA, Andreotti F, et al. Optimal timing of coronary invasive strategy in non-ST-segment elevation acute coronary syndromes: a systematic review and meta-analysis. Ann Intern Med. 2013;158(4):261-70.
47. Mehta SR, Granger CB, Boden WE, et al. Early vs. delayed invasive intervention in acute coronary syndromes. N Engl J Med. 2009;360(21):2165-75.
48. Greenhalgh J, Hockenhull J, Rao N, et al. Drug-eluting stents vs. bare metal stents for angina or acute coronary syndromes. Cochrane Data-base Syst Rev. 2010(5):CD004587.
49. Andersen HR, Nielsen TT, Rasmussen K, et al. A comparison of coronary angioplasty with fibrinolytic therapy in acute myocardial infarction. N Engl J Med. 2003;349(8):733-42.
50. Dalby M, Bouzamondo A, Lechat P, Montalescot G. Transfer for primary angioplasty vs. immediate thrombolysis in acute myocardial infarction: a meta-analysis. Circulation. 2003;108(15):1809-14.
51. Hochman JS, Sleeper LA, Webb JG, et al. Early revascularization in acute myocardial infarction complicated by cardiogenic shock. SHOCK Investigators. Should We Emergently Revascularize Occluded Coronaries for Cardiogenic Shock. N Engl J Med. 1999;341(9):625-34.
52. Jolly SS, Yusuf S, Cairns J, et al. Radial vs. femoral access for coronary angiography and intervention in patients with acute coronary syndromes (RIVAL): a randomised, parallel, multicentre trial. Lancet. 2011;377(9775):1409-20.
53. Romagnoli E, Biondi-Zoccai G, Sciahbasi A, et al. Radial vs. femoral randomized investigation in ST-segment elevation acute coronary syndrome: the RIFLE-STEACS (Radial vs. Femoral Randomized Investigation in ST-Elevation Acute Coronary Syndrome) study. J Am Coll Cardiol. 2012;60(24):2481-89.
54. Baklanov DV, Kaltenbach LA, Marso SP, et al. The prevalence and outcomes of transradial percutaneous coronary intervention for ST-segment elevation myocardial infarction: analysis from the National Cardiovascular Data Registry (2007 to 2011). J Am Coll Cardiol. 2013;61(4):420.
55. Nordmann AJ, Hengstler P, Harr T, et al. Clinical outcomes of primary stenting vs. balloon angioplasty in patients with myocardial infarction: a meta-analysis of randomized controlled trials. Am J Med. 2004;116(4):253-62.
56. Stone GW, Grines CL, Cox DA, et al. Comparison of angioplasty with stenting, with or without abciximab, in acute myocardial infarction. N Engl J Med. 2002;346(13):957-66.
57. Stone GW, Witzenbichler B, Guagliumi G, et al. Heparin plus a glycoprotein IIb/IIIa inhibitor vs. bivalirudin monotherapy and paclitaxel-eluting stents vs. bare-metal stents in acute myocardial infarction (HORIZONS-AMI): final 3-year results from a multicentre, randomised controlled trial. Lancet. 2011;377(9784):2193-2204.
58. Kalesan B, Pilgrim T, Heinimann K, Raber L, et al. Comparison of drug-eluting stents with bare metal stents in patients with ST-segment elevation myocardial infarction. Eur Heart J. 2012;33(8):977-87.
59. Nakazawa G, Finn AV, Vorpahl M, et al. Coronary responses and differential mechanisms of late stent thrombosis attributed to first-generation sirolimus- and paclitaxel-eluting stents. J Am Coll Cardiol. 2011;57(4).
60. Hofma SH, Brouwer J, Velders MA, et al. Second-generation everolimus-eluting stents vs. first-generation sirolimus-eluting stents in acute myocardial infarction. 1-year results of the randomized XAMI (XienceV Stent vs. Cypher Stent in Primary PCI for Acute Myocardial Infarction) trial. J Am Coll Cardiol. 2012;60(5):381-7.
61. Sabate M, Cequier A, Iniguez A, et al. Everolimus-eluting stent vs. bare-metal stent in ST-segment elevation myocardial infarction (EXAMINATION): 1 year results of a randomised controlled trial. Lancet. 2012;380(9852):1482-90.
62. Raber L, Kelbaek H, Ostojic M, et al. Effect of biolimus-eluting stents with biodegradable polymer vs. bare-metal stents on cardiovascular events among patients with acute myocardial infarction: the COMFORTABLE AMI randomized trial. JAMA. 2012;308(8):777-87.
63. Sabate M, Raber L, Heg D, et al. Comparison of Newer-Generation Drug-Eluting With Bare-Metal Stents in Patients With Acute ST-Segment Elevation Myocardial Infarction: A Pooled Analysis of the EXAMINATION (clinical Evaluation of the Xience-V stent in Acute Myocardial INFARCTION) and COMFORTABLE-AMI (Comparison of Biolimus Eluted from an Erodible Stent Coating with Bare Metal Stents in Acute ST-Elevation Myocardial Infarction) Trials. JACC Cardiovasc Interv. 2014;7(1):55-63.
64. Vlaar PJ, Svilaas T, vander Horstl C, et al. Cardiac death and reinfarction after 1 year in the Thrombus Aspiration during Percutaneous coronary intervention in Acute myocardial infarction Study (TAPAS): a 1-year follow-up study. Lancet. 2008;371(9628):1915-20.
65. Sardella G, Mancone M, Bucciarelli-Ducci C, et al. Thrombus aspiration during primary percutaneous coronary intervention improves myocardial reperfusion and reduces infarct size: the EXPIRA (thrombectomy with export catheter in infarct-related artery during primary percutaneous coronary intervention) prospective, randomized trial. J Am Coll Cardiol. 2009;53(4):309-15.
66. De Luca G, Dudek D, Sardella G, et al. Adjunctive manual thrombectomy improves myocardial perfusion and mortality in patients undergoing primary percutaneous coronary intervention for ST-elevation ESC/EACTS Guidelines myocardial infarction: a meta-analysis of randomized trials. Eur Heart J. 2008;29(24):3002-10.
67. Costopoulos C, Gorog DA, Di Mario C, Kukreja N. Use of thrombectomy devices in primary percutaneous coronary intervention: a systematic review and meta-analysis. Int J Cardiol. 2013;163(3):229-41.
68. De Luca G, Navarese EP, Suryapranata H. A meta-analytic overview of thrombectomy during primary angioplasty. Int J Cardiol. 2013;166(3):606-12.
69. Bavry AA, Kumbhani DJ, Bhatt DL. Role of adjunctive thrombectomy and embolic protection devices in acute myocardial infarction: a comprehensive meta-analysis of randomized trials. Eur Heart J. 2008;29(24):2989-3001.
70. Frobert O, Lagerqvist B, Olivecrona GK, et al. Thrombus aspiration during ST-segment elevation myocardial infarction. N Engl J Med. 2013;369(17):1587-97.

71. Politi L, Sgura F, Rossi R, Monopoli D, Guerri E, Leuzzi C, Bursi F, Sangiorgi GM, Modena MG. A randomised trial of target-vessel vs. multivessel revascularisation in ST-elevation myocardial infarction: major adverse cardiac events during long-term follow-up. Heart. 2010;96(9):662-7.
72. Wald DS, Morris JK, Wald NJ, Chase AJ, Edwards RJ, Hughes LO, Berry C, Oldroyd KG. Randomized trial of preventive angioplasty in myocardial infarction. N Engl J Med. 2013;369(12):1115-23.
73. Subramanian S, Sabik JF 3rd, Houghtaling PL, Nowicki ER, Blackstone EH, Lytle BW. Decision-making for patients with patent left internal thoracic artery grafts to left anterior descending. Ann Thorac Surg. 2009;87(5):1392-8; discussion 1400.
74. Zhao DX, Leacche M, Balaguer JM, Boudoulas KD, Damp JA, Greelish JP, Byrne JG. Writing Group of the Cardiac Surgery CA, Interventional Cardiology Groups at the Vanderbilt H, Vascular I, Ahmad RM, Ball SK, Cleator JH, Deegan RJ, Eagle SS, Fong PP, Fredi JL, Hoff SJ, Jennings HS 3rd, McPherson JA, Piana RN, Pretorius M, Robbins MA, Slosky DA, Thompson A. Routine intraoperative completion angiography after coronary artery bypass grafting and 1-stop hybrid revascularization results from a fully integrated hybrid catheterization laboratory/operating room. J Am Coll Cardiol. 2009;53(3):232-41.
75. Laflamme M, DeMey N, Bouchard D, Carrier M, Demers P, Pellerin M, Couture P, Perrault LP. Management of early postoperative coronary artery bypass graft failure. Interact Cardiovasc Thorac Surg. 2012;14(4):452-6.
76. Sabik JF 3rd, Blackstone EH, Houghtaling PL, Walts PA, Lytle BW. Is reoperation still a risk factor in coronary artery bypass surgery? Ann Thorac Surg. 2005;80(5):1719-27.
77. Yap CH, Sposato L, Akowuah E, Theodore S, Dinh DT, Shardey GC, Skillington PD, Tatoulis J, Yii M, Smith JA, Mohajeri M, Pick A, Seevanayagam S, Reid CM. Contemporary results show repeat coronary artery bypass grafting remains a risk factor for operative mortality. Ann Thorac Surg. 2009;87(5):1386-91.
78. Morrison DA, Sethi G, Sacks J, Henderson WG, Grover F, Sedlis S, Esposito R. Investigators of the Department of Veterans Affairs Cooperative Study AWESOME. Percutaneous coronary intervention vs. repeat bypass surgery for patients with medically refractory myocardial ischemia: AWESOME randomized trial and registry experience with post-CABG patients. J Am Coll Cardiol. 2002;40(11):1951-4.
79. Harskamp RE, Beijk MA, Damman P, Kuijt WJ, Woudstra P, Grundeken MJ, Kloek JJ, Tijssen JG, de Mol BA, de Winter RJ. Clinical outcome after surgical or percutaneous revascularization in coronary bypass graft failure. J Cardiovasc Med (Hagers- town). 2013;14(6):438-45.
80. Sabik JF 3rd, Raza S, Blackstone EH, Houghtaling PL, Lytle BW. Value of internal thoracic artery grafting to the left anterior descending coronary artery at coronary reoperation. J Am Coll Cardiol. 2013;61(3):302-10.
81. Coolong A, Baim DS, Kuntz RE, O'Malley AJ, Marulkar S, Cutlip DE, Popma JJ, Mauri L. Saphenous vein graft stenting and major adverse cardiac events: a predictive model derived from a pooled analysis of 3958 patients. Circulation. 2008;117(6):790-7.
82. Roffi M, Mukherjee D, Chew DP, Bhatt DL, Cho L, Robbins MA, Ziada KM, Brennan DM, Ellis SG, Topol EJ. Lack of benefit from intravenous platelet glycoprotein IIb/IIIa receptor inhibition as adjunctive treatment for percutaneous interventions of aortocoronary bypass grafts: a pooled analysis of five randomized clinical trials. Circulation. 2002;106(24):3063-7.
83. Baim DS, Wahr D, George B, Leon MB, Greenberg J, Cutlip DE, Kaya U, Popma JJ, Ho KK, Kuntz RE, Saphenous vein graft Angioplasty Free of Emboli Randomized Trial I. Randomized trial of a distal embolic protection device during percutaneous intervention of saphenous vein aorto-coronary bypass grafts. Circulation. 2002;105(11):1285.
84. Stone GW, Rogers C, Hermiller J, Feldman R, Hall P, Haber R, Masud A, Cambier P, Caputo RP, Turco M, Kovach R, Brodie B, Herrmann HC, Kuntz RE, Popma JJ, Ramee S, Cox DA, FilterWire EXREI. Randomized comparison of distal protection with a filter-based catheter and a balloon occlusion and aspiration system during percutaneous intervention of diseased saphenous vein aorto-coronary bypass grafts. Circulation. 2003;108(5):548-553.
85. Mauri L, Cox D, Hermiller J, Massaro J, Wahr J, Tay SW, Jonas M, Popma JJ, Pavliska J, Wahr D, Rogers C. The PROXIMAL trial: proximal protection during saphenous vein graft intervention using the Proxis Embolic Protection System: a randomized, prospective, multicenter clinical trial. J Am Coll Cardiol. 2007;50(15):1442-9.
86. Naidu SS, Turco MA, Mauri L, Coolong A, Popma JJ, Kereiakes DJ. Contemporary incidence and predictors of major adverse cardiac events after saphenous vein graft intervention with embolic protection (an AMEthyst trial substudy). Am J Cardiol. 2010;105(8):1060-4.
87. Frobert O, Schersten F, James SK, Carlsson J, Lagerqvist B. Long-term safety and efficacy of drug-eluting and bare metal stents in saphenous vein grafts. Am Heart J. 2012;164(1):87-93.
88. Wiisanen ME, Abdel-Latif A, Mukherjee D, Ziada KM. Drug-eluting stents vs. bare-metal stents in saphenous vein graft interventions: a systematic review and meta-analysis. JACC Cardiovasc Interv. 2010;3(12):1262-73.
89. Brilakis ES, Lichtenwalter C, Abdel-karim AR, de Lemos JA, Obel O, Addo T, Roesle M, Haagen D, Rangan BV, Saeed B, Bissett JK, Sachdeva R, Voudris VV, Karyofillis P, Kar B, Rossen J, Fasseas P, Berger P, Banerjee S. Continued benefit from paclitaxel-eluting compared with bare-metal stent implantation in saphenous vein graft lesions during long-term follow-up of the SOS (Stenting of Saphenous Vein Grafts) trial. JACC Cardiovasc Interv. 2011;4(2):176-82.
90. Hakeem A, Helmy T, Munsif S, Bhatti S, Mazraeshahi R, Cilingiroglu M, Effat M, Leesar M, Arif I. Safety and efficacy of drug eluting stents compared with bare metal stents for saphenous vein graft interventions: a comprehensive meta-analysis of randomized trials and observational studies comprising 7,994 patients. Catheter Cardiovasc Interv. 2011;77(3):343-55.
91. Mamas MA, Foley J, Nair S, Wiper A, Clarke B, El-Omar M, Fraser DG, Khattar R, Neyses L, Fath-Ordoubadi F. A comparison of drug-eluting stents vs. bare metal stents in saphenous vein graft PCI outcomes: a meta-analysis. J Interv Cardiol. 2011;24(2): 172-80.
92. Ko DT, Guo H, Wijeysundera HC, Zia MI, Dzavik V, Chu MW, Fremes SE, Cohen EA, Tu JV. Long-term safety and effectiveness of drug-eluting stents for the treatment of saphenous vein grafts disease: a population-based study. JACC Cardiovasc Interv. 2011;4(9):965-73.
93. Mehilli J, Pache J, Abdel-Wahab M, Schulz S, Byrne RA, Tiroch K, Hausleiter J, Seyfarth M, Ott I, Ibrahim T, Fusaro M, Laugwitz

KL, Massberg S, Neumann FJ, Richardt G, Schomig A, Kastrati A. Drug-eluting vs. bare-metal stents in saphenous vein graft lesions (ISAR-CABG): a randomised controlled superiority trial. Lancet. 2011;378(9796):1071-8.

94. Nauta ST, Van Mieghem NM, Magro M, Deckers JW, Simsek C, Van Geuns RJ, Van Der Giessen WJ, De Jaegere P, Regar E, Van Domburg RT, Serruys PW. Seven-year safety and efficacy of the unrestricted use of drug-eluting stents in saphenous vein bypass grafts. Catheter Cardiovasc Interv. 2012;79(6):912-18.
95. Alam M, Bandeali SJ, Virani SS, Jneid HM, Shahzad SA, Ramanathan KB, Kar B, Kleiman NS, Lakkis N. Clinical outcomes of percutaneous interventions in saphenous vein grafts using drug-eluting stents compared to bare-metal stents: a comprehensive meta-analysisof all randomized clinical trials. Clin Cardiol. 2012;35(5):291-6.
96. Brilakis ES, Lasala JM, Cox DA, Berger PB, Bowman TS, Starzyk RM, Dawkins KD. Outcomes after implantation of the TAXUS paclitaxel-eluting stent in saphenous vein graft lesions: results from the ARRIVE (TAXUS Peri-Approval Registry: A Multicenter Safety Surveillance) program. JACC Cardiovasc Interv. 2010;3(7):742-50.
97. Chechi T, Vecchio S, Vittori G, Giuliani G, Lilli A, Spaziani G, Consoli L, Baldereschi G, Biondi-Zoccai GG, Sheiban I, Margheri M. ST-segment elevation myocardial infarction due to early and late stent thrombosis a new group of high-risk patients. J Am Coll Cardiol. 2008;51(25):2396-2402.
98. Alfonso F, Dutary J, Paulo M, Gonzalo N, Perez-Vizcayno MJ, Jimenez-Quevedo P, Escaned J, Banuelos C, Hernandez R, Macaya C. Combined use of optical coherence tomography and intravascular ultrasound imaging in patients undergoing coronary interventions for stent thrombosis. Heart. 2012;98(16):1213-20.
99. Armstrong EJ, Feldman DN, Wang TY, Kaltenbach LA, Yeo KK, Wong SC, Spertus J, Shaw RE, Minutello RM, Moussa I, Ho KK, Rogers JH, Shunk KA. Clinical presentation, management, and outcomes of angiographically documented early, late, and very late stent thrombosis. JACC Cardiovasc Interv. 2012;5(2):131-40.
100. Wiviott SD, Braunwald E, McCabe CH, Montalescot G, Ruzyllo W, Gottlieb S, Neumann FJ, Ardissino D, De Servi S, Murphy SA, Riesmeyer J, Weerakkody G, Gibson CM, Antman EM. Prasugrel vs. clopidogrel in patients with acute coronary syndromes. N Engl J Med. 2007;357(20):2001-15.
101. Kastrati A, Mehilli J, von Beckerath N, Dibra A, Hausleiter J, Pache J, Schuhlen H, Schmitt C, Dirschinger J, Schomig A. Sirolimus-eluting stent or paclitaxel-eluting stent vs. balloon angioplasty for prevention of recurrences in patients with coron- ary in-stent restenosis: a randomized controlled trial. JAMA. 2005;293(2):165-71.
102. Mehilli J, Byrne RA, Tiroch K, Pinieck S, Schulz S, Kufner S, Massberg S, Laugwitz KL, Schomig A, Kastrati A. Randomized trial of paclitaxel- vs. sirolimus-eluting stents for treatment of coronary restenosis in sirolimus-eluting stents: the ISAR-DESIRE 2 (Intracoronary Stenting and Angiographic Results: Drug Eluting Stents for In-Stent Restenosis 2) study. J Am Coll Cardiol. 2010;55(24):2710-16.
103. Alfonso F, Perez-Vizcayno MJ, Hernandez R, Bethencourt A, Marti V, Lopez-Minguez JR, Angel J, Mantilla R, Moris C, Cequier A, Sabate M, Escaned J, Moreno R, Banuelos C, Suarez A, Macaya C. A randomized comparison of sirolimus-eluting stent with balloon angioplasty in patients with in-stent restenosis: results of the Restenosis Intrastent: Balloon Angioplasty vs. Elective Sirolimus-Eluting Stenting (RIBS-II) trial. J Am Coll Cardiol. 2006;47(11):2152-60.
104. Alfonso F, Zueco J, Cequier A, Mantilla R, Bethencourt A, Lopez-Minguez JR, Angel J, Auge JM, Gomez-Recio M, Moris C, Seabra-Gomes R, Perez-Vizcayno MJ, Macaya C. A randomized comparison of repeat stenting with balloon angioplasty in patients with in-stent restenosis. J Am Coll Cardiol. 2003; 42(5):796-805.
105. Dibra A, Kastrati A, Alfonso F, Seyfarth M, Perez-Vizcayno MJ, Mehilli J, Schomig A. Effectiveness of drug-eluting stents in patients with bare-metal in-stent restenosis: meta-analysis of randomized trials. J Am Coll Cardiol. 2007;49(5):616-23.
106. Scheller B, Clever YP, Kelsch B, Hehrlein C, Bocksch W, Rutsch W, Haghi D, Dietz U, Speck U, Bohm M, Cremers B. Long-term follow-up after treatment of coronary in-stent restenosis with a paclitaxel-coated balloon catheter. JACC Cardiovasc Interv. 2012;5(3):323-330.
107. Scheller B, Hehrlein C, Bocksch W, Rutsch W, Haghi D, Dietz U, Bohm M, Speck U. Treatment of coronary in-stent restenosis with a paclitaxel-coated balloon catheter. N Engl J Med. 2006;355(20):2113-24.
108. Unverdorben M, Vallbracht C, Cremers B, Heuer H, Hengstenberg C, Maikowski C, Werner GS, Antoni D, Kleber FX, Bocksch W, Leschke M, Ackermann H, Boxberger M, Speck U, Degenhardt R, Scheller B. Paclitaxel-coated balloon catheter vs. paclitaxel-coated stent for the treatment of coronary in-stent restenosis. Circulation. 2009;119(23):2986-94.
109. Rittger H, Brachmann J, Sinha AM, Waliszewski M, Ohlow M, Brugger A, Thiele H, Birkemeyer R, Kurowski V, Breithardt OA, Schmidt M, Zimmermann S, Lonke S, von Cranach M, Nguyen TV, Daniel WG, Wohrle J. A randomized, multicenter, single-blinded trial comparing paclitaxel-coated balloon angioplasty with plain balloon angioplasty in drug-eluting stent restenosis: the PEPCAD-DES study. J Am Coll Cardiol. 2012;59(15):1377-82.
110. Habara S, Mitsudo K, Kadota K, Goto T, Fujii S, Yamamoto H, Katoh H, Oka N, Fuku Y, Hosogi S, Hirono A, Maruo T, Tanaka H, Shigemoto Y, Hasegawa D, Tasaka H, Kusunose M, Otsuru S, Okamoto Y, Saito N, Tsujimoto Y, Eguchi H, Miyake K, Yoshino M. Effectiveness of paclitaxel-eluting balloon catheter in patients with sirolimus-eluting stent restenosis. JACC Cardiovasc Interv. 2011;4(2):149-54.
111. Byrne RA, Neumann FJ, Mehilli J, Pinieck S, Wolff B, Tiroch K, Schulz S, Fusaro M, Ott I, Ibrahim T, Hausleiter J, Valina C, Pache J, Laugwitz KL, Massberg S, Kastrati A. Paclitaxel-eluting balloons, paclitaxel-eluting stents, and balloon angioplasty in patients with restenosis after implantation of a drug-eluting stent (ISAR- DESIRE 3): a randomised, open-label trial. Lancet. 2013;381(9865):461-7.
112. Indermuehle A, Bahl R, Lansky AJ, Froehlich GM, Knapp G, Timmis A, Meier P. Drug-eluting balloon angioplasty for in-stent restenosis: a systematic review and meta-analysis of randomised controlled trials. Heart. 2013;99(5):327-33.
113. Stone GW, Gao R, Kimura et al. 1-year outcomes with the Absorb bioresorbable scaffold in patients with coronary artery disease: a patient- level pooled meta-analysis. Lancet. 2016.
114. Ormiston JA, Serruys PW, Regar E, Dudek D, Thuesen L, Webster MW, Onuma Y, Garcia-Garcia HM, McGreevy R, Veldhof S. A

bioabsorbable everolimus-eluting coronary stent system for patients with single de-novo coronary artery lesions (ABSORB): a prospective open-label trial. Lancet. 2008;371(9616): 899-907.

115. Serruys PW, Ormiston JA, Onuma Y, Regar E, Gonzalo N, Garcia-Garcia HM, Nieman K, Bruining N, Dorange C, Miquel-Hebert K, Veldhof S, Webster M, Thuesen L, Dudek D. A bioabsorbable everolimus-eluting coronary stent system (ABSORB): 2-year outcomes and results from multiple imaging methods. Lancet. 2009;373(9667):897-910.
116. Haude M, Erbel R, Erne P, Verheye S, Degen H, Bose D, Vermeersch P, Wijnbergen I, Weissman N, Prati F, Waksman R, Koolen J. Safety and performance of the drug-eluting absorbable metal scaffold (DREAMS) in patients with de-novo coronary lesions: 12 month results of the prospective, multicentre, first-in-man BIOSOLVE-I trial. Lancet. 2013;381(9869):836-44.
117. Bondesson P, Lagerqvist B, James SK, Olivecrona GK, Venetsanos D, Harnek J. Comparison of two drug-eluting balloons: a report from the SCAAR registry. Euro- Intervention. 2012;8(4):444-9.
118. Scheller B, Hehrlein C, Bocksch W, Rutsch W, Haghi D, Dietz U, Bohm M, Speck U. Treatment of coronary in-stent restenosis with a paclitaxel-coated balloon catheter. N Engl J Med. 2006;355(20):2113-24.
119. Maier LS, Maack C, Ritter O, Bohm M. Hot line update of clinical trials and registries presented at the German Cardiac Society meeting 2008. (PEPCAD, LokalTax, INH, German ablation registry, German device registry, DES.DE registry, DHR, Reality, SWEETHEART registry, ADMA, GERSHWIN). Clin Res Cardiol. 2008;97(6):356-63.
120. Unverdorben M, Vallbracht C, Cremers B, Heuer H, Hengstenberg C, Maikowski C, Werner GS, Antoni D, Kleber FX, Bocksch W, Leschke M, Ackermann H, Boxberger M, Speck U, Degenhardt R, Scheller B. Paclitaxel-coated balloon catheter vs paclitaxel-coated stent for the treatment of coronary in-stent restenosis. Circulation. 2009;119(23):2986-94.
121. Rittger H, Brachmann J, Sinha AM, Waliszewski M, Ohlow M, Brugger A, Thiele H, Birkemeyer R, Kurowski V, Breithardt OA, Schmidt M, Zimmermann S, Lonke S, von Cranach M, Nguyen TV, Daniel WG, Wohrle J. A randomized, multicenter, single-blinded trial comparing paclitaxel-coated balloon angioplasty with plain balloon angioplasty in drug-eluting stent restenosis: the PEPCAD-DES study. J Am Coll Cardiol. 2012;59(15):1377-82.
122. Habara S, Mitsudo K, Kadota K, Goto T, Fujii S, Yamamoto H, Katoh H, Oka N, Fuku Y, Hosogi S, Hirono A, Maruo T, Tanaka H, Shigemoto Y, Hasegawa D, Tasaka H, Kusunose M, Otsuru S, Okamoto Y, Saito N, Tsujimoto Y, Eguchi H, Miyake K, Yoshino M. Effectiveness of paclitaxel-eluting balloon catheter in patients with sirolimus-eluting stent restenosis. JACC Cardiovasc Interv. 2011;4(2):149-54.
123. Fischer D, Scheller B, Schafer A, Klein G, Bohm M, Clever Y, Cremers B. Paclitaxcel-coated balloon plus bare metal stent vs. sirolimus-eluting stent in de novo lesions: an IVUS study. EuroIntervention. 2012;8(4):450-55.
124. Belkacemi A, Agostoni P, Nathoe HM, Voskuil M, Shao C, Van Belle E, Wildbergh T, Politi L, Doevendans PA, Sangiorgi GM, Stella PR. First results of the DEB-AMI (drug eluting balloon in acute ST-segment elevation myocardial infarction) trial: a multicenter randomized comparison of drug-eluting balloon plus bare-metal stent vs. bare-metal stent vs. drug-eluting stent in primary percutaneous coronary intervention with 6-month angiographic, intravascular, functional, and clinical outcomes. J Am Coll Cardiol. 2012;59(25):2327-37.
125. Latib A, Colombo A, Castriota F, Micari A, Cremonesi A, De Felice F, Marchese A, Tespili M, Presbitero P, Sgueglia GA, Buffoli F, Tamburino C, Varbella F, Menozzi A. A randomized multicenter study comparing a paclitaxel drug-eluting balloon with a paclitaxel-eluting stent in small coronary vessels: the BELLO (Balloon Elution and Late Loss Optimization) study. J Am Coll Cardiol. 2012;60(24):2473-80.
126. Byrne RA, Neumann FJ, Mehilli J, Pinieck S, Wolff B, Tiroch K, Schulz S, Fusaro M, Ott I, Ibrahim T, Hausleiter J, Valina C, Pache J, Laugwitz KL, Massberg S, Kastrati A. Paclitaxel-eluting balloons, paclitaxel-eluting stents, and balloon angioplasty in patients with restenosis after implantation of a drug-eluting stent (ISAR- DESIRE 3): a randomised, open-label trial. Lancet. 2013;381(9865):461-7.

CHAPTER

26

Future of Angioplasty

Tiny Nair, K Krishnakumar

Medical field is moving from disease based medicine to P4 medicine (personalized, predictive, preventive, participatory)

–Josep Brugada, Barcelona, Spain

In 1985, Wilhelm Conrad Rontgen discovered X-ray, formally inaugurating the science of imaging; a science that over the years grew by massive proportions. Catheter based interventions piggybacked on angiogram and changed the face of cardiovascular (CV) therapeutics. With more than 3 million angioplasty procedures done annually worldwide,[1] percutaneous coronary intervention (PCI) has become a gold standard of therapy in obstructive coronary artery disease.

This review tries to look into the future of angioplasty, not merely a utopian crystal ball gazing, but a realistic view of what is likely to come.

LUMINOGRAM TO PLAQUE CHARACTER

On October 30, 1958 Dr F Mason Sones, working at the Cleveland Clinic, Ohio performed the first 'unintentional' coronary angiography when the catheter meant for aortic root injection accidentally slipped into the right coronary sinus.[2] This marked the beginning of a new era in diagnostic and subsequently interventional cardiology. Quickly, coronary angiogram became the gold standard of diagnosis in obstructive coronary artery disease, because of its clarity and ease. Over time, the cath-lab graduated from a film based system to completely digital platform with huge amount of post processing capability.

The fact that it is just a coronary luminogram and that it gave away only limited information about the severity of coronary blockages was quickly understood, but that did not deter its spread and progress. Coronary angiogram had several caveats; it did not identify the nature and severity of obstructive plaque, plaque vulnerability or the total plaque burden. It also did not give information regarding the health of the perfusing myocardium (viability). This made angiogram a poor tool to prognosticate future CV events. Subsequently, new techniques like intravascular ultrasound (IVUS), optical coherence tomography (OCT), virtual histology, multislice computerized tomography (MSCT) and cardiac magnetic resonance (CMR) gave us more information about plaque character. Positron emitting tomography-computed tomography (PET-CT) set a new standard in diagnosis of myocardial viability, clearing another blind spot of coronary angiogram. Coronary angiogram also did not give information on the physiologic and hemodynamic characters of the block, making decision-making difficult in borderline blockages. The Doppler wire technology gave us fractional flow reserve (FFR), which could now document pressure difference across a coronary block to decide whether or not to stent a lesion. Further, MSCT coupled with noninvasive FFR gave us a combination of information of coronary anatomy, physiology as well as plaque morphology, noninvasively.

More powerful MR systems, and thinner IVUS catheter, more sensitive OCT with virtual histology and faster multislice CTA are being introduced every year to improve accuracy of diagnosis, operator ease and patient comfort. Newer sharper and more precise imaging modalities might come but the real future perhaps is somewhere else, and that may be 'integration' of imaging modalities.

INTEGRATED IMAGING

Today's diagnostic flow chart in ischemic heart disease is fairly streamlined. Symptomatic angina patients directly go to coronary angiogram, while milder or asymptomatic patients have a stress test (induced by adenosine, dobutamine or physical exercise) and objective ischemia is recorded (by either perfusion imaging, echocardiographic wall motion abnormality or by an ECG change). Sometimes a coronary calcium score (CCS) or a CTA precedes a coronary angiogram, in intermediate risk cases. Despite today's advances in imaging, most high tech coronary imaging options start with coronary angiogram and depending on the results, further work up including IVUS, OCT, FFR or CMR are done. But in future perhaps we are going to see an integration of all the imaging modalities.[3]

The concept of integrated imaging of the future is not just availability of all imaging modalities in one room, but integrating them to get information to make decision making more precise and relevant. This is a transition from present 'first see-then do' approach to 'see-as-you-do' approach (Fig. 26.1).

The integrated imaging center of future would have an integrated MSCT with noninvasive FFR, a CMR. Even before the first puncture is performed, the interventional cardiologist would be aware of the scale of problem, and what exactly to address. Once a 'multipurpose' catheter goes in, it would record every invasive modality including IVUS, OCT, virtual histology. The outputs of all these multimodality images would be superimposed and computed to give the operator an insight into the anatomy, physiology, hemodynamics of the block, details of the histology and dynamic behavior of the plaque as well as the state of the perfusing myocardium. This would take the guessing game out of diagnosis and give clarity on therapeutic options. A repeat integrated imaging post intervention would not only define success of the procedure but also give a precise prognosis of the disease. The interventional cardiologist would go in knowing what exactly to do, how to do and to what extent.

Despite improvement in intervention, no reflow and viability assessment remain a challenging problem in PCI. Integrating PET-CT into the integrated imaging center is likely to reduce the problem burden. The challenge of incorporating PET CT (size and cost) would certainly be solved out in the future.

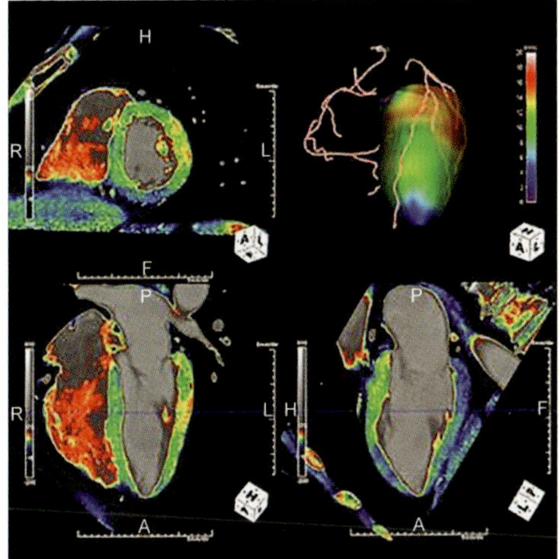

Fig. 26.1 CT myocardial perfusion image (Vital Image Inc.)

MINIATURIZATION

With miniaturization and nanotechnology firmly setting foot in every arena of science, angioplasty would also see tremendous change in miniaturization of hardware in the future. Twenty years back 8 to 10 French guide catheters were standard for intervention, while today up to 3 French catheters are being introduced for newer drug eluting stents and devices.[4] Miniaturization would give us the advantage of minimal invasiveness, less access site complications, patient comfort as well as less operator stress.

Outpatient procedures and same day discharges are no longer a novelty and have become the norm and are likely to become standard of care tomorrow, even for the most complex procedures.

HYBRID PROCEDURES

Hybrid strategy is defined as one in which a surgical procedure like coronary artery bypass grafting (CABG) is combined with a percutaneous procedure to reduce surgical time, hence surgical complications are reduced. These are done in patients with comorbidities to minimize procedural time (e.g. on-pump time). Presently patients go from cath lab to the operating room or vice-versa. In the 'hybrid rooms', the operating room and cath lab are one combined room where both procedures are done.

But the future 'hybrid suite' would be a combination of integrated imaging to the hybrid suit to enable creation of an all-in-one 'single window' cardiac station, that would offer all cardiac and diagnosis under one roof, electrophysiology (EP) lab and percutaneous valve implantations inclusive. The challenge of such futuristic therapy would be cost effectiveness and economic viability.

ROBOTICS AND NAVIGATION

Twisting and turning of a catheter at the operator's end and trying to translate the torque and thrust to the inside of coronary artery will no longer be necessary in the future (Fig. 26.2). Improved navigation system with advanced electro- mechanical, hydraulic and magnetic control at the catheter tip would enable the operator to simply use a trackball or a touch pad to direct and command the system to 'home-in' to the necessary coronary artery, and get past even the most difficult lesions. The tip of the catheter would sense and send back tactic feel to the operator.[5] The fact that the operator sits on a remote location would provide him safety from harmful doses of radiation (Fig. 26.3).

The system would first generate an individual specific 3D image of the patient's coronary artery by obtaining 3 or more views simultaneously and form a 3D map of the

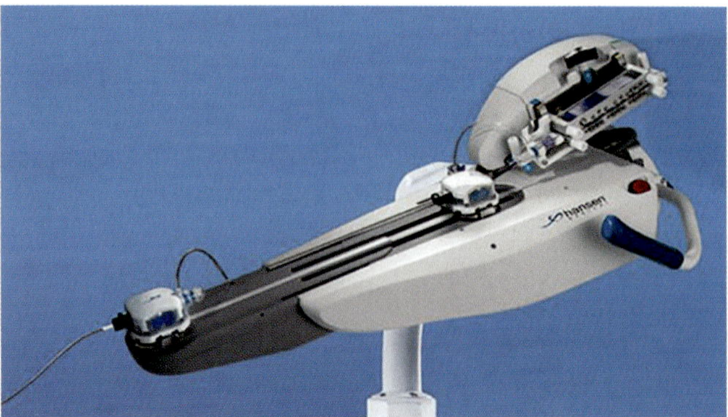

Fig. 26.2 Hansen medicals Magellan 10 French robotic catheter

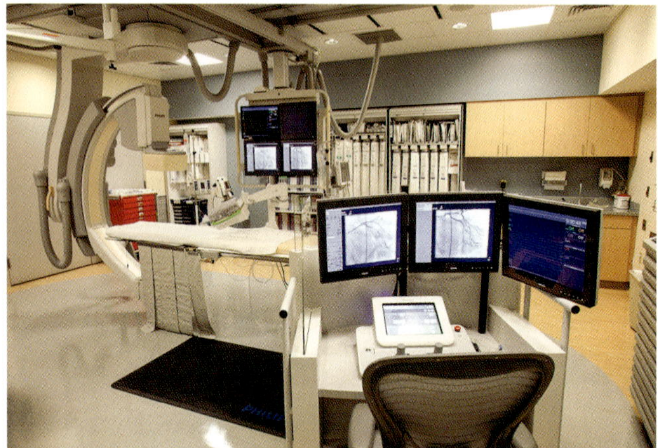

Fig. 26.3 The CorPath 200 system is a robotic cath lab where the operator sits in a radiation shielded operating cockpit and controls the catheter and hardware movement with a joystick. A table mounted robotic arm, connected via a cassette transmits these movements precisely at steps of 1 mm to the catheter tip. The learning curve of the system is said to be good when compared to nonrobotic systems

coronary artery (like a Google navigation). This would enable a catheter or a guidewire to home-in and reach the desired location despite difficult lesions (akin to bad roads). Dynamic multipurpose guidewires would change shape and glide effortlessly through the most uncross-able lesions. Perforation of coronary wires would relegate itself to the history of angioplasty. Like an experienced operator, the system would reset catheter negotiation speed, depending on tip feedback, like an automatic gearshift, thus reducing time.

HARDWARE

Drug eluting stents have already given way to biovascular scaffolds. Future scaffolds would have different dissolution

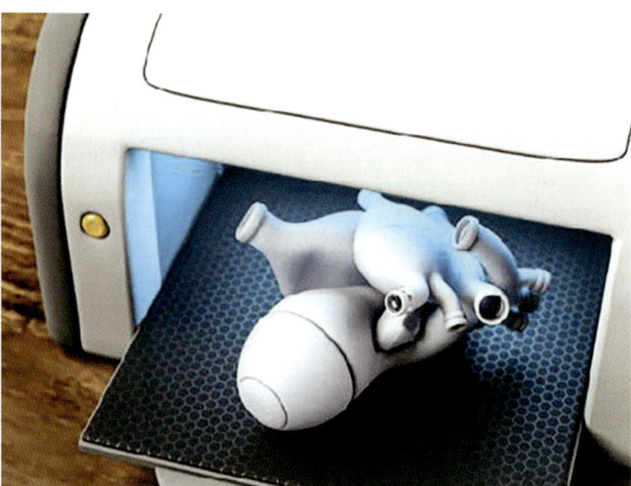

Fig. 26.4 Heart model being printed in a 3D printer

profiles, some of which may be programmed from outside later. The exact 'time-to- dissolve' of the stent could be programmed postimplant. A burst of magnetic field or a radiofrequency would alter the dissolution profile as needed. The biovascular platforms of the future would be virtually free from stent thrombosis and restenosis, needing reduction or elimination of antiplatelet drug dosage and consequential long term bleeding complications. Simple things like inflation of the balloon would not be a vague, elective decision, but a computer controlled feedback loop driven algorithm enabling maximizing inflation pressure with minimal tissue damage. Postprocedure, as the access catheter (sheath) is removed, the automated sealing device would deploy, making sure that the patients does not suffer the pain of prolonged compression while access site bleedings are reduced to the minimum. The intelligent stretch sensitive plaster would warn the staff early if there is any hematoma despite these methods. This would make even femoral access patients to be discharged on the same day.

PRINTABLE HARDWARE

With 3D printing technology pervading every aspect of life, the future cath lab will depend heavily on 'on-site' 3D printing of majority of hardware (Fig. 26.4) 3D printed heart model for teaching purpose as well as implantables are already being printed (Fig. 26.5).

The future cath lab will not stockpile huge volumes of hardware of different shapes and sizes, but would print them as necessary. A sheet of bioabsorbable material would be fed into the printer to 3D print an exact tailor-made stent or device right at the lab. The advantage of printing on site would be an exact sized stent that the patient needs, and not one that the manufacturer supplies as standard.

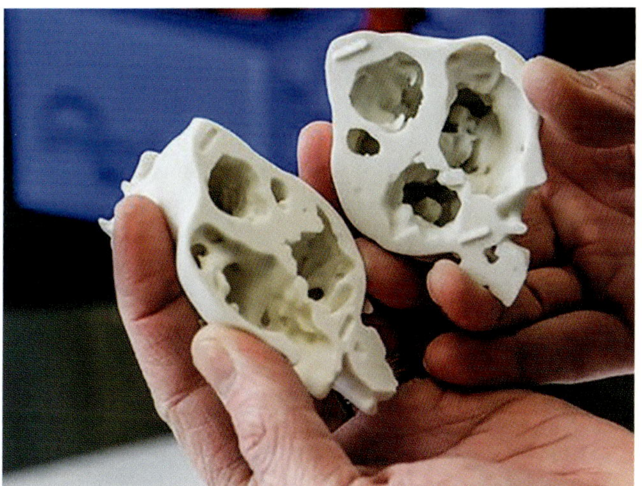

Fig. 26.5 3D printed heart model for teaching

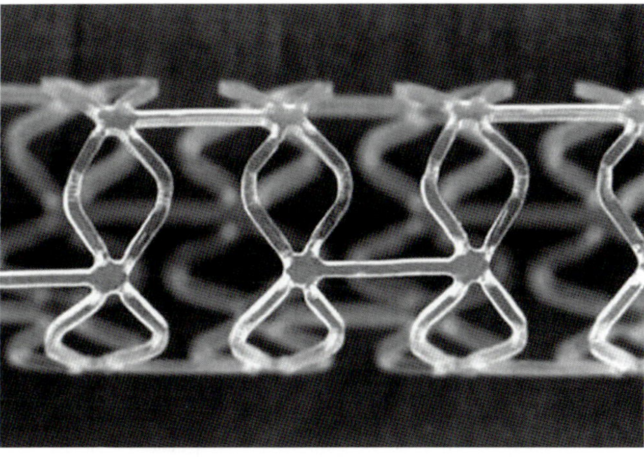

Fig. 26.6 Bioabsorbable stent platform

CLOSURE DEVICE

Automated closure devices are already in extensive use. The future cath lab would see a more extensive usage of this technology. The future systems would deploy automatically when the sheath is removed. Bioabsorbable closure devices have already hit the market and are likely to become more popular, offering more variants and sizes (Figs 26.6 and 26.7).

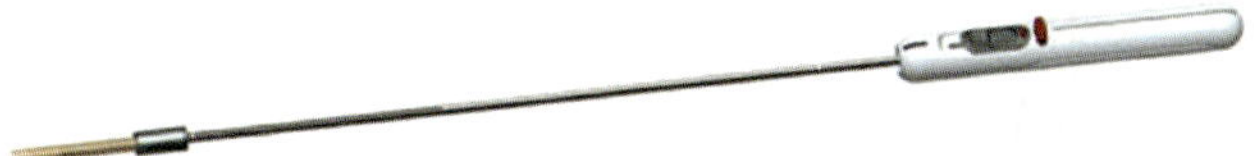

Fig. 26.7 Vivasure bioabsorbable closure device is available for large bore arteriotomies like TAVR

ECONOMICS AND COST

Dream of integrated diagnostic suits are good, (like the birthing suits) as concept. In fact, people have envisaged all-in-one suit to integrate diagnostics. The main concern in this regard is the cost. The cost involved in setting up such a unit would be huge. So a common patient needing an angiogram just to rule out a coronary artery disease would have to needlessly pay for the huge amount of money to offset the cost of setting up a high tech integrated imaging lab. Today in India, diagnostic angiograms could be done at a cost as low as ₹ 5000 (less than USD 100). Such low-cost angiograms would perhaps not be possible till the cost of technology comes down.

LOCATING HARDWARE IN THE LAB

Today's cath-labs have already become huge storehouse of large number of hardware. With hundreds of different types of hardware, wires, guides, catheters and stents, locating one in a busy cath lab is a challenge, especially when time is critical. Physical knowledge of location of hardware is not easy. Checking 'location-logs' slow down process. Absence of a critical cath lab tech, who knows the location of such device, is no longer feasible. Standardized radiofrequency analysis (RFA) tagging of hardware enable the cath lab technicians to quickly track down necessary hardware quickly. In the future cath lab, the operator has to speak to the voice activated command system, which would immediately show the location of the particular device or hardware in a lab-map. Fast 3D printers would manufacture patient specific hardware instantly.

RADIATION SAFETY

Complex procedures need exposure to more radiation, both for the patient and the operator. Seating the operator away from the radiation source is today a reality, and Corpath 200 lab is the first step in that direction. Better radiation shields that are comfortable to wear are already there and are likely to become more fashionable and trendy. With more and more talented young operators joining the bandwagon and spending more time in the cath lab, cath lab fashion needs to be changing with time while being 100% radiation safe. The radiation safe dress would be equipped with sensor that change color once the radiation dosage nears the safe limits, thus warning the operator and the supporting staff the need for a radiation holiday. Systems producing less radiation, keeping the operation to a remote location and using

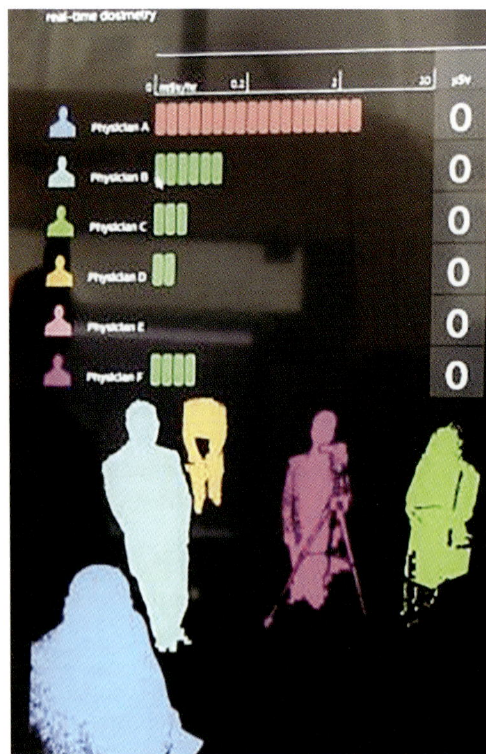

Fig. 26.8 Radiation sensitive video recorder

nonradiation imaging options are the future of angioplasty. Radiation sensitive video recorder that 'color-codes' everyone in the lab and shows (labels) their individual radiation exposure is ready for market (Fig. 26.8).

MYOCARDIAL VIABILITY

Integrated imaging lab of the future is also likely to have viability imaging by way of stress echo, myocardial perfusion imaging or PET-CT.

DATA NETWORK

Patients are unlikely to be tethered to one hospital, or even one medical chain. In today's world people travel from place to place, and expect their medical records to be available to every hospital they go, but with full confidence and privacy. The challenge of widespread availability coupled with privacy entails that there needs to be extensive data encryption at the same time real-time connected network that is easy to access and fast but secure for the patient. Every angiogram, every PCI, recorded even the remotest corners of the world would be uploaded instantly and available anywhere for review, interpretation and analysis. Such database would also help creating registries with flawless statistics for planning population-based strategies.

CONCLUSION

The future of angioplasty looks bright and shining, with a promise to improve quality of life with minimal complication, discomfort and risk. It promises to be the pit stop of cardiac care in the modern fast paced race of human life.

REFERENCES

1. Y Gerber, C Rihal, TR Sundt, J Killian, S Weston, T Therneau, et al. Coronary revascularization in the community. A population-based study, 1990 to 2004. J Am Coll Cardiol. 2007;50:1223-9.
2. Ryan TJ. The coronary angiogram and its seminal contribution to cardiovascular medicine over five decades. Circulation. 2002;106:752-6.
3. Zaidi H, Montandon ML, Alavi A. The clinical role of fusion imaging using PET, CT, and MR imaging. Magn Reson Imaging. Clin N Am. 2010;18:133-49.
4. Goldstein JA. Coronary intervention with miniaturized guiding systems: Is smaller necessarily better? Catheter Cardiovasc Interv. 2010;75:989-90.
5. Lemoine P, Gutierrez M, Vexo F, Thalmann D. Mediators: Virtual interfaces with haptic feedback. Available at: *http://citeseerx.ist.psu.edu/viewdoc/download.*

CHAPTER

27

Rotablation in Coronary Artery Disease

Chandrashekhar Makhale, Varun Nivargi

INTRODUCTION

Andreas Gruentzig performed the first successful percutaneous transluminal coronary angioplasty on a human on September 16, 1977 at University Hospital, Zurich. The procedure was initially limited to the fewer than 10% of patients with symptomatic coronary artery disease (CAD) who had a single, focal, noncalcified lesion in a proximal coronary vessel. As equipment design and operator experience evolved over the next decade, the use of percutaneous coronary interventions (PCI) expanded to encompass an increasing spectrum of coronary anatomy—including multivessel CAD, total occlusions, diseased saphenous vein grafts (SVGs), and acute ST-segment elevation myocardial infarction (STEMI), among other complexities.

The year 2012 marked the 25th year since Jerome Ritchie, David Auth, and colleagues[1] introduced rotational atherectomy (RA) as a technique for the endovascular treatment of obstructive atherosclerotic disease. RA emerged in the 1990s as one of several tools to treat luminal obstruction via physical removal of plaque. Although initially explored as an alternative to balloon angioplasty, RA proved complementary, facilitating angioplasty and, later, stenting of complex lesions, particularly those affected by heavy calcification. Beyond immediate procedural success, however, data have not shown a consistent long-term benefit of lesion modification by RA for restenosis and major adverse cardiovascular events (MACE). Today, RA use is infrequent. At one time, RA was involved in up to 10% of percutaneous coronary interventions (PCI).[2] In more recent series, RA use has fallen to 3–5% in select high-volume centers and <1% in others.[3] Though uncommon, RA maintains purpose in the modern cardiac catheterization laboratory.

Since, the development of rotational coronary atherectomy in the early 80s the indications for the procedure have changed. In complex coronary lesions no difference in the rate of restenosis at 6 months was evident when rotational atherectomy was compared with conventional percutaneous transluminal coronary angioplasty (PTCA), but procedural complications were somewhat higher with rotablation.[4,5] The single center excimer rotablator balloon angioplasty comparison (ERBAC) study of 685 patients compared excimer laser, rotational atherectomy and PTCA in complex lesions and demonstrated a higher procedural success rate for rotational atherectomy but higher target lesion revascularization (TLR) rates.[6] The multicenter COBRA trial demonstrated higher procedural success rates with rotational atherectomy compared to PTCA, but no difference in clinical outcomes.[7] The use of rotational atherectomy has continued as a lesion preparation tool for better delivery and implantation of coronary stents,[8] especially drug-eluting stents (DES).[9,10] Debulking complex atherosclerotic lesions prior to stenting resulted in higher luminal gain and smaller late luminal loss.[11] Rotational atherectomy may also be used to treat restenosis.[12,13] The success of the intervention depends on the rotablation technique (burr-to-artery ratio, revolutions per minute) and operator experience.[14,15] In a comparison of rotational atherectomy with coronary artery bypass grafting (CABG) for patients with failed conventional PCI, there was no significant difference in major cardiovascular events but rotational atherectomy carried a lower risk of periprocedural complications and a higher rate of target vessel revascularization.[16]

The European Society of Cardiology recommends using rotational atherectomy to prepare lesions that cannot be crossed with the balloon catheter or adequately dilated (recommendation class I, evidence level C).[17]

NEED FOR ROTABLATION

Long, calcific and tubular lesions cannot be addressed by simple balloon inflations, use of cutting/scoring balloons. Balloon dilatation although will give an angiographically good flow but the crossing of stent and stent expansion will be hampered because of the sheer volume of calcification in the lesion. Hence, the need for debulking with rotablation.

Benefits

- Minimizes vessel wall stretch and elastic recoil
- Eliminates vessel barotrauma
- Removes all plaque morphologies, soft, fibrotic and calcified
- Produces a smooth lumen channel.

Principles

- Differential cutting
- The orthogonal displacement of friction.

Differential Cutting (Fig. 27.1)

- The ability to selectively ablate one material while sparing the other
- The elliptical burr differentiates the healthy elastic vessel wall from the plaque
- All diseased plaque is inelastic.

Example

Scraping a knife gently on one's skin and then across a fingernail.

Shaving: A razor will cut inelastic whiskers but will not cut the healthy underlying elastic skin (Figs 27.2A and B)

A nail file on your skin will not cut your skin, but when applied to the nail,will cut the nail.

Orthogonal Displacement of Friction

- Friction occurs when sliding surfaces are in contact
- Friction is minimized by a sliding motion perpendicular or orthogonal to the contact surface
- The faster something is turned the more the friction is reduced.

Example (Fig. 27.3)

- Removal of a cork from a wine bottle. If a cork is twisted as it is pulled, the friction is reduced and the cork can be withdrawn easily.
- Removal of a ring from a finger. If, it is twisted the removal can be much easier.

Plaque is ablated into small particles called microparticles.

The size of the microparticles is less than 5 μ (smaller than a red blood cell).

The microparticles are picked up by the RES (reticulo-endotheliel system) (Fig. 27.4)

Fundamental Elements of Optimal RA Technique

- Single burr with burr-to-artery ratio of 0.5–0.6
- Rotational speed of 140,000–150,000 rpm
- Gradual burr advancement using a pecking motion
- Short ablation runs of 15–20 s
- Avoidance of decelerations >5,000 rpm
- Final polishing run.

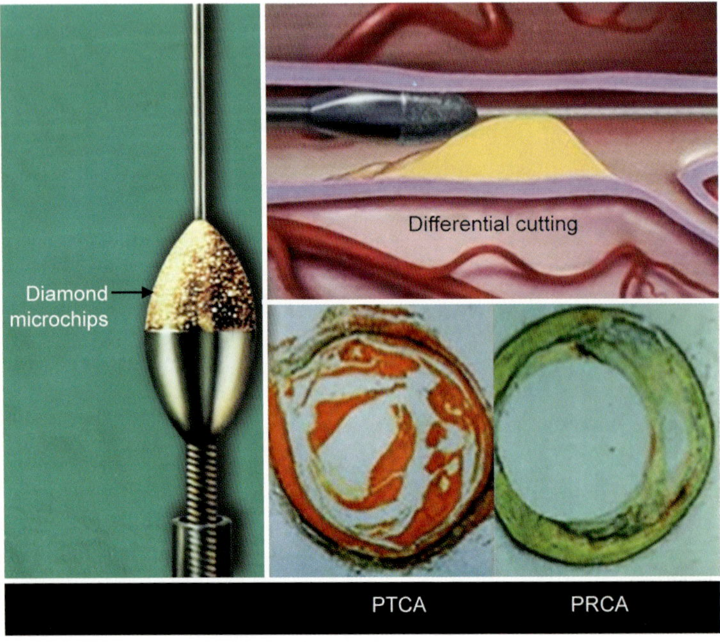

Fig. 27.1 Atherectomy: Differential cutting

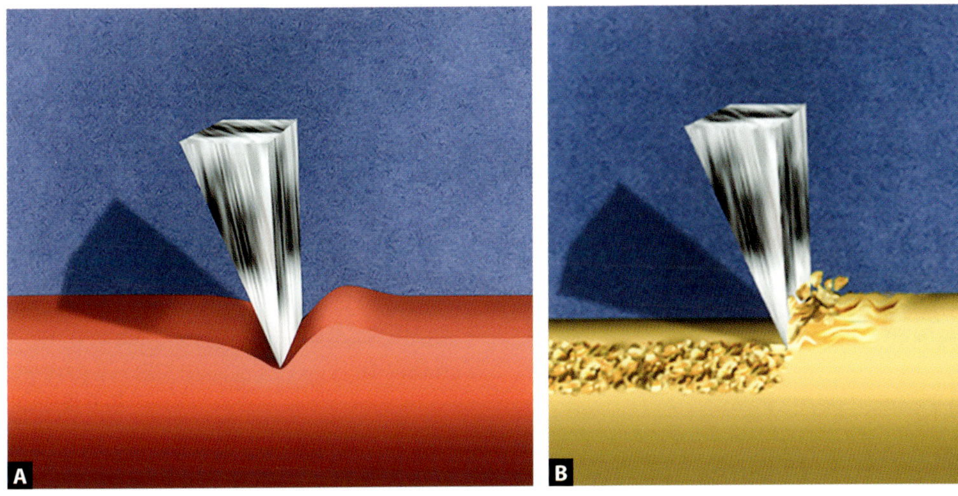

Figs 27.2A and B (A) Elastic tissue; (B) Inelastic tissue

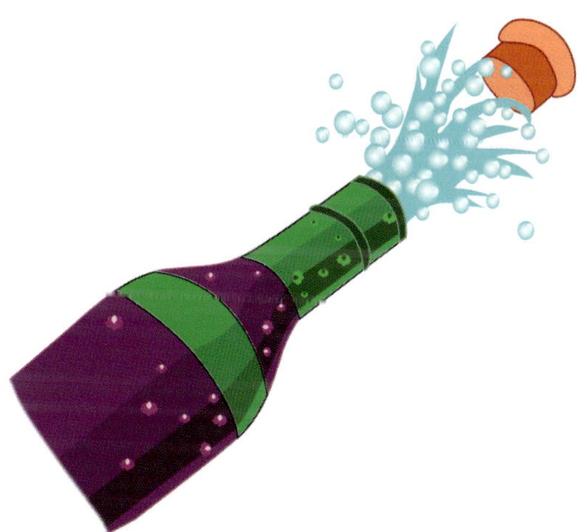

Fig. 27.3 Orthogonal displacement

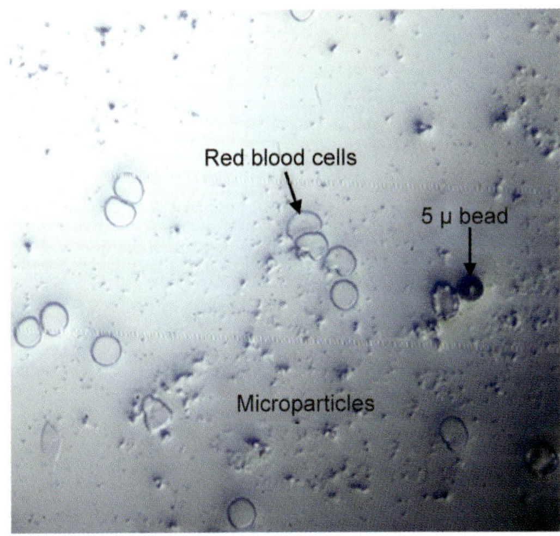

Fig. 27.4 Atherectomy debris

INDICATIONS

- DeNovo calcific lesions
- Restenotic lesions
- Single vessel or multivessel lesions
- Long calcific lesions
- Bifurcated lesions
- Vessels not suitable for stenting (less than 2.0 mm)
- Pre-stent deployment (debulking).

OTHER FREQUENT USES

- In-stent restenosis
- Ostial lesion
- Rota stent
- Long diffuse/calcific disease
- Total occlusions
- Unprotected/protected left main
- Anastomosis sites of SVGs
- "Train wrecks" with no other treatment options and surgeons refuse.

CONTRAINDICATIONS

- Thrombus
- Compromised left ventricular function
- Saphenous vein grafts
- Dissection
- Occlusions not passable with a guidewire.

ROTABLATOR PRODUCTS AND SYSTEM COMPONENTS (FIGS 27.5 TO 27.10)

Burr

- Elliptical shaped with 2,000–3,000 microscopic diamond crystals on the leading edge
- The proximal surface is smooth
- The burr is nickel coated
- The diamond crystals are 20 microns in size, with only 5 microns extruding from the nickel coating (Like an iceberg in a sea of nickel).

Irrigating the Rota Burr

See Figure 27.6.

Air Supply Set Up

Dual Gauge Regulator

- Pressure regulator (relieving type is preferred) capable of delivering at least 5 scfm (140 liter/min or 0.1 m^3/min) at 620–758 kPa (90–100 psi or 6.5–7.5 bar or 6.3–7.7 atm). Pressure of the gas supplied to the air or nitrogen connector does not exceed 758 kPa (110 psi or 7.6 bar).

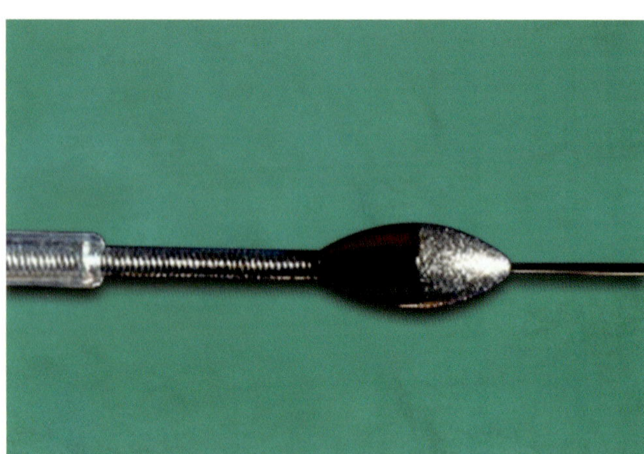

Fig. 27.5 Burr

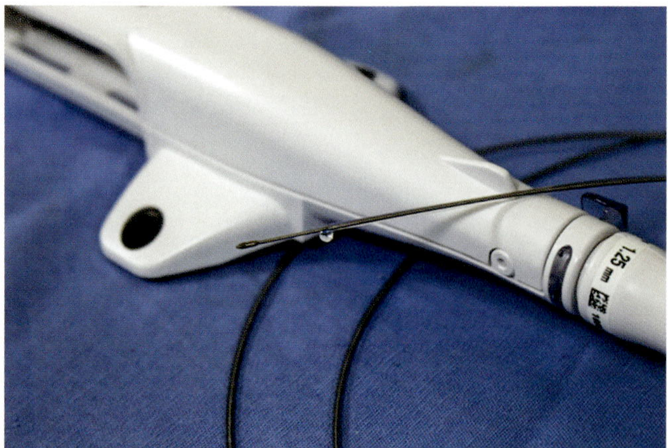

Fig. 27.6 Irrigation tip

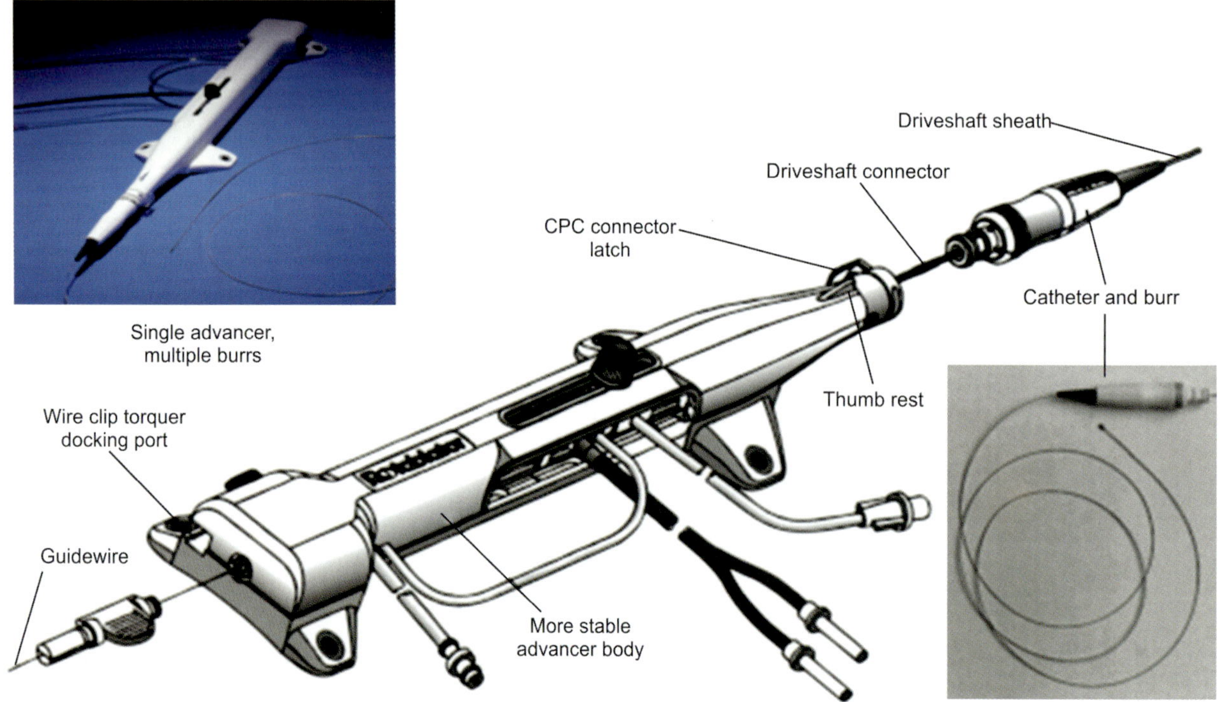

Fig. 27.7 Rotablator

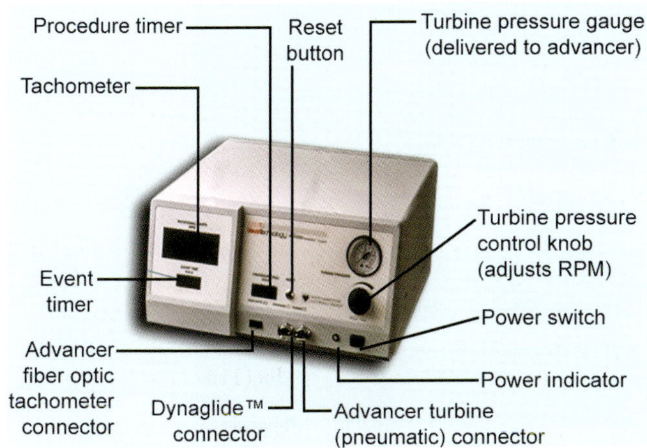

Fig. 27.8 Rotablator console

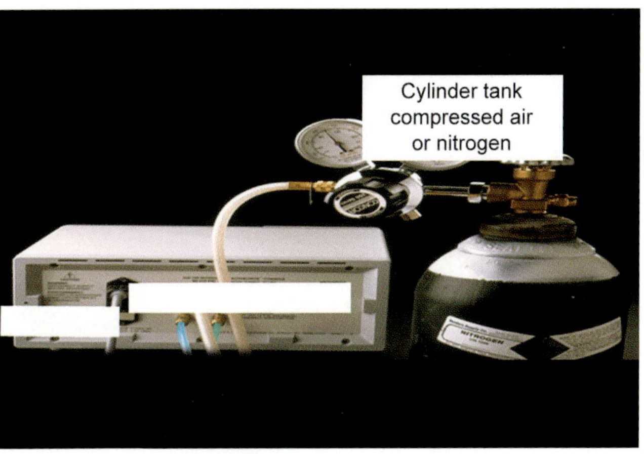

Fig. 27.9 Air supply set up

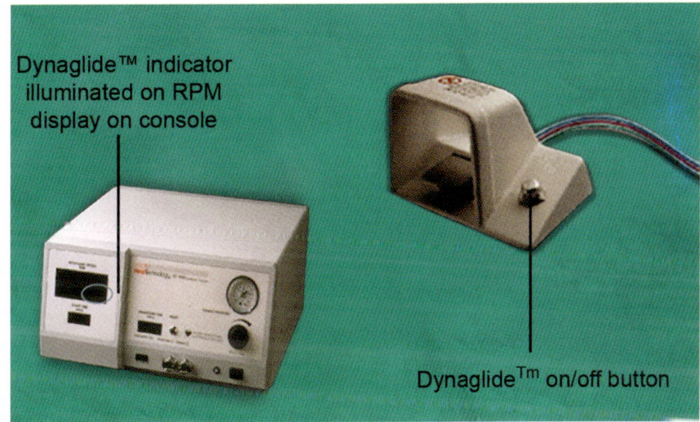

Fig. 27.10 Foot pedal

- If the pressure in the tank is below 6,205–6,894 kPa (900–1000 psi or 63.3–70.3 atm) consider changing tanks before the procedure begins.

FIRST-GENERATION GUIDEWIRES (FIG. 27.11)

- Stainless steel
- 0.009" diameter
- 0.017" diameter spring tip
- 325 cm in length
- Always require back loading.

SECOND-GENERATION WIRES: FLOPPY AND EXTRA SUPPORT (FIG. 27.12)

- Stainless steel
- 0.009" diameter
- 0.014" diameter spring tip
- 325 cm in length
- Always require back loading.

WIRE CLIP TORQUER FEATURES (FIG. 27.13)

- Side mount grip mechanism (clam shell)
- Acts as a secondary brake

PROCEDURE

Preprocedural Evaluation

- Clinical history
- 12 lead electrocardiogram
- Echocardiography as patients with low ejection fraction are at very high risk
- Radionuclide study for viability
- Biochemistry

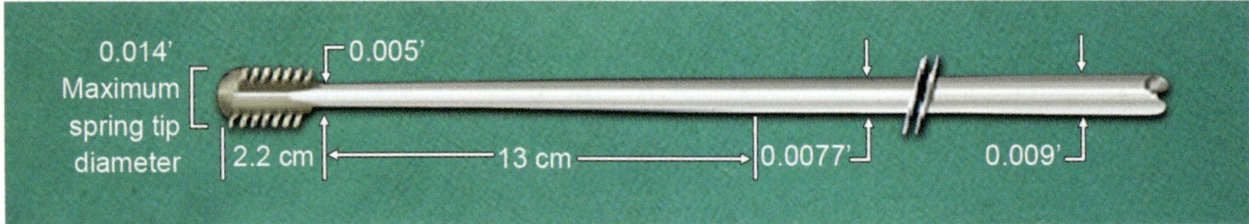

Fig. 27.11 Rotawire floppy

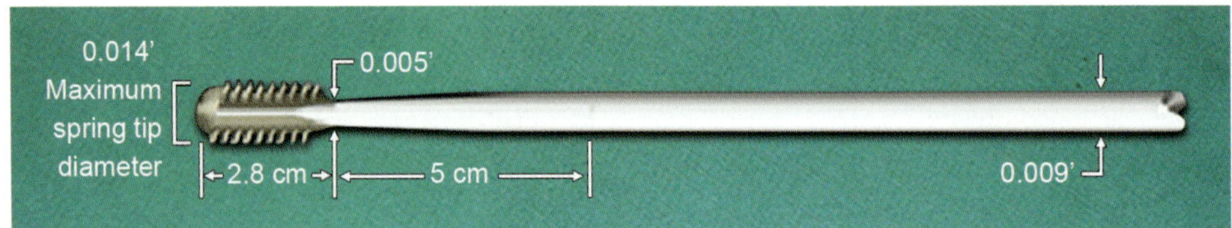

Fig. 27.12 Rotawire extra support

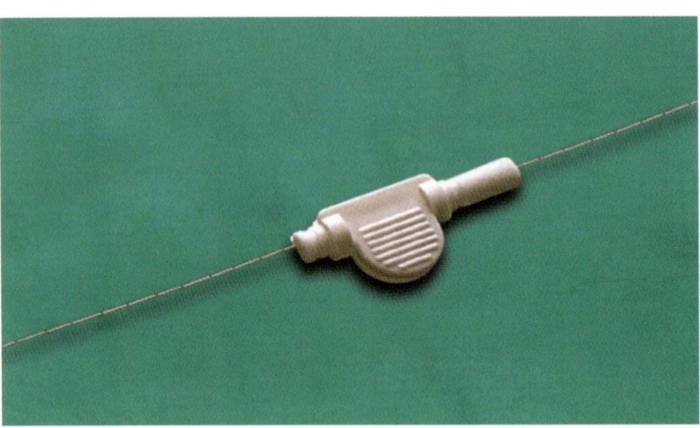

Fig. 27.13 Wire clip torquer

Table 27.1 Burr selection and treatment strategies

Millimeter	*Burr diameter inches*	*Recommended guide catheter (French)*	*Minimum ID required (Inches)*
1.25	0.049	6.0	0.060
1.50	0.059	6.0	0.063
1.75	0.069	7.0	0.073
2.00	0.079	8.0	0.083
2.15	0.085	8.0	0.089
2.25	0.089	9.0	0.093
2.38	0.094	9.0	0.098
2.50	0.098	9.0	0.102

- Angiographic evaluation—to assess the calcification pattern, tortuosity, severity of the lesion
- IVUS—to look for intimal calcification as adventitial calcification is not amenable to rotablation, minimal lumen diameter, minimal lumen area
- Optical coherence tomography—to look for calcification pattern.

Preprocedure Checklist (DRAW)

Before advancing the Burr in to the guiding catheter perform DRAW test

D = Drip rate increases

R = Rpm's or Burr Speed set

A = Advancer, move the advancer knob forward and back and lock down 1" forward from back

W = Wire Clip Torquer on and confirm brake activation

To prevent the vasospasm during the procedure, all the patients have to be pretreated with oral calcium antagonist and the vasodilators such as nitroglycerin and/or verapamil should be added to flush solution (Rotaflush). Other procedural management is similar to POBA. Administration of platelet glycoprotein IIb/IIIa inhibitors is reported to reduce the incidence of slow flow or no reflow during the procedure.[17]

Guide Catheter Selection

In the Rotablator, the selection and the positioning of the guide catheter are important for the ease of advancement of the burr and the trajectory of the guidewire which orients the burr and affects the direction of ablation plane. Coaxial alignment of the guide catheter and guidewire has to be verified before ablation.

The inner diameter of the guide catheter has to be 0.004 inch larger than the final burr. Most 8 Fr, 9 Fr and 10 Fr guide catheters permit passage of up to a 2.15 mm, 2.38 mm and 2.50 mm burr, respectively (Table 27.1).

Rotablator-alone strategy (primary therapy) is to achieve a satisfactory result with the use of a single large burr or, alternatively, with the use of several burrs by stepwise increments until a satisfactory angiographic results has been obtained. In this strategy, the noncompliant oversized balloon (less than 1 atm) was applied for the bailout from an angiographic complication or for the relief of vasospasm. The burr-to-artery ratio in these cases is in the range of 0.7-0.9. Therefore, the lesion morphologies that are applicable to this strategy are limited to those without severe angulation and with good distal runoff.

Burr-balloon strategy is commonly used approach. In this strategy, the Rotablator is used to improve the lesion characteristics (lesion modification) in order to apply the conventional balloon. This proposes the use of an undersized burr (burr-to-artery ratio 0.6–0.75) with minimal risk, followed by adjunctive balloon angioplasty. In the recent literatures, it is recommended to use the noncompliant oversize balloon with minimal pressure (1 atm).[18] Therefore, this strategy is safer than Rotablator-alone strategy. Rota-stent strategy is to put the stents after the pretreatment by the Rotablator and adjunctive balloon angioplasty. In the heavily calcified lesion, it is sometimes difficult to put the stent even after the preballoon dilation. In that case, the passage of the stent can be easy by the pretreatment using the Rotablator. Also stent expansion and apposition are supposed to be improved after the use of Rotablator.[19]

Guidewire Selection

The guidewire in the Rotablator is not simply a device for burr delivery but has an integral role in ablation. Therefore, the position, tension, and stiffness of guidewire are important to do safe and effective ablation. The divergence from the central axis of the vessel is referred to as guidewire bias. Usually, guidewire bias is unfavorable because it resulted in preferential cutting along one wall of the vessel and if the force exceeds the elastic threshold of the vessel, normal tissue will be ablated. However, guidewire bias can be favorable when it orients the burr toward the lesion and may result in larger luminal achievement than the size of burr.

Our Technique

While inserting the burr over the rotawire the wire has to be kept taut and straight not allowing any kinks all along the length of the wire. If the wire is not straight or has any kinks it can lead to:

- Accidental dislodgement of the guidewire out of the coronary artery
- Looping of the guidewire between the guide catheter and the coronary artery ostia

Usually a soft hydrophilic wire is crossed into the distal vessel past the lesion, then a microcatheter is passed over it, followed by exchange of the hydrophilic wire with the rotawire. On certain occasions the microcatheter wont cross the lesion, in such cases:

- Do a low pressure balloon dilatation with 1 mm balloon – this is to prevent dissections and facilitate the easy crossing of the microcatheter
- Keep microcatheter at the site of lesion where it is not crossing then insert the rotawire through it and with the help of the torquer guide it into the distal vessel.

Burr Speed and Burr Advancement

The knob movement should be with fingers like playing a guitar and not forceful with wrist or forearm. It is not mandatory to ablate entire length in one go but one should do it incrementally in few millimeter. This avoids burr entrapment. The burr speed is adjusted according to burr size and the recommended speed for smaller burr (less than 2.0 mm) is 180,000 rpm and that for larger burr (more than 2.15 mm) is 170,000 rpm. However, the recent experimental study revealed that the reduction of burr speed to the minimal approved level (140,000 rpm) much reduced the platelet aggregation due to heat generation[20] This low speed treatment may be beneficial for the reduction of slow flow or no reflow which is often complicated with the treatment in the lesion with highly complex morphology, especially in the long lesion. On the other hand, it takes longer ablation time and needs more refined hands. During the ablation, excessive deceleration (more than 5,000 rpm) must be avoided because it results in improper ablation and increases the risk of vessel injury, the formation of large particles, and ischemic complications related to excessive heat generation.[21]

Pecking Method

"Pecking" technique is used, where the burr is moved forward and backward the lesion, avoiding crossing the entire lesion during the initial passage.

"Pecking" motion prevents "trenching" into arterial wall, allows wire to reposition as vessel compliance changes with debulking.

Use of Temporary Pacemaker

At our institute prophylactic use of temporary pacemaker is done in all the rotablation cases.

Use of GP2B3A Inhibitors

Frequently used at our institute.

Rotaglide Solution

It is used to reduce the friction between the drive shaft and the guidewire. Some hospitals utilize a cocktail consisting of verapamil (10 mg/L), nitroglycerin (4 mg/L), and heparin (2,000 units/L), which was developed to prevent spasm and *in situ* thrombosis with rotational atherectomy.[22]

Should not be used in people allergic to egg products or olive oil.

Rotaglide may further reduce heat generation and the amount of force required to advance the burr.

Sources of Heat

- Advancement of burr/tortuous anatomy
- Between vessel wall and burr
- Between guidewire and burr
- Long run times (excess of 45 seconds)

In patients with *de novo* calcified lesions for whom PCI is indicated clinically, lesion modification via rotational or orbital atherectomy is appropriate in order to facilitate procedural success when calcification is severe. If calcification severity is intermediate or indeterminate by angiography, intravascular imaging with IVUS or OCT may be useful for reclassification (Flow chart 27.1).

Postprocedural Evaluation

- Microvascular angina due to debris created by rotablation
- Perforation
- Access site complication
- Arrhythmia (complete heart block)

Flow chart 27.1 Use of rotational or orbital atherectomy in management of *de Novo* calcified lesions

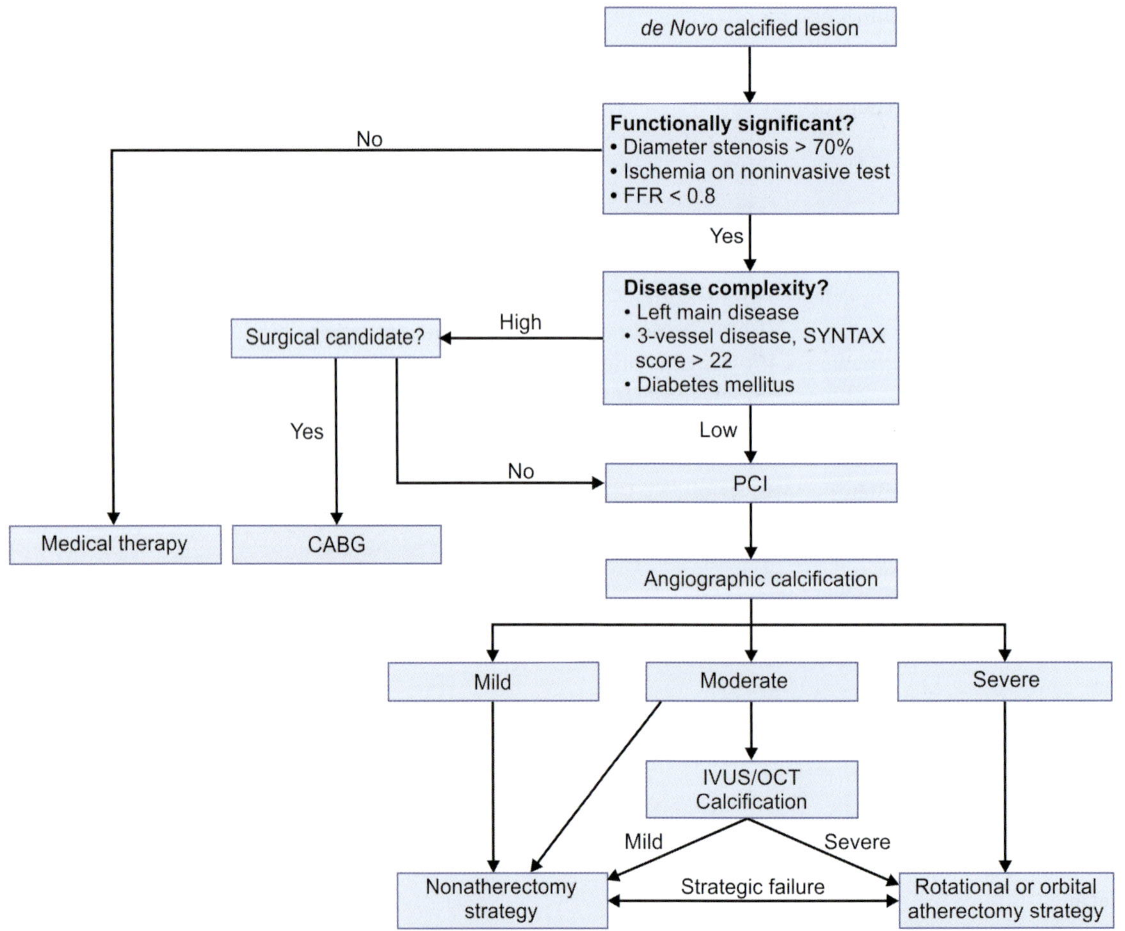

Source: Tomey MI, Kini AS, Sharma SK. Current status of rotational atherectomy. J Am Coll Cardiol Intv. 2014;7(4):345-353. doi:10.1016/j.jcin.2013.12.196

Abbreviations: CABG, coronary artery bypass graft surgery; FFR, fractional flow reserve; IVUS, intravascular ultrasound; OCT, optical coherence tomography; PCI, percutaneous coronary intervention.

Complications (Tables 27.2 to 27.4)

Rotablator system failure:

- Burr entrapment
- Burr detachment
- Burr stalling
- Rota guidewire fracture

Others, Like–

- Bradycardia and AV blocks
- Slow flow or no reflow and vasospasm
- Dissection
- Perforation
- Side branch occlusion
- Hypotension

Mechanism of Burr Entrapment

The rotablator device is an olive-shaped, front-cutting, diamond-coated and tipped burr for antegrade ablation. The back side (proximal part) of this burr is smooth and does not allow cutting when pulling back. Spinning displaces friction orthogonally, reducing forward friction and allowing the burr to advance slowly, debulking the lesion as it moves forward.

The proposed mechanisms of burr entrapments are

- Spasm.
- Advancement of a small burr beyond a calcified lesion.
- Under-deployed stents, or in-stent stenosis without sufficient ablation.
- Popping the device through unprepared lesions may lead to distal entrapment. The absence of retrograde debulking is a limitation to removal at this point.
- The device can get stuck at a bend in a calcified vessel due to coronary spasm or incomplete atherectomy of calcium.

Use of a smaller burr, with high speed, minimal forward pressure while advancing the burr, slow advancement of the burr, and avoidance of deceleration helps to prevent this complication.

Table 27.2 Potential mechanisms of slow-flow/no-reflow during RA and associated strategies for prevention and treatment

Mechanism	*Therapeutic strategy*
Atheromatous debris embolism	Small burr sizing Intermittent ablation Avoidance of significant decelerations
Platelet activation aggregation, and lysis	Optimal antiplatelet therapy including use of a glycoprotein IIb/IIIa inhibitor
Microcirculatory vasospasm	Vasodilators liberal use of flush solution
Neurohumoral reflex bradycardia	Atropine temporary venous pacemaker (especially for lesions in a dominant right coronary artery)
Intraprocedural hypotension	Vasopressors (in particular, phenylephrine) intra-aortic balloon counterpulsation

Abbreviation: RA, rotational atherectomy

Table 27.3 Reported complications of RA and DES implantation

Trial/First Author	*Year*	*N*	*Deah %*	*MI %*	*Urgent CABG, %*	*Vascular %*	*Dissection %*	*Perforation %*	*Acute closure, %*	*Side branch loss, %*	*Slow flow/no reflow %*
ROTAXUS	2013	120	1.7	1.7	0.8	5.8	3.3	1.7	—	—	0.0
Abdel-Wahab et al.	2013	205	1.5	2.4	—	—	4.4	0.5	—	—	2.0
Naito et al.	2012	233	0.0	1.3	—	—	1.7	0.4	—	—	—
Benezet et al.	2011	102	1.0	1.0	—	—	2.9	0.0	—	—	—
Dradas et al.	2011	184	0.0	—	—	—	—	—	—	—	—
Garcia de Lara et al.	2010	50	4.0	14.0	0.0	—	2.0	2.0	2.0	4.0	0.0
Rathore et al.	2010	391	1.0	6.9	0.0	—	5.9	2.0	0.3	3.6	2.6
Vaquerizo et al.	2010	63	0.0	3.2	0.0	1.6	—	—	1.6	—	—
Furuichi et al.	2009	95	0.0	3.2	—	—	2.1	1.1	—	—	1.1
Clavijo et al.	2006	81	0.0	19.8	—	—	1.9	—	—	—	—

Abbreviations: CABG, coronary artery bypass graft surgery; DES, drug-eluting stents; MI, myocardial infarction; RA, rotational atherectomy
Source: J Am Coll Cardiol Intv. 2014;7(4):345-353. doi:10.1016/j.jcin.2013.12.196

Table 27.4 Long-term outcomes after RA and DES implantation

First author	*Year*	*Patients*	*Follow-up*	*MACE, %*	*Repeat revascularization, %*	*ST, %*
Abdel-Wahab et al.	2013	205 DES	15 months	17.7	9.9 TVR, 6.8 TLR	1.0
Mangiacapra et al.	2012	104 DES	1 Year	12.0	5 TVR	3.0
		83 BMS		23.5	12.3 TVR	4.9
Naito et al.	2012	179 SES	630 days	14.8	6.8 TVR, 4.9 TLR	
		54 PES	625 days	13.7	11.8 TVR, 9.8 TLR	
Benezet et al.	2011	102 DES	15 months	12.7	8.8 TLR	2.9
Dardas et al.	2011	184 DES	49 months	14.9	3.3 TVR, 2.8 TLR	
Fujimoto et al.	2010	54 DES	12 months			
		26 RA+			11.5 TLR	0
		28 RA–			35.7 TLR	7.1
Garcia de Lara et al.	2010	50 DES	1 year	6 (CV death)	6 TLR	
Rathore et al.	2010	391 DES	6–9 months		10.6 TLR*	0.8
		125 BMS			25.0 TLR	0.8
Vaquerizo et al.	2010	63 DES	15 months	9.5	4.8 TLR	2.8
Furuichi et al.	2009	96 DES	15 months	15.8	11.6 TVR, 9.5 TLR	4.2
Tamekiyo et al.	2009	79 DES	2 years	30.1	25.0 TLR	
		144 BMS		43.1	39.1 TLR	
Clavijo et al.	2006	150 DES	6 months	(Death)		
		81 RA+		6.8	4.2	
		69 RA–		7.9	4.9	

Source: J Am Coll Cardiol Intv. 2014;7(4):345-53. doi:10.1016/j.jcin.2013.12.196

Table 27.5 Retrieval techniques and related complications

Retrieval techniques	*Limitations/complications*
• Manual traction of the rota burr	• Proximal vessel injury • Shaft fracture due to high force
• Speed up rotablator with advancement to distal lumen and retrieval while spinning	• Stalled Rotablator may not spin • No backward cutting from Rotablator
• Guidewire and balloon advancement and inflation around the device	• Upsize to 8 French to accommodate both Rota and balloon
• Cut the Rota shaft, sleeve removal, advance guidewire and balloon (with existing 6 French guide)	
• Second guide catheter engagement in "ping pong" fashion with guidewire and balloon inflation around the device	• New access site
• Utilization of snare around the device	
• GuideLiner (Vascular Solutions), "child" catheter, micro- catheter advancement near the stuck device	
• Laser atherectomy device	

Retrieval Techniques

Manual traction on the rota burr is the easiest method with off-on low speed rotation in DynaGlide mode. However, careful monitoring of traction on the vessel and avoiding deep seating of the guide are necessary in order to avoid vessel injury. Excessive traction on the shaft may result in shaft fracture (Table 27.5).

Advancing the burr into the distal lumen and retrieving it, all while rotating it, may allow for retrieval.

Passing a guidewire distal to the lesion and passing a small balloon alongside the stuck device with serial balloon inflations may allow successful removal. However, guide size is a limitation for this technique. The shaft of the rotablator is 4.3 French and most balloon catheters are 3 French, so utilization of an 8 French guide may be necessary. Upsizing of the guide can be done after cutting off the advancer sheath (but will not allow any further spinning of the burr). Alternatively, a separate access and guide catheter may be needed to pass the wire and balloon.

Drive shaft sheath removal after cutting off near the advancer and insertion of a second guide wire/balloon through the 6 French guide is another innovative method.[23]

As another way to remove the device, passing the snare over the shaft, after cutting the shaft as described above, and snaring the shaft just proximal to the burr may allow retraction of the burr and guide catheter in a controlled fashion.

Advancement of a mother and child catheter after cutting the shaft as above and applying traction on the burr and anti-traction to the daughter catheter can provide a large, local force to retrieve the burr.[24] The daughter catheter will prevent proximal vessel damage and can be helpful if dissection/perforation at the stuck site occurs.

Laser coronary atherectomy can be used for successful retrieval by modifying and softening the calcified lesion/plaque behind the entrapped device.

IVUS IN ROTABLATION

Role of IVUS in calcified lesions: Unable to cross the lesion-rotablator, scoring balloon or conventional balloon with buddy wire (Figs 27.14A1 to C2).

Check location and distribution of calcium:

- Superficial—Rotablator
- Deep—Predilatation with balloon

Check position of the IVUS catheter within the lumen to understand the guidewire bias for effective debulking with rotablator.

IVUS finding postrotablation:

- Morphological changes of calcium
- If calcium was adequately ablated, IVUS demonstrates smooth surface and round shape calcium with reverberation behind calcium.

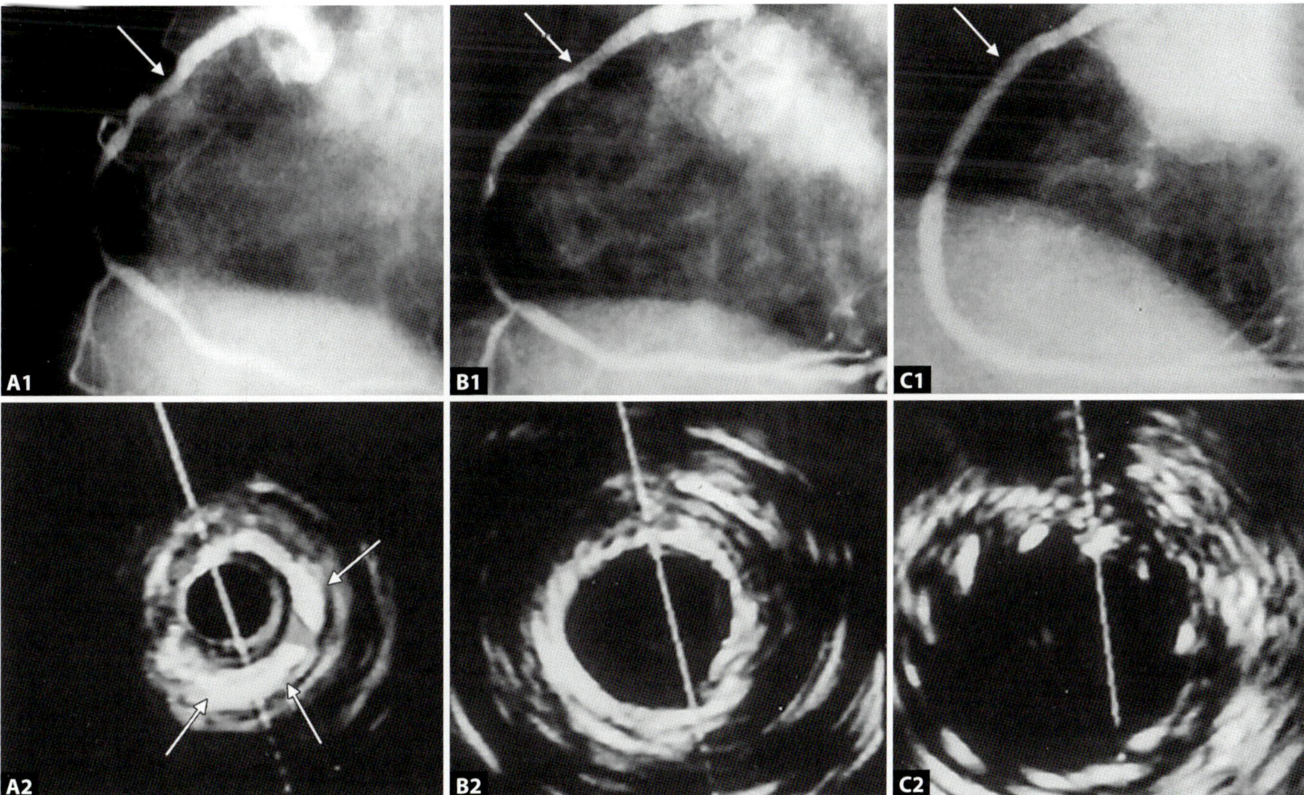

Figs 27.14A1 to C2 (A1) Baseline coronary angiogram showing right coronary artery with midcalcified lesion (arrow); (A2) IVUS cross section through the culprit lesion; note 360° calcifications (small white arrows); (B1) Coronary angiogram showing right coronary artery and culprit lesion (arrow) after rotablation and PTCA; (B2) IVUS cross section through culprit lesion after rotablation and PTCA; (C1) Coronary angiogram showing culprit lesion poststenting (arrow); (C2) IVUS cross section through culprit lesion; note symmetrical and complete expansion of the stent

- It is important to check the position of the IVUS catheter within the lumen and the location of calcium, that help you determine to use bigger size of a burr.

OCT IN ROTABLATION

See Figures 27.15 and 27.16.

High resolution (10–20 μm) of the OCT images allow for accurate characterization of atherosclerotic lesions, which are classified as fibrous (hyperintense), lipidic (hypointense, with undefined edges), and calcified (hypointense, with well-defined borders).[25] In addition, in the context of PCI, it allows the identification of dissections, plaque prolapse through the stent struts, malapposition and neointimal tissue

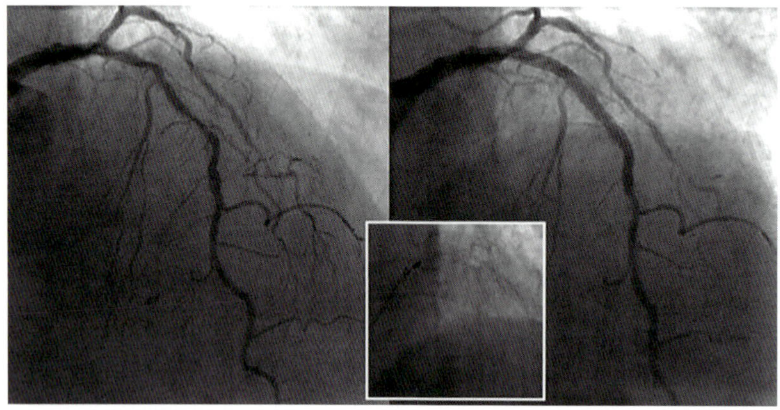

Fig. 27.15 Angiographic image of the calcified lesion on the descending anterior (left) artery and of the result after the intervention (right)

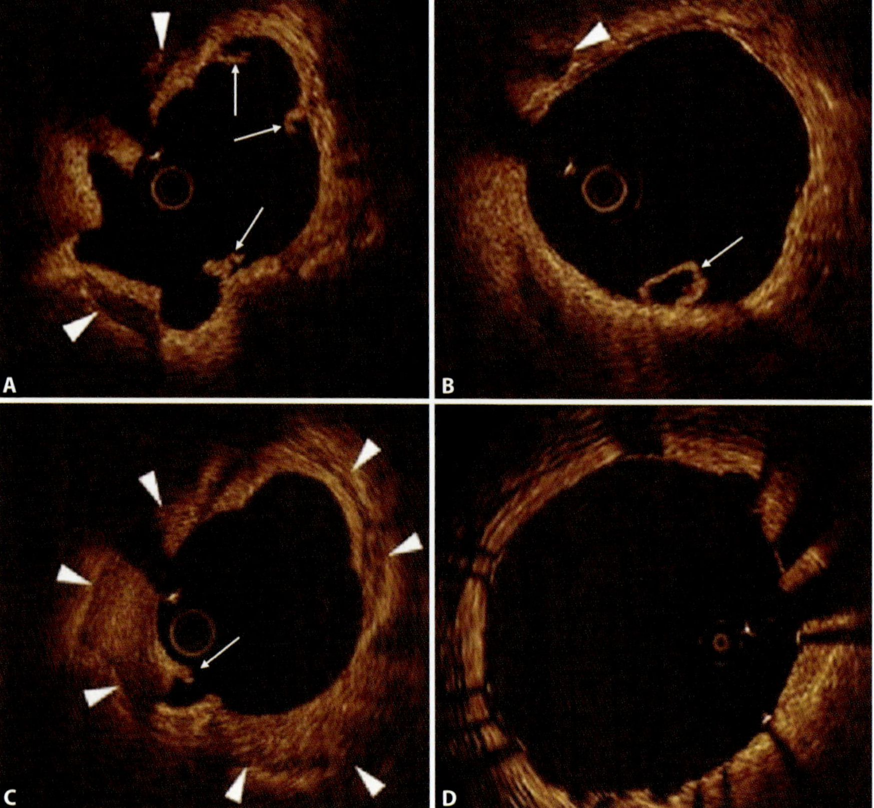

Figs 27.16A to D Optical coherence tomography following rotational atherectomy. (A and B) Calcified lesion (arrowheads) and multiple intimal microdissections (arrows); (C) Circumferential calcification area; (D) Result after stent implantation

with an elevated sensibility,[26,27] better than intracoronary ultrasound. The main limitation is the need to displace the blood from inside the vessel during the acquisition of images. An "occlusive" technique is usually used, with a proximal occlusion balloon and an injection of saline through its lumen,[28] which results technically complex and causes transitory ischemia. The alternative "non-occlusive" technique simplifies the procedure considerably.[29]

Rotablator atherectomy is still a procedure of choice in selected cases.

It definitely increases success of complex PCI.

There is a steep learning curve.

The acute success of calcific lesions and debulking is helpful for stent tracking, however this equipment should be used judiciously and all steps have to be followed.

REFERENCES

1. Ritchie JL, Hansen DD, Intlekofer MJ, Hall M, Auth DC. Rotational approaches to atherectomy and thrombectomy. Z Kardiol. 1987;76(Suppl 6):59-65.
2. Lasala JM, Reisman M. Rotablator plus stent therapy (rotastent). Curr Opin Cardiol. 1998;13:240-7.
3. Mota P, Santos R, Pereira H, et al. Facts on rotational atherectomy for coronary artery disease: multicentric registry (abstr). Paper presented at: Euro PCR; May 21, 2013; Paris, France.
4. Villanueva EV, Wasiak J, Petherick ES. Percutaneous transluminal rotational atherectomy for coronary artery disease. Cochrane Database Syst Rev. 2003(4): p. CD003334.
5. Bittl JA, et al. Meta-analysis of randomized trials of percutaneous transluminal coronary angioplasty versus atherectomy, cutting balloon atherotomy, or laser angioplasty. J Am Coll Cardiol. 2004;43(6): 936-42.
6. Reifart N, et al. Randomized comparison of angioplasty of complex coronary lesions at a single center. Excimer Laser, Rotational Atherectomy, and Balloon Angioplasty Comparison (ERBAC) Study. Circulation. 1997;96(1):91-8.
7. Dill T, et al. A randomized comparison of balloon angioplasty versus rotational atherectomy in complex coronary lesions (COBRA study). Eur Heart J. 2000;21(21):1759-66.
8. Niccoli G, et al. Directional atherectomy before stenting versus stenting alone in percutaneous coronary interventions: a meta-analysis. Int J Cardiol. 2006;112(2):178-83.
9. Clavijo LC, et al. Sirolimus-eluting stents and calcified coronary lesions: clinical outcomes of patients treated with and without rotational atherectomy. Catheter Cardiovasc Interv. 2006;68(6):873-8.
10. Khattab AA, et al. Drug-eluting stents versus bare metal stents following rotational atherectomy for heavily calcified coronary lesions: late angiographic and clinical follow-up results. J Interv Cardiol. 2007; 20(2):100-6.
11. Bramucci E, et al. Adjunctive stent implantation following directional coronary atherectomy in patients with coronary artery disease. J Am Coll Cardiol. 1998;32(7):1855-60.
12. Goldberg SL, et al. Rotational atherectomy or balloon angioplasty in the treatment of intrastent restenosis: BARASTER multicenter registry. Catheter Cardiovasc Interv. 2000;51(4):407-13.
13. Sharma SK, et al. Randomized trial of Rotational Atherectomy Versus Balloon Angioplasty for Diffuse In-stent Restenosis (ROSTER). Am Heart J. 2004;147(1):16-22.
14. Hinohara T. Percutaneous coronary intervention: current perspective. Keio J Med, 2001;50(3):152-60.
15. Whitlow PL, et al. Results of the study to determine rotablator and transluminal angioplasty strategy (STRATAS). Am J Cardiol. 2001; 87(6):699-705.
16. Brambilla N, et al. Directional coronary atherectomy plus stent implantation vs left internal mammary artery bypass grafting for isolated proximal stenosis of the left anterior descending coronary artery. Catheter Cardiovasc Interv. 2005;64(1):45-52.
17. Wijns W, Kolh P, Danchin N, et al. Guidelines on myocardial revascularization. Eur Heart J. 2010;31:2501-2555. [PubMed]
18. Kini A, et al. Rotational atherectomy: improved procedural outcome with evolution of technique and equipment. Single-center results of first 1,000 patients. Catheter Cardiovasc Interv. 1999;46(3):305-11.
19. Braden G, et al. Restenosis following minimally traumatic rotational atherectomy: the acute and long-term results of the Rotablator and restenosis (R&R) study. J Am Coll Cardiol, 1998;31(Suppl); 378A.
20. Moussa I, et al. Coronary stenting after rotational atherectomy in calcified and complex lesions. angiographic and clinical follow-up results. Circulation, 1997;96(1):128-36.
21. Reisman M, et al. Analysis of low-speed rotational atherectomy for the reduction of platelet aggregation. Cathet Cardiovasc Diagn, 1998;45(2):208-14.
22. Cohen BM, Weber VJ, Blum RR, et al. Cocktail attenuation of rotational ablation flow effects (CARAFE) study: Pilot Cathet Cardiovasc Diagn. 1996;3:69-72.
23. Sakakura K, Ako J, Momomura S. Successful removal of an entrapped rotablation burr by extracting drive shaft sheath followed by balloon dilatation. Catheter Cardiovasc Interv. 2011; 78(4):567-70.
24. Cunnington M, Egred M. Guide Liner, a child-in-a-mother catheter for successful retrieval of an entrapped rotablator burr. Catheter Cardiovasc Interv. 2012;79(2):271-3.
25. Cavusoglu E, Kini AS, Marmur JD, Sharma SK. Current status of rotational atherectomy. Catheter Cardiovasc Interv. 2004;62: 485-98.
26. Díaz-Sandoval LJ, Bouma BE, Tearney GJ, Jang IK. Optical coherence tomography as a tool for percutaneous coronary interventions. Catheter Cardiovasc Interv. 2005;65:492-6.
27. Bouma BE, Tearney GJ, Yabushita H, Shishkov M, Kauffman CR, deJoseph D, et al. Evaluation of intracoronary stenting by intravascular optical coherence tomography.Heart. 2003;89: 317-20.
28. Yamaguchi T, Terashima M, Akasaka T, Hayashi T, Mizuno K, Muramatsu T, et al. Safety and feasibility of an intravascular optical coherence tomography image wire system in the clinical setting. Am J Cardiol. 2008;101:562-7.
29. Prati F, Cera M, Ramazzotti V, Imola F, Giudice R, Albertucci A. Safety and feasibility of a new non-occlusive technique for facilitated intracoronary optical coherence tomography acquisition in various clinical and anatomical scenarios. Eurointerv. 2007;3:365-70.

CHAPTER

28 Hardware for Chronic Total Occlusion

Jaskaran Singh Dugal, Ajit Mehta

The holy grail of interventional cardiology has been to open chronic total occluded coronary arteries. The inability to be predictably successful has been a leading cause of why patients are referred to surgery or medical therapy rather than receiving percutaneous revascularization. In the last 15 years, with the introduction of stiffer guideline retrograde techniques and new antegrade dissection and re-entry, the "holy grail" is now being achieved by a growing number of interventional cardiologist around the globe.

One of the most frequently asked questions about chronic total occlusion (CTO) is:

What equipment do I really need?

Most operators would like to have everything available. The reality is that equipment cost and space limitation require prioritizing. At least one item that is required for chronic total occlusion percutaneous coronary intervention (CTO PCI) steps should be available[1] (e.g. septal crossing wires, support catheter, channel dilators wire externalization and snaring) At the same time operator should be familiar with equipment that is required during complications like covered stents and coils.

There are 10 categories of equipment required.[2-5] These are further divided into two categories; first one is must have and the second one is good to have!

SHEATHS

All the sheaths should be available. Most of the procedures are done with 7F or 8F sheath. If radial approach is used, 6F sheath is used. The disadvantage of 6F sheath for CTO PCI are:

- Weaker support of 6F guiding catheter than larger catheters.
- Inability to use such equipment as trapping technique, Anchor technique, simultaneously use of intravascular ultrasound (IVUS) catheter and support catheter like tornus, cross-boss catheter and Stingray balloon

A sheathless guide system (Asahi intecc) allows CTO PCI with 8.5 guides through arterial puncture equivalent to 6F sheath. It is good to have long 45 cm sheath, which allows sheaths to reach the level of diaphragm and they straighten iliac tortuosity, and thereby guiding catheter manipulation becomes easier.

GUIDE CATHETERS

Diameter, Length and Shape

Diameter

Dual 8F catheter provides good support and visualization. However, even with femoral approach, the 8F catheter are used for antegrade approach and 6F catheter for retrograde approach which allow use of corsair and also decrease the risk of coronary dissection.

Length

Generally 100 cm guiding catheters are used, but it is good to have 80 cm long, which helps in retrograde approach.

Shapes

It is must to have catheter which provides support such as XB, EBU, AL in different sizes (like 0.75, 1, 2, 3, 3.5 and 4) for left coronary and AL and JR 4.0 for right coronary artery.

Shortening of Guiding Catheter

If short guiding catheter are not available, a 100 cm long guide catheter can be shortened using the technique mentioned below:

- We must know the length of the catheter inside. For this the guide catheter is inserted into the body of the patient to engage the target coronary vessel and to ascertain the length which is outside the femoral sheath. The length is marked.

- The guiding catheter is removed and the length/segment is cut as per the measurement taken.
- A sheath is taken 1Fr smaller than the guiding catheter used (that is 7Fr for 8Fr guiding catheter). It is cut so as to have 4 cm of the connecting segment. Both ends of the connecting segment are flared with the dilator 1Fr bigger than the cut sheath.
- The connecting sheath segment is used to connect the proximal and distal connector pieces.

Side Holes

Chronic total occlusion (CTO) involving right coronary artery side holes are preferred (more so for proximal occlusion) as they prevent damping, may allow antegrade flow to the vessel and also prevent hydraulic dissection. Nevertheless, they provide false sense of security and dissection may still occur and contrast use is higher.

As far left system is concerned, especially for unprotected left main coronary artery, side hole should be avoided. If no side hole guides are available, they can be made using 18G needle. This however leads to weakening of the catheter and may cause kinking.

Y Connector with Hemostatic Valves

As CTO PCI is a lengthy procedure, using a hemostatic valve such as Copilot (Abbott vascular), or Guardian (Vascular solution) are helpful as compared to rotating valves as blood loss in these procedures can be minimized.

MICROCATHETERS (TABLE 28.1)

Chronic total occlusion (CTO) crossing should always be attempted using over the wire balloon or microcatheter because of the following:

- They provide better support and also increase wire tip stiffness.
- Allows wire exchange and escalation.
- Allows reshaping of wires.
- As the microcatheter has marker at the tip, it provides accurate assessment of its location in the vasculature as compared to over the wire balloon.
- Microcatheters are more flexible and track better.
- Microcathers have less tendency to kink than over the wire balloons.
- Several microcatheters are available.

Corsair

It was developed as (ASAHI INTECC) channel dilator to facilitate retrograde angioplasty.[6] It has SHINKA shaft constructed with 8 thin wires and two large wires which help in torque transmission. Its inner lining is coated with polymer that enables contrast injection as well as wire advancements. The distal shaft (60 cm) has hydrophilic polymer to improve its crossing. The tip is tapering and soft with tungsten coating to improve its visibility (Figs 28.1A to C).

Corsair: Tips and tricks

- Two lengths are available (135 and 150 cm) 135 cm is generally used for antegrade approach and 150 for retrograde approach.
- The catheter is advanced by rotating and pushing in counter clock and clockwise rotation.
- Contrast can be injected to visualize the pathway of advancement. The catheter should be flushed to avoid stickiness.
- Catheter may be exchanged with a new one if there is catheter fatigue or if its tip becomes flared.
- If wire externalization is performed, the tip of antegrade balloon and stent should never come in contact.
- New Corsair is available in Japan which has better trackability and pushability.

Other companies also make, i.e. vascular solutions, Spectra Medics and Volcano.

Finecross

Finecross (Terumo) and Valet (Volcano) microcatheters are the lowest crossing profile microcatheters currently available (1.8Fr distal tip). The fine cross catheter has a stainless steel braid (to enhance torqueability) and a distal marker located at 0.7 mm from the tip (Fig. 28.2).

Finecross catheter tips and tricks

- The finecross catheter is very flexible and navigates well through tortuosity.

Table 28.1 Microcatheters

1	Termo	a. Prograet b. Finecross MG	110 cm 130 cm 130 cm 150 cm	2.4 and 2.7 Fr 1.8 Fr
2	ASAHI INTECC	a. Tornus b. Corsair c. Caravel	135 cm 135cm 150 cm	2.1 Fr 2.6 Fr
3	Boston Scientific	a. Renegade 18 b. Tracker excel 14 c. Excels 18	105 cm 115 cm 135 cm 150 cm 150 cm	2.5 1.5 2.0
4	Cordis	a. Transit b. Prowler	135 cm 150 cm	2.5 1.5 Fr

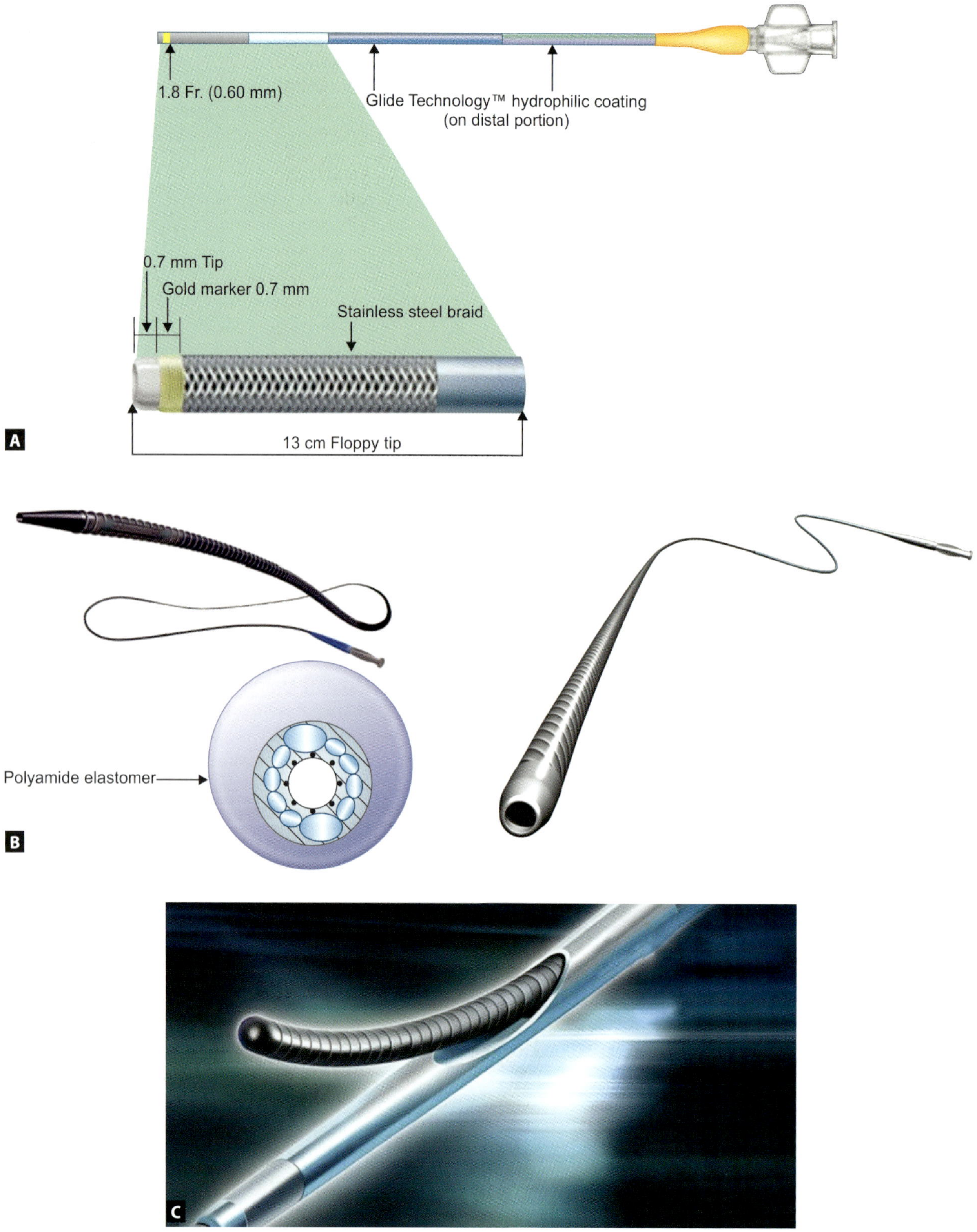

1.8 Fr. (0.60 mm)

Glide Technology™ hydrophilic coating (on distal portion)

0.7 mm Tip

Gold marker 0.7 mm

Stainless steel braid

13 cm Floppy tip

A

Polyamide elastomer

B

C

Figs 28.1A to C Microcatheters

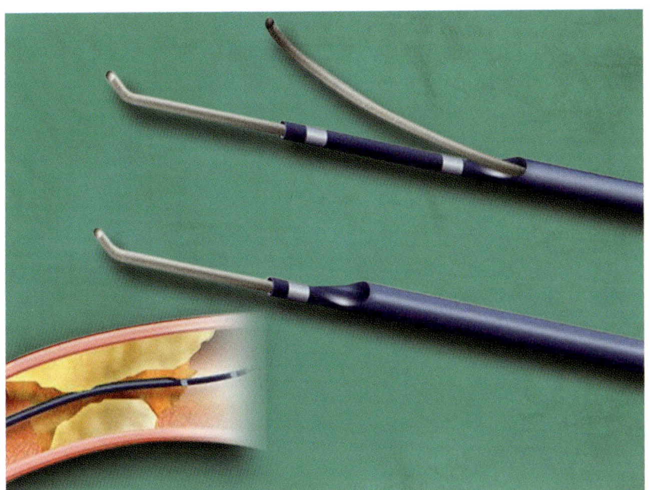

Fig. 28.2 Twinpass catheters

- Although this catheter is mainly advanced using forward push, many operators are using a combination of push and rotation to facilitate advancement.
- The fine cross catheter cannot be used for delivery of coils.
- Coil delivery requires larger microcathcters such as Progreat (Terumo) and Renegade (Boston) and Transit (Cordis).

Venture

The Venture catheter by vascular solutions has an 8 mm radiopaque torquable distal tip that has a bend radius of 2.5 mm. The tip can be deflected 90° by clockwise rotation of a thumb wheel on the external handle, steering in all planes is possible. This goes over 0.014 wire and is compatible with 6F guide catheter (Fig. 28.3).[7]

GUIDEWIRES

This area has the largest number of options, as well as personal preferences. High volume operators limit options down to few must:

- Fielder XT, XTA, XT-R, XTFC which is polymer jacket tapered and nontapered wire for initial antegrade crossing via microchannels.
- *GAIA First, Second and Third*: These are new wires having composite structures. They are available in different tip loads and have very good torque response and are used more and more in antegrade approach.

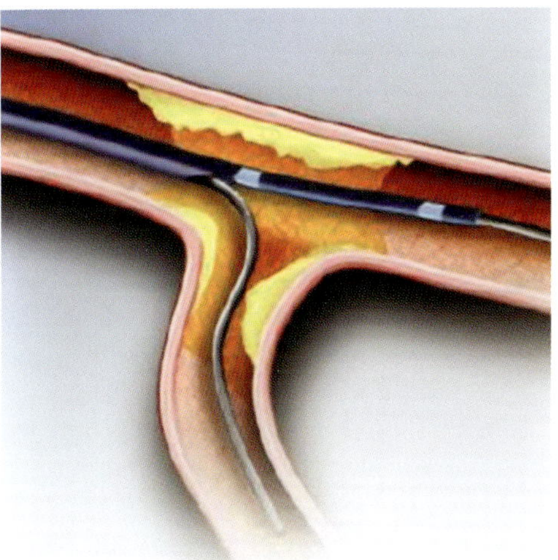

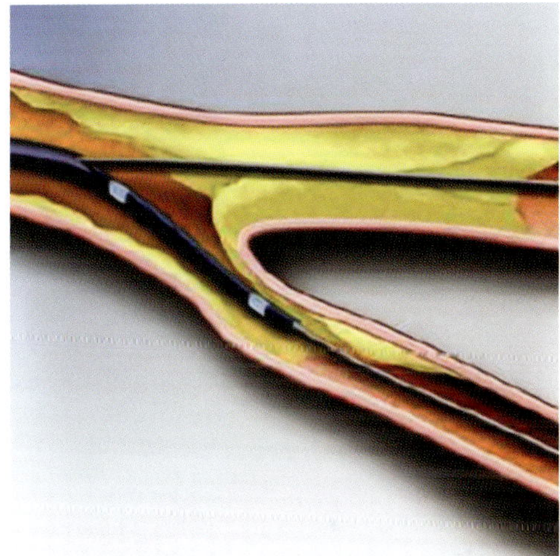

Fig. 28.3 Crusade catheters for bifurcation

GAIA Wires

GAIA		Diameter	Tip load
	First	0.010–0.014	1.7 gmf
	Second	0.011–0.014	3.5 gmf
	Third	0.012–0.014	4.5 gmf

- *Miracle and Confianza family of wires*: They are stiff wires up to 12 g distal stiffness and high penetrating power. They are nonhydrophilic and are favored for delivering gear to chronic total occlusion (CTO) segments, caps or spaces as they are less likely to slip out of spaces. The Confinaza are stiff but also have tapered tip.

  Tips and tricks of use:

- Confianza pro is very useful in penetrating proximal cap.
- It is also useful when there is a large side branch.
- Also helpful in entering true lumen in antegrade approach.

- *Pilot family of wires*: They are polymer jacketed wires with increasing stiffness.The pilot 200 has a 4.1 g tip load and is preferred wire for antegrade approach, if initial CTO crossing wire with soft polymer jacket fails. These wires are also used in knuckle formation in both antegrade and retrograde dissection.
- *Sion wires*: They have composite core technology and provide excellent transmission and resistance to deformation.
- *Externalization guidewire*: They are long wires used in externalization during retrograde approach.
  - Viper advance wire
  - R350 vascular solution
  - RG3.

Externalization tips:

- Externalization is done when Corsair is advanced into antegrade guiding catheter.
- One should avoid kinking.
- Administration of small amount of Rota glide solution (Boston scientific) through the microcatheter is helpful.
- The wire introducer should be used through the hemostatic valve of antegrade catheter to tread the externalization wire followed by reattachment of the Y connection to the guiding catheter.
- The wire should be pulled only when inside the catheter, otherwise causes tissue injury.
- Managing the loop between the guides and actively maintaining the guide catheter position is critical.

Description of Coronary Guide Wires Commonly Utilized in CTO PCI

See Table 28.2.

DISSECTION/REENTRY EQUIPMENT

Although wires with knuckle can be used, it is profitable to use Cross boss catheter and Stingray balloon as they improve success ratio and efficiency of the procedure.

CrossBoss Catheter

The CrossBoss catheter is a stiff over the wire catheter with 1 mm blunt rounded hydrophilic coated distal tip that can advance through the occlusion when the catheter is rotated rapidly using a torque device. If it enters the sub intimal space using sting ray balloon and guidewire, the distal true lumen can be reentered (Figs 28.4 and 28.5).

Stingray Balloon and Guidewire

This balloon is a flat balloon having a length of 10 mm and has 2.5 mm width. It is inflated at 2–4 atmosphere, it orients itself automatically to true lumen. The guidewire is stiff and has 20 cm distal opaque segment and a 0.009 inch tapered tip and 0.0035 inch distal prong. It is directed towards one of the two side ports of the Stingray balloon to enter the true lumen (Figs 28.6A and B).

SNARES

Snares are often used for gathering the retrograde wire into antegrade catheter. The three-loop (tulip) snares, such as Ensnare (merit) and Atrieve (angiotech), are more effective for capturing the guidewire as compared to Amplatzer Goosneck snare (Figs 28.7 and 28.8).

UNCROSSABLE AND UNDILATABLE LESION EQUIPMENT

The second most common reason for CTO PCI failure is failure to dilate the lesion after crossing. For this the following equipment should be available.

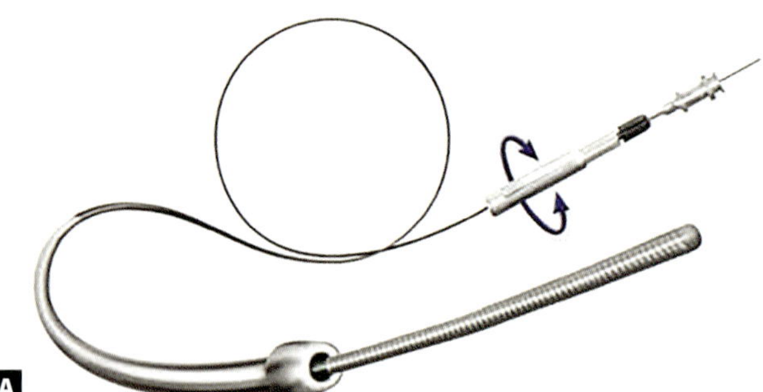

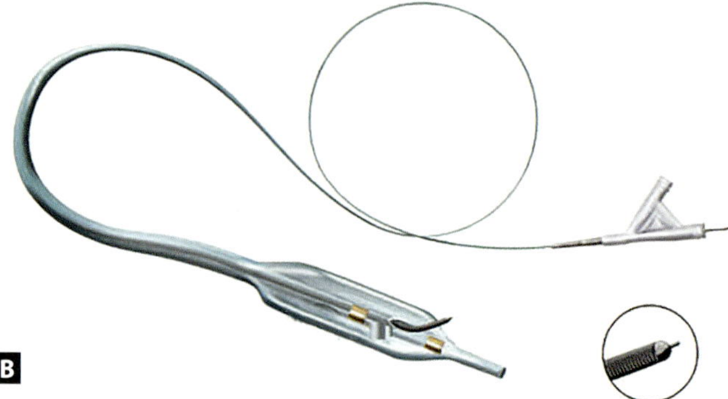

Figs 28.4A and B (A) CrossBoss catheter; (B) Stringray catheter

Table 28.2 Description of coronary guidewires commonly utilized in CTO-PCI

Wire category	*Tip style*	*Commercial name*	*Tip stiffness*	*Manufacturer*	*Properties*
Polymer covered					
	Tapered	Fielder XT[a] XT-A XT-R	1.2 g 1.0 g 0.6 g	Asahi Intecc	Frontline wire for antegrade crossing. Can also be used for knuckle wire formation and for retrograde crossing.
	Straight (non-tapered) Low tip stiffness	Fielder FC[a] Whisper LS, MS,ES Pilot 50 Choice PT Floppy.	1.6 g 0.8,1.0,1.2 g 1.5 g 2.1 g	Asahi Intecc Abott Vascular Abott Vascular Boston Scientific	Used to cross through collateral vessels during retrograde approach
	Straight (non-tapered), high tip stiffness	Pilot 150, 200[a] Cross wire NT PT graphics intermediate PT2 Moderate support Shinobi Shinobi Plus	2.7 g, 4.1 g 7.7 g 1.7 g 2.9 g 7.0 g 6.8 g	Abott Vascular Terumo Boston Scientific Boston Scientific Cordis Cordis	Antegrade crossing, especially when the course of the occluded vessel is unclear. Also useful for knuckle wire formation and for re-entry into true lumen during LAST technique
Open coil (no polymer jacket)					
	Straight, low tip stiffness	SION (hydrophilic)[a] SION BLUE SION BLACK	0.7 g 0.5 g 0.8 g	Asahi Intecc	First choice guidewire for retrograde crossing. Well balanced workhorse Sliding performance
	Tapered, low tip stiffness	Cross-it 100XT(0.010 in.) Runthrough NS Tapered (0.008 in.)	1.7 g 1.0 g	Abott Vascular Terumo	
	Tapered, high tip stiffness, Hydrophilic coating	Confianza Pro9,12[a] (0.009") PROGRESS 140T, 200T (0.0105", 0.009") Persuader 9 (0.011") ProVia 9, 12 (0.009") MiracleBros 3, 4.5,6	9.3,12.4 g 12.5,13.3 g 9.1g 11.8,13.5 g 3.9, 4.4, 8.8 g	Asahi intecc Abott Vascular Medtronic Medtronic Asahi intecc	Antegrade crossing when vessel course is known. Antegrade crossing when vessel course is known.
	Straight tip, high tip stiffness	MiracleBross 12 PROGRESS 40, 80, 120 Persuader 3,6 (-phillic and – phobic) Provia 3, 6 6 (-phillic and – phobic)	13.0 g 5.5, 9.7, 13.9 g 5.1, 8.0 g 8.3, 9.1 g	Asahi intecc Abott Vascular Medtronic Medtronic	
	Tapered, high tip stiffnes, hydrobhobic coating	Confianza 9 (hydrophobic) Persuader 9 (hydrophobic) ProVia 9, 12 (hydrophobic)	8.6 g 9.1g 11.8g, 13.5g	Asahi intecc Medtronic Medtronic	Antegrade crossing when vessel course is known.
Externalization Wires		Viper (0.014 tip)[a] RG 3 RotaWire floppy and extra support R 350	 3.6 g	CSI Asahi intecc Boston Scientific Vascular solutions	335 cm in length 330 cm in length 325 cm in length 350 cm in length
New GAIA		1 2 3	1.7g 3.5g 4.5g	Asahi intecc	Torque and tip flexibility.

[a] most commonly utilized guidewires

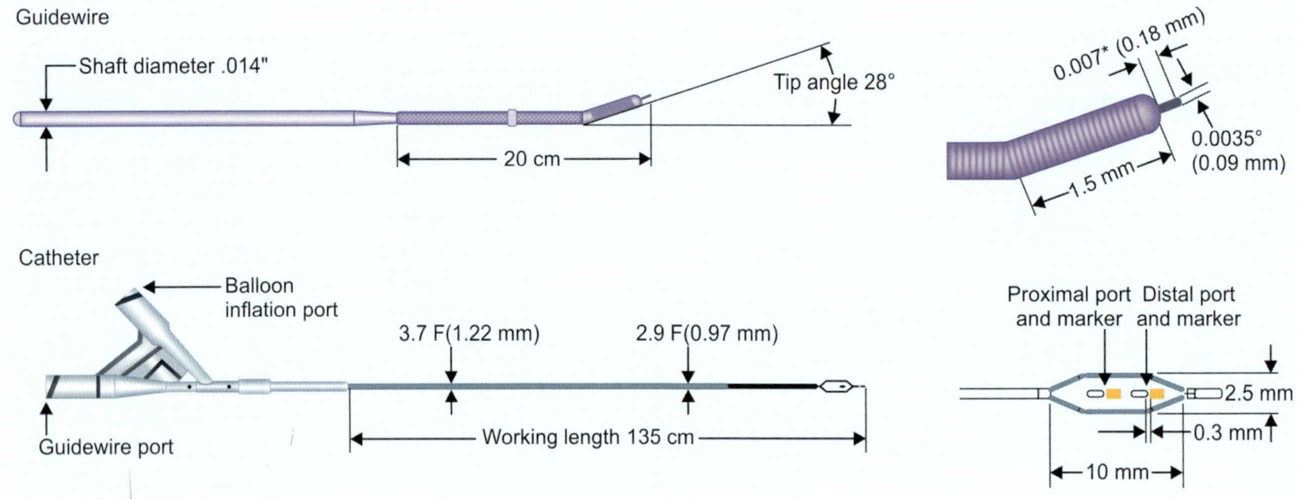

Fig. 28.5 Stingray balloon and guidewire

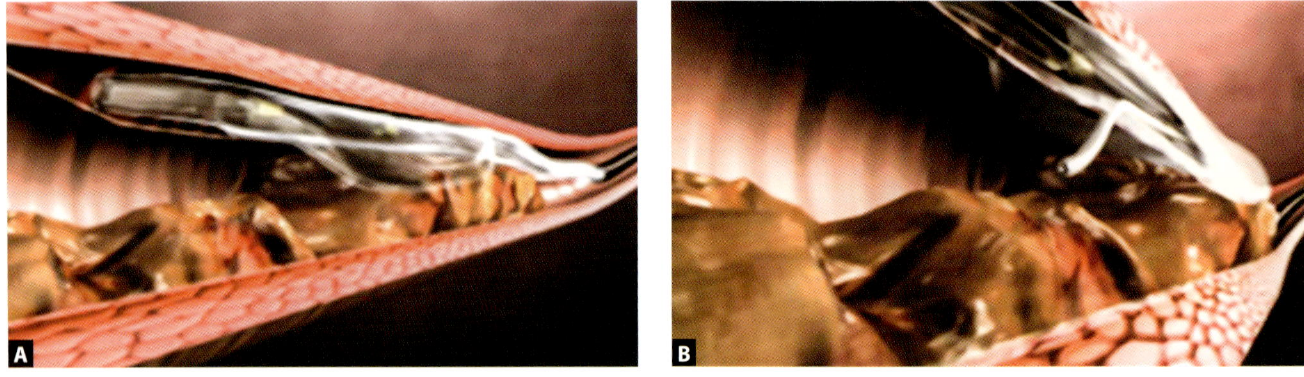

Figs 28.6A and B Re-entry into true lumen

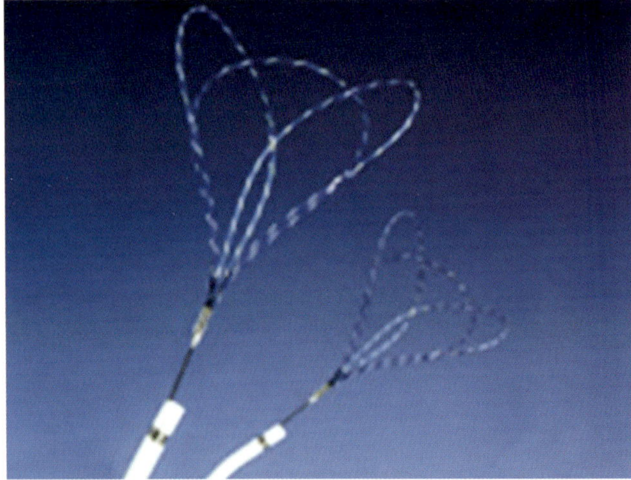

Fig. 28.7 Three-loop snares

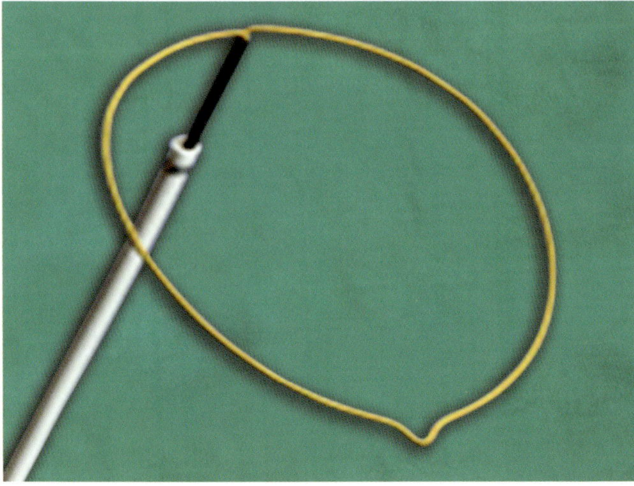

Fig. 28.8 Amplatzer Goosneck snare

Tornous catheter 2.1Fr and 2.6Fr: This is advanced over the wire by counter clock wise rotation but it should not be more than 20 turns. It is withdrawn by clockwise turns.[8] It does not have inner polymer unlike Crosair and therefore injection of contrast cannot be made. The tornous catheter consists of 8 stainless steel wire stranded in a coil (Fig. 28.9).

Guide Catheter Extension

Two guidewire extensions are currently available in India:

1. Guideliner (Vascular solutions) (Fig. 28.10)
2. Guidezilla (Boston scientific) (Fig. 28.11)
   - The guideliner is available in 4 sizes : 5.5, 6, 7 and 8 Fr that fits into small 6, 6, 7, 8 Fr guide catheter respectively resulting in 1 Fr smaller lumen than the guide catheter. It is 145 long and 25 cm single lumen cylinder that enters the coronary vessel.[9]
   - The guidezilla catheter is also a rapid exchange mother and child guide catheter extension that has been FDA approved in March 2013 and available in one size 6F. It is similar to guideliner but has large internal diameter (1.45 vs 1.42 mm).

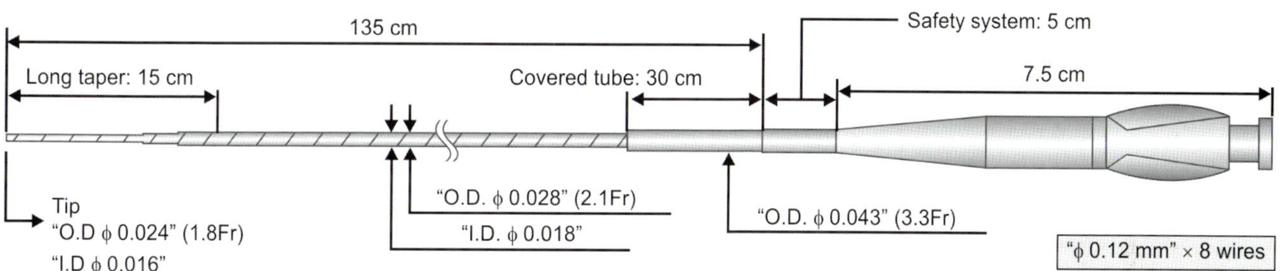

Fig. 28.9 Tornus catheter

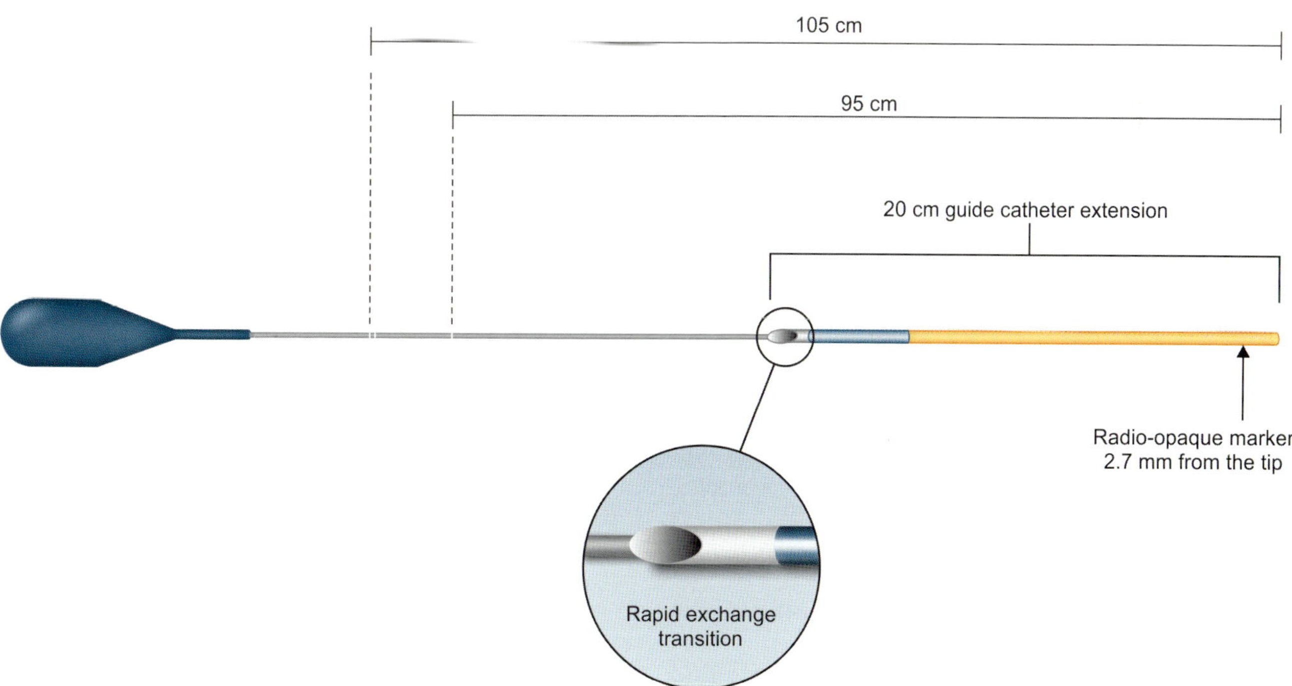

Fig. 28.10 The guideliner catheter. This consists of a flexible 20 cm straight guide extension connected to a stainless steel push tube

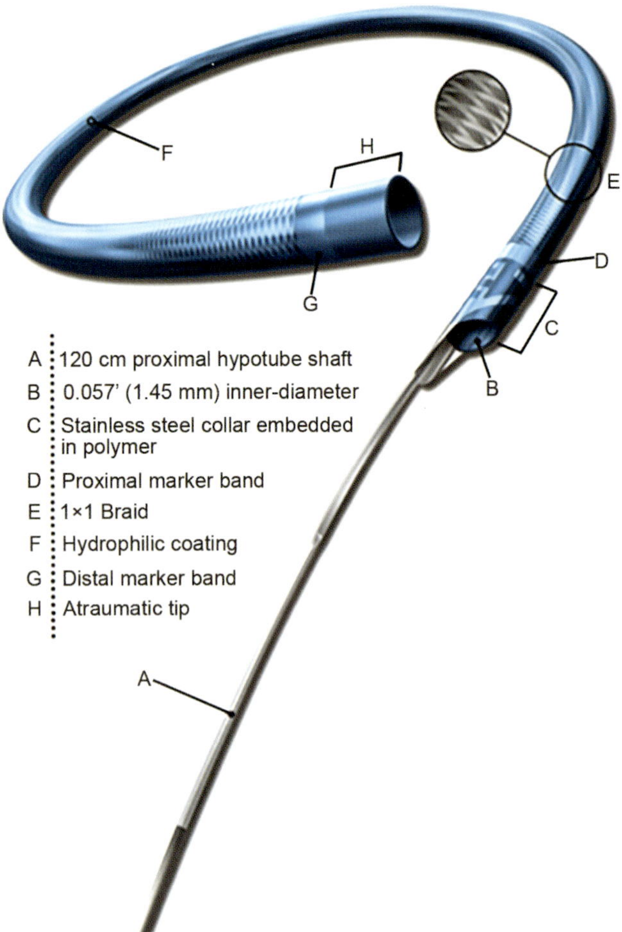

Fig. 28.11 Guidezilla catheter

Tips

- Deformation of equipment and stents can occur while advancing and while withdrawing the equipment.
- Deep advance of guidewire extension can cause dissection.
- Guidewire extension can be used in reverse CART, Reverse Controlled Antegrade and Retrograde tracking and dissection.
- One should avoid pressure damping while using guide catheter extension.
- Although distal to proximal stenting is preferred, but reverse can be done.
- Advance of guide catheter extension is done better while using balloon or microcatheter.
- It is also helpful when coaxial alignment of catheter is not possible, though preferred.
- The proximal portion of the guide catheter extension should not be advanced outside the guide catheter.

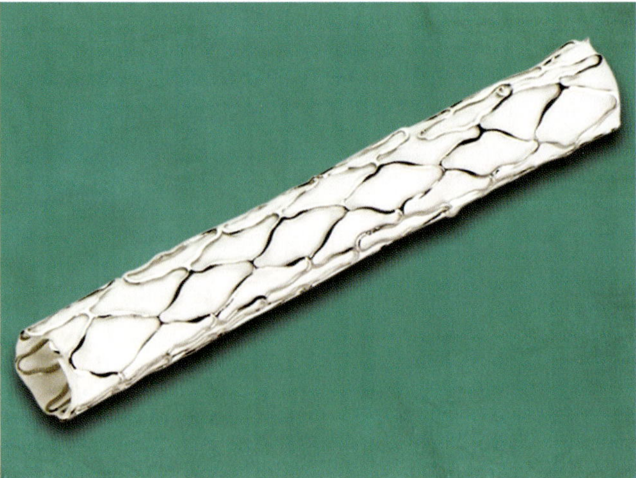

Fig. 28.12 Covered stent

- During its use, special attention should be paid to activated clotting time.

INTRAVASCULAR ULTRASOUND

It is helpful in the following situations:

- Identify the lesion proximal cap in cases of proximal cap ambiguity.
- Confirm antegrade wire has engaged the lesion.
- Confirm that retrograde wire has entered the true lumen before externalization.
- Determine the approximate size of the balloon/stents for controlled antegrade and retrograde subintimal tracking (CART) and reverse CART.

COMPLICATION MANAGEMENT EQUIPMENT

1. Covered stents (Fig. 28.12)
2. Coils
3. Pericardiocentesis tray

- Covered Stent:[10] Till recently, the covered stent that was available was Jostent Graftmaster but now another one is available from Biotronic - PK Papyrus, having, very small profile. They are used for perforation and as they tend to shorten on expansion therefore adequate coverage should be done. The Jostent required very high atmospheric pressure more than 14 atmosphere for adequate expansion.
- Coils: They are used for distal coronary perforation. Coils are usually made of stainless steal with Dacron fiber attached along the length of wire once advanced or pushed into distal target vessel, they attain their preformed shape, sealing the perforation.[11]

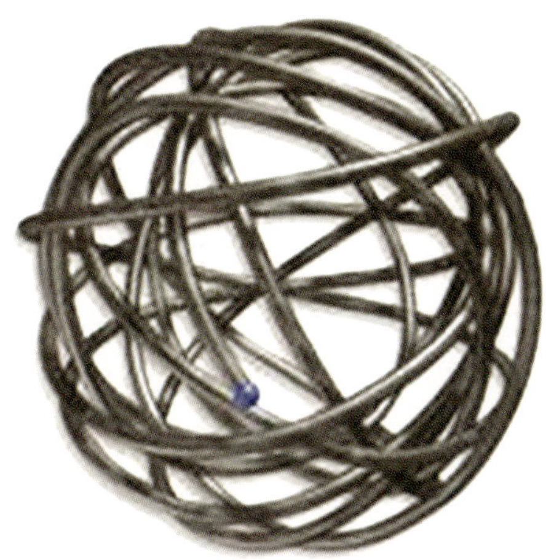

Fig. 28.13 Coils

It is important to know coils are not delivered through the catheters we use for chronic total occlusion like fine cross or corsair. We require larger lumen catheter and one should have either Transit, Prograde or Renegrade Microcatheters in the laboratory (Fig. 28.13).

- Pericardiocentesis tray: A tray having the following should be available:
  - 0.018 needle
  - J wire
  - Pigtail catheter

RADIATION PROTECTION

As chronic total occlusion (CTO) procedures are long procedures, all protection available should be used.

To conclude, different equipment can be used in chronic total occlusion percutaneous coronary intervention (CTO-PCI) there is no universal or standard CTO-PCI equipment and it is a matter of personal preference of the individual operator. Having proper tool for each step can simplify the procedure and increase the success rate in CTO-PCI.

REFERENCES

1. Brikalis ES. Manual of Coronary total Occlusion Intervention: A Step by Step approach, 1st edn. Waltham MA Elsevier; pp.19-66.
2. Brikalis ES. The essential equipment for CTO interventions. Cardilol Today's Interv. 2013 [May June 2013].
3. Joyal D, Thomsons CA, Grantham JA, Buller CEH, Rinfret S. The retrograde technique for recanalization of chronic total occlusions: a step by step approach. JACC Cadivasc Interv. 2012;5:1-11.
4. Brikalis ES, Grantham JA, Thompson CA, et al. The retrograde approach to coronary artery chronic total conclusion: a practical approach. Catheter Cardiovasc Interv. 2012;79:3-19.
5. Brilakis ES, Grantham JA, Rinfret S, et al. A percutaneous treatment algorithm for crossing coronary chronic total occlusion. JACC Cardiovasc Interv. 2012;79:3-19.
6. Tsuchikane E, Katoh O, Kimura M, Nasu K, Kinoshita Y, Suzuki T. The first clinical experience with a novel catheter for collateral channel tracking in retrograde approach for chronic coronary occlusion. JACC Cardiovasc Interv. 2010;3:165-71.
7. Mclure SJ, Wahr DW, Webb JG. Venture wire control catheter. Catheter Cardiovasc Intern. 2005;66:346-50.
8. Fang HY, Lee Ch, Fang CY, et al. Applications of penetration device (Tornus) for percutaneous coronary intervention in balloon un-crossable chronic total conclusion-procedure outcomes, complications and predictors of device success. Catheter Cardiovasc Interv. 2011;78:356-62.
9. Papayannis AC, Micheal TT, Brikalis ES. Challenges associated with use GuideLiner catheter in percutaneous coronary interventions. J invasive Cardilol. 2012;24:370-1.
10. Rogumera R, Waksman R. Covered stent for coronary perforations: Is there enough evidence? Catheter Cardiovasc Interv. 2011;78:246-53.
11. Pershad A, Yarkoni a, Biglari D. Management of distal coronary perforations. J Invasive Cardilol. 2008;20:E187-91.

Index

Page numbers followed by *f* refer to figure and *t* refer to table

D

E

M

N

O

P

Q

R

V

W

Y

Z